Evidence-Based Psychotherapies
for Children and Adolescents

OKANAGAN UNIVERSITY COLLEGE
LIBRARY
BRITISH COLUMBIA

Evidence-Based Psychotherapies for Children and Adolescents

Edited by

ALAN E. KAZDIN
JOHN R. WEISZ

THE GUILFORD PRESS
New York   London

© 2003 The Guilford Press
A Division of Guilford Publications, Inc.
72 Spring Street, New York, NY 10012
www.guilford.com

All rights reserved

No part of this book may be reproduced, translated, stored in a retrieval system,
or transmitted, in any form or by any means, electronic, mechanical, photocopying,
microfilming, recording, or otherwise, without written permission from the Publisher.

Printed in the United States of America

This book is printed on acid-free paper.

Last digit is print number: 9 8 7 6 5 4 3 2

Library of Congress Cataloging-in-Publication Data

Evidence-based psychotherapies for children and adolescents / edited by
Alan E. Kazdin, John R. Weisz.
     p. cm.
Includes bibliographical references and index.
   ISBN 1-57230-683-1
  1. Child psychotherapy.   2. Adolescent psychotherapy.   3.
Evidence-based medicine.   I. Kazdin, Alan E.   II. Weisz, John R.
RJ504.E95 2003
618.92′89142—dc21   2002156031

To Fran, a model of courage, rationality, and caring
—A. E. K.

To Jenny, loving advocate for children and families
—J. R. W.

About the Editors

Alan E. Kazdin is Director of the Child Study Center and John M. Musser Professor of Psychology at Yale University School of Medicine. He is also Director of the Yale Child Conduct Clinic, an outpatient treatment service for children and their families. He received his PhD in clinical psychology from Northwestern University (1970). Prior to coming to Yale, Dr. Kazdin was on the faculty of the Pennsylvania State University and the University of Pittsburgh School of Medicine. He has been a fellow of the Center for Advanced Study in the Behavioral Sciences, President of the Association for Advancement of Behavior Therapy, and Chairman of the Department of Psychology at Yale University. He has been recipient of the Distinguished Scientific Contribution and Distinguished Professional Contribution awards in clinical psychology. Dr. Kazdin has served as Editor of various journals—*Journal of Consulting and Clinical Psychology, Behavior Therapy, Psychological Assessment,* and *Clinical Psychology: Science and Practice*—and currently is Editor of *Current Directions in Psychological Science.* His books and articles focus on psychotherapy, child and adolescent disorders, and methodology and research design.

John R. Weisz is a Professor in the Departments of Psychology and Psychiatry and Biobehavioral Sciences at the University of California at Los Angeles, where he has served as Director of the Graduate Program in Clinical Psychology and Director of the Psychology Clinic. He received his BA degree from Mississippi College (1967), subsequently served in the U.S. Peace Corps (in Kenya), and later studied at Yale University, where he received a PhD in clinical and developmental psychology (1975). Before his appointment at UCLA, he was on the faculty at Cornell University and at the University of North Carolina at Chapel Hill. Dr. Weisz has served as President of the Society of Clinical Child and Adolescent Psychology (a division of the American Psychological Association) and is currently President of the International Society for Research in Child and Adolescent Psychopathology. His books and articles focus on youth problem behavior and disorders, cultural factors in development and dysfunction, and psychotherapy for children and adolescents.

Contributors

Arthur D. Anastopoulos, PhD, Department of Psychology, University of North Carolina at Greensboro, Greensboro, North Carolina

Sasha G. Aschenbrand, MA, Child and Adolescent Anxiety Disorders Clinic, Temple University, Philadelphia, Pennsylvania

Paula M. Barrett, PhD, School of Applied Psychology, Griffith University—Mt. Gravatt Campus, Brisbane, Australia

Tammy D. Barry, PhD, Department of Psychology, University of Alabama, Tuscaloosa, Alabama

David A. Brent, MD, Western Psychiatric Institute and Clinic, University of Pittsburgh School of Medicine, Pittsburgh, Pennsylvania

Mary Y. Brinkmeyer, MS, Department of Clinical and Health Psychology, University of Florida, Gainesville, Florida

Lauren I. Brookman, MA, Autism Research and Training Center, Graduate School of Education, University of California, Santa Barbara, California

Patricia Chamberlain, PhD, Oregon Social Learning Center, Eugene, Oregon

Bruce F. Chorpita, PhD, Department of Psychology, University of Hawaii at Manoa, Honolulu, Hawaii

Gregory N. Clarke, PhD, Kaiser Permanente Center for Health Research, Portland, Oregon

Jennifer Connor-Smith, PhD, Department of Psychology, Oregon State University, Corvallis, Oregon

Giuseppe Costantino, PhD, Lutheran Medical Center, Brooklyn, New York

Lynn L. DeBar, PhD, Kaiser Permanente Center for Health Research, Portland, Oregon

Kristen Pollack Dorta, PhD, Department of Psychiatry, College of Physicians and Surgeons of Columbia University, New York, New York

Leonard H. Epstein, PhD, Department of Pediatrics, University at Buffalo School of Medicine and Biomedical Sciences, Buffalo, New York

Sheila M. Eyberg, PhD, Department of Clinical and Health Psychology, University of Florida, Gainesville, Florida

Suzanne E. Farley, MA, Department of Psychology, University of North Carolina at Greensboro, Greensboro, North Carolina

Elizabeth A. Franks, MA, Department of Psychology, Loyola University Chicago, Chicago, Illinois

Elana B. Gordis, PhD, Department of Psychology, University of Southern California, Los Angeles, California

Rachel Neff Greenley, MA, Department of Psychology, Loyola University Chicago, Chicago, Illinois

Scott W. Henggeler, PhD, Department of Psychiatry and Behavioral Sciences, Medical University of South Carolina, Charleston, South Carolina

Olga E. Hervis, MSW, Department of Psychiatry and Behavioral Sciences, University of Miami School of Medicine, Miami, Florida

Kimberly Hoagwood, PhD, New York State Psychiatric Institute, Columbia University, New York, New York

Grayson N. Holmbeck, PhD, Department of Psychology, Loyola University Chicago, Chicago, Illinois

Arthur C. Houts, PhD, Department of Psychology, University of Memphis, Memphis, Tennessee

Jennifer L. Hudson, PhD, Department of Psychology, Macquarie University, Sydney, Australia

Alan E. Kazdin, PhD, Child Study Center, Yale University School of Medicine, New Haven, Connecticut

Philip C. Kendall, PhD, Child and Adolescent Anxiety Disorders Clinic, Temple University, Philadelphia, Pennsylvania

Robert L. Koegel, PhD, Autism Research and Training Center, Graduate School of Education, University of California, Santa Barbara, California

Lynn Kern Koegel, PhD, Autism Research and Training Center, Graduate School of Education, University of California, Santa Barbara, California

Terry Lee, MD, Hawaii Department of Health, John A. Burns School of Medicine, University of Hawaii, Honolulu, Hawaii

Peter M. Lewinsohn, PhD, Oregon Research Institute, Eugene, Oregon

John E. Lochman, PhD, Department of Psychology, University of Alabama, Tuscaloosa, Alabama

O. Ivar Lovaas, PhD, Department of Psychology, University of California at Los Angeles, Los Angeles, California

Robert G. Malgady, PhD, Department of Teaching and Learning, New York University, New York, New York

Victoria B. Mitrani, PhD, Department of Psychiatry and Behavioral Sciences, University of Miami School of Medicine, Miami, Florida

Laura Mufson, PhD, Department of Psychiatry, College of Physicians and Surgeons of Columbia University, New York State Psychiatric Institute, New York, New York

Dustin A. Pardini, MA, Department of Psychology, University of Alabama, Tuscaloosa, Alabama

M. Jamila Reid, PhD, Parent Clinic, University of Washington, Seattle, Washington

Michael S. Robbins, PhD, Department of Psychiatry and Behavioral Sciences, University of Miami School of Medicine, Miami, Florida

Arthur L. Robin, PhD, Department of Psychiatry and Behavioral Neurosciences, Wayne State University School of Medicine, Detroit, Michigan

Daniel A. Santisteban, PhD, Department of Psychiatry and Behavioral Sciences, University of Miami School of Medicine, Miami, Florida

Seth J. Schwartz, PhD, Department of Psychiatry and Behavioral Sciences, University of Miami School of Medicine, Miami, Florida

Alison L. Shortt, PhD, School of Psychology, University of Queensland, St. Lucia, Australia

Dana K. Smith, PhD, Oregon Social Learning Center, Eugene, Oregon

Tristram Smith, PhD, Department of Pediatrics (Psychology), University of Rochester School of Medicine and Dentistry, Rochester, New York

Michael A. Southam-Gerow, PhD, Department of Psychology, Virginia Commonwealth University, Richmond, Virginia

José Szapocznik, PhD, Department of Psychiatry and Behavioral Sciences, University of Miami School of Medicine, Miami, Florida

Carolyn Webster-Stratton, PhD, Department of Family and Child Nursing, University of Washington, Seattle, Washington

V. Robin Weersing, PhD, Child Study Center, Yale University School of Medicine, New Haven, Connecticut

John R. Weisz, PhD, Departments of Psychology and Psychiatry and Biobehavioral Sciences, University of California at Los Angeles, Los Angeles, California

Preface

The treatment of social, emotional, and behavioral problems of children and adolescents has developed remarkably in the past decade. The effects are felt in current research, clinical practice, and training of mental health professionals. Perhaps the main development pertains to issues surrounding the effectiveness of treatment. Reviews of the evidence have consistently found that many treatments for children and adolescents produce therapeutic change, and that these changes are marked. The development of effective treatments has progressed perhaps in part due to the broad interest in treatment from different perspectives. Those involved in research and clinical practice are among the key parties concerned with interventions and their effects, yet there has been increased concern among the public (e.g., parents of children with disorders) and those who oversee clinical practice (e.g., third-party payers) about the accountability of treatment. Some of this has been driven by economic considerations, but it would be a mistake to consider advances in research, practice, and training as a mere response to strong external forces. Indeed, it is easy to argue the reverse—budding advances in empirical research underscore the importance of increased accountability. What is being used in treatment can only come into question when emerging evidence suggests that something else should be used instead.

Central to current developments is interest in and movement toward "evidence-based treatments." Broadly conceived, the term refers to those interventions that have evidence in their behalf. Many different approaches have been used to identify these treatments, with criteria differing slightly from one approach to the next. Most significant is the common ground: There is considerable consensus across various approaches that to be considered evidence-based, treatments must use replicable procedures (e.g., treatments codified in manuals), must be evaluated in well-controlled experiments, and must show replication of the effects so there are assurances that any seemingly wonderful effect or outcome in fact can be reproduced, ideally by others. A substantial number of current treatments meet these criteria in varying degrees. Perhaps as important, there are many research programs in place that are developing treatments, identifying treatments that may be effective, and evaluating more intricate questions about how, why, and for whom treatment works. This means that, in addition to palpable advances evident in current research, investigators are investing in the future as well so that, in the not too distant future, the "present" state of treatments for children and adolescents will be even brighter.

There are important reasons to consolidate contemporary gains by identifying evidence-based treatments and attending to the kinds of work needed for continued progress. For example, it is still the case that most of the treatments in clinical practice have little or no evidence in their behalf. And it is still the case that the great majority of the 200 disorders in the fourth edition of the *Diagnostic and Statistical Manual of Mental Disorders* that can be applied to children and adolescents lack evidence-based treatments that can be used with young people. Also, most training programs in the major mental health professions—clinical psychology, child psychiatry, social work, counseling, and pediatrics—still provide little or no training in evidence-based psychotherapies. All this is changing, of course, but the changes may best be supported by efforts to identify, describe, and highlight the relevant treatments and the evidence supporting them.

The purpose of this book is to present a set of treatments that are supported by evidence and to capture facets of the historical, theoretical, scientific, ethical, and policy climate within which the treatments exist. The treatment descriptions provide greater detail than is ordinarily available to convey what the treatments are, how they are implemented, and what resources are available to researchers and clinicians interested in the treatments. Contributors were asked to provide a review of research to convey the status of the treatments but to do so concisely. Thus, the chapters are unique in providing a crisp statement of the evidence in behalf of the treatments. Much of each chapter is devoted to describing details of the treatment sessions themselves, who administers the treatment, and the training and supervision required for implementation. Chapter contents allow the reader to see the progression of research over time. Contributors describe a sequence of studies and research progress over time. To that end, we have asked contributors to discuss the next set of questions on which they are working and the challenges that need to be addressed in the future.

The book ought to be of keen interest to professionals and policymakers concerned with the mental health and care of children and adolescents. In addition, researchers and clinicians interested in current evidence for psychotherapies for children and adolescents will find the format informative and useful. For those considering research on treatment for children, the chapters will be useful in describing how one selects participants, codifies treatments, trains therapists, and moves from study to study to develop treatment and ask increasingly finer-grained questions. For those interested in extensions of treatment to clinical practice, the chapters provide details of the contents and themes of sessions, problems of actually implementing treatment, and the clients to whom treatment is likely to be suited.

Although we have emphasized the focus of the chapters, it would be a mistake not to underscore what we perceive to be the highlight of the book—the contributors. We were extremely fortunate in obtaining senior investigators whose works and contributions are already widely recognized.

We are pleased to acknowledge several sources of support for our own research that we received during the period in which this book was prepared. These sources include the John D. and Catherine T. MacArthur Foundation, the National Institute of Mental Health, the State of Connecticut Department of Social Services, and the William T. Grant Foundation. We are both especially indebted to our thoughtful colleagues and graduate students, continuing sources of intellectual stimulation and sheer fun. One of the editors, who shall go nameless, wishes to acknowledge what a pleasure it has been to work with the other editor, who will also go nameless. Perhaps more than any other set of people, we are both very grateful to the contributors, whose work we admire greatly. Finally, Seymour Weingarten, Editor-in-Chief of The Guilford Press, played a major role in the conceptualization of this book and the impetus in bringing it to fruition. We are pleased to have had the opportunity to work with him.

ALAN E. KAZDIN
JOHN R. WEISZ

Contents

III. CONCLUSIONS AND FUTURE DIRECTIONS

I

FOUNDATIONS OF CHILD AND ADOLESCENT THERAPY RESEARCH

1

Introduction

Context and Background of Evidence-Based Psychotherapies for Children and Adolescents

ALAN E. KAZDIN AND JOHN R. WEISZ

Psychotherapy has a long and remarkable history. Precisely how long and remarkable depends in part on how therapy is defined. A defensible place to begin would be with the work of Aristotle (384–322 BCE), who emphasized the role of catharsis in tragic drama, comedy, and the arts more generally in arousing and alleviating emotional states (*Poetics,* 350 BCE; *Politics* VIII, 350 BCE).[1] The paths from Aristotle to today could readily be charted by tracing medicine, religion, spiritualism, and less easily classified disciplines that have used such practices as suggestion, hypnosis, and assorted quasi medical or expectancy-based interventions directed toward the alleviation of stress, maladjustment, and a broad scope of maladies (Shapiro & Shapiro, 1998). The formal delineation of psychotherapy as an area of study and clinical work can be traced to the past 100 years or so (Freedheim, 1992). In this context, therapy grew directly from efforts to intervene to address impaired mental (psychiatric) function and problems of maladjustment.

Discussions of therapy and its development focus almost exclusively on therapy for adults. Attention to children and adolescents is more recent. For example, much of contemporary therapy is traced to psychoanalysis and the contributions of Sigmund Freud (1856–1939). Freud's treatment of a little boy (Hans) by consulting with the father or the psychoanalysis of his own daughter, Anna Freud (1895–1982), are de rigueur points to mention in the development of child therapy. Anna Freud made a significant leap in developing child therapy by studying children and adapting psychoanalytic concepts and treatment to them (e.g., A. Freud, 1946, 1965). Her work began in the 1920s and reached a high point in the 1960s at a clinic in London. The clinic, originally named the Hampstead Clinic and later renamed the Anna Freud Centre, continues to be quite active.

Research on therapy, as distinguished from clinical work with children, has a more recent and more easily traced history. Reviews of the therapy literature that mark a useful beginning point (Levitt, 1957, 1963) identified a small number of treatment studies that included children or adolescents. For example, the 1957 reviews 18 studies identified; the 1963 review, identified; 22 additional studies. The reviews concluded that therapy did not seem to be more effective than the passage of time, that is, no therapy. The rate of improvement among children (67–73%) was about the same whether or not treatment was provided. This conclusion was similar to the one reached by Eysenck (1952) in his highly influential review of adult therapy. In revised and expanded versions, Eysenck (1960, 1966) included therapies for children, adolescents, and adults and reached the same conclusion as in his original review, namely, there was no firm evidence that treatment led to greater improvements than the mere passage of time (no treatment).

These reviews exerted important influence. The conclusions, even though quite consistent among the different reviews, were debatable at the time. In almost all cases, the studies on which the conclusions were based were methodologically weak, the samples were small, and the treatments were not well specified. For example, randomized controlled trials of treatment, the methodological Esperanto of all disciplines that evaluate interventions, were rarely conducted. In the past 40 years, the number of studies one can bring to bear on the effects of psychotherapy has become huge. As important, the methodological rigor of these studies has evolved. Indeed, a major impetus for this book is to feature exemplary research to illustrate the substantive advances and methodological quality of the research on which these advances are based.

CONDITIONS THAT WARRANT OR PRECIPITATE TREATMENT

The need for effective treatments stems in part from the range of conditions that children and adolescents experience. We provide an overview of the range of problems to convey the scope of the challenges of identifying and developing treatments. For the purpose of presentation, the dysfunctions are grouped into three categories: social, emotional, and behavioral problems; problem and at-risk behaviors; and delinquency.

Social, Emotional, and Behavioral Problems

We include in this category a broad range of problems that fall within the domain of mental health, that are associated with impairment in functioning, and that often serve as the basis for treatment. Within this category are dysfunctions referred to as psychiatric or mental disorders. These disorders refer to patterns of behavior that are associated with distress, impairment, or significantly increased risk of suffering, death, pain, disability, or an important loss of freedom. Various diagnostic systems, such as the fourth edition of the *Diagnostic and Statistical Manual of Mental Disorders* (DSM-IV; American Psychiatric Association, 1994) and the *International Classification of Diseases* (ICD-10; World Health Organization [WHO], 1992) enumerate the range of psychological dysfunctions or disorders that individuals can experience. DSM is the dominant system in use (Maser, Kaelber, & Weise, 1991) and recognizes several disorders that arise in infancy, childhood, or adolescence. Table 1.1 lists these disorders, grouped into 10 categories.

Many disorders that can arise over the lifespan and hence are not unique to childhood and adolescence are omitted from the table. The diagnostic criteria for these disorders are similar or identical at any age. Major examples include anxiety, mood, eating, substance-related, schizophrenia, sexual and gender identity, and adjustment disorders. Table 1.2 highlights specific disorders within these categories to illustrate some of the

TABLE 1.1. Categories of Major Disorders First Evident in Infancy, Childhood, or Adolescence

Mental retardation: Significant subaverage general intellectual functioning (Intelligence Quotient [IQ] of approximately < 70) associated with deficits or impairments in adaptive behavior (e.g., communication, self-care, social skills, and functional academic or work skills). Onset is before the age of 18. Degrees of severity are distinguished based on intellectual impairment and adaptive functioning.

Learning disorders: Achievement that is substantially below normative levels, based on the individual's age, schooling, and level of intelligence. Separate disorders are distinguished based on the domain of dysfunction and include disorders of reading, mathematics, and written expression.

Motor skills disorder: Marked impairment in the development of motor coordination that interferes with academic achievement or activities of daily living and that cannot be traced to a general medical condition.

Communication disorders: Impairment in the use of language that is substantially below normative levels of performance. The impairment interferes with daily functioning (e.g., at school). Separate disorders are distinguished and include disorders of expressive language, mixed receptive-expressive language, phonological (use of speech sounds) disorders, and stuttering.

Pervasive developmental disorders: Severe and pervasive impairment in several areas of development including social interactions, language and communication, and play (stereotyped behaviors, interests, and activities). These are usually evident in the first years of life. Separate disorders are distinguished based on the scope of impairment and time of onset and include autistic disorder, Rett's, Asperger's, and childhood disintegrative disorders.

Attention-deficit and disruptive behavior disorders: Behaviors associated with inattention, impulsivity, overactivity, oppositionality and disobedience, provocative, aggressive, and antisocial behavior. Separate disorders are distinguished including attention-deficit/hyperactivity, conduct, and oppositional defiant disorders.

Feeding and eating disorders of infancy or early childhood: Persistent eating and feeding disturbances such as eating nonnutritive substances (pica), repeated regurgitation and rechewing of food (rumination disorder), and persistent failure to eat adequately, resulting in significant failure to gain weight or weight loss (feeding disorder of infancy or early childhood).

Tic disorders: Sudden, rapid, and recurrent stereotyped motor movement or vocalizations. Separate disorders are distinguished based on scope of the tics (e.g., motor and vocal) and their duration and include Tourette's syndrome, chronic motor or vocal, and transient tic disorders.

Elimination disorders: Dysfunction related to urination or defecation in which these functions appear to be uncontrolled and beyond the age in which control has usually been established. Two disorders, enuresis and encopresis, are distinguished and require the absence of medical condition in which these symptoms would emerge.

Other disorders of infancy, childhood, or adolescence: A collection of other disorders that are not covered elsewhere and include separation anxiety, selective mutism, reactive attachment, and stereotypic movement disorders.

*Note.*The disorders within each category have multiple inclusion and exclusion criteria related to the requisite symptoms, severity and duration, and patterns of onset (see American Psychiatric Association, 1994). Details of the diagnoses are beyond the scope of this chapter.

more common diagnoses, particularly for children and adolescents. Listing major disorders does not convey their complexities. A given type of disorder (e.g., anxiety or eating) may have different versions, depending on its onset and symptoms. Also, some disorders may emerge at any time; others emerge only during childhood or adolescence. It is useful to consider the list as a way to identify various types of dysfunctions in childhood and adolescence.

Psychiatric disorders refer to specific diagnostic entities. It is useful to expand the category to encompass social, emotional, and behavioral problems more generally for

TABLE 1.2. Examples of Disorders That May Be Evident at Any Point over the Lifespan

Major depressive disorder: The appearance of depressed mood or loss of interest that lasts for at least 2 weeks and is associated with at least four additional symptoms including a change in appetite or weight, sleep, and psychomotor activity; feelings of worthlessness or guilt; diminished energy; difficulty thinking, concentrating, or making decisions; and recurrent thoughts of death or suicidal ideation, plans, or attempts.

Posttraumatic stress disorder: Development of symptoms of anxiety after exposure to an extreme traumatic event involving actual or threatened injury or witnessing an event that involves death, injury, or a threat to the physical integrity of another person, or learning about these events experienced by a family member. The events may include personal assault (e.g., sexual, physical, and robbery), accidents, life-threatening illness, a disaster (e.g., loss of one's home after a hurricane or tornado). Key symptoms involve intense fear, helplessness, horror, reexperience of the event (e.g., thoughts and dreams), avoidance of stimuli associated with the event, and numbing of general responsiveness (e.g., detachment and restricted affect), persistent symptoms of increased arousal (difficulty falling or remaining asleep).

Eating disorders: A disorder in which the individual does not maintain minimal normal body weight (< 85% of normal body weight), is intensely afraid of gaining weight, and exhibits a significant disturbance in the perception of his or her body. Many methods of weight loss may be adopted such as self-induced vomiting, misuse of laxatives, and increased or excessive exercise.

Substance abuse disorder: A set of disorders (depending on the substance) characterized by a maladaptive use of the substance as evident in recurrent and significant adverse consequences (e.g., failure to fulfill role obligations at school, work, or home, and social and interpersonal problems). A period of 12 months of use and continued use after untoward consequences (e.g., in role performance, legal problems, and school expulsion) have occurred is required for the diagnosis.

Schizophrenia: A disorder that lasts at least 6 months and includes two or more of these symptoms: delusions, hallucinations, disorganized speech, grossly disorganized catatonic behavior, and negative symptoms such as flat affect, poverty of speech (brief, empty replies), and inability to initiate or persist in goal-directed behavior. Significant dysfunction occurs in one or more areas of functioning including interpersonal relations, work, school, or self-care.

Adjustment disorder: Development of clinically significant emotional or behavioral symptoms in response to an identifiable psychological stressor or stressors. The symptoms develop within 3 months of the event and are associated with marked distress or a reaction in excess of what might be expected within the context or culture. The symptoms of many other disorders may emerge (e.g., anxiety, depressed mood, and conduct problems).

Other conditions: A set of problems are included that are not mental disorders but may serve as the focus of clinical attention. These may include relational problems (e.g., between parent and child or between spouses), physical or sexual abuse of an adult or child, isolated antisocial behavior, bereavement, and many others that are not considered mental disorders but are brought to the attention of mental health professionals.

two reasons. First, treatment research often focuses on symptom severity on specific measures rather than on diagnoses. Thus, children might be included in a treatment trial because their level of anxiety, depression, or aggression meets a particular cutoff. Second, diagnoses themselves among children who are referred for treatment are often not sharply delineated. Children may have multiple symptoms for a given set of disorders or multiple disorders. These comments do not in any way gainsay the utility of diagnoses but underscore that research, as well as clinical referrals, often focuses on symptoms, symptom severity, and dysfunction whether or not subsequent assessment of diagnosis is made.

Most of the clinical problems that are brought to psychotherapy are encompassed by the terms "externalizing disorders" and "internalizing disorders." Externalizing disorders are problems directed toward the environment and others. Primary examples include oppositional, hyperactive, aggressive, and antisocial behaviors and are encompassed by the psychiatric diagnostic category, attention-deficit and disruptive behavior disorders (in Table 1.1). Internalizing disorders are problems directed toward inner experience. Primary examples include anxiety, withdrawal, and depression. Externalizing disorders dominate as the primary basis for referring children and adolescents to inpatient and outpatient treatment.

Several studies spanning different geographical locales (e.g., the United States, Puerto Rico, Canada, and New Zealand) have yielded rather consistent results on the prevalence of disorders among children and adolescents (i.e., ages 4–18 years old). Between 17 and 22% suffer significant developmental, emotional, or behavioral problems (e.g., U.S. Congress, 1991; WHO, 2001). The high prevalence rates of psychiatric disorder (approximately one of five children) are likely to underestimate the range of mental disorders and impairment. Children who fail to meet the cutoff for a diagnosis because of the severity, number, or duration of symptoms can nonetheless suffer significant impairment and untoward long-term prognoses (Boyle et al., 1996; Gotlib, Lewinsohn, & Seeley, 1995; Lewinsohn, Solomon, Seeley, & Zeiss, 2000; Offord et al., 1992). Clearly, prevalence rates, when based on meeting criteria for diagnoses, provide a conservative estimate of child impairment and the need for treatment.

The scope of the problem is further misrepresented by suggesting that children may have only one of the problems highlighted previously. Many individuals meet criteria for two or more diagnoses, a phenomenon referred to as *comorbidity* (see Angold, Costello, & Erkanli, 1999; Clark, Watson, & Reynolds, 1995). Among community samples, comorbidity rates are relatively high. For example, among youth who meet criteria for one disorder, approximately half also meet criteria for another disorder (Cohen et al., 1993; Greenbaum, Foster-Johnson, & Petrila, 1996). Among clinically referred samples, the rates of comorbidity are much higher. For example, among adolescents with a diagnosis of substance abuse, most (e.g., $\geq 70\%$) meet criteria for other disorders (Milin, Halikas, Meller, & Morse, 1991; Weinberg, Rahdert, Colliver, & Glantz, 1998). Thus, a challenge of treatment is to address multiple problems that are often present.

Problem and At-Risk Behaviors

There are problems other than psychiatric disorders that warrant intervention. During adolescence, there is an increase in a number of activities referred to as problem or at-risk behaviors (see DiClemente, Hansen, & Ponton, 1996; Ketterlinus & Lamb, 1994; US Congress, 1991). Examples include use of illicit substances, truancy, school suspensions, stealing, vandalism, and precocious and unprotected sex. These are referred to as at-risk behaviors because they increase the likelihood of adverse psychological, social, and health outcomes. For example, alcohol abuse is associated with the three most frequent forms of mortality among adolescents: automobile accidents, homicides, and suicide (Windle, Shope, & Bukstein, 1996); approximately 90% of automobile accidents among adolescents involve the use of alcohol.

Many youth with problem behaviors might well meet criteria for a psychiatric disorder (e.g., substance abuse disorder). However, there is a larger group that would not—that is, they engage in problem behaviors, fit in with their peers, and manage daily functioning (e.g., at school). The prevalence rates of problem behaviors are relatively high. For example, in one survey 50.8% of 12th-grade students reported some alcohol use in the 30 days prior to the survey; 31.3% reported being drunk at least once; and 4.9% reported using marijuana daily or almost daily (Johnston, 1996). Other studies paint a similar picture, even though estimates of substance abuse vary as a function of the age of the sample, the types of substances (e.g., inhalants), the time frame (use in past week, month, year), the assessment method (e.g., self-report vs. medical emergency visits), and the impact of many other factors (e.g., social class, ethnicity, and neighborhood). Even so, the rates of abuse and use are alarming. Moreover, current data suggest that rates of substance use are increasing, a trend that began in the early 1990s (Weinberg et al., 1998).

Substance abuse is merely one example of at-risk behavior. Other examples include unprotected sexual activity and its risk for sexually transmitted diseases (including human immunodeficiency virus [HIV]) and teen pregnancy; delinquent, antisocial, and violent behavior; dropping out of school; and running away from home (DiClemente et al., 1996; Dryfoos, 1990). Multiple problem behaviors often go together (see Ketterlinus & Lamb, 1994), so that a youth identified with one of the behaviors (e.g., early sexual activity) is likely to have higher rates of other problem behaviors (substance use and abuse, delinquent acts).

Delinquency

Delinquency is a legal designation that includes behaviors that violate the law such as robbery, drug use, and vandalism. Some of the acts are illegal for both adults and juveniles (referred to as index offenses) and encompass such serious offenses as homicide, robbery, aggravated assault, and rape. Other acts (referred to as status offenses) are illegal only because of the age at which they occur, namely, only for juveniles. Examples include underage drinking, running away from home, truancy from school, and driving a car.

Delinquent acts overlap with the psychiatric disorders and problem behaviors mentioned previously. Indeed, the distinction between delinquency and mental disorder is not always sharp, and individuals can readily meet criteria for both based on the same behaviors (e.g., conduct disorder symptoms). Moreover, individuals identified as delinquent often have high rates of diagnosable psychiatric disorders. Up to 50–80% of delinquent youth may show at least one diagnosable psychiatric disorder—with conduct, attention deficit, and substance abuse disorders being the most common (see Kazdin, 2000).

The prevalence rates of delinquency in the population at large vary as a function of how delinquency is measured. Arrest records, surveys of victims, and reports of individuals about their own criminal activities are among the most common methods of measurement. Because much crime goes unreported and undetected, self-report has often been used and detects much higher rates than official records. A large percentage of adolescents (70%) engage in some delinquent behavior, usually status rather than index offenses (Elliott, Huizinga, & Ageton, 1985; Farrington, 1995). Most of these individuals do not continue criminal behavior into adulthood. A much smaller group (20–35%) engages in more serious offenses (robbery and assault) and may be identified through arrest or contact with the courts. There is a small group (5%) of persistent or career criminals who engage in many different and more severe delinquent activities and are responsible for approximately half of the officially recorded offenses (Farrington, 1995; Moffitt, 1993; Tracy, Wolfgang, & Figlio, 1990).

General Comments

In highlighting the scope of the problems that children and adolescents experience, four conclusions are worth underscoring:

1. Children and adolescents experience many different types of problems,
2. They often experience multiple problems concurrently (e.g., comorbid disorders, multiple problem behaviors, academic and learning problems,
3. These problems can emerge at many different points over the course of development, and
4. Several million children and adolescents and are in need of and could profit from some intervention.

Mentioned previously was an estimate of prevalence of 20% of children and adolescents who evince some form of psychiatric disorder. Even without adding problem behaviors and delinquent acts, the scope of problems in need of intervention is great. Psychotherapy is one of many interventions to address social, emotional, and behavioral problems. Other interventions (e.g., preventive interventions, school educational programs, and medication), beyond the scope of this book, are also pertinent to the problems.

PSYCHOTHERAPY DEFINED

The focus of the book is on psychotherapy, a broad term. In the context of adult therapy, psychotherapy is defined as a special interaction between two (or more) individuals in which one person (the patient or client) has sought help for a particular problem and in which another person (the therapist) provides conditions to alleviate that person's distress and to improve functioning in everyday life (Garfield, 1980; Walrond-Skinner, 1986). A more recent definition in the context of evaluating child and adolescent treatment defines therapy as any intervention that is designed to alleviate distress, reduce maladaptive behavior, or enhance adaptive functioning and that uses means that include counseling and structured or planned interventions (Weisz, Weiss, Han, Granger, & Morton, 1995).

The interaction is designed to alter the feelings, thoughts, attitudes, or actions of the person who has sought or been brought to treatment. Typically, special conditions define the interactions of therapist and client. The client usually describes his or her difficulties and life circumstances and the reasons for seeking help. The therapist provides conditions (e.g., support, acceptance, and encouragement) to foster the interpersonal relationship and systematic experiences (e.g., new ways of behaving through practice, role-playing, homework assignments, and advice) designed to produce change. The definition is modified slightly in relation to children and adolescents. For example, children usually do not seek help but someone responsible for them seeks treatment, and in some cases the therapist may work more directly with responsible others (i.e., parents) than with the child.

The goals of therapy and the means to obtain them help clarify what uniquely defines psychotherapy. The *goals* consist of improving adjustment and functioning in both intrapersonal and interpersonal spheres and reducing maladaptive behaviors and various psychological and often physical complaints. *Intrapersonal* adjustment reflects such areas as how one views or feels about oneself and courses of action one pursues. *Interper-*

sonal functioning refers to how one adapts to and interacts with others (e.g., relatives, significant others, peers, and colleagues). The *means* by which the goals are achieved are primarily interpersonal contact; for most treatments this consists of verbal interaction. In child therapy, the means can include talking, playing, rewarding new behaviors, or rehearsing activities with the child. Also, the persons who carry out these actions may include therapists, parents, teachers, or peers. A variety of therapeutic aids such as puppets, games, and stories may be used as the means through which treatment goals are sought.

The definition of psychotherapy is restricted to psychosocial interventions in which the means rely primarily on various interpersonal sources of influence such as learning, persuasion, social support, discussion, and similar processes. The focus is on some facet of how clients feel (affect), think (cognitions), and act (behaviors). The definition is necessarily general because of the range of approaches and techniques that need to be accommodated. Thus, the definition includes a variety of treatments subsumed under many general rubrics such as individual, group, family, insight-oriented, behavioral, and cognitive therapies.

Excluded from the definition of psychotherapy are interventions that use biological and medical means of producing change, such as medication, diet, exercise, megavitamins, and psychosurgery. These latter interventions are often directed toward improved psychological functioning (e.g., medication to control hyperactivity or electroconvulsive shock to ameliorate recalcitrant depression). However, the methods, theoretical rationales, and clinical–research issues differ from those raised by psychosocial procedures. Also excluded are interventions directed toward educational objectives, such as various tutorial, school, and counseling programs singularly directed to enhance achievement and academic performance. Omitted from the standard definitions of psychotherapy are activities such as chatting with relatives and friends; engaging in hobbies, sports, or other individual or group activities (e.g., dancing, singing, and fishing); and participating in religion. All these can be therapeutic (i.e., can improve adjustment and functioning), but they are not formally regarded as psychotherapy. By tradition, the definition of therapy is restricted to a large class of psychosocial interventions, as we have noted. These interventions are also those studied by the mental health professions (psychology, psychiatry, counseling, and social work) and professions in which mental health services can play a major role (pediatrics, nursing).

SPECIAL CHALLENGES OF TREATING CHILDREN AND ADOLESCENTS

Treating children and adolescents raises special challenges that affect the administration and evaluation of treatment and have direct implications for research. Salient challenges pertain to identifying what problems warrant treatment, assessing child functioning, deciding the focus of treatment, and issues related to child and family participation in treatment.

Identifying Dysfunction

The initial task of identifying problems worthy of treatment raises special issues. Extreme and pervasive departures from normative functioning, by definition, are readily identifiable as in need of special intervention. Examples include autism and more severe forms of mental retardation. These are pervasive developmental disorders and are relatively easily recognizable, at least when compared to anxiety, depression, and hyperactivity. While more easily recognizable, the pervasive disorders are not usually the focus of psychotherapy for children and adolescents.

The social, emotional, and behavioral problems that are most frequently seen in treatment are externalizing (e.g., oppositional, conduct, and hyperactivity) and internalizing (anxiety, depression, withdrawal) behaviors, as mentioned previously. Most of the symptoms that comprise these problems are relatively common to some degree as a part of normative development. For example, fears, fighting, lying, difficulty in concentrating, and social withdrawal are symptoms of recognized disorders. They are also relatively common at different points in development. The clinically severe versions are more extreme, but they are not always easy to discern. Separation fears in young children, for example, can be upsetting to the "normal" child and can disrupt the child's and parents' lives (e.g., interfere with attending or remaining in day care or add to marital conflict). Many problems that warrant treatment are present in smaller or less intense doses in everyday life, which raises the question of when to treat. Identifying a pattern of behavior as a problem worthy of intervention is a difficult task for parents, teachers, and physicians who are often responsible for referring cases to treatment.

The difficulty of identifying a problem or dysfunction worthy of treatment is that it may not be the behavior or characteristic of the child that is deviant or significant at all. Rather, the significance of the behavior may stem from when the problem occurs over the course of development. For example, the implications and long-term outcome of a behavioral pattern (e.g., fighting and bedwetting) depend on the age of the child (e.g., 2 vs. 10 years old). Bed-wetting in middle and later childhood but not in early childhood (before age 5) is a risk factor for later psychopathology (Rutter, Yule, & Graham, 1973). One ought to evaluate and intervene in middle to late childhood but probably not in early childhood.

With maturation and socialization, many problem behaviors, emotional reactions, and maladaptive cognitions subside. For example, most adults are toilet trained, do *not* suck their thumbs, and do *not* cry themselves to sleep because of the darkness or monsters that are about in the bedroom. The specific age or point in development at which some problem behaviors emerge and subside can be identified only approximately. Although one can identify points at which behaviors clearly are problematic and impair functioning, many instances are not so easily identified. Thus, one of the challenges of child and adolescent treatment is deciding whether the qualitative or quantitative characteristics of the behavior are maladaptive or are within the normative range for the period of development of the child.

Assessing Dysfunction

Measuring clinical problems in children and adolescents raises special challenges that affect treatment and treatment research. Children and adolescents are often asked to report on their own dysfunction. Measures often ask subtle questions about the onset, duration, and intensity of specific symptoms. Many children can report on their symptoms and their functioning in everyday life, but their ability and willingness to do so depends on the nature of the problem and the characteristics of the children, their age and developmental level, and the precise method of assessment.

As a guideline, children are usually not considered to be reliable reporters in early childhood (<5 years of age) on self-report measures (interviews, paper-and-pencil measures with items read to the child). For children ages 8–9 and older, considerable re-search indicates validity of child report (e.g., La Greca, 1990; Mash & Terdal, 1997). Evidence suggests that adapting the format of self-report in a more user- and develop-mentally friendly way can assess clinical dysfunction and associated features in young children. For example, asking children to identify which of two puppets is more like them, as the puppets playfully self-disclose various characteristics, including social, emo-tional, and behavioral problems, yields information that is unlikely to emerge from sim-ply asking the questions directly (Measelle, Ablow, Cowan, & Cowan, 1998).

Parents are usually the primary source of information regarding child functioning because they are knowledgeable about the child's behavior over time and across situa-tions and usually play a central role in the referral of children for treatment. Social, emo-tional, and behavioral problems often reflect a departure from behavior as usual for the child (e.g., not interacting with friends and loss of interest in activities). Parents are in a unique position to comment on change. Parent evaluations are often obtained on stan-dardized rating scales (e.g., Behavior Problem Checklist and Child Behavior Checklist) that assess several domains of child functioning (e.g., aggression, hyperactivity, anxiety, and depression); on measures, parents typically rate the extent to which their child shows a particular behavior or problem on a 3-point scale (e.g., 0 = not at all, 2 = often). In standardized diagnostic interviews (e.g., Diagnostic Interview Schedule for Children), parents typically report on whether their child shows symptoms of various disorders (e.g., diminished interest in activities as a symptom of major depressive disorder) and with what frequency, severity, and duration. Scores of studies have attested to the utility and validity of parent reports well beyond the confines of treatment research.

The information parents provide about their child's functioning raises its own inter-pretive problems. For example, parent (usually maternal) perceptions of child adjustment and functioning may be related to parental culture and the associated expectations, be-liefs, and standards that form the context for the parent reports (Weisz, McCarty, East-man, Chaiyasit, & Suwanlert, 1997). Moreover, parent perceptions and reports are also related to parent psychopathology (especially anxiety and depression), marital discord, stressors, and social support outside the home (see Kazdin, 1994). Parents with their own psychopathology or who are experiencing stress are more likely to rate their children as more deviant, even when other, independently obtained evidence, suggests that the chil-dren are no more deviant than children of parents with fewer symptoms or stressors. Thus, parent reports of child deviance are shaded by parental culture, parental dysfunc-tion, and no doubt other aspects of what parents bring to the judgments they make. This is a rather unique issue for child treatment and evaluation of child functioning. Child im-provement at the end of treatment may reflect actual changes in the child, changes in the parent's perspective on how the child should behave, reductions in parental stress, or some combination. Similarly, lack of improvement on parent-completed measures may reflect either a failure by the child to show specific culturally valued changes or contin-ued or increased parent stress, even though the child may have actually improved. In short, parent perspectives and functioning may influence how deviant a child appears be-fore and after treatment, at least on parent-report measures. Because parent-report mea-sures are the most frequently used means of treatment evaluation, this is an issue and concern within child therapy.

The use of multiple informants and multiple methods of assessment (e.g., self-report, other report, and direct observation) is routinely endorsed as a strategy for treatment outcome evaluation. Parent, teacher, and child or adolescent reports, perhaps supple-mented with other measures (e.g., physiological measures of anxiety and school or arrest records), might be used. A challenge is that measures often do not correspond well in the information they provide about the child (Achenbach, McConaughy, & Howell, 1987; Kazdin, 1994). This means, of course, that children who appear deviant or to have problems on measures obtained from one source (e.g., parents) may not appear to have problems on measures obtained from another source (e.g., teachers) (see Kazdin 1989; Offord et al., 1996). Also, therapeutic change at the end of treatment may be reflected on one measure or set of measures (e.g., those completed by the parent) but not on another set (e.g., those completed by the teacher). A challenge is interpretation of the results. It is possible that therapeutic changes are restricted to a set of measurement domains due to the specific effects and limited impact of therapy, characteristics of assessment, or both in varying degrees.

Focus of Treatment

Obviously, or so it would seem, the child is brought to treatment because he or she has a problem or significant impairment. This being the case, it would seem natural to focus on the child as the target of treatment. Yet children, like the rest of us, function in a context or set of systems (Bronfenbrenner, 1979; Lerner, 1991). *Context,* for purposes of the present discussion, refers to the environmental factors in which the child functions, and encompasses interpersonal relations (e.g., with parents, peers, and siblings), systems (e.g., family and school), and settings (e.g., neighborhoods). Although we all depend on our contexts, our dependence of children on adults makes them particularly vulnerable to influences over which they have little control.

Many adverse contextual influences affect child functioning and have direct implications for child adjustment and psychopathology. Familiar examples include poor prenatal care and nutrition, prenatal substance abuse by the mother, physical and sexual abuse, and neglect of the child. Contextual influences can affect attendance to, participation in, and effects of treatment. For example, among children and adolescents with externalizing problems, socioeconomic disadvantage, high levels of stress, parent psychopathology, and marital discord can influence the likelihood that families will attend treatment and, among those who do attend, the extent to which the children will improve and maintain their improvements over time (Kazdin, 2001).

The child's dependence on parent and family influences and evidence that many of these influences are somehow involved in the child's problems raise questions about the appropriate focus of treatment. To whom should the treatment be directed? Major options include the child, parents, the family (as a unit), teachers, peers, and siblings. Of course, at a broader level it would be reasonable as well to target neighborhoods, cities, and society at large (e.g., through legislation or social policy) to reduce clinical dysfunction. In clinical work, treatment of child or adolescent dysfunction usually incorporates the parent, family, and teacher in some way (Kazdin, Siegel, & Bass, 1990; Koocher & Pedulla, 1977), which may entail involving parents in the sessions with the child, seeing parents separately, meeting with the family, and using the teacher to assess or intervene at school (e.g., a behavior modification program in the classroom). The entire matter of where to intervene is especially complex in relation to child treatment in general in light of the range of options.

If children are particularly dependent on the parent and family, perhaps the parent and family are the best place to intervene. This focus could be justified on one of two grounds. First, it could be that several of the forces or influences that promote or sustain the child's problems are within the family or interpersonal context. In other words, contextual influences could be considered pertinent to the onset and maintenance of the problem. Second, contextual influences could be considered a valuable way to alter child functioning. That is, no matter how the problem came about, changing aspects of the context might be an excellent way to effect change.

Contexts and their influence change over the course of development. Thus, in relation to treatment, it might make sense to involve the parents extensively in the treatment of young children. For adolescents, perhaps peers might need to be involved in treatment given their critical influence on behavior. At an abstract and "overview" level, it is easy to say that treatment may need to consider contextual influences. From the perspective of providing treatment clinically or investigating treatment, involving others in the child's treatment raises its own challenges and obstacles. Compliance with treatment is likely to be a function of the complexity of the precise demands that are made but also in the number of individuals (e.g., child, parents, and teachers) who are asked to participate in the treatment.

Motivation for and Participation in Treatment

In almost all cases, children and adolescents do not refer themselves for treatment or identify themselves of their own volition as experiencing stress, symptoms, or problems. Young children may not have the perspective to identify their own psychological impairment and its impact on daily functioning, nor to consider the possibility that therapy is a viable means to help. This may explain why, when referred for treatment and asked to identify the problems for which they need help, children tend to note problems that differ from those identified by their parents (Yeh & Weisz, 2001). Also, problems most commonly referred for treatment among children and adolescents involve externalizing or disruptive behavior (e.g., aggression, and hyperactivity). In such cases, it is likely that adults experience the child as disturbing. Indeed, a cliché of child treatment is that much of therapy focuses on *disturbing* rather than *disturbed* behavior. Reports from adults (parents, teachers) serve as the impetus for treatment, so the focus may in part be someone else's stress rather than the child's. Children are less likely to report dysfunction or a problem in relation to their own experience. This is, of course, much less true of adolescents, although here too behavioral patterns that parents would see as problematic (e.g., behaviors related to substance use and abuse, unprotected sex, vandalism, talk of killing oneself, or excessive concern with body image and extreme dieting) are not usually considered by adolescents as in need of any intervention.

The tendency of children and adolescents either to perceive no problem or to identify problems different from those their parents have targeted for treatment affects motivation for seeking and remaining in treatment and for engaging in the tasks that the particular treatment approach requires. Getting the child to come to treatment is a significant obstacle. Although the parent is "in control" of the decision to come to treatment and to begin the treatment process, it is likely that the child may be much more interested in staying after school for soccer practice than using the time for therapy sessions.

Once at the treatment sessions, the therapist will implement the various techniques he or she considers to be the means of achieving the treatment goals. The techniques could involve talk, play, role-play, games, or a meeting with the entire family. Getting the child to participate in these activities is a challenge. Many therapists want the child to grasp the point of the activities. Yet, there is little motivation, interest, or incentive for the child even to be in treatment, particularly when contrasted with the other activities (hanging out, being with friends) that he or she is sacrificing. Similarly, parents often are concerned if the child is removed from school to participate in treatment.

Assume for a moment that the child and parent come willingly to treatment. Retaining children and families in treatment is a significant challenge. Among children who begin treatment, 40–60% drop out prematurely and against the advice of the clinician (Kazdin, 1996; Wierzbicki & Pekarik, 1993). Perhaps the reasons can be deduced from points already highlighted. Thus, if the child is not motivated to come to treatment or the parent is ambivalent about activities (class, sports) that compete with the time therapy is scheduled, problems in attending and continuing in treatment could easily be created.

Many factors influence whether families will remain in treatment. For example, among oppositional, aggressive, and antisocial children, dropping out of treatment is predicted by many adverse contextual factors mentioned previously (e.g., socioeconomic disadvantage, high stress, parent psychopathology, severity of dysfunction of the child, and perceived obstacles associated with coming to treatment (e.g., Garcia & Weisz, 2002; Kazdin, Holland, & Crowley, 1997; Kazdin, Stolar, & Marciano, 1995). The context in which child dysfunction is embedded plays a role in remaining in treatment. Consequently, even if one is not focusing on the parents or family in ways that are intended to improve child functioning, parent and family factors may need to be addressed to ensure that families remain in treatment (Prinz & Miller, 1994; Santisteban et al., 1996).

General Comments

We mention the challenges of providing treatment to place into context research covered in subsequent chapters. The challenges of providing therapy heighten the significance of the advances of child and adolescent therapy research. Execution, completion, and analyses of controlled trials could be readily undermined by the challenges that are more likely to occur with treatment of children and adolescents as compared with adults. These challenges arise in addition to those common to treatment researchers in general, such as recruiting sufficient numbers of cases for a study and conducting follow-up assessment among those families that do complete treatment.

Although this book focuses on treatment outcome research, the "challenges" we have identified are areas of research in their own right. For example, assessment of child dysfunction and therapeutic change is a vast area of research that includes measurement development and validation, identifying criteria on various assessment devices that reflect important or clinically significant change. Also, retaining children and families in treatment has been a separate focus of research. We mention these lines of work merely to note that the advances in treatment to which this book is devoted have depended on related areas of research that we cannot cover.

GOALS OF THIS BOOK

The book presents psychotherapies for children and adolescents that have strong evidence in their behalf and illustrates the type of research needed to place treatment on a strong empirical footing. There have been separate and somewhat independent efforts to identify such treatments by different professional organizations and committees spanning different countries (e.g., *Evidence-Based Mental Health*, 1998; Nathan & Gorman, 2000; Roth & Fonagy, 1996; Task Force on Promotion and Dissemination of Psychological Procedures, 1995). These efforts have used different terminology to delineate treatments that have evidence in their behalf and different criteria for making this delineation. Among the terms that have been used are "empirically validated treatments," "empirically supported treatments," "evidence-based treatments," "evidence-based practice," and "treatments that work." The criteria have varied too but often include use of randomized controlled trials to demonstrate treatment effects, replication of treatment effects by an independent investigator or investigative team, use of clinical samples, and others.

The chapters of this book encompass many treatments that have been delineated as evidence based. However, we did not invoke a set of criteria to delineate what would and would not be covered in the book. Rather, we selected interventions and programs of research we felt would be exemplary and where palpable progress has been made in controlled studies. As the reader will note, many of the chapters cover treatments that have been well established in controlled trials and with multiple replications. The book is designed to highlight advances among such evidence-based treatments. In addition, we have presented treatments in various stages of development, including treatments that may have only one well-controlled trial but for which programmatic studies are well under way. Although the book is intended to display the rich yield from years of research the chapters also nicely illustrate the process of programmatic research. The purpose of this feature of the book is to help researchers who are developing treatment and contemplating careers in intervention research by providing examples of research programs.

The majority of chapters that follow are devoted to specific treatment techniques. For these chapters, contributors were asked to provide an overview of the clinical problem they have been studying, the model or underlying assumptions of treatment, and the goals of treatment. Chapters include details of the intervention so the reader can discern the content of the treatment sessions, the sequence of material covered in the sessions, and the skills or tasks emphasized in treatment. Such details are not permitted in the usual publication outlets for research such as journal publication so we as readers are often persuaded that a given intervention might work but do not really have an idea of what the intervention really was in any detail. Contributors were encouraged to describe the intervention, to discuss how it is implemented, what treatment manuals they used and are available, and who serves as therapists, how therapists are trained and supervised, and other details.

Contributors were also asked to provide the scope of the evidence for their treatment. The contributors are seasoned investigators with remarkable programs of research. Consequently, asking them to present the outcome results in a brief space ranges somewhere between cruel and unfair. Even so, contributors met the challenge and provided us with a concise statement of the outcome evidence for the treatment they have covered and the questions that research has addressed in relation to that treatment. The chapters provide a concise statement of what the treatment is, to whom it is applied, the evidence in support of the treatment, and the key questions that remain to be researched.

Not all the chapters focus on specific treatment techniques. The book begins with chapters that address broad issues on which treatment research heavily depends. First, developmental issues relate directly to the design, implementation, and evaluation of treatment and consequently these issues are presented. Second, ethical and legal issues provide the context for how research can and ought to be designed and conducted. Third, issues regarding evidence-based treatments are also critical. The many issues relate to what it means to be designated as an evidence-based treatment, how these treatments are defined, and how they are implemented and evaluated.

NOTE

1. Tracing therapy back to Aristotle is not much of a stretch. Aristotle spoke about emotional states and how people suffering from emotional outbreaks can be cured by cathartic songs (*Politics* VIII 7.1342a4–16). Yet the connection is even more explicit in developing or charting a history of therapy. For example, Jacob Bernays (1824–1881), a relative of Freud by marriage, drew on Aristotle to note further that the cathartic benefits obtained via tragic drama are similar to a process of psychological healing (Bernays, 1857).

REFERENCES

Achenbach, T. M., McConaughy, S. H., & Howell, C. T. (1987). Child/adolescent behavioral and emotional problems: Implications of cross-informant correlations for situational specificity. *Psychological Bulletin, 101*, 213–232.

American Psychiatric Association. (1994). *Diagnostic and statistical manual of mental disorders* (4th ed.). Washington, DC: Author.

Angold, A., Costello, E., & Erkanli, A. (1999). Comorbidity. *Journal of Child Psychology and Psychiatry, 40*, 55–87.

Bernays, J. (1857). *Zwei Abhandlungen uber die aristolische Theorie des Drama: I. Grundzüge der verlorenen Abhandlung des Aristoteles über Wirkung der Tragödie; II. Ergänzung zu Aristoteles' Poetik.* Berlin, 1880. (Part I first published Breslau, 1857).

Boyle, M. H., Offord, D., Racine, Y. A., Szatmari, P., Fleming, J. E., & Sanford, M. N. (1996). Identifying thresholds for classifying psychiatric disorder: Issues and prospects. *Journal of the American Academy of Child and Adolescent Psychiatry, 35*, 1440–1448.

Bronfenbrenner, U. (1979). *The ecology of human development: Experiments by nature and design.* Cambridge, MA: Harvard University Press.

Clark, L. A., Watson, D., & Reynolds, S. (1995). Diagnosis and classification of psychopathology: Challenges to the current system and future directions. *Annual Review of Psychology, 46*, 121–152.

Cohen, P., Cohen, J., Kasen, S., Velez, C. N., Hartmark, C., Johnson, J., Rojas, M., Book, J., & Streuning, E. L. (1993). An epidemiological study of disorders in late childhood and adolescence I. Age- and gender-specific prevalence. *Journal of Child Psychology and Psychiatry, 34*, 851–867.

DiClemente, R. J., Hansen, W. B., & Ponton, L. E. (Eds.). (1996). *Handbook of adolescent health risk behavior.* New York: Plenum Press.

Dryfoos, J.G. (1990). *Adolescents at risk: Prevalence and prevention.* New York: Oxford University Press.

Elliott, D. S., Huizinga, D., & Ageton, S. S. (1985). *Explaining delinquency and drug use.* Beverly Hills, CA: Sage.

Evidence-Based Mental Health (1998). [A journal devoted to evidence-based treatments and linking research to practice.] Volume 1, number 1.

Eysenck, H. J. (1952). The effects of psychotherapy: An evaluation. *Journal of Consulting Psychology, 16*, 319–324.

Eysenck, H. J. (1960). The effects of psychotherapy. In H. J. Eysenck (Ed.), *Handbook of abnormal psychology: An experimental approach.* London: Pitman.

Eysenck, H. J. (1966). *The effects of psychotherapy.* New York: International Science Press.

Farrington, D. P. (1995). The development of offending and antisocial behaviour from childhood: Key findings from the Cambridge study in delinquent development. *Journal of Child Psychology and Psychiatry, 36*, 929–964.

Freedheim, D. K. (Ed.). (1992). *History of psychotherapy: A century of change.* Washington, DC: American Psychological Association.

Freud, A. (1946). *The psychoanalytical treatment of children: Technical lectures and essays.* London: Imago.

Freud, A. (1965). *Normality and pathology in childhood: Assessment of development*. New York: International Universities Press.

Garcia, J. A., & Weisz, J. R. (2002). When youth mental health care stops: Therapeutic relationship problems and other reasons for ending outpatient treatment. *Journal of Consulting and Clinical Psychology, 70*, 439–443.

Garfield, S. L. (1980). *Psychotherapy: An eclectic approach*. New York: Wiley.

Gotlib, I. H., Lewinsohn, P. M., & Seeley, J. R. (1995). Symptoms versus a diagnosis of depression: Differences in psychosocial functioning. *Journal of Consulting and Clinical Psychology, 63*, 90–100.

Greenbaum, P. E., Foster-Johnson, L., & Petrila, A. (1996). Co-occurring addictive and mental disorders among adolescents: Prevalence research and future directions. *American Journal of Orthopsychiatry, 66*, 52–60.

Johnston, L. D. (1996, December). *The rise of drug use among American teens continues in 1996. Monitoring the Future study*. Ann Arbor: University of Michigan Press.

Kazdin, A. E. (1989). Identifying depression in children: A comparison of alternative selection criteria. *Journal of Abnormal Child Psychology, 17*, 437–455.

Kazdin, A. E. (1994). Informant variability in the assessment of childhood depression. In W. M. Reynolds & H. Johnston (Eds.), *Handbook of depression in children and adolescents* (pp. 249–271). New York: Plenum Press.

Kazdin, A. E. (1996). Dropping out of child therapy: Issues for research and implications for practice. *Clinical Child Psychology and Psychiatry, 1*, 133–156.

Kazdin, A.E. (2000). Adolescent development, mental disorders, and decision making of delinquent youths. In T. Grisso & R. Schwartz (Eds.), *Youth on trial: A developmental perspective on juvenile justice* (pp. 33–84). Chicago: University of Chicago Press.

Kazdin, A. E. (2001). Treatment of conduct disorders. In J. Hill & B. Maughan (Eds.), *Conduct disorders in childhood and adolescence* (pp. 408–448). Cambridge, UK: Cambridge University Press.

Kazdin, A. E., Holland, L., & Crowley, M. (1997). Family experience of barriers to treatment and premature termination from child therapy. *Journal of Consulting and Clinical Psychology, 65*, 453–463.

Kazdin, A. E., Siegel, T. C., & Bass, D. (1990). Drawing upon clinical practice to inform research on child and adolescent psychotherapy: A survey of practitioners. *Professional Psychology: Research and Practice, 21*, 189–198.

Kazdin, A. E., Stolar, M. J., & Marciano, P. L. (1995). Risk factors for dropping out of treatment among White and Black families. *Journal of Family Psychology, 9*, 402–417.

Ketterlinus, R. D., & Lamb, M. E. (Eds.). (1994). *Adolescent problem behaviors: Issues and research*. Hillsdale, NJ: Erlbaum.

Koocher, G. P., & Pedulla, B. M. (1977). Current practices in child psychotherapy. *Professional Psychology, 8*, 275–287.

La Greca, A. M. (Ed.). (1990). *Through the eyes of the child: Obtaining self-reports from children and adolescents*. Needham Heights, MA: Allyn & Bacon.

Lerner, R. M. (1991). Changing organism–context relations as the basic process of development: A developmental contextual perspective. *Developmental Psychology, 27*, 27–32.

Levitt, E. E. (1957). The results of psychotherapy with children: An evaluation. *Journal of Consulting Psychology, 21*, 189–196.

Levitt, E. E. (1963). Psychotherapy with children: A further evaluation. *Behaviour Research and Therapy, 60*, 326–329.

Lewinsohn, P. M., Solomon, A., Seeley, J. R., & Zeiss, A. (2000). Clinical implications of "subthreshold" depressive symptoms. *Journal of Abnormal Psychology, 109*, 345–351.

Maser, J. D., Kaelber, C., & Weise, R. E. (1991). International use and attitudes toward DSM-III and DSM-III-R: Growing consensus in psychiatric classification. *Journal of Abnormal Psychology, 100*, 271–279.

Mash, E. J., & Terdal, L. G. (Eds.). (1997). *Assessment of childhood disorders* (3rd ed.). New York: Guilford Press.

Measelle, J. R., Ablow, J. C., Cowan, P. A., & Cowan, C. P. (1998). Assessing young children's views of their academic, social, and emotional lives: An evaluation of the self-perception scales of the Berkeley Puppet Interview. *Child Development, 69,* 1556–1576.

Milin, R., Halikas, J. A., Meller, J. E., & Morse, C. (1991). Psychopathology among substance abusing juvenile offenders. *Journal of the American Academy of Child and Adolescent Psychiatry, 30,* 569–574.

Moffitt, T. E. (1993). Adolescence-limited and life-course persistent antisocial behavior: A developmental taxonomy. *Psychological Review, 100,* 674–701.

Nathan, P. E., & Gorman, J. M. (Eds.). (2000). *Treatments that work* (2nd ed.). New York: Oxford University Press.

Offord, D., Boyle, M. H., Racine, Y. A., Fleming, J. E., Cadman, D. T., Blum, H. M., Byrne, C., Links, P. S., Lipman, E. L., MacMillan, H. L., Rae Grant, N. I., Sanford, M. N., Szatmari, P., Thomas, H., & Woodward, C. A. (1992). Outcome, prognosis, and risk in a longitudinal follow-up study. *Journal of the American Academy of Child and Adolescent Psychiatry, 31,* 916–923.

Offord, D., Boyle, M. H., Racine, Y. A., Szatmari, P., Fleming, J. E., Sanford, M. N., & Lipman, E. L. (1996). Integrating assessment data from multiple informants. *Journal of the American Academy of Child and Adolescent Psychiatry, 35,* 1078–1085.

Prinz, R. J., & Miller, G. E. (1994). Family-based treatment for childhood antisocial behavior: Experimental influences on dropout and engagement. *Journal of Consulting and Clinical Psychology, 62,* 645–650.

Roth, A., & Fonagy, P. (1996). *What works for whom?: A critical review of psychotherapy research.* New York: Guilford Press.

Rutter, M., Yule, W., & Graham, P. (1973). Enuresis and behavioural deviance: Some epidemiological considerations. In I. Kolvin, R. MacKeith, & S. R. Meadow (Eds.), *Bladder control and enuresis: Clinics in developmental medicine* (Vol. 48/49). London: Heinemann/SIMP.

Santisteban, D. A., Szapocznik, J., Perez-Vidal, A., Kurtines, W. H., Murray, E. J., & LaPerriere, A. (1996). Efficacy of intervention for engaging youth and families into treatment and some variables hat may contribute to differential effectiveness. *Journal of Family Psychology, 10,* 35–44.

Shapiro, A. K., & Shapiro, E. (1998). *Powerful placebo: From ancient priest to modern physician.* Baltimore: Johns Hopkins University Press.

Task Force on Promotion and Dissemination of Psychological Procedures. (1995). Training in and dissemination of empirically validated psychological treatments: Report and recommendations. *The Clinical Psychologist, 48*(1), 3–23.

Tracy, P. E., Wolfgang, M. E., & Figlio, R. M. (1990). *Delinquency careers in two birth cohorts.* New York: Plenum Press.

U.S. Congress, Office of Technology Assessment. (1991). *Adolescent health* (OTA-H-468). Washington, DC: U.S. Government Printing Office.

Walrond-Skinner, S. (1986). *Dictionary of psychotherapy.* London: Routledge & Kegan Paul.

Weinberg, N. Z., Rahdert, E., Colliver, J. D., & Glanz, M. D. (1998). Adolescent substance abuse: A review of the past 10 years. *Journal of the American Academy of Child and Adolescent Psychiatry, 37,* 252–261.

Weisz, J. R., McCarty, C. A., Eastman, K. L., Chaiyasit, W. & Suwanlert, S. (1997). Developmental psychopathology and culture: Ten lessons from Thailand. In S. S. Luthar, J. A. Burack, D. Cicchetti, & J. R. Weisz (Eds.), *Developmental psychopathology: Perspectives on adjustment, risk, and disorder* (pp. 568–592). Cambridge, UK: Cambridge University Press.

Weisz, J. R., Weiss, B., Han, S. S., Granger, D. A., & Morton, T. (1995). Effects of psychotherapy with children and adolescents revisited: A meta-analysis of treatment outcome studies. *Psychological Bulletin, 117,* 450–468.

Wierzbicki, M., & Pekarik, G. (1993). A meta-analysis of psychotherapy dropout. *Professional Psychology: Research and Practice, 24,* 190–195.

Windle, M., Shope, J. T., & Bukstein, O. (1996). Alcohol use. In R. J. DiClemente, W. B. Hansen,

& L. E. Ponton (Eds.), *Handbook of adolescent health risk behavior* (pp. 115–159). New York: Plenum Press.

World Health Organization. (1992). *International classification of diseases and health-related problems*. Geneva, Switzerland: Author.

World Health Organization. (2001). The world health report: 2001: Mental health: New understanding, new hope. Geneva, Switzerland: Author.

Yeh, M., & Weisz, J. R. (2001). Why are we here at the clinic? Parent-child (dis)agreement on referral problems at outpatient treatment entry. *Journal of Consulting and Clinical Psychology, 69*, 1018–1025.

2

Developmental Issues and Considerations in Research and Practice

Grayson N. Holmbeck, Rachel Neff Greenley,
and Elizabeth A. Franks

An interesting and potentially challenging aspect of providing treatment to children as well as conducting research on treatment effectiveness is the fact that recipients of such treatment are developmental "moving targets." The course of developmental change also varies across individuals, such that two children who are the same age may differ dramatically with respect to cognitive, emotional, physical, and social functioning (Eyberg, Schuhmann, & Rey, 1998). Moreover, there are developmental and age variations in the nature and frequency of child symptomatology, with the same behaviors that are developmentally normative at a younger age becoming developmentally atypical at a later age (e.g., temper tantrums; Kazdin, 1993). We also know that the same underlying psychopathology may be expressed differently at different stages of development (i.e., heterotypic continuity) and that two children who exhibit the same level of psychopathology may have reached that level of pathology along different pathways (i.e., equifinality; Cicchetti & Rogosch, 2002). Given such developmental variation and change, it seems reasonable to postulate that outcomes of child and adolescent psychotherapy will be enhanced if clinicians attend to developmental issues in designing and evaluating their treatment strategies (Holmbeck et al., 2000; Kendall, Lerner, & Craighead, 1984; Shirk, 1988, 1999, 2001; Silverman & Ollendick, 1999; Weisz, 1997; Weisz & Hawley, 2002).

In this chapter, we emphasize the importance of considering a child's developmental level within the context of the therapeutic intervention. What do we mean by "developmental level"? A child's developmental level can be conceptualized as a snapshot at one point in time of the accumulation of predictable age-related changes that occur in an individual's biological, cognitive, emotional, and social functioning (Feldman, 2001). Although developmental level comprises all these domains of functioning, researchers in the area of child treatment have largely focused on the cognitive domain, as many treatments designed for children and adolescents are predicated on the assumption that altering one's thinking is an important precursor to more adaptive functioning in emotional, behavioral, or social domains (Shirk, 2001). Later in the chapter, we provide examples of how cognitive developmental level has been or could be operationalized in treatment and/or research.

What makes a given treatment developmentally oriented? As we discuss in more detail, such a treatment takes into account the critical developmental tasks and milestones relevant to a particular child's or adolescent's presenting problems (e.g., development of age-appropriate same-sex friendships, self-control, and emotion regulation in early and middle childhood; pubertal development and development of behavioral autonomy and social perspective-taking during adolescence). Such a treatment would also be flexible enough that therapists could choose which presenting symptoms to prioritize, depending on the degree to which each of the symptoms is developmentally atypical (Weisz & Hawley, 2002). For example, an adolescent might present with inappropriately low levels of behavioral self-control (e.g., poor anger management and high levels of risk-taking) as well as moderate levels of parent–adolescent conflict. The therapist might determine that the former is more developmentally atypical and problematic than the latter, thus necessitating a focus on self-control difficulties in treatment.

A developmentally sensitive treatment would also be tailored to take into account the developmental level of the child or adolescent (Forehand & Wierson, 1993); in fact, different versions of the same treatment may be needed to serve children over a wide age range. For example, it may be that a less complex version of a treatment is provided for children at lower cognitive developmental levels, with a more sophisticated version being provided for those at higher levels (Shirk, 2001). Indeed, many cognitive-behavioral treatments require that children be able to evaluate and change their own thought processes as well as consider links between their own thinking and their subsequent emotional states—skills that require more advanced cognitive abilities (Shirk, 2001). Finally, a treatment that is developmentally oriented would take a child's current social context into account (Forehand & Wierson, 1993). Thus, in early childhood, parents may be incorporated into the treatment, whereas during adolescence, relations with peers are more likely to be considered.

Are current child and adolescent treatments developmentally oriented? In general, the answer to this question is "no" (Holmbeck et al., 2000; Weisz & Hawley, 2002). But this is not to say that such adevelopmental treatments have been ineffective. As reviewed by Weisz and Hawley (2002), meta-analyses suggest that treatments for children and adolescents demonstrate medium to large effect sizes. It is our contention that effect sizes would be even larger if treatment was tailored to the developmental level of the child, although more research is needed on this issue.

The goal of this chapter is to discuss ways that developmental issues can be incorporated into the treatment of children and adolescents. First, we examine the degree to which developmental issues have been considered in the design and implementation of child psychotherapy. Evidence that treatment effects vary as a function of age and developmental level are reviewed. Second, we discuss how developmental level can serve as a moderator or a mediator of treatment effects on outcome. Third, we argue that knowledge of certain developmental issues will likely improve the quality of treatment manuals and the effectiveness of child psychotherapy. Finally, we provide recommendations for therapists and researchers who wish to incorporate "development" into their work.

PAST WORK ON DEVELOPMENTAL ISSUES
AND PSYCHOLOGICAL TREATMENTS

Are Current Treatments Developmentally Oriented?

In this section, we target literature reviews on the developmental sensitivity of treatments for adolescents, given that comprehensive reviews from a developmental perspective have not yet been conducted for other age groups. Holmbeck et al. (2000) conducted a review of recent treatment outcome studies employing cognitive-behavioral therapy (CBT) with adolescents. Of the 34 studies reviewed, only 26% (9 of 34) considered developmental issues when discussing the design or evaluation of the treatment. Of these 9 studies, only one examined a developmental variable (age) as a moderator of treatment effects. Some of these "developmentally oriented" studies considered various adolescent developmental issues in the design of the treatments (e.g., the advantages and disadvantages of parental involvement in treatment and the use of outcome measures developed specifically for adolescents) whereas others included developmentally oriented interpretations of treatment outcome findings.

Authors of book chapters, literature reviews, and meta-analyses were more likely than authors of empirical papers to consider developmental issues when discussing the literature on CBT (43%; 20 of 46 review articles; see Holmbeck et al., 2000). Although many authors suggest possible adaptations of treatment manuals to make them more developmentally sensitive, few provide methods for doing so (Weisz & Hawley, 2002). Several authors recommend that the therapist assess an adolescent's cognitive-developmental level; again, little advice has been forthcoming for how to do this (although see Bierman, 1988, for an exception). Finally, almost half the authors of literature reviews and book chapters discuss developmental variability in relation to the course of psychopathology (e.g., child and adolescent depression); unfortunately, little guidance is provided for how this information can be taken into account when designing treatments. In summary, most of those who study outcomes of CBT for adolescent clients do not mention developmental issues. Of those who do, there is little information regarding how such issues could be incorporated into the treatment process.

In their comprehensive review of the literature on the treatment of adolescents, Weisz and Hawley (2002) examined 25 empirically supported psychotherapies that have been used with children and adolescents. According to these authors, 14 of the 25 therapies have been shown to be effective with adolescents. Interestingly, 7 are downward adaptations of treatments originally designed for adults and 6 are upward adaptations of treatments originally designed for children, leaving only 1 that was developed specifically for adolescents (Henggeler, Schoenwald, Borduin, Rowland, & Cunningham, 1998). In other words, few of the 14 empirically supported treatments that have been used with adolescents take into account the primary developmental tasks of adolescence. Thus, at least in the literature on adolescents, little attention has been paid to developmental issues in the design, implementation, or evaluation of treatments.

Impact of Development on Treatment Outcome: Meta-Analyses

Meta-analyses have focused on the age of children or adolescents (a proxy for cognitive-developmental level) as a potential moderator of the effectiveness of CBT (e.g., Durlak, Fuhrman, & Lampman, 1991; Dush, Hirt, & Schroeder, 1989; also see Weisz, Weiss, Han, Granger, & Morton, 1995). In general, the techniques of CBT emphasize self-reflection and metacognition (thinking about one's thinking), consequential thinking (reflecting on the outcome of a particular pattern of thinking), and consideration of future possibilities (thinking about how changes in one's thinking might affect one's life in the future). In other words, the techniques of CBT are based on complex symbolic processes, which require a high level of cognitive development. As such, proponents of cognitive and cognitive-behavioral theories maintain that interventions will be more effective for those functioning at more advanced levels of cognitive development (e.g., Shirk, 2001).

Results of meta-analyses focusing on CBT are consistent with this contention (Durlak et al., 1991; Dush et al., 1989); effect sizes for adolescents (presumably those in the formal operational stage of Piagetian development) are nearly twice the magnitude of effect sizes for younger children (those in the preoperational or concrete operational stages of development; although see Keating, 1990, and Moshman, 1998, for critiques of Piaget's stage theory). Of course, there are disadvantages to using age as a proxy for cognitive-developmental level (Durlak et al., 1991; Kazdin, 1993; Weisz & Hawley, 2002). For example, it is possible that developmental variables other than cognitive-developmental level (which differ across age) could account for these findings. Moreover, age is likely a weak proxy for cognitive-developmental level given the vast heterogeneity in cognitive development, even within adolescents the same age (Keating, 1990). But, given that few researchers who evaluate outcomes of CBT actually include measures of cognitive-developmental level in their research protocols, meta-analysts have not had access to data on more sophisticated measures of developmental level and have, therefore, chosen to rely on age as an approximation.

Impact of Development on Treatment Outcome: Empirical Examples

In addition to the meta-analyses, researchers have attempted to assess the impact of developmental level on treatment outcome. In general, this body of research has focused on the impact of cognitive, behavioral, or cognitive-behavioral interventions across different domains of child and adolescent adjustment. Rather than attempting to provide an exhaustive review of this literature, a few programs of research are highlighted. Although each line of research presented in the following pages is sensitive to the impact of developmental factors on treatment outcome, the studies differ in the particular area of development with which they are most concerned, as well as the manner by which they incorporate developmental variables.

Age Differences in the Effects of Parent Training

Researchers have considered the impact of developmental factors on the effectiveness of parent training programs in reducing disruptive behavior disorders (Dishion & Patterson, 1992; Forehand & Wierson, 1993; Ruma, Burke, & Thompson, 1996). Developmental theory suggests that the effectiveness of parent training may differ across early childhood, middle childhood, and adolescence for several reasons (Forehand & Wierson, 1993). First, as children progress through middle childhood and adolescence, the peer group takes on an increasingly significant role (Holmbeck et al., 2000). Indeed, a large body of literature has documented the salience of the peer group as both a motivator and reinforcer of behavior during adolescence. Moreover, comparatively less time is spent with parents during this period. Second, the period of adolescence is characterized by an increased desire for autonomy as children traverse the early adolescent developmental period (i.e., increases in emotional and behavioral autonomy; Holmbeck et al., 2000).

Based on such developmental changes, it might be anticipated that traditional parent-training programs would be less effective for older children and adolescents who are attempting to consolidate their own identity compared with those in early childhood, who are still highly reliant on their parents and lack the same drive toward independence.

Guided by the foregoing theoretical predictions, investigators have tested these hypotheses empirically (Dishion & Patterson, 1992; Ruma et al., 1996). Dishion and Patterson (1992) focused on two groups of children with behavioral problems, those in early childhood (ages 2 years, 6 months to 6 years, 6 months) and those in middle childhood (ages 6 years, 6 months to 12 years, 5 months). Results of their investigation suggested that, although the effectiveness of the parent training did not vary as a function of the child's age, younger children demonstrated more clinically significant change than did older children, even after eliminating subjects who were in the subclinical range prior to treatment. Moreover, early termination from treatment was more common in the older group.

Extending these findings, Ruma et al. (1996) examined the impact of parent training on three groups of children with disruptive behavior disorders: those in early childhood (2–5 years), those in middle childhood (6–11 years), and those in adolescence (12–16 years). Results of their investigation supported Dishion and Patterson's (1992) previous work such that more young children fell in the subclinical range following intervention, although adolescents evidenced the most severe problems relative to the other groups at pretreatment.

Cognitive Developmental Level as a Moderator of Treatment Outcome

A separate line of research conducted by Schleser and colleagues has focused on measures of cognitive developmental level as moderators of CBT effectiveness (Borden, Brown, Wynne, & Schleser, 1987; Schleser, Cohen, Meyers, & Rodick, 1984; Schleser, Meyers, & Cohen, 1981). These researchers argued that the impact of their self-instructional training program should be greater in children functioning at higher levels of cognitive development because more cognitively sophisticated children would be better able to systematically apply problem-solving strategies and employ recursive thought processes (Forehand & Wierson, 1993).

Schleser et al. (1981, 1984) found support for their central thesis in samples of preoperational and concrete operational normal children. Specifically, both groups of children benefited from training and made gains in terms of their problem-solving skills, but children who had more advanced levels of cognitive development evidenced significantly better performance on perceptual perspective-taking tasks and were better able to generalize their learning to different perspective-taking tasks after being coached in appropriate self-instructions. Borden et al. (1987) extended Schleser's previous work to a population of children diagnosed with attention problems. Contrary to predictions, preoperational children benefited most from the training. The authors explain this counter-intuitive and unexpected finding by suggesting that younger children had more to gain from treatment because they were lacking in the metacognitive skills targeted by the intervention, whereas older children were not.

Treatment of Developmentally Relevant Social Behavior in Socially-Withdrawn Maltreated Children

In contrast to studies that conceptualized developmental factors as moderators of treatment outcome, Fantuzzo et al. (1996) considered a critical social developmental milestone by targeting children's peer play in the treatment of socially withdrawn, maltreated preschool children. Play activities were the focus of this program because peer play is the primary means by which preschoolers learn rules for social behavior; such learning may be less well developed in withdrawn children. For this treatment, socially withdrawn children were paired with peers who exhibited well-developed adaptive play skills. Findings suggested that relative to controls, children in the treatment condition (regardless of maltreatment status) evidenced gains in their prosocial behaviors and self-concept, as well as decreases in their antisocial behavior. Such findings highlight the potential utility of considering developmental issues when designing a treatment.

DEVELOPMENTAL LEVEL AS A MEDIATOR AND/OR MODERATOR OF TREATMENT EFFECTIVENESS

As noted previously, developmental level may play a role in determining the effectiveness of a treatment intervention. In this section, we explain differences between mediator and moderator effects (see Baron & Kenny, 1986; Hinshaw, 2002; Holmbeck, 1997, 2002; Kraemer, Stice, Kazdin, Offord, & Kupfer, 2001). A moderator is a variable that specifies conditions under which a given predictor is or is not related to an outcome (see top of Figure 2.1). For example, it may be that the impact of a given intervention on a given outcome varies as a function of some moderator (developmental level, age, gender, social class, etc.). In this way, the treatment may be more effective at one level of the moderator than at another level. A significant mediator is a variable that specifies a mechanism by

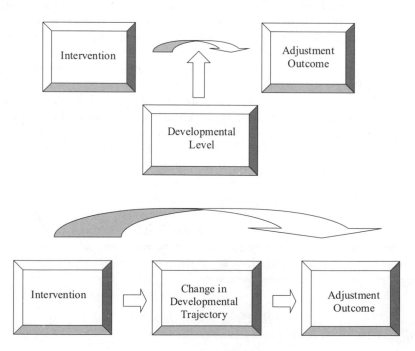

FIGURE 2.1. Moderational (top) and mediational (bottom) models of treatment outcome: The role of developmental level.

which a predictor has an impact on an outcome (see bottom of Figure 2.1). With mediation, the predictor (e.g., treatment condition) is associated with the mediator (e.g., change in developmental level), which is, in turn, associated with the outcome (e.g., adjustment). The mediator accounts for a significant portion of the relationship between predictor and outcome.

Developmental Level as a Moderator

By examining *moderators* of treatment effectiveness, we are interested in isolating conditions that determine when a treatment is particularly effective or ineffective (Figure 2.1). A relevant moderator, highlighted previously, is cognitive-developmental level. The examples discussed earlier focused primarily on differences between children with preoperational and concrete operational abilities. Turning now to older children, Piaget (1972) identified adolescence as the period in which formal operational thinking typically emerges; adolescents who have achieved such abilities are able to think more complexly, abstractly, and hypothetically and to take the perspective of others and employ future-oriented thinking.

Although there is general agreement that a shift in thinking occurs during the transition from childhood to adolescence, critics of the Piagetian approach have suggested alternatives (Moshman, 1998). Proponents of the information-processing perspective, for example, have sought to isolate specific changes in cognitive activity that may account for advances in thinking. They maintain that there are significant advances in processing capacity or efficiency, knowledge base, and cognitive self-regulation (Keating, 1990). A third approach to cognitive development during adolescence is the contextualist perspective. Vygotsky (1978) suggested that psychological processes have a social basis. Of interest here are the child's socially relevant cognitions such as one's understanding of significant others and their behaviors. The development of role-taking and empathy skills, the role of affect in understanding people, attributional processes in social situations, and prosocial behavior are a few of the social cognitive-developmental tasks that may influence progress in therapy (Nelson & Crick, 1999).

Given this list of cognitive changes during childhood and adolescence, it seems reasonable to propose that the degree to which a child has developed these skills will enhance or limit the potential effectiveness of a given psychotherapeutic intervention (Bierman, 1988; Downey, 1995; Forehand & Wierson, 1993; Wasserman, 1984; Weisz, Rudolph, Granger, & Sweeney, 1992). It is even possible that more advanced cognitive abilities may exacerbate some types of psychopathology (e.g., depressogenic cognitions; Eyberg et al., 1998). Research on cognitive-developmental moderator variables can be of use to those who develop new cognitively oriented treatments or to those who wish to develop alternative versions of treatments tailored to the needs of individuals at different developmental levels.

How might therapists assess the cognitive-developmental level of their adolescent clients? Unfortunately, a straightforward, user-friendly method of assessing level of cognitive development across different cognitive subdomains is not available. On the other hand, researchers in the area of cognitive development have been successful in developing several measures, some of which may be relevant within the therapeutic context. Some examples are as follows: (1) Fischhoff's measure of perceived consequences of risky behaviors (Beyth-Marom, Austin, Fischhoff, Palmgren, & Jacobs-Quadrel, 1993); (2) the Youth Decision-Making Questionnaire that assesses social decision making in various peer and parent approval conditions (Ford, Wentzel, Wood, Stevens, & Siesfeld, 1989);

(3) the Selection Task (Chapell & Overton, 1998), which requires evaluation of 10 conditional "if . . . then" propositions that assess deductive reasoning abilities; (4) the Similarities subtest of the WISC-III (Wechsler, 1991), which assesses abstract reasoning abilities; and (5) Dodge's measures of social information processing (Dodge Laird, Lochman, Zelli, & Conduct Problems Prevention Research Group, 2002; also see Nelson & Crick, 1999, for similar measures). Other more complex measures are also available but may be more useful to researchers than to clinicians (e.g., Flavell's and Selman's measures of role-taking, perspective-taking, and friendship development; Flavell, 1968; Selman, 1981).

Of course, cognitive-developmental variables are not the only developmentally oriented variables that can serve as moderators of treatment impact. Weisz and Hawley (2002; also see Shirk, 2001) highlight a different psychological moderator, namely, motivation. Here the focus is on the motivation to engage in treatment and the motivation for therapeutic change. This variable is "developmental" insofar as children of different ages may exhibit differing levels of motivation. As noted by Weisz and Hawley (2002), motivation may be lower in adolescence and particularly for those who are more peer-oriented (vs. adult/parent-oriented). On the other hand, therapists who work with adolescents may be more successful in using "future benefits" as a motivator than those who work with children (Piacentini & Bergman, 2001). Regarding biological development, interventions focusing on early sexual risk behaviors may prove to be more effective with adolescents who have begun to experience the changes of puberty because such interventions may be viewed as more salient by this subset of adolescents (although we know that there are certain preventive benefits to providing such interventions in prepubertal children).

Change in Developmental Level as a Mediator

Examining developmental level as a *mediator* addresses a different set of questions (Figure 2.1). If one has already established that a given treatment affects a given outcome, one is likely to pose questions regarding possible mechanisms by which the treatment affects the outcome of interest (Kazdin, 1997). From this perspective, a mediator is assumed to account for at least a portion of the treatment effect. Also, the mediator is viewed as causally antecedent to the outcome, such that change in the mediator is expected to be associated with subsequent changes in the outcome.

Interestingly, some may prefer to focus on the mediator (rather than the adjustment outcome) as the preferred target of treatment because of some known causal connection between the mediator and the outcome. For example, Treadwell and Kendall (1996) found that negative self-statements (or, more accurately, change in self-statements) mediated the effect of treatment on anxiety severity. In this way, self-statements accounted for a portion of the treatment effect. Moreover, self-statements were not only a target of the treatment but were also viewed as causally antecedent to anxiety severity. Perhaps more relevant to our discussion regarding developmental level, Guerra and Slaby (1990) found that change in problem-solving ability was associated with positive outcomes in delinquent behavior. Arbuthnot and Gordon (1986) have found similar results with moral reasoning as a mediator. Finally, changes in parenting skills (Forgatch & DeGarmo, 1999; Martinez & Forgatch, 2001), family relations (Eddy & Chamberlain, 2000; Huey, Henggeler, Brondino, & Pickrel, 2000), and deviant peer affiliation (Eddy & Chamberlain, 2000; Huey et al., 2000) have been examined as mediators of treatment → adjustment effects.

Examining mediator models in the context of treatment outcome studies is a particularly useful research strategy because of the experimental (i.e., random assignment) aspects of the design. As noted by Collins, Maccoby, Steinberg, Hetherington, and Bornstein (2000), if the manipulated variable (i.e., treatment) is associated with change in the mediator which is, in turn, associated with change in the outcome, there is significant support for the hypothesis that the mediator is a causal mechanism. To further support this hypothesis, it would be important to demonstrate (via the research design) that changes in the mediator precede changes in the treatment outcome (Kraemer et al., 2001).

An important corollary of these findings and speculations is that developmental level can be the focus of treatment (Figure 2.1; Eyberg et al., 1998; Shirk, 1999). That is, if research suggests that children who have failed to master certain developmental tasks or successfully navigate certain developmental milestones are more likely to exhibit certain symptoms, the developmental level of the child could be the target of the intervention. Returning to our example involving cognitive-developmental changes, adolescents may benefit from treatment that initially focuses on changing or accelerating cognitive-developmental processes (Shirk, 1999; Temple, 1997), particularly if lack of development in this domain has been linked with subsequent increases in symptoms. For example, treatment that affects children's perspective-taking abilities or their development of social–cognitive hostile attribution biases may ultimately produce a decrease in a child's level of aggression (Aber, Jones, Brown, Chaudry, & Samples, 1998). Aiding adolescents in developing more intimate relationships with their same-age peers may affect their level of social anxiety. In the area of substance use, treatments that focus on an adolescent's level of decision-making autonomy or future-oriented thinking may facilitate their ability to make decisions that reduce health risks. Finally, for externalizing symptoms and attention-deficit/hyperactivity disorder (ADHD), level of impulse control and self-regulation may be an appropriate mediator of treatment impact (Mezzacappa, Kindlon, & Earls, 1999).

Moderated mediation is also possible. For example, it may be that increased perspective taking is a significant mediator of treatment effectiveness for aggression, *but* only for adolescent-age participants. In this way, the mediational model is moderated by age. What are the implications of such a finding? Perhaps a different treatment is needed for younger children, or it may be that this treatment works for younger children but the mechanism by which the treatment has an effect differs across age. Or, it may be that both are true; different treatments may be needed at different ages because the mediational mechanisms vary with age. For example, if we are attempting to treat externalizing symptoms in younger and older children, we may find that parent training works well with younger children and that change in parenting quality is a significant mediating mechanism. With older children, however, we may find that use of a cognitively oriented approach works well and that a cognitive-developmental mediator (e.g., self-regulation) is a significant intervening causal mechanism. Despite the plausibility of these speculations, it is important to note that time-limited child treatments may not have dramatic affects on "development" (although see Keating, 1990, for an alternative perspective). If this is found to be the case, the mediational role of developmental level would need to be reconsidered.

In models that include moderated mediation, the mediator could be nondevelopmental and the moderator could be developmental. For example, as noted earlier, Treadwell and Kendall (1996) found that negative self-statements mediated the impact of treatment on outcome (see Weersing & Weisz, 2002, for an extended discussion of nondevelopmental mediators of treatment effects). It could be that this mediational model is moderated by a cognitive-developmental variable such as metacognitive ability (i.e., thinking about one's own thinking). That is, it may be that the most favorable outcomes are found for those who possess more well-developed metacognitive skills, as such skills would likely enhance children's ability to identify their own negative self-statements (S. Shirk, personal communication, April, 2002).

CONSIDERATION OF DEVELOPMENTAL FACTORS WHEN CONDUCTING THERAPY

Developmental Level, Milestones, and Norms

In Figure 2.2, we review important developmental stages and milestones that are relevant at different ages and developmental periods (based on Arnett, 2000; Feldman, 2001; Forehand & Wierson, 1993; Holmbeck et al., 2000). One implication of this list of milestones is that therapists who work with children and adolescents may need to address not only a client's presenting symptoms (e.g., ADHD and aggressiveness) but also the normative skills (e.g., self-control, emotion regulation) that the child failed to develop as a consequence of having a severe behavior problem (Shirk, 1999). It is also clear that the context and targets of treatment change dramatically as one moves across the first two decades of life. For example, whereas cognitive factors and peer relationships are less relevant when applying parent training in families of preschool children, such factors become highly salient in the treatment of those in middle childhood and adolescence (Forehand & Wierson, 1993).

As noted by Henggeler and Cohen (1984), when discussing different treatment options for children and adolescents who have experienced trauma (e.g., sexual abuse), consideration of developmental stage is critical when selecting an appropriate treatment. For example, when working with an adolescent who has experienced a traumatic event, it is important that the therapist distinguish between recent traumatic events *versus* events that occurred during childhood which are now being revisited anew during adolescence. With a previously experienced event, an adolescent may view the event from a new perspective (e.g., he or she can comprehend the injustice of the events). Such a new perspective on an "old" event may necessitate additional therapeutic attention. Indeed, treatment for a given trauma (e.g., early child abuse and marital disruption) may need to be administered *intermittently* at different critical periods as the original trauma is "re-experienced" at new developmental stages. For example, new issues may arise for the adolescent who was sexually abused as a child as he or she develops physically and begins developing opposite-sex friendships (see Figure 2.2).

Knowledge of developmental norms serves as a basis for making sound diagnostic judgments (and avoiding over and underdiagnosis). Unfortunately, the system according to the *Diagnostic and Statistical Manual of Mental Disorders* (DSM) tends to ignore developmental issues when providing diagnostic criteria, despite evidence that symptoms of most child psychopathologies vary with age. For example, although young children often display obsessive–compulsive symptoms as part of normal development (March & Mulle, 1998), such obsessive–compulsive behaviors are not typical of adolescents. Knowledge of normative behavior also has implications for decisions about treatment necessity and selecting the appropriate treatment. For example, strategies that focus on self-control may be more useful with older adolescents than behavioral programs that involve parents in the intervention.

With respect to developmental level, Weisz and Weersing (1999) detailed ways in which cognitive-developmental level affects the process of therapy and the types of treatments that are selected. A child's cognitive-developmental level may limit (or enhance) the degree to which the child understands the purpose and process of therapy. Similarly, the degree to which a child is able to employ abstract reasoning or perspective-taking skills may determine, in part, whether certain cognitive or insight-oriented techniques as well as strategies that require hypothetical thinking (e.g., role-playing exercises) can be implemented (Weisz, 1997). If a child does not have such skills, other therapeutic tech-

Infancy (0–2 years)	• Infants explore world via direct sensory–motor contact • Emergence of emotions • Object permanence and separation anxiety develop • Critical attachment period: secure parent–infant bond promotes trust and healthy growth of infant; insecure bonds create distrust and distress for infant • Initial use of sounds and words to communicate • Piaget's Sensorimotor stage
Toddler/preschool years (2–6 years)	• Use of multiple words and symbols to communicate • Learns self-care skills • Mainly characterized by egocentricity, but preschoolers appreciate differences in perspectives of others • Use of imagination, engagement in "pretend" play • Increasing sense of autonomy and control of environment • Develops school readiness skills • Piaget's Preoperational stage
Middle childhood (6–10 years)	• Social, physical, and academic skills develop • Logical thinking and reasoning develops • Increased interaction with peers • Increasing self-control and emotion regulation • Piaget's Concrete Operational stage
Adolescence (10–18 years)	• Pubertal development; sexual development • Development of metacognition (i.e., use of higher-order strategizing in learning; thinking about one's own thinking) • Higher cognitive skills develop, including abstraction, consequential thinking, hypothetical reasoning, and perspective taking • Transformations in parent–child relationships; increase in family conflicts • Peer relationships increasingly important and intimate • Making transition from childhood to adulthood • Developing sense of identity and autonomous functioning • Piaget's Formal Operations stage
Emerging adulthood (18–25 years)	• Establishment of meaningful and enduring interpersonal relationships • Identity explorations in areas of love, work, and worldviews • Peak of certain risk behaviors • Obtaining education and training for long-term adult occupation

FIGURE 2.2. Developmental milestones and stages across childhood, adolescence, and emerging adulthood.

niques may be necessary (e.g., therapists may need to demonstrate how to identify mal-adaptive thoughts by talking aloud during role-plays; Piacentini & Bergman, 2001). Finally, knowledge of developmental level may guide the stages of treatment. When teaching a child increasingly complex levels of social interaction as part of social skills training, for example, the therapist can follow the developmental sequencing and stages of social play and social relationships (Selman, 1981). As noted earlier, "development" can be the target of treatment.

Developmental Psychopathology

Developmental psychopathology is an extension of developmental psychology insofar as the former is concerned with variations in the course of normal development (Rutter & Garmezy, 1983). Research based on a developmental psychopathology perspective has informed us about the developmental precursors and future outcomes of child and adolescent psychopathology. Moreover, the field of developmental psychopathology has provided us with a vocabulary with which to explain phenomena that are relevant to therapists and that researchers seek to explain empirically (e.g., risk and protective processes, cumulative risk factors, equifinality, multifinality, heterotypic continuity, resilience, developmental trajectories, distinctions between factors that produce symptom onset vs. those that serve to maintain or exacerbate existing symptoms; Cicchetti & Rogosch, 2002; Olin, 2001). Developmental psychopathologists have also informed us about boundaries between normal and abnormal and how such distinctions are often blurred at certain stages of development for certain symptoms (e.g., substance abuse vs. normative experimentation with substances; Cicchetti & Rogosch, 2002). In fact, some symptoms may even be reflections of children's attempts to negotiate normative developmental tasks (Siegel & Scoville, 2000).

Research indicates that the frequency and nature of most disorders varies as a function of age. Regarding changes in frequencies, Loeber, Farrington, Stouthamer-Loeber, and Van Kammen (1998) have documented age shifts in the prevalence of certain disorders (delinquency, substance use, sexual behaviors, etc.). Loeber and his colleagues have also documented important differences between children and adolescents with early-onset problem behavior (i.e., life-course persistent delinquency; Moffitt, 1993) versus those with later-onset problem behaviors (i.e., adolescent-limited delinquency). Rutter (1980) reviewed changes that occur in behavior disorders from childhood to adolescence and concluded that roughly half of all adolescent disorders are continuations of those seen in childhood. Those that emerge during adolescence (e.g., anorexia) tend to be quite different than those that began during childhood (e.g., ADHD), with the symptomatology of most child and adolescent disorders being manifestations of particular stages of development (e.g., for anorexia, pubertal and body image concerns during adolescence; for ADHD, self-regulation concerns during early childhood). The field of developmental psychopathology also addresses issues of continuity/discontinuity. Antisocial behavior tends toward continuity insofar as antisocial adults have almost always been antisocial children (Loeber et al., 1998), but many depressed adults tend not to have been depressed children (Rutter, 1980). Similarly, schizophrenia is often not preceded by psychotic disorders during childhood (Rutter, 1980).

A clinician's knowledge of developmental predictors has a number of implications for the treatment of children and adolescents, as illustrated by the following examples. First, if we know, based on longitudinal studies, that a specific set of behavioral deficits in early childhood (e.g., externalizing behavior symptoms and oppositional defiant disorder) is related to more serious pathology later in the individual's life (e.g., delinquency and conduct disorder), we can then treat the less severe antecedent disturbance before having to deal with the more serious subsequent disturbance. Early intervention is critical, because children with behavioral difficulties often "choose" environments that exacerbate psychopathology. Second, some children with certain developmental trajectories (e.g., girls who experience early pubertal development) may be at risk for subsequent behavioral symptoms (e.g., early sexual risk behaviors), and these individuals could be the targets of intervention. Third, the literature on peer relationships and later personal adjustment suggests that poor peer relationships early in childhood (e.g., peer rejection, aggressiveness, shyness, and social withdrawal) place children at risk for developing later adjustment difficulties. Although individuals such as those just described are often the focus of both universal and targeted *group* prevention efforts, the at-risk status of a given individual is also relevant within the context of *individual* treatment. In addition to focusing on behaviors that are most likely to place the individual at risk for future psychopathology, therapists can also identify opportunities for "protection" in the child's life (e.g., the availability of supportive, nonparental adults) that can buffer the at-risk child from developing later adaptational difficulties.

The terms "equifinality," "multifinality," and "heterotypic continuity" are also likely to be useful to the clinician who works with children and adolescents. Interestingly, it appears that equifinality and multifinality are more the rule than the exception (Cicchetti & Rogosch, 2002). Specifically, equifinality is the process by which a single disorder is produced via different developmental pathways ("children may share the same diagnosis but not the same pathogenic process" [Shirk, 1999, p. 65]). For example, it is likely that two depressed adolescents will have different etiological factors present in their backgrounds. Multifinality involves the notion that the same developmental events may lead to different adjustment outcomes (some adaptive, some maladaptive). For example, two young children who are sexually abused at the same level of severity may exhibit different developmental trajectories over time. Given past research support for the concepts of equifinality and multifinality (Cicchetti & Rogosch, 2002), it appears that therapists are best served by gathering as much developmental and historical information as possible about a given child (in addition to what the therapist already knows about the etiology of the disorder in question). Put another way, if equifinality proves to be an adequate explanatory model for most child psychopathologies, then treatments that are based on single causal/mediational models will likely not be effective for sizable proportions of affected children (Cicchetti & Rogosch, 2002). Finally, heterotypic continuity involves the notion that a given pathological process will be exhibited differently with continued development. For example, behavioral expression of an underlying conduct disorder may change over time even though the underlying disorder and meaning of the behaviors remain relatively unchanged (Cicchetti & Rogosch, 2002).

In sum, a therapist working with children and adolescents would want to have knowledge of developmental norms and milestones as well as developmental psychopathology to aid in generating hypotheses about the course of a given child's disturbance. With such knowledge, one would be in a better position to answer questions such as the following: In the absence of treatment, is it likely that this child's disturbance will change, abate, or stay the same over time? Is the observed disturbance typical of the problems that are usually seen for a child of this age? Without answers to these questions, the therapist may misdiagnose, be prone to apply inappropriate treatments, or be overly concerned about the presence of certain symptoms.

RECOMMENDATIONS FOR THERAPISTS AND RESEARCHERS

In this section, we provide recommendations for therapists and researchers who seek to incorporate developmental principles into their work.

Recommendations for Therapists

1. *Stay current with the developmental literature* (Holmbeck & Updegrove, 1995). It is recommended that therapists subscribe to journals such as *Development and Psychopathology, Child Development, Developmental Psychology,* and the *Journal of Research on Adolescence.* Interestingly, all these journals regularly publish papers that examine clinical issues within a developmental context. Similarly, outlets such as the *Journal of Consulting and Clinical Psychology* often publish papers that integrate developmental and clinical issues. Also, the American Psychological Association publishes abstracts from developmental and clinical journals as part of its PsycSCAN series (PsycSCAN: Developmental Psychology and PsycSCAN: Clinical Psychology). Therapists are more likely to stay current with the developmental literature if training programs integrate their clinical child programming with offerings from a developmental program.

2. *Use developmentally-sensitive techniques.* Researchers who conduct interventions with young children (ages 4–8) often have success using techniques such as videotape modeling strategies or life-size puppets rather than strict cognitive approaches (Eyberg et al., 1998). Most young children are unable to distinguish between different types of emotions; thus, drawings and pictures from media publications may be useful. The degree to which children are motivated by the possibility of acquiring future benefits of treatment also varies as a function of age and should be considered when addressing motivational issues (Piacentini & Bergman, 2001).

3. *Focus on developmental tasks and milestones* that the child is attempting to master (e.g., self-control and social skills; Forehand & Wierson, 1993; Weisz, 1997). Weisz and Hawley (2002) have argued that developmental research may not always be useful in guiding the treatment of individuals, because group trends that emerge in developmental research may not apply to a specific case. On the other hand, these authors also provide some useful suggestions for ways to incorporate knowledge of developmental tasks into one's clinical work. First, they suggest that knowledge of developmental findings can *alert* the therapist to specific domains of functioning that are likely salient at a given age. In this way, the knowledgeable therapist is aware of what developmental issues to assess in an individual child client. Second, findings from developmental research can aid therapists in *prioritizing* certain presenting complaints over others, depending on which are most developmentally atypical or pathological. Finally, developmental research data can help the therapist in *selecting* treatment strategies or modules (from a more comprehensive set of treatments) that may be developmentally appropriate for a given individual.

4. When working with older children and adolescents, *think multisystemically* and consider a child's context (Forehand & Wierson, 1993; Henggeler et al., 1998; Kazdin, 1997; Reid, 1993). Working with adolescents, Henggeler and colleagues (1998) have documented the importance of attending to the multiple systems (family, peer, school) in which a child interacts. Similarly, if a family-oriented CBT approach is deemed optimal, the adjustment of parents and the quality of parenting should be assessed prior to including the parents as part of the intervention (Shirk, 1999). Incorporating peers and/or teachers as "therapists" may be a particularly useful strategy (Holmbeck et al., 2000), if age-appropriate.

5. *Help parents (and other relevant adults, such as teachers) to become developmentally sensitive* (Forehand & Wierson, 1993; Holmbeck & Updegrove, 1995). Parents are likely to manage their children differently if they know, for example, that increases in parent–child conflict over certain issues is normative during the transition to adolescence than if they did not have this knowledge.

6. To prevent exacerbation of symptomatology, *anticipate future developmental tasks and milestones* (Forehand & Wierson, 1993). For example, therapists can discuss the normative tasks of adolescence with a family seeking treatment for a pre-adolescent. Discussing how such future tasks may affect a particular child with certain vulnerabilities could be helpful.

7. *Consider the concept of equifinality* when conducting treatment (Cicchetti & Rogosch, 2002; Shirk, Talmi, & Olds, 2000). As noted earlier, different developmental pathways may lead to the same psychopathological outcome (i.e., equifinality). In keeping with this perspective, Shirk et al. (2000) have suggested that treatment not be guided exclusively by diagnostic status. Indeed, treatments may be unsuccessful for some children because the developmental precursors for their symptoms differ from the precursors of symptoms for children exhibiting successful treatment outcomes. Some researchers have isolated developmentally oriented typologies for certain psychopathologies that will be useful in matching treatment with pathology subtype (e.g., substance abuse and delinquency; Cicchetti & Rogosch, 2002).

8. *Consider alternative models of treatment delivery.* Kazdin (1997) has provided a useful discussion of how different types of psychopathology may require different types of treatment delivery. Indeed, it is likely that most children will not derive maximum benefits from traditional time-limited treatment. Kazdin (1997) describes six such models of treatment delivery, which vary with respect to dosage, the number of systems targeted, and the degree to which the treatment is continuous or intermittent. He draws parallels between treatment for psychological symptoms and treatments for various medical conditions. Some psychopathologies may require continued care, much like ongoing treatment for diabetes. Treatment is modified over time but is never discontinued. Other psychopathologies may be best treated with a "dental model." With this approach, treatment is discontinued, but the child is monitored at regular intervals (particularly during important developmental transition points). Such treatment delivery models differ from the more standard notion of "booster" sessions. Booster sessions are typically used to reinforce treatment already provided; the types of care Kazdin (1997) is advocating are entirely different from treatment as usual.

9. *Begin to fill your therapeutic "toolbox" with empirically supported treatment "modules"* that can be used as needed (Shirk et al., 2000; Weisz & Hawley, 2002). In the area of neuropsychological assessment, both fixed battery and flexible assessment strategies have been advocated, with the latter becoming increasingly popular (Sattler, 2002). An analogy can be drawn between such neuropsychological assessment strategies and the treatment of children and adolescents. If an individual presents with a specific neuropsychological difficulty and a fixed battery approach is used, it is likely that many of the tests administered are irrelevant to the presenting symptoms. Moreover, because of the time required to administer the complete battery, certain areas of functioning that are relevant to the presenting problems may be underassessed. Advocates of the module/toolbox approach view treatment of children in a similar manner. Rather than using a more rigidly defined set of therapeutic techniques, it may make more sense to have a set of empirically supported techniques that can be used (or not used) as indicated (see Weisz & Hawley, 2002, for an example involving youth depression).

Recommendations for Researchers

1. *Know your disorder.* Prior to developing or evaluating a treatment, it is critical that an investigator generate a thorough developmentally oriented conceptualization of the disorder in question. In this way, the investigator comes to understand developmental antecedents in relation to the onset, maintenance, and escalation of the disorder; the developmental course of the symptoms; and any subtypes (Kazdin, 1997; see Conduct Problems Prevention Research Group, 1992; Weisz et al., 1992, for examples). Such an analysis will provide initial hypotheses concerning types of treatments that may be effective as well as mediational mechanisms that may account for significant treatment effects.

2. *Include measures of developmental level in treatment outcome studies and use them to evaluate moderational effects.* If evaluations of age differences in treatment outcome were to become the norm, this would be progress for the field. But it would be even better if researchers began to include measures of developmental level, so that the moderational effects of these variables could be assessed. Examples of variables that could be included are as follows (names of measures that could be used are included with references): pubertal development (Pubertal Development Scale; Petersen, Crockett, Richards, & Boxer, 1988), social skills and friendship quality (Social Skills Rating Scale; Gresham & Elliott, 1990; see Bierman, 1988, for methods of assessing conceptions of social relationships), cognitive-developmental level (e.g., metacognition, decision-making, and problem-solving abilities; abstract reasoning; social information processing; executive functioning; see earlier list), emotion regulation and self-control (Child Affect Questionnaire; Garber, Braafladt, & Weiss, 1995; also see Greenberg, Kusche, Cook, & Quamma, 1995, for other measures of emotion regulation), autonomy development (Decision-Making Questionnaire; Steinberg, 1987), and change in parent–child relationships (Issues Checklist; a measure of parent–child conflict; Robin & Foster, 1989). Of course, the types of variables included would vary depending on the treatment under investigation.

User-friendly measures of various cognitive-developmental constructs are sorely needed. For example, a measure of metacognition would be useful to clinicians attempting to select the best-fitting CBT strategies. Clinician-friendly measures of social perspective taking, empathy skills, self-control, future-oriented thinking, and decision making would also have considerable utility, although it is important to note that paper-and-pencil measures may provide somewhat limited and less ecologically valid assessments of cognitive skills than would observations of real-life encounters (e.g., self-reports of decision-making strategies vs. decision making in an actual peer relationship situation).

3. *Examine mediators of treatment effects.* Knowledge of mediational processes informs us about mechanisms through which treatments have their effects. Developmentally oriented variables, such as those just noted, could be examined as intervening causal mechanisms. Such developmental variables could also be examined as moderators of mediational treatment models (Weersing & Weisz, 2002).

4. *Begin to examine the efficacy and effectiveness of alternative modes of treatment.* As noted by Kazdin (1997), most studies of treatment outcome examine time-limited interventions. As reviewed earlier, there are other ways that we could conduct our treatments (e.g., continued care vs. intervention followed by regular monitoring). The effectiveness of these strategies should be compared with traditional treatments.

5. *Build "development" into treatment strategies.* When discussing mediational effects, it was noted that developmental variables could be the target of treatment efforts.

An example of this strategy is the Promoting Alternative Thinking Strategies (PATHS) program developed by Greenberg et al. (1995). The focus of their work is on increasing a child's ability to express and understand emotions in both low- and high-risk samples.

SUMMARY AND CONCLUSIONS

Although it appears that most treatments for children and adolescents are not developmentally oriented (with most of them being downward or upward extensions of treatments for individuals of ages other than the target population), there is great potential for the integration of developmental research with clinical practice. Ways in which developmental variables could serve as mediators or moderators of treatment effects were highlighted. We also reviewed various types of developmental research that could be informative to therapists who work with children and adolescents or researchers who develop new treatments or evaluate existing ones. Knowledge of normative development can aid the therapist in formulating appropriate treatment goals, provide a basis for designing alternate versions of the same treatment, and guide the stages of treatment. We have provided a number of recommendations for clinicians and researchers who wish to integrate developmental principles into their work. Although we argued that the quality of treatment is likely to be enhanced if therapists attend to developmental issues, this argument is mostly speculation as this point (Weisz, 1997). We hope that this chapter will serve as a "call" for more research on ways that "development" can influence treatment effectiveness.

ACKNOWLEDGMENTS

Completion of this chapter was supported in part by research grants from the March of Dimes Birth Defects Foundation (12-FY01-0098) and the National Institute of Mental Health (R01-MH50423). We wish to thank Stephen Shirk and Joseph Durlak for comments on an earlier version of this chapter.

REFERENCES

Aber, J. L., Jones, S. M., Brown, J. L., Chaudry, N., & Samples, F. (1998). Resolving conflict creatively: Evaluating the developmental effects of a school-based violence prevention program in neighborhood and classroom context. *Development and Psychopathology, 10,* 187–213.

Arbuthnot, J., & Gordon, D. A. (1986). Behavioral and cognitive effects of a moral reasoning development intervention for high-risk behavior-disordered adolescents. *Journal of Consulting and Clinical Psychology, 54,* 208–216.

Arnett, J. J. (2000). Emerging adulthood: A theory of development from the late teens through the twenties. *American Psychologist, 55,* 469–480.

Baron, R. M., & Kenny, D. A. (1986). The moderator-mediator variable distinction in social psychological research: Conceptual, strategic, and statistical considerations. *Journal of Personality and Social Psychology, 51,* 1173–1182.

Beyth-Marom, R., Austin, L., Fischhoff, B., Palmgren, C., & Jacobs-Quadrel, M. (1993). Perceived consequences of risky behaviors: Adults and adolescents. *Developmental Psychology, 29,* 549–563.

Bierman, K. L. (1988). The clinical implications of children's conceptions of social relationships. In S. R. Shirk (Ed.), *Cognitive development and child psychotherapy* (pp. 247–272). New York: Plenum Press.

Borden, K. A., Brown, R. T., Wynne, M. E., & Schleser, R. (1987). Piagetian conservation and response to cognitive therapy in attention deficit disordered children. *Journal of Child Psychology and Psychiatry and Allied Disciplines, 28,* 755–764.

Chapell, M. S., & Overton, W. F. (1998). Development of logical reasoning in the context of parental style and test anxiety. *Merrill-Palmer Quarterly, 44,* 141–156.

Cicchetti, D., & Rogosch, F. A. (2002). A developmental psychopathology perspective on adolescence. *Journal of Consulting and Clinical Psychology, 70,* 6–20.

Collins, W. A., Maccoby, E. E., Steinberg, L., Hetherington, E. M., & Bornstein, M. H. (2000). Contemporary research on parenting: The case for nature and nurture. *American Psychologist, 55,* 218–232.

Conduct Problems Prevention Research Group. (1992). A developmental and clinical model for the prevention of conduct disorder: The FAST Track Program. *Development and Psychopathology, 4,* 509–527.

Dishion, T. J., & Patterson, G. R. (1992). Age effects in parent training outcome. *Behavior Therapy, 23,* 719–729.

Dodge, K. A., Laird, R., Lochman, J. E., Zelli, A., & Conduct Problems Prevention Research Group. (2002). Multidimensional latent-construct analysis of children's social information-processing patterns: Correlations with aggtessive behavior problems. *Psychological Assessment, 14,* 60–73.

Downey, J. (1995). Psychological counseling of children and young people. In R. Woolge & W. Dryden (Eds.), *The handbook of counseling psychology* (pp. 308–333). Thousand Oaks, CA: Sage.

Durlak, J. A., Fuhrman, T., & Lampman, C. (1991). Effectiveness of cognitive-behavior therapy for maladapting children: A meta-analysis. *Psychological Bulletin, 110,* 204–214.

Dush, D. M., Hirt, M. L., & Schroeder, H. E. (1989). Self-statement modification in the treatment of child behavior disorders: A meta-analysis. *Psychological Bulletin, 106,* 97–106.

Eddy, J. M., & Chamberlain, P. (2000). Family management and deviant peer association as mediators of the impact of treatment condition on youth antisocial behavior. *Journal of Consulting and Clinical Psychology, 68,* 857–863.

Eyberg, S., Schuhmann, E., & Rey, J. (1998). Psychosocial treatment research with children and adolescents: Developmental issues. *Journal of Abnormal Child Psychology, 26,* 71–81.

Fantuzzo, J. W., Sutton-Smith, B., Atkins, M., Meyers, R., Stevenson, H., Collahan, K., Weiss, A., & Manz, P. (1996). Community-based resilient peer treatment of withdrawn maltreated preschool children. *Journal of Consulting and Clinical Psychology, 64,* 1377–1386.

Feldman, R. S. (2001). *Child development* (2nd ed.). Upper Saddle River, NJ: Prentice-Hall.

Flavell, J. H. (1968). *The development of role-taking and communication skills in children.* New York: Wiley.

Ford, M. E., Wentzel, K. R., Wood, D., Stevens, E., & Siesfeld, G. A. (1989). Processes associated with integrative social competence: Emotional and contextual influences on adolescent social responsibility. *Journal of Adolescent Research, 4,* 405–425.

Forehand, R., & Wierson, M. (1993). The role of developmental factors in planning behavioral interventions for children: Disruptive behavior as an example. *Behavior Therapy, 24,* 117–141.

Forgatch, M. S., & DeGarmo, D. S. (1999). Parenting through change: An effective prevention program for single mothers. *Journal of Consulting and Clinical Psychology, 67,* 711–724.

Garber, J., Braafladt, N., & Weiss, B. (1995). Affect regulation in depressed and nondepressed children and young adolescents. *Development and Psychopathology, 7,* 93–115.

Greenberg, M. T., Kusche, C. A., Cook, E. T., & Quamma, J. P. (1995). Promoting emotional competence in school-aged children: The effects of the PATHS curriculum. *Development and Psychopathology, 7,* 117–136.

Gresham, F. M., & Elliott, S. N. (1990). *Social skills rating system: Manual.* Circle Pines, MN: American Guidance Service.

Guerra, N. G., & Slaby, R. G. (1990). Cognitive mediators of aggression in adolescent offenders: II. Intervention. *Developmental Psychology, 26,* 269–277.

Henggeler, S. W., & Cohen, R. (1984). The role of cognitive development in the family-ecological systems approach to childhood psychopathology. In B. Gholson & T. I.. Rosenthal (Eds.), *Applications of cognitive-developmental theory* (pp. 173–189). New York: Academic Press.

Henggeler, S. W., Schoenwald, S. K., Borduin, C. M., Rowland, M. D., & Cunningham, P. B. (1998). *Multisystemic treatment of antisocial behavior in children and adolescents*. New York: Guilford Press.

Hinshaw S. P. (2002). President's message: Explanation in treatment research: Moderators and mediators. *Clinical Child and Adolescent Psychology Newsletter, 17,* 1–3.

Holmbeck, G. N. (1997). Toward terminological, conceptual, and statistical clarity in the study of mediators and moderators: Examples from the child-clinical and pediatric psychology literatures. *Journal of Consulting and Clinical Psychology, 65,* 599–610.

Holmbeck, G. N. (2002). Post-hoc probing of significant moderational and mediational effects in studies of pediatric populations. *Journal of Pediatric Psychology, 27,* 87–96.

Holmbeck, G. N., Colder, C., Shapera, W., Westhoven, V., Kenealy, L., & Updegrove, A. (2000). Working with adolescents: Guides from developmental psychology. In P. C. Kendall (Ed.), *Child and adolescent therapy: Cognitive-behavioral procedure* (pp. 334–385). New York: Guilford Press.

Holmbeck, G. N., & Updegrove, A. L. (1995). Clinical-developmental interface: Implications of developmental research for adolescent psychotherapy. *Psychotherapy, 32,* 16–33.

Huey, S. J., Henggeler, S. W., Brondino, M. J., & Pickrel, S. G. (2000). Mechanisms of change in multisystemic therapy: Reducing delinquent behavior through therapist adherence and improved family and peer functioning. *Journal of Consulting and Clinical Psychology, 68,* 451–467.

Kazdin, A. E. (1993). Psychotherapy for children and adolescents: Current progress and future research directions. *American Psychologist, 48,* 644–657

Kazdin, A. E. (1997). A model for developing effective treatments: Progression and interplay of theory, research, and practice. *Journal of Clinical Child Psychology, 26,* 114–129.

Keating, D. P. (1990). Adolescent thinking. In S. S. Feldman & G. R. Elliott (Eds.), *At the threshold: The developing adolescent* (pp. 54–89). Cambridge, MA: Harvard University Press.

Kendall, P. C., Lerner, R. M., & Craighead, W. E. (1984). Human development and intervention in childhood psychopathology. *Child Development, 55,* 71–82.

Kraemer, H. C., Stice, E., Kazdin, A., Offord, D., & Kupfer, D. (2001). How do risk factors work together? Mediators, moderators, and independent, overlapping, and proxy risk factors. *American Journal of Psychiatry, 158,* 848–856.

Loeber, R., Farrington, D. P., Stouthamer-Loeber, M., & Van Kammen, W. B. (1998). *Antisocial behavior and mental health problems: Explanatory factors in childhood and adolescence.* Mahwah, NJ: Erlbaum.

March, J. S., & Mulle, K. (1998). *OCD in children and adolescents: A cognitive-behavioral treatment manual.* New York: Guilford Press.

Martinez, C. R., & Forgatch, M. S. (2001). Preventing problems with boys' noncompliance: Effects of a parent training intervention for divorcing mothers. *Journal of Consulting and Clinical Psychology, 69,* 416–428.

Mezzacappa, E. , Kindlon, D., & Earls, F. (1999). Relations of age to cognitive and motivational elements of impulse control in boys with and without externalizing behavior problems. *Journal of Abnormal Child Psychology, 27,* 473–483.

Moffitt, T. E. (1993). Adolescent-limited and life-course-persistent antisocial behavior: A developmental taxonomy. *Psychological Review, 100,* 674–701.

Moshman, D. (1998). Cognitive development beyond childhood. In D. Kuhn & R. S. Siegler (Eds.), *Handbook of child psychology: Vol. 2. Cognition, perception, and language,* (pp. 957–978). New York: Wiley.

Nelson, D. A., & Crick, N. R. (1999). Rose-colored glasses: Examining the social information-processing of prosocial young adolescents. *Journal of Early Adolescence, 19,* 17–38.

Olin, S. (2001). Blueprint for change: Research on child and adolescent mental health. *The Child, Youth, and Family Services Advocate, 24,* 1–5.

Petersen, A. C., Crockett, L., Richards, M., & Boxer, A. (1988). A self-report measure of pubertal status: Reliability, validity, and initial norms. *Journal of Youth and Adolescence, 13,* 93–111.

Piacentini, J., & Bergman, R. L. (2001). Developmental issues in cognitive therapy for childhood anxiety disorders. *Journal of Cognitive Psychotherapy, 15,* 165–182.

Piaget, J. (1972). Intellectual evolution from adolescence to adulthood. *Human Development, 15,* 1–12.

Reid, J. B. (1993). Prevention of conduct disorder before and after school entry: Relating interventions to developmental findings. *Development and Psychopathology, 5,* 243–262.

Robin, A. L., & Foster, S. L. (1989). *Negotiating parent–adolescent conflict: A behavioral-family systems approach.* New York: Guilford Press.

Ruma, P. R., Burke, R. V., & Thompson, R. W. (1996). Group parenting training: Is it effective for children of all ages? *Behavior Therapy, 27,* 159–169.

Rutter, M. (1980). *Changing youth in a changing society: Patterns of adolescent development and disorder.* Cambridge, MA: Harvard University Press.

Rutter, M., & Garmezy, N. (1983). Developmental psychopathology. In P. H. Mussen (Series Ed.), & E. M. Hetherington, Vol. Ed.), *Handbook of child psychology* (Vol. IV, pp. 775–912). New York: Wiley.

Sattler, J. M. (2002). *Assessment of children: Behavioral and clinical applications* (4th ed.). San Diego, CA: Author.

Schleser, R., Cohen, R., Meyers, A., & Rodick, J. D. (1984). The effects of cognitive level and training procedures on the generalization of self-instructions. *Cognitive Therapy and Research, 8,* 187–200.

Schleser, R., Meyers, A. W., Cohen, R. (1981). Generalization of self-instructions: Effects of general versus specific content, active rehearsal, and cognitive level. *Child Development, 52,* 335–340.

Selman, R. L. (1981). The child as friendship philosopher. In S. R. Asher, & J. M. Gottman (Eds.), *The development of children's friendships* (pp. 242–272). Cambridge, UK: Cambridge University Press.

Shirk, S. R. (Ed.). (1988). *Cognitive development and child psychotherapy.* New York: Plenum Press.

Shirk, S. R. (1999). Developmental therapy. In W. K. Silverman & T. H. Ollendick (Eds.), *Developmental issues in the clinical treatment of children* (pp. 60–73). Boston: Allyn & Bacon.

Shirk, S. R. (2001). Development and cognitive therapy. *Journal of Cognitive Psychotherapy, 15,* 155–163.

Shirk, S., Talmi, A., & Olds, D. (2000). A developmental psychopathology perspective on child and adolescent treatment policy. *Development and Psychopathology, 12,* 835–855.

Siegel, A. W., & Scovill, L. C. (2000). Problem behavior: The double symptom of adolescence. *Development and Psychopathology, 12,* 763–793.

Silverman, W. K., & Ollendick, T. H. (Eds.). (1999). *Developmental issues in the clinical treatment of children.* Boston: Allyn & Bacon.

Steinberg, L. (1987). Impact of puberty on family relations: Effects of pubertal status and pubertal timing. *Developmental Psychology, 23,* 451–460.

Temple, S. (1997). *Brief therapy for adolescent depression.* Sarasota, FL: Professional Resource Press.

Treadwell, K. R. H., & Kendall, P. C. (1996). Self-talk in youth with anxiety disorders: States of mind, content specificity, and treatment outcome. *Journal of Consulting and Clinical Psychology, 64,* 941–950.

Vygotsky, L. (1978). *Mind in society: The development of higher psychological processes.* Cambridge, MA: Harvard University Press.

Wasserman, T. H. (1984). The effects of cognitive development on the use of cognitive behavioral techniques with children. *Child and Family Behavior Therapy, 5,* 37–50.

Wechsler, D. (1991). *Wechsler Intelligence Scale for Children—Third edition.* San Antonio: Psychological Corporation.

Weersing, V. R., & Weisz, J. R. (2002). Mechanisms of action in youth psychotherapy. *Journal of Child Psychology and Psychiatry, 43,* 3–29.

Weisz, J. R. (1997). Effects of interventions for child and adolescent psychological dysfunction: Relevance of context, developmental factors, and individual differences. In S. S. Luthar, J. A. Burack, D. Cicchetti, & J. R. Weisz (Eds.), *Developmental psychopathology: Perspectives on adjustment, risk, and disorder* (pp. 3–22). Cambridge, UK: Cambridge University Press.

Weisz, J. R., & Hawley, K. M. (2002). Developmental factors in the treatment of adolescents. *Journal of Consulting and Clinical Psychology, 70,* 21–43.

Weisz, J. R., Rudolph, K. D., Granger, D. A., & Sweeney, L. (1992). Cognition, competence, and coping in child and adolescent depression: Research findings, developmental concerns, therapeutic implications. *Development and Psychopathology, 4,* 627–653.

Weisz, J. R., & Weersing, V. R. (1999). Developmental outcome research. In W. K. Silverman & T. H. Ollendick (Eds.), *Developmental issues in the clinical treatment of children* (pp. 457–469). Boston: Allyn & Bacon.

Weisz, J. R., Weiss, B., Han, S. S., Granger, D. A., & Morton, T. (1995). Effects of psychotherapy with children and adolescents revisited: A meta-analysis of treatment outcome studies. *Psychological Bulletin, 117,* 450–468.

3

The Frontier of Evidence-Based Practice

The last 10 years have seen a revolution in practice development, accompanied by a new emphasis on principles of science, improvements in clinical research, and the connection of practice with the latest evidence. Dozens of groups have been involved in these new debates about what constitutes appropriate empirical support for a particular intervention, and more importantly, about the implications of such support for practice (e.g., Chambless & Hollon, 1998; Weisz, Hawley, Pilkonis, Woody, & Follette, 2000). These efforts have raised numerous issues central to understanding and facilitating continued improvements in practice and have at the same time informed new ways of conducting and interpreting research. Nevertheless, it can be argued that many of the issues connecting evidence with real-world practice remain unexplored (Kazdin, 2001; Weisz, Donenberg, Han & Weiss, 1995). The "frontier of evidence-based practice" is yet to be mapped, and much still stands in the way of forging sustainable connections between research and clinical service.

Many of the recent developments regarding evidence-based practice stemmed from the important work by the Task Force on Psychological Intervention Guidelines of the American Psychological Association (APA Task Force; 1995), whose charge was to develop recommendations for research-based practice guidelines following the ascendance of managed care. These well-known guidelines emphasized the dimensions of (1) efficacy (i.e., how well a treatment is known to bring about change in a target syndrome in research) and (2) effectiveness (i.e., how well an intervention is expected to perform in a "real world" setting). Soon thereafter, the APA Division 12 Task Force on Promotion and Dissemination of Psychological Procedures outlined a more detailed definition of efficacy and developed a list of those psychosocial interventions judged to possess the greatest empirical support. The Division 12 Task Force issued the first major list of empirically supported treatments in 1995, and has since published several updates (Chambless et al., 1996; 1998). Numerous additional efforts have served to clarify or extend this work at various levels (e.g., Chorpita et al., 2002; Nathan & Gorman, 1998; Weisz et al., 2000). As noted previously, such work has been revolutionary with respect to the manner in which stakeholders now talk about practice and policy. The term "evidence-based practice"—though perhaps not always well understood or agreed on—is now ubiquitous.

Interestingly, the ambiguity of the term "evidence-based" is emblematic of the issues and controversies facing a scientific approach to practice development. For example, the Division 12 Task Force originally proposed the term "empirically validated" to describe treatments supported by specific research criteria, and the term met quickly with criticism due to the unintended implications that the status of these interventions was finalized (e.g., Chambless & Hollon, 1998; Garfield, 1996). The term was subsequently changed to "empirically supported" (e.g., Chambless & Hollon, 1998), and along the way, some scholars have begun to use the terms "evidence-based" and "empirically supported" seemingly interchangeably, even though the latter term has connotations specific to Division 12 Task Force criteria, whereas the former term does not. It is a central theme of this chapter that the promotion of a scientific approach to practice will require even more careful and focused attention to this vexing issue of defining evidence (cf. Rosen & Davison, in press; Weisz et al., 2000). Kazdin (1996) offered an apt analogy: "Everyone seemed to agree with Socrates that justice was a good thing, but there was a complete lack of consensus on the definition of justice." (p. 216)

THE CONNECTION OF EVIDENCE WITH PRACTICE

To fully understand the importance of this issue of defining evidence, it is first necessary to outline a model to propose how evidence—however defined—will ultimately connect with practice. Figure 3.1 outlines such an association of elements. In the figure, the ele-

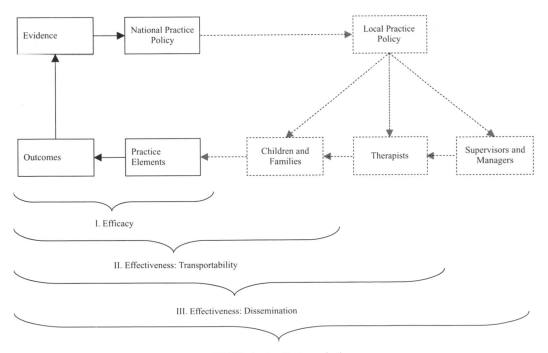

FIGURE 3.1. A model for the connection between evidence and practice.

ments and connections already developed are drawn in a darker shade, and less developed elements are drawn in a lighter shade. The first darker pathway shows the connection between practice elements and outcomes established by investigators, whose collective work has shown that particular interventions and protocols are comparatively likely to lead to positive outcomes. These observations have contributed to a body of evidence, a distillation of which has been the source of recently issued practice policy at the national level (e.g., Division 12 Task Force). It is tempting to think that these established elements are sufficient, but as the figure implies, many more steps are involved before one can close the loop. In fact, even those who have developed evidence-based criteria and guidelines acknowledge that policy alone is not likely to change the elements of practice that are delivered in real-world settings (Chambless & Hollon, 1998; Persons, 1995; Schoenwald & Hoagwood, 2001). Rather, the initial APA Task Force work was intended mainly as a demonstration to managed care and other policymakers that some psychological procedures had established efficacy at a time at which such information was critical to produce (Barlow, 1994). In terms of actually changing practice, there would indeed be more ground to cover.

It is proposed here that a first step in addressing the obstacles likely requires the engagement of organizations controlling local practice policy (e.g., managed care organizations, state mental health systems, public schools, and private provider networks). Here, the term "local" is not so much geographic as organizational. For example, a practice policy board in a large national managed care organization would be considered "local," even though its policies might have implications across many states. These local practice policies then need to be connected to all levels of the organization in which the new practice standards are to be implemented, as the downward arrows imply. Such connections would optimally involve at least three processes: (1) engagement, or the development of interest in the parties being addressed by the policy; (2) transmission of information (e.g., training), and (3) the use of supportive tools and technology (e.g., treatment manuals, flowcharts, and computer software). The understanding of these processes is limited, owing to the comparatively little research attention at the level of practice organizations (although see Glisson & Hemmelgarn, 1996).

Some examples can help clarify these connections. At the level of children and families, for example, engagement is an extremely important issue (Cunningham & Henggeler, 1999; McKay, McCadam, & Gonzales, 1996). Ideally, consumers of mental health services should be interested in the most promising interventions and seek them out. For this to happen, information about these interventions has to be presented to the public in some credible yet high-impact manner, for example through well-crafted articles in popular magazines or through ambitious public lectures (Persons, 1995). In that sense, training and engagement go hand in hand. Building further on this process, technology and tools to support this type of public education could take the form of such things as informational brochures and web sites. Ideally, all three proposed avenues (engagement, training, and technology) would correspond closely to the local policy to be implemented, to maximize the fit between consumer expectation and actual practice.

All three processes are equally important at the level of the therapist as well. Therapist engagement is presumably a prerequisite to any change in therapist practice. A system or organization therefore has to provide incentives for change and must maintain an organizational climate that ensures fidelity to the local practice policy. The value of the practice policy must therefore be made obvious to those who will implement it in their work (which is not often the case). Assuming this interest is established, there must be training in the new interventions, which can take any number of forms, from readings to workshops to mentorship. Finally, the training should ideally be supported through the use of technology and tools (e.g., manuals or clinical decision flowcharts). Multisystemic therapy, for example, encourages therapists to carry a card in their wallet outlining the major principles of the intervention (Henggeler, Schoenwald, Borduin, Rowland, & Cunningham, 1998). Such tools, when used properly, presumably amplify and sustain the effects of well-conducted training.

Finally, systems must also be addressed at the level of case managers and supervisors. The former are often most often involved in the selection of services (Burns, Farmer, Angold, Costello, & Behar, 1996). If case managers are not engaged, trained, and supported regarding evidence-based practice policy, their selection of services for a child might be based solely on nonpractice factors (e.g., proximity of a therapist to a family's home). Thus, local policy organizations need to demonstrate the value of these interventions, train managers to know how to critically evaluate them, and provide the tools and supports that facilitate their selection in any mental health system.

The same set of issues is true for supervisors. Although not often discussed in the outcome literature, supervisors are presumably a primary influence on therapist adherence to a protocol (Weisz & Hawley, 1998), and so too must be interested, knowledgeable, and well-supported regarding evidence-based protocols and policy. Further, supervisors are yet another pathway to therapist engagement and therapist practice knowledge (i.e., starting down the path from supervisors to outcomes in Figure 3.1), and thus play a doubly important role in the model.

Under ideal circumstances, then, case managers would select services that are evidence-based, their supervisors would be skilled and interested in supporting adherence to the treatment elements, therapists would be skilled and interested in implementing the protocol, and families would be engaged with the therapist and comfortable with the particular evidence-based approach. Assuming all these elements are in place, the psychological outcome research implies that particular practice elements should lead to positive results.

Were it only so simple. As the lightened shading implies, such connections are typically not in place, and thus it is important to identify the obstacles to their formation. As implied earlier, some of these connections await a better understanding of the most promising methods of engaging, training, and supporting new practice. However, one important theme of this chapter, noted previously, is that many of the problems in crossing this frontier stem from the nature of the outcome research and the resulting definition of evidence. For that reason, it is important to consider some different types of research and their implications for system engagement (i.e., their influence on the viability of the connection from national to local practice policy in Figure 3.1). Simply put, there are many ways to think about research and about the evidence it yields.

THE EVIDENCE BASE: FOUR TYPES OF RESEARCH

Type I: Efficacy

As shown in Figure 3.1, the accumulation of laboratory-based efficacy research has established the connection between practice elements and outcomes. This type of research is labeled here as Type I research, commonly known as efficacy research (e.g., Chambless & Hollon, 1998). In Type I research, the "upstream" elements are typically controlled in some way (i.e., children and families are carefully screened and selected, therapists are highly trained and have explicit allegiance to the investigator, and supervision is intensive and often provided by a national expert). Under conditions that maximize these upstream elements, we have some confidence that fidelity to a particular protocol matched to a certain problem is related to positive results. This is essentially the evidence base from efficacy research, and it allows us to say such things as "studies show that parent training is efficacious for oppositional youth."

Type II: Transportability

Although the prevailing terminology for outcome research suggests a dichotomy of methods (efficacy research and effectiveness research), it is argued here that our research methods exist more on a punctuated continuum—with multiple points along a dimension—and that effectiveness research can thereby take at least three forms. The first, labeled here as Type II research, involves the study of interventions in laboratory conditions, without the exclusionary criteria typical in most Type I research. For example, this strategy is used in our laboratory at the University of Hawaii and involves an externally controlled referral stream with no exclusionary criteria for participation in treatment outcome research. For the purposes of research, no children are screened out. Schoenwald and Hoagwood (2001) termed this type of effectiveness research "transportability" research, as it speaks to whether a particular intervention might be promising for delivery into a true practice setting. Essentially, Type II research allows for inferences about the performance of a protocol under a wider range of client conditions that closely approximate or are equivalent to client conditions in true practice settings but at the same time still maxime therapist and supervisor performance in a contrived laboratory setting. This approach would allow us to say, "parent training is a promising approach for real world cases of oppositional youth."

Type III: Dissemination

Moving up another level, Type III research involves the use of system employees (e.g., school counselors and private practitioners) as therapists. Schoenwald and Hoagwood (2001) termed this approach "dissemination" research, in that it relates to the performance of a protocol once deployed into a system. This research is (perhaps) what is most commonly referred to when one encounters the term "effectiveness," and it allows for inferences about the performance of the intervention under highly naturalistic conditions (e.g., Henggeler et al., 1998). Nevertheless, in such research the supervision is still provided by the investigator team, and thus questions remain about whether the same practice standards would be maintained after the investigator team withdrew from the system. From this research we could nevertheless state something like "parent training is a promising approach for school-based therapists serving oppositional youth."

Type IV: System Evaluation

The final question regarding system independence can only be addressed directly by Type IV research, which could be referred to as "system evaluation," in which the system to be evaluated and the investigator team are fully independent. This strategy would allow the final inference to be made: whether practice elements can lead to positive outcomes when a system stands entirely on its own. Although studies of entire systems do exist (Bickman, 1996; Bickman, Lambert, Andrade, & Penaloza, 2000; Burns et al., 1996), these do not truly represent Type IV research, because they have not specified evidence-based interventions in one of the experimental conditions but, rather, compare different arrangements of "usual care." Consequently, the outcomes of these studies primarily show differences in practice patterns (e.g., access to system and dropout rates) but are unsupportive with respect to differential outcomes at the level of the child (Bickman, 1999). This absence of child outcomes is perhaps due to the fact that such "systems" studies have not controlled and specified all the elements in the chain outlined in Figure 3.1 but, rather, have focused only on such things as supervision practice or case management practice. Without monitoring the "downstream" elements in the investigation, there is no guarantee that strategies at the higher level will not be neutralized by poor strategies at the lower level (cf. Weisz, Han, & Valeri, 1997). Thus, it is expected that for Type IV research to demonstrate substantive differences in child outcomes, the experimental condition will need to specify not only the supervision and case management practice but also the specific intervention to be used by the therapist.

Good examples of such studies do not exist, probably because they await a greater accumulation of Type II and III investigations that speak to the promise of transportability and successful deployment of various interventions. Further, system evaluation of practice organizations becomes an exercise in permutation in that the independent variable in efficacy research—practice elements—is now crossed with a variety of other factors. These all need to be fixed and varied in various orders, depending on the questions of interest. Assuming three interventions, two referral streams, two different therapist training methods, presence and absence of programmatic supervision, and the presence and absence of case managers, a balanced design would require 48 different arms and well in excess of 2,000 children. Obviously, this means that findings from smaller, unbalanced designs must accumulate over time to sketch out the important patterns in practice systems, all the while keeping a closer eye on the interventions themselves.

At this point in time, then, the evidence base is understandably skewed in favor of Type I research, and examples of Type II, III, and IV are, respectively, less frequent than examples of each previous type. Were one to graph the frequency of these four types of studies, the trend would move sharply downward from left to right. Interestingly, were one to graph the ability of these four types of studies to allow for reliable inferences about real-world practice, the trend would arguably move upward from left to right—in the opposite direction. Thus, because of the necessary sequential nature of outcome research, we have an immature evidence base that contains the fewest examples of the studies needed most. This fact may be in large part responsible for the absence of a strong connection between national practice policy and local practice policy. That is, the evidence that exists may not be considered fully relevant to systems that seek to use such evidence to shape practice policy (Persons, 1991). To speak of evidence-based interventions to practice systems inherently privileges some types of evidence and discounts others, and can thereby provide a misleading seal of approval, when those systems have had little to say about how evidence should in fact be defined. Connecting evidence with practice might therefore require a broader definition of evidence itself, which involves rethinking current methods of reviewing both efficacy and effectiveness in all their forms.

DEFINING EVIDENCE: EFFICACY

> The values of science and the values of democracy are concordant,
> in many cases indistinguishable.
>   —SAGAN (1996, p. 38)

Defining evidence is not a simple task (Chambless & Hollon, 1998; Hoagwood, Burns, Kiser, Ringeisen, & Schoenwald, 2001), and yet the arguments outlined thus far suggest that the definition of evidence may in fact make or break the connection to local practice policy, which in turn can drive systems to change or not to change their practice. To date, APA Division 12 efforts have emphasized efficacy—the scientific validity of the outcome research—as the major component of evidence in evaluating most promising interventions. Even within that domain defined by researchers themselves, there is controversy (Chambless & Hollon, 1998; Fensterheim & Raw, 1996; Garfield, 1996; Persons, 1991). Many of the arguments focus on the relevance to real-world practice of the criteria and methodology used to distill and summarize the efficacy research (Chorpita et al., 2002). Some of these arguments will be outlined here.

Levels of Evidence

One of the most central questions regarding the definition of efficacy involves where one chooses to draw the line separating supported and unsupported interventions. The issue of creating boundary lines between best, good, and poor evidence is essentially a signal detection task, one of maximizing specificity and sensitivity of the criteria that define efficacy. Make the definition too conservative, and there are few or no choices of interventions for a particular area, thus defeating the purpose of a system designed to allow informed choices. Make the definition too relaxed, and hundreds of interventions have similar levels of support, again defeating the purpose of a system designed to allow informed choices.

The prevailing methodology of Division 12 defines two levels of empirical support: "well established," and "probably efficacious" (Chambless & Hollon, 1998, later referred to three levels: "possibly efficacious," "efficacious," and "efficacious and specific;" however, the prevailing convention has been to retain the formal 1995 Task Force definitions). The criteria for these classifications are spelled out in detail elsewhere (Task Force on Promotion and Dissemination of Psychological Procedures, 1995) but essentially require at least two independent randomized clinical trials with active controls for the higher status of support (i.e., "well established"), and one randomized clinical trial with an active control or two trials with wait-list controls for the lower status of support (i.e., "probably efficacious"). More recent efforts by the Division 12 Committee on Science and Practice have considered collapsing these to a single level, such that interventions are simply either supported or not (Weisz et al., 2000). Although there are many advantages in terms of the simplicity of such as system, there are also some costs, mainly involving these boundary issues. With a single rather than multiple cut points between good and poor empirical support, the task of drawing the line in the proper place becomes even more demanding, perhaps impossible in some cases. This task is further challenged when there is a uniform standard imposed, because research in some areas will show a large number of interventions passing a given threshold, whereas research in other areas will show no interventions that pass that same threshold.

One example involves the area of autism, for which the Task Force on Empirically Supported Psychosocial Interventions for Children (Lonigan, Elbert, & Bennett Johnson, 1998) found no interventions supported at either level using Division 12 criteria (Rogers, 1998). From the standpoint of the local policymaker, supervisor, case manager, or consumer, such a method of defining and classifying evidence offers no help in the discrimination among interventions. For example, applied behavior analysis, facilitated communication, or dolphin therapy would be considered equivalent under such a system, and yet there is strong professional consensus and reasonable experimental evidence that the first approach is helpful and the second two are not.

This method also raises a troubling semantic issue: The taxonomy of support states that interventions failing to pass an empirical threshold are not "evidence-based," implying indiscriminately and sometimes falsely that such interventions have no supportive evidence—even when the evidence is in fact comparatively substantial as in the autism example of applied behavior analysis. Suggestions to handle such issues were proposed by the APA Task Force's (1995) somewhat dimensional view of efficacy, which suggested the following hierarchy of evidence (in decreasing order of strength): comparative treatment trials, placebo-controlled trials, no-treatment control trials, quantified clinical observations, strongly positive clinical consensus, mixed clinical consensus, strongly negative clinical consensus, and evidence of harmful effects. These multiple levels would allow for the approval of some weaker forms of evidence, which would solve some of the problems inherent in summarizing the evidence based successfully. More will be said on the topic of multiple levels later.

Recommendations of the APA Task Force (1995) also underscored another troubling issue that prevailing definitions of evidence do not address: the lack of a means for classifying interventions with known harmful effects. From the standpoint of the consumer, knowledge about what interventions might be harmful can be the some of the most important information of all.

Time Series Penalty

Other equally important issues come into play in terms of defining evidence with regard to particular problem areas. For example, Division 12 criteria and even the APA Task Force recommendations reflect an emphasis on between-group, randomized research designs that are less easily implemented with children than with adults. This choice is reasonable, as between-group designs do indeed represent the most internally valid means of examining treatment effects (Kazdin, 1993). However, a great deal of child research cannot involve inactive control conditions for ethical reasons, and children are not as capable of giving truly informed consent about the possibility of being assigned to a control condition. This design issue is particularly problematic in such areas as autism and mental retardation, for which few parents want their child to be at risk of being assigned to a control group. Although time series design, are allowable under Division 12 criteria, they are held to a higher standard than between-group designs in that an active (e.g., alternative treatment) control condition is required for time series designs but not for all between-group designs. Research areas that involve proportionally greater use of time series designs are then penalized in their efforts to identify promising interventions. This highlights the challenge of crafting a single definition of evidence that will apply across multiple problems and populations.

Defining Control

An even more troubling issue involves identifying a "good" design (Weisz et al., 2000), one particular challenge of which involves the notion of defining appropriate control groups. The child literature is replete with quasi-experimental designs involving nonrandom group assignment, buffered by tests showing no pretreatment differences on demographic and symptom measures. Some of these are considered among the strongest trials in a particular area (e.g., Lovaas, 1987), yet a strict definition of experimental control once again discounts or discards these sources of evidence. To reiterate, it is not so simple an issue as merely including quasi experimental research—that may in many areas "open the floodgates" and lead to the overidentification of interventions in which there is comparatively little confidence. The presumed goal is to draw a line that allows for some differentiation in quality among the thousands of studies of child interventions—as noted earlier, an issue that is perhaps best solved through the use of multiple levels.

A related example with respect to experimental control involves a comparative trial for which the experimental treatment condition lasts for a greater length of time than the control condition, stemming from the ethical considerations that are paramount in child research as discussed previously (e.g., Kendall, 1994). How do these issues get resolved? Most groups have so far considered the first example insufficient control and the latter example sufficient control. These are clearly issues that APA's Division 12 and 53 Committees on Science and Practice are working hard to resolve by operationalizing and reliably measuring all of these parameters, but the challenge is daunting, and its implications are mighty.

DEFINING EVIDENCE: EFFECTIVENESS

All that said, the foregoing so far addresses only half the issues regarding evidence. A second source of evidence involves the external validity of intervention research. Such considerations were also emphasized by the APA Task Force (1995), which articulated a variety of parameters relevant to the dissemination of interventions. Formal efforts to identify these types of information in published trials have been proposed by the Division 12 and 53 Committees on Science and Practice (Weisz et al., 2000) and have been conducted by at least one local practice organization (Chorpita et al., 2002). Of note here is that harnessing such information, or evidence, regarding effectiveness need not await research of Types II through IV noted earlier. Much of this information can already be drawn from the existing evidence base of laboratory intervention research, albeit with some limitations. Table 3.1 represents a summary of these parameters that are important to consider in any outcome research, organized according to the APA Task Force's (1995) three broad areas of feasibility, generalizability, and cost/benefit. Many of these parameters are the same or similar to those originally recommended by the APA Task Force (1995).

The first broad area, feasibility, refers to the possibility that an intervention will be successful or possible under real-world conditions (Task Force on Psychological Intervention Guidelines, 1995). Acceptance speaks directly to this issue, in that interventions that are successful cannot be feasible if few or no children agree to participate. As noted in the table, characterization of the nature of acceptance and refusal would be informative. The rate of dropouts represents similar information, and thus should be summarized and classified. Finally, information about training is also highly relevant to feasibility. For an intervention to be introduced into a system, it has to be packaged for maximum efficiency. It is arguable that most practice organizations cannot afford to train staff in the manner that therapists in laboratory clinical trials are trained: long-term expert supervision in a specialized university or medical school setting, often using observation, audio or videotaping, or a trained cotherapist. Thus, the availability of treatment manuals and training curricula (e.g., slide shows, workshop notes, videotapes, and manualized training protocols) speaks directly to whether an intervention can be adopted quickly by a particular system.

Generalizability refers to whether the findings regarding an intervention might be applicable to a broader range of conditions, and it has typically been one of the most

TABLE 3.1. Effectiveness Parameters of Interest in Published Research

Parameter	Examples
Feasibility	
Acceptance rate	Refusals who do not want to participate in research, refusals for other reasons (e.g., do not want to participate in either therapy offered); acceptance by ethnicity associations should be reported when possible
Dropouts	Therapist initiated (e.g., client too dangerous to self); client initiated (clients dissatisfied with therapy); dropout by ethnicity associations should be reported when possible
Trainability	Manual available (yes/no), other training materials available (e.g., video), nature of training in study (e.g., workshop; ongoing supervision, cotherapy), length of training
Generalizability	
Therapist characteristics	Training degree (e.g., graduate student, MA, MD, and PhD), years of experience, ethnicity, first language, gender, and age
Supervision	Hours administered; group versus individual
Supervisor characteristics	Training degree (e.g., graduate student, MA, MD, and PhD), years of experience supervising, years of experience practicing, ethnicity, first language, gender, and age
Contact variables	Frequency (e.g., weekly and daily), duration (e.g., 3 months and 6 months), number of meetings/sessions, total number of hours, use of booster sessions
Setting	University clinic, community clinic, inpatient, residential, home, school, special home (e.g., therapeutic foster home), special school (e.g., day treatment)
Referral sources	Proportions from teachers, parents, pediatricians, etc.
Payment	Sliding scale, insurance, and other fee information
Recruitment	Newspaper ad, yellow pages, agency as part of managed care of other system of care
Sample definition	Defined by extreme scores, diagnosis on structured interview, unstructured interview, or other characteristics (sexual abuse, substance abuse, motor vehicle accident, parental divorce, etc.)
Demographics	Number of parents/caretakers in home, parent marital status, parent education level, family income, type of neighborhood (e.g., urban/rural), public/private school, sex, age, grade, primary ethnicity, language spoken at home
Prior experience with therapy	Number of contacts, number of years, perceived success and failures
Cost and benefit	
Cost	Cost to state, insurance company, or individual; costs of withholding treatment (e.g., missed schooldays)
Effect size	Within subjects, between subjects

contested areas regarding the promotion of evidence-based treatments to date. Central issues in this domain include information about supervisor and therapist background and the nature of supervision. Knowledge about practice structure is also important and includes information not only about the schedule of client contacts but also about the setting, fee basis, and manner in which individuals or families enter the system. All these variables help define the nature of the practice organization, which could range from publicly provided school-based services delivered daily to special education students to traditional outpatient, clinic-based, fee-for-service weekly therapy. Especially important is information on how participants are recruited, as these avenues in many ways define the population to which the results generalize.

This information of course leads to one of the most important aspects of generalizability: characteristics of the children and families themselves. Almost uniformly, research reports give a clear indication of age and gender. However, Chorpita et al. (2002) found that reporting of ethnicity, parent education, and family income varied considerably across the child intervention literature, and more detailed information on aspects of culture (e.g., neighborhood and language spoken in the home) was absent from the majority of research reports. Such variables speak not only to the possibility of success across different population but also to therapist engagement with evidence-based approaches more generally. To the extent that information on culture, ethnicity, and family variables is minimized in research reports, practice organizations are less likely to see the relevance of such reports to their own mission.

Finally, it is important to provide information on the cost and benefits of an intervention. For a system to adopt a new approach to service delivery, it must be able to forecast the fiscal impact and the clinical benefits of that approach. For example, a public school system seeking to implement classroom behavior management programs for attention-deficit/hyperactivity disorder would need to know the costs of training and service delivery relative to the expected benefits for the child, teacher, and classmates-preferably in comparison with similar information on stimulant medication interventions. However, the lack of effect size reporting in the child outcome literature is surprising; within- or between-group effect sizes rarely appear in original research and are limited almost exclusively to meta-analytic reviews (e.g., Weisz et al., 1995). Although recent changes in APA editorial policy require thr reporting of effect sizes, there is still no convention requiring reporting of both within-group (pre–post) and between-group (differences at post) effects. Furthermore, APA controls reporting in only a handful of research journals, and even among them the policies are not uniformly enforced.

WHAT EVIDENCE GETS EXAMINED

Even when the definition of evidence is broadened to include both elements of efficacy and effectiveness, it does not in any way guarantee that all relevant and appropriate information is summarized to guide practice. A number of other considerations remain regarding what areas of evidence are examined in the first place, and just a few of the relevant arguments are outlined here.

One issue that has received some of the greatest attention involves the notion of how practice elements are defined. The prevailing convention is to define interventions at the levels of manuals (e.g., Chambless & Hollon, 1998). However, it raises a number of potential problems, not the least of which is that manuals are somewhat unpopular among practicing clinicians (Addis & Krasnow, 2000). A more fine-grained question concerns the definition of a manual itself. For example, an investigator might choose to make minor improvements to a manual between two clinical trials. One might therefore ask whether the second trial is a completely new test or a replication (Weisz & Hawley, 1998). A possible solution could be to define practice elements at the level of techniques or procedures rather than manuals (e.g., Kazdin, 1995; Rosen & Davison, in press). For example, by a hypothetical criterion, "time out," and "rewards" could be considered evidence-based techniques.

This issue is important because however narrowly or broadly one chooses to define practice, there will be a direct impact on the interpretation of the existing evidence base. For example, rather than defining interventions at the level of manuals, one could consider interventions sharing a majority of components with similar strategies and theoretical underpinnings to be the same for the purposes of evaluation. Using this approach, different treatments for depression that involved self-monitoring, identifying problem thoughts, developing coping thoughts or problem-solving strategies, and accompanying behavioral exercises would be collectively labeled "cognitive-behavioral therapy" (CBT) and evaluated together. This collective approach would yield a high degree of support for CBT, given the large number of manuals each having a small number of supportive trials (Kaslow & Thompson, 1998). Were each manual to be evaluated alone, the evidence might not appear so strong, but viewed together the suggestion is that CBT is efficacious and robust to its many variations across protocols. Of course, this suggestion requires defining the boundaries of a particular type of intervention (e.g., how to decide what is and is not considered CBT), an undertaking that can be fraught with subjectivity. This issue could perhaps be addressed through the analysis of judges' agreement on classification of interventions, although such procedures would be time-intensive.

A second major issue involves the somewhat diagnostic focus of evidence-based treatment reviews (Lonigan et al., 1998), which might not be so appropriate for children as it is for adults. In addition to dealing with diagnosable conditions, many systems handle "juvenile delinquents," "sexually abused youth," "foster children," "truants," and so on. To begin with, a disorder-based approach to defining populations and classifying interventions stands in contrast to child psychopathology literature implicating the ecological nature of most child problems (e.g., Bronfenbrenner, 1986). More important, although a diagnostic approach is likely to facilitate deployment in medical systems and managed care organizations, it may hinder dissemination in school and public service settings whose staff may not organize children according to disorder. One needs to ask whether strategies exist to review studies of school aggression, teenage pregnancy, or vandalism, all of which are of considerable interest to child service organizations.

A third issue is the comparatively greater focus of evidence-based policy on "outpatient" versus "services" strategies. Some of this imbalance is driven by the comparative strength of the child outcome literature on office-based interventions. However, some controlled trials of foster care, residential treatment centers, and case management practice do exist (Burns et al., 1996; Chamberlain & Reid, 1998). Broadening the definitions of interventions to be evaluated as evidence-based is of particular importance given that the majority of children receiving mental health services do not get them from outpatient clinics (Hoagwood et al., 2001; U.S. Department of Health and Human Services, 1999). For example, in a recent study of service utilization, Burns et al. (1995) found that schools are the largest provider of child mental health services. If there is to be a connection of evidence to practice, all practice-relevant sources of evidence need to be included (Weisz et al., 2000).

A fourth issue concerns the lack of emphasis on evaluating the evidence on prevention programs. Again, this issue may stem from a methodology that was perhaps better designed for reviewing outcome research with adults. Excellent controlled tests of prevention programs exist (Greenberg, Domitrovich, & Bumbarger, 2001), but they are more difficult to identify using current methodology for reviewing evidence-based strategies. Many schools and state public health programs, however, have a greater interest in identifying and serving children at risk than in providing traditional interventions only after problems emerge.

Finally, it is worth asking whether the focus on evaluating evidence should rely entirely on deficits and symptoms. Development of strengths and competencies might be equally important goals of interventions and may be of considerable interest to practice organizations. For example, the number of classes attended, number of friends, school grades, and number of hobbies are all variables that often represent the interest of parents and teachers, perhaps more so than the number of symptoms of a given disorder. Because effects sizes for these more distal variables might be smaller, it would be important to summarize both symptom reduction evidence and evidence regarding broader aspects of strengths and functioning when reviewing treatment outcome research (Kazdin, 2001; National Advisory Mental Health Council Workgroup on Child and Adolescent Mental Health Intervention Development and Deployment, 2001).

LOOKING AT ALL THE EVIDENCE: INTERVENTIONS IN THE CONTEXT OF SYSTEMS

> In all uses of science, it is insufficient-indeed it is dangerous-to produce only a small, highly competent, well-regarded priesthood of professionals. Instead, some fundamental understanding of the findings and methods of science must be available on the broadest scale.
>
> —SAGAN (1996, p. 37)

Consideration of the aforementioned issues suggests reexamination of the definition of evidence, where it comes from, and how and by whom it is summarized. Consideration must go beyond the link between interventions and outcomes to include the broader set of organizational variables relevant to practice systems. Fortunately, these ideas are being recognized and supported as part of a national research agenda that aims to promote the relevance and utility of intervention research (National Advisory Mental Health Council, 2001). University-based research will always play an important role in understanding and advancing the theoretical underpinnings of interventions, yet there is an emerging need to develop new "laboratories" at the level of mental health systems (Bickman, 1999; Chorpita, 2002). With the laboratory being the system itself, planned constraints and controls would allow important inferences about the sequence of effects connecting system practice policy to child outcomes (see Figure 3.1). We can then begin to map the frontier in detail.

Space permits the brief illustration of one such example. In the wake of a major reorganization due to a federal lawsuit, the Child and Adolescent Mental Health Division (CAMHD) of the Hawaii Department of Health is an organization that has begun to take these very steps. It has sought to build and infrastructure to facilitate practice innovation and to implement efficacy-based interventions within a system of care. These developments have come on many fronts.

As noted in Figure 3.1, establishing a local practice policy organization is regarded as a critical bridge to influencing system practice standards. To address the need for improvement of the services delivered within its mental health system, the Hawaii Department of Health organized the Task Force on Empirical Basis to Services (EBS) in October 1999 (see Chorpita et al., 2002; Task Force on Empirical Basis to Services, 2000). The group received a small amount of state funding to support a library search assistant but was otherwise composed of volunteers. The EBS Task Force conducted a multidisciplinary evaluation of psychosocial interventions for common disorders of childhood and adolescence based on a formal and scientific literature review of controlled studies in psychology, psychiatry, and related mental health disciplines. As implied by the figure, the primary methodology, procedures, and criteria for evaluating treatment studies were adapted from the guidelines published in previous national efforts (i.e., APA Division 12). Over 2 years later, the EBS Task Force continues to meet monthly, serving as a standing body for evidence review, practice development, and the design of state practice guidelines and performance standards. Topics related to any mental health service can be nominated for review and trigger a literature search, distribution of readings, and the cataloguing of evidence by independent raters. All these procedures are in accordance with a structured methodology that was designed when the group was established. The methods are open to periodic revision as is found necessary by the group and supported by consensus (e.g., suspending the need for a clearly defined population when evaluating the efficacy of seclusion and restraint procedures).

In bridging this connection to the local level, the EBS Task Force adapted and extended national practice policy to fit local needs. Such adaptations included using a five-level system to classify the efficacy of interventions, which adequately addressed the problem of identification of an appropriate array of services and also compensated for the "time series penalty" noted above (see Chorpita et al., 2002, for a detailed review of methodology). The second major adaptation has been to include a review of the effectiveness parameters similar to those outlined in Table 3.1. Thus, for the controlled outcome studies in which such information was reported, the EBS Task Force summarized all effectiveness information and distributed the findings to individuals working in the system (cf. Chambless & Hollon, 1998; Weisz et al., 2000).

With such a bridge having been established, the next steps involve the mechanisms of support just described: engagement, training, and technological supports for the local policy. To maximize system engagement, there has been a strong emphasis on inclusion of all relevant stakeholders in the process. Thus, membership in Hawaii's EBS Task Force remains open and admission criteria require only regular attendance and a willingness to read and review studies. Members include university faculty, practitioners, parents, administrators, employees from the Departments of Health and Education, and other community members. Professional disciplines represented have included psychiatry, psychology, social work, nursing, and law. This inclusion has increased system engagement in two ways. First, the policies and standards resulting from the reviews are less likely to be perceived as coming strictly from managers and academicians (Hayes, Barlow, & Nelson-Gray, 1999), in that the reviews are a completely open process. Second, the methodology of the group—while remaining strictly science-based—has been influenced by multiple constituencies and consequently achieves an optimal balance, satisfying a diversity of interests. Any group that has a stake in the system has been invited to have a voice in the process by which evidence is defined and distilled locally. It was in fact the interests of parents and practitioners—who voiced the greatest concerns about the relevance of laboratory research—that paved the way to the extend reviews beyond mere efficacy in the outcome literature.

Education is the second strategy that has been important for encouraging the use of evidence-based interventions in the Hawaii child mental health system. Along these lines, the state has funded free workshops on both practice policy and intervention techniques. Over 20 state-funded trainings have been conducted in the past 2 years to describe the development of the EBS Task Force, its methodology, its results, and their implications. Participants have included families, practitioners, supervisors, case managers, teachers, health and education administrators, and lawmakers. This particular training has a primary effect of increasing the public knowledge base regarding evidence-based approaches but also serves to strengthen engagement further by allowing dialogue with all system members. For example, questions, comments, and reactions at trainings are taken back to the EBS Task Force and serve as a barometer of the relevance and quality of the Task Force endeavors. When topics of interest or debate arise, they are quickly brought to the group for evaluation. Over time, the group has become a recognized resource for open review of the scientific basis regarding any policy—few decisions are made now without first requesting a review of the latest literature. To keep things in check, these endeavors are balanced with an openness regarding what is not known and an emphasis on inclusion of interventions and identification of promising approaches rather than exclusion of particular types of practice (with the exception of potentially harmful interventions). All this is, of course, common sense to the behaviorist: Better to reward appropriate activities than to punish inappropriate ones.

Workshops—paid for by the state—are also conducted for practitioners and supervisors on the identified interventions themselves. This allows all service providers to become more knowledgeable about interventions whose use is most encouraged by local practice standards. These trainings so far number in the dozens and have reached hundreds of child practitioners.

Finally, technology has been developed to support these practice innovations. Some tools are relatively simple. For example, Hawaii's CAMHD has developed a single-page matrix of interventions and child problems, known locally as the "blue menu" (printed on blue paper), whose function is to concisely summarize the efficacy review by the EBS Task Force. Often in the context of training, the menu has been distributed statewide to all case managers in health centers and public schools as a tool to facilitate procurement of the most promising interventions. Supervisors and therapists have been provided with the menu as well to assist in the review and selection of techniques and interventions. Anecdotal signs of the enthusiasm for evidence-based practice in Hawaii's child mental health system are the commonly sighted menus conspicuously taped up on office walls.

Building on these strategies, the Hawaii CAMHD is designing software modules for its case managers that allow electronic interface with the menu, which links to providers trained in those specific services. Thus, case managers should be able to select therapists or agencies that can offer the appropriate evidence-based approaches using an electronic decision support system, whose algorithm derives directly from local evidence review by the EBS Task Force. Similar technology is being developed for supervision in a partnership between the Hawaii Departments of Health and Education, so that supervisors can track the use of evidence-based approaches and their contribution to positive outcomes. Clearly, the plans are ambitious and much remains to be done, but the goals are clearly in sight.

SUMMARY AND CONCLUSIONS

Overall, a gulf remains between mental health policy and practice. The assumption that better guidelines will lead to better practice is perhaps not a safe one. There is now a need for researchers and policymakers to evaluate more closely the many unexamined links between the evidence base and line-level practice. These efforts might include increasing the research focus on effectiveness parameters, such as those detailed in Table 3.1, thereby increasing the relevance of the knowledge in the accumulating evidence base. Local efforts to digest and transform evidence into policy are also important but must be supported by training, engagement, and technology, as outlined earlier. As systems begin to detail these connections, research should track and test each link in the chain to determine the relative and collective merit of a variety of practice development strategies.

Hawaii's child mental health system is but one example of an attempt to build such an organizational connection between evidence and practice. The methods in Hawaii are certainly not uniformly relevant to other practice organizations but only illustrate one attempt at the marriage of efficacy-based research findings with practice systems—and on a broader scale connecting science with public knowledge (Sagan, 1996). In many ways conquering this frontier represents the next great challenge to all mental health disciplines (Barlow, 2000; Weisz et al., 1995), and it is maintained that this challenge will require increasing scrutiny on the definition of evidence itself, from inside and out. However we choose to define evidence, it has already become the primary criterion by which we must measure practice standards, and there is no turning back. The frontier that lies ahead is formidable, and there will certainly be wrong turns and missteps. However, a definition of evidence in which everyone has a voice will ultimately point the way.

ACKNOWLEDGMENTS

Preparation of this chapter was supported in part by National Institute of Mental Health Grant R03 MH60134, an award from the University of Hawai'i Research Council, and an award from the Hawai'i Department of Health.

REFERENCES

Addis, M. E., & Krasnow, A. D. (2000). A national survey of practicing psychologists' attitudes toward psychotherapy treatment manuals. *Journal of Consulting and Clinical Psychology, 68,* 331–339.

Barlow, D. H. (1994). Psychological interventions in the era of managed competition. *Clinical Psychology: Science and Practice, 1,* 109–122.

Barlow, D. H. (2000). Evidence based practice: A world view. *Clinical Psychology: Science and Practice, 7,* 241–242.

Bickman, L. (1996). A continuum of care: More is not always better. *American Psychologist, 51,* 689–701.

Bickman, L. (1999). Practice makes perfect and other myths about mental health services. *American Psychologist, 54,* 965–977.

Bickman, L., Lambert, E. W., Andrade, A. R., & Penaloza, R. V. (2000). The Fort Bragg continuum of care for children and adolescents: Mental health outcomes over 5 years. *Journal of Consulting and Clinical Psychology, 68,* 710–716.

Bronfenbrenner, U. (1986). Ecology of the family as a context for human development: Research perspectives. *Developmental Psychology, 22,* 723–742.

Burns, B. J., Costello, E. J., Angold, A., Tweed, D., Stangl, D., Farmer, E. M. Z., & Erkanli, A. (1995). Children's mental health service use across service sectors. *Health Affairs (Millwood), 14,* 147–159.

Burns, B. J., Farmer, E. M. Z., Angold, A., Costello, E. J., & Behar, L. (1996). A randomized trial of case management for youths with serious emotional disturbance. *Journal of Clinical Child Psychology, 25,* 476–486.

Chamberlain, P., & Reid, J. B. (1998). Comparison of two community alternatives to incarceration for chronic juvenile offenders. *Journal of Consulting and Clinical Psychology, 66,* 624–633.

Chambless, D. L., Baker, M. J., Baucom, D. H., Beutler, L. E., Calhoun, K. S., Crits-Christoph, P., Daiuto, A., DeRubeis, R., Detweiler, J., Haaga, D. A. F., Bennett Johnson, S., McCurry, S., Mueser, K. T., Pope, K. S., Sanderson, W. C., Shoham, V., Stickle, T., Williams, D. A., Woody, S. R. (1998). Update on empirically validated therapies II. *The Clinical Psychologist, 51,* 3–16.

Chambless, D. L., & Hollon, S. D. (1998). Defining empirically supported therapies. *Journal of Consulting and Clinical Psychology, 66,* 7–18.

Chambless, D. L., Sanderson, W. C., Shoham, V., Johnson, S. B., Pope, K. S., Crits-Christoph, P., Baker, M., Johnson, B., Woody, S. R., Sue, S., Beutler, L., Williams, D. A., McCurry, S. (1996). An update on empirically validated therapies. *The Clinical Psychologist, 49,* 5–18.

Chorpita, B. F. (2002). Treatment manuals for the real world: Where do we build them? *Clinical Psychology: Science and Practice, 9,* 431–433.

Chorpita, B. F., Yim, L. M., Donkervoet, J. C., Arensdorf, A., Amundsen, M. J., McGee, C., Serrano, A., Yates, A., & Morelli P. (2002). Toward large-scale implementation of empirically supported treatments for children: A review and observations by the Hawaii Empirical Basis to Services Task Force. *Clinical Psychology: Science and Practice, 9,* 165–190.

Cunningham, P. B., & Henggeler, S. W. (1999). Engaging multiproblem families in treatment: Lessons learned throughout the development of multisystemic therapy. *Family Process, 38,* 265–286.

Fensterheim, H., & Raw, S. (1996). Psychotherapy research is not psychotherapy practice. *Clinical Psychology: Science and Practice, 3,* 168–171.

Garfield, S. L. (1996). Some problems associated with "validated" forms of psychotherapy. *Clinical Psychology: Science and Practice, 3,* 218–234.

Glisson, C., & Hemmelgarn, A. (1996). The effects of organizational climate and interorganizational coordination on the quality and outcomes of children's service systems. *Child Abuse and Neglect, 22,* 401–421.

Greenberg., M. T., Domitrovich, C., & Bumbarger, B. (2001). The prevention of mental disorders in school-aged children: Current state of the field. *Prevention and Treatment: Special Issue, 4.*

Hayes, S. C., Barlow, D. H., & Nelson-Gray, R. O. (1999). The scientist practitioner: Research and accountability in the age of managed care (2nd ed.). Boston: Allyn & Bacon.

Henggeler, S. W., Schoenwald, S. K., Borduin, C. M., Rowland, M. D., & Cunningham, P. B. (1998). *Multisystemic treatment of antisocial behavior in children and adolescents.* New York: Guilford Press.

Hoagwood, K., Burns, B. J., Kiser, L., Ringeisen, H., & Schoenwald, S. K. (2001). Evidence-based practice in child and adolescent mental health services. *Psychiatric Services, 52,* 1179–1189.

Kaslow, N. J., & Thompson, M. P. (1998). Applying the criteria for empirically supported treatments to studies of psychosocial interventions for child and adolescent depression. *Journal of Clinical Child Psychology, 27,* 146–155.

Kazdin, A. E. (1993). *Research design in clinical psychology* (2nd ed.). Boston: Allyn & Bacon.

Kazdin, A. E. (1995). Scope of child and adolescent psychotherapy research: Limited sampling of dysfunctions, treatments, and client characteristics. *Journal of Clinical Child Psychology, 24,* 125–140. Kazdin, A. E. (Ed.). (1996). Validated treatments: Multiple perspectives and issues [special section]. *Clinical Psychology: Science and Practice, 3,* 216–267.

Kazdin, A. E. (2001). Bridging the enormous gaps of theory with therapy research and practice. *Journal of Clinical Child Psychology, 30,* 59–66.

Kendall, P. C. (1994). Treating anxiety disorders in children: Results of a randomized clinical trial. *Journal of Consulting and Clinical Psychology, 62,* 100–110.

Lonigan, C. J., Elbert, J. C., & Bennett Johnson, S. (1998). Empirically supported psychosocial interventions for children: An overview. *Journal of Clinical Child Psychology, 27,* 138–145.

Lovaas, O. I. (1987). Behavioral treatment and normal educational and intellectual functioning in young autistic children. *Journal of Consulting and Clinical Psychology, 55*, 3–9.

McKay, M. M., McCadam, K., & Gonzales, J. J. (1996). Addressing the barriers to mental health services for inner city children and their caretakers. *Community Mental Health Journal 32*, 353–361.

Nathan, P. E., & Gorman, J. M. (Eds.). (1998). *A guide to treatments that work.* New York: Oxford University Press.

National Advisory Mental Health Council Workgroup on Child and Adolescent Mental Health Intervention Development and Deployment. (2001). *Blueprint for change: Research on child and adolescent mental health.* Washington, DC: Author.

Persons, J. B. (1991). Psychotherapy outcome studies do not accurately represent current models of psychotherapy: A proposed remedy. *American Psychologist, 46*, 99–106.

Persons, J. B. (1995). Why practicing psychologists are slow to adopt empirically-validated treatments. In S. C. Hayes, V. M. Follette, R. M. Dawes, & K. E. Grady. (Eds.), *Scientific standards of psychological practice: Issues and recommendations* (pp. 141–157). Reno, NV: Context Press.

Rogers, S. (1998). Empirically supported comprehensive treatments for young children with autism. *Journal of Clinical Child Psychology, 27*, 168–179.

Rosen, G. M., & Davison, G. C. (in press). Psychology should list empirically supported principles of change (ESPs) and not credential trademarked therapies or other treatment packages. *Behavior Modification.*

Sagan, C. (1996). The demon-haunted world: Science as a candle in the dark. New York: Ballantine.

Schoenwald, S. K. & Hoagwood, K. (2001). Effectiveness, transportability, and dissemination of interventions: What matters when. Psychiatric Services, 52, 1190–1197.

Task Force on Empirical Basis to Services. (2000, August). *Report on the most promising treatments for child and adolescent disorders.* Honolulu, HI: Child and Adolescent Mental Health Division, Department of Health.

Task Force on Promotion and Dissemination of Psychological Procedures, Division of Clinical Psychology, American Psychological Association. (1995). Training in and dissemination of empirically-validated psychological treatments: Report and recommendations. *The Clinical Psychologist, 48*, 3–23.

Task Force on Psychological Intervention Guidelines of the American Psychological Association. (1995). *Template for developing guidelines: Interventions for mental disorders and psychosocial aspects of physical disorders.* Washington, DC: American Psychological Association.

U.S. Department of Health and Human Services. (1999). *Mental health: A report of the Surgeon General.* Rockville, MD: U.S. Department of Health and Human Services, Substance Abuse and Mental Health Services Administration, Center for Mental Health Services, National Institutes of Health, National Institute of Mental Health.

Weisz, J. R., Donenberg, G. R., Han, S. S., & Weiss, B. (1995). Bridging the gap between laboratory and clinic in child and adolescent psychotherapy. *Journal of Consulting and Clinical Psychology, 63*, 688–701.

Weisz, J. R., Han, S. S., & Valeri, S. M. (1997). More of what? Issues raised by the Fort Bragg Study. *American Psychologist, 52*, 541–545.

Weisz, J. R., & Hawley, K. M. (1998). Finding, evaluating, refining, and applying empirically supported treatments for children and adolescents. *Journal of Clinical Child Psychology, 27*, 206–216.

Weisz, J. R., Hawley, K. M., Pilkonis, P. A., Woody, S. R., & Follette W. C. (2000). Stressing the (other) three Rs in the search for empirically supported treatments: Review procedures, research quality, relevance to practice and the public interest. *Clinical Psychology: Science and Practice, 7*, 243–258.

4

Ethical Issues in Child and Adolescent Psychosocial Treatment Research

KIMBERLY HOAGWOOD

Ethical issues in research on mental health are occasionally treated as an afterthought—as an idea for a symposium topic, an academic seminar, or an after-dinner conversation, interesting but peripheral to scientific inquiry. Yet analysis of ethical issues in research cuts to the scientific core, revealing the *raison d'être* for a study as well as the dialectical tensions between empirical inquiry and the study *of* human beings *by* human beings.

Ethical dilemmas arise when harm to research participants—however small, unforeseen, or tenuous—enters into the design or implementation of a study, or is experienced by a research participant during the course of a study. Such harm may occur inadvertently because of an unanticipated consequence from a procedure, measure, or process. Or it may be an explicitly stated risk about which a participant is informed in advance of entering into a protocol. In either case, however, the responsibility for estimating the potential for harm and for building safeguards into the protocol to protect research participants falls directly on the investigators, and, consequently, such estimates have to be made prior to embarking on a study.

The key defense against vulnerability to harm through participation in research, as described in more detail later, is the concept of informed consent. If participants knowingly enter into a study in which the potential for harm to them is clearly listed, then the presumption exists that any untoward consequences were voluntarily entertained and that therefore the investigator has met his or her obligation. Yet, as will be seen, the clarity of this presumption is made much more problematic in studies involving children and adolescents, especially those who also experience mental health problems.

The essential dialectic between scientific inquiry and social obligation is revealed perhaps most starkly in the field of child and adolescent mental health, where unevenness in the scientific knowledge base and urgent public health concerns about the status of children's mental health are in sharp relief. The lack of a strong scientific foundation concerning, for example, the effects of psychotropic drug treatments on children with mental illnesses creates an ethical problem. Prescriptions for such treatments and in particular the combination of such treatments are rapidly rising (Bhatara, Feil, Hoagwood,

Vitiello, & Zima, 2002; Zito et al., 2000), but the knowledge base on the safety, efficacy, and long-term impact of the majority of the commonly prescribed medications does not yet exist (Jensen 1998; Jensen, Bhatara, et al., 1999). Clearly there is a need for strengthening knowledge about the effects of these medications, especially given the increase in their use. However, at the same time, constructing basic science studies on the safety and efficacy of psychotropic treatments, which may involve the use of these agents with normal controls, can introduce unforeseen harm to participants. A similar dilemma exists for psychosocial treatments, in which the lack of a knowledge base, combined with widespread use of non-evidence-based treatments, creates a tension between the need to accelerate study of the efficacy and effectiveness of treatments and the lack of even basic understanding of what constitutes risk to research participants.

Added to this central ethical tension is the fact that the prevalence rates of unmet need for mental health services among children and adolescents with impairing forms of emotional, behavioral, or brain disorders are as high now as they were 20 years ago (National Advisory Mental Health Council, 2001; Roberts, Atkisson, & Rosenblatt, 1998; U.S. Public Health Service, 2000). From a public health standpoint, the urgency of strengthening the science base on effective treatments has never been stronger. Yet equally urgent is the need to attend to a range of ethical issues that will inevitably arise when studying children and adolescents with mental health needs. Consequently, investigators embarking on studies of treatments for children's mental disorders have to shoulder an enormous responsibility to ensure that potential harm is considered, that such harm is minimized, and, simultaneously, that scientifically valuable and valid knowledge is created.

This chapter helps investigators define and examine a range of ethical issues that may arise in studies of psychosocial treatments for youth. The chapter first describes the boundaries between ethical issues and legal regulations and the reasons why these categories are becoming increasingly indistinguishable. It then describes the primary federal regulations that guide approaches to studies of children and adolescents. This chapter also describes some of the common research processes in which ethical dilemmas may arise, which include obtaining informed consent, weighing risks and benefits, engaging families or community stakeholders in studies, providing clinical feedback, offering incentives, and ensuring confidentiality.

BOUNDARIES BETWEEN ETHICAL ISSUES AND LEGAL ISSUES

In research on child and adolescent mental health and illness, the boundaries between ethical issues (i.e., the application of philosophically derived moral principles to questions of right and wrong) and legal issues (i.e., questions of what is or is not lawful) are often blurred. In fact, one can find articles about ethical issues in research that do little more than describe federal regulations (Vitiello, 2002).

It is easy to see why the boundaries between ethical and legal issues in research have become indistinguishable in many discussions about human subjects' protections. The historical starting point within the federal government that precipitated attention to ethical principles in research with human subjects was the Belmont Report, issued by the National Commission for the Protection of Human Subjects of Biomedical and Behavioral Research (National Commission, 1979) and from which the Code of Federal Regulations was later derived. In this report, the Commission described three major principles that presumably dictate ethical practice in research with human beings.

1. *Respect for persons.* This principle prescribes that all individuals should be treated as autonomous and should be protected from risk. Protection is especially important for persons with diminished autonomy, including children and adolescents. Research issues related to informed consent, confidentiality, and voluntariness of participation are derived from this principle.
2. *Beneficence.* This principle reflects the perspective that not only must persons' decisions be respected and protected from harm but efforts to secure their well-being must also be made. Beneficence (i.e., maximizing good and minimizing harm to individuals or to society) is thus an obligation.
3. *Justice.* This principle dictates that the benefits and burdens of research must be distributed fairly and equitably and that research participants should be chosen for reasons related to scientific inquiry, not for reasons of accessibility or convenience. In addition, persons with disabilities should not be asked to bear a disproportionate share of the burden.

All biomedical research must be guided by these three principles. Shortly after the Belmont Report was released in 1979, the first regulatory guidelines were issued. Called the Code of Federal Regulations on the Protection of Human Subjects (or CFR), this code was explicitly written to establish the basic beneficence-related requirements for research. These requirements are discussed later. However, the point here is that these guidelines essentially laid out the parameters of federal policy with respect to the ethical study of children and adolescents and thus from the outset combined regulatory language with issues of right and wrong.

An additional set of issues has led to the intermingling of ethical and legal perspectives on mental health research, which involves the nature of psychological and psychiatric research itself. Because the focus of study often involves individuals with emotional or mental impairments, legal issues often arise by necessity. For example, laws governing consent, custody, or involuntary commitment may enter into the implementation of a study protocol even if such issues are not a primary or even secondary focus of the project. Legal considerations can dictate parameters of studies that may not have been previously anticipated.

Finally, there are anecdotal reports that ethical and legal concerns may increasingly be vying for ascendancy within university-based institutional review boards (IRBs). The current increase in lawsuits directed against universities involved in research with human subjects has led to a climate wherein concerns about the protection of these subjects are weighed against concerns about potential litigation within the review deliberations that occur in IRBs. This is an inevitable result of the mixed purposes of academic institutions, in which attracting large research grants leads to institutional accreditation, credibility, and stature; however, large-scale scientific projects, especially in new or untested areas of science (e.g., genetic therapies, therapeutic development of new agents, or therapies with high-risk patients, such as those who are suicidal) also entail increased potential for harm to research subjects and increased likelihood of litigation against the university if harm occurs.

GUIDELINES AND FEDERAL REGULATIONS

Guidelines

Though the foundational principles underpinning protection of human subjects in research has remained unchanged since the 1970s, the application of these principles to subpopulations and their interpretation is dynamic and changeable (Hoagwood, Jensen, & Fisher, 1996). Research ethics involving children and adolescents with mental health needs has been the subject of recent federal attention (Arnold et al., 1995; Charney, 2000; Shore & Hyman, 1999). In 1998, the National Bioethics Advisory Commission issued its report on Research Involving Persons with Mental Disorders that May Affect Decision-making Capacity. In 1999, the National Institute of Mental Health (NIMH) created a workgroup of the National Advisory Mental Health Council to provide additional safeguards and reviews of human subjects' concerns for grant applications involving challenging designs, methods, or techniques. In 2000, the National Human Research Protections Advisory Committee (NHRPAC) met to review ethical issues inherent in research involving children and formed a workgroup to examine the adequacy of the existing regulations in Subpart D (described later). In 2000, the National Institutes of Health (NIH) issued new requirements governing the education of clinical investigators in the protection of research subjects. The NIMH has also issued program announcements specifically targeting studies of research ethics (NIH, 1999). All these activities reflect the heightened awareness at the federal level of the need to attend carefully to issues of human subjects' protection while ensuring the growth and solidity of the scientific foundation on issues of public health significance.

From a public health scientific standpoint, in addition to the three principles defined in the Belmont Report (National Commission, 1979), there are several fundamental requirements without which the ethical grounding of a scientific study can be questioned. The first is that the potential yield of the study must be significant in its promise of improving public health. Investigators have been cautioned to focus on scientific issues of genuine significance, rather than questions that may be interesting but trivial or unrelated to general societal benefit (Hyman, 1999). Second, the experimental design must be sound, and alternative designs should be considered carefully with respect to both ethical and practical concerns (Vitiello, Jensen, & Hoagwood, 1999). In addition, the balance between risk and potential benefit should be weighed favorably toward the study participants. Finally, research participants must be fully informed of the risks, benefits, implications, and alternatives to participation.

Federal Regulations

The specific policy that sets the standards for federally funded research was first issued in 1983 as the Code of Federal Regulations on the Protection of Human Subjects. Within CFR were requirements for the establishment of IRBs, criteria for IRB approval, criteria for determining the hierarchy of risks, circumstances under which parental permission is needed or waivers obtainable, and special protections for children involved as subjects in research. The CFR was revised in 1991, and the revision included more specific discussion of the protection of children and adolescents as research subjects (U.S. Department of Health and Human Services [DHHS], 1991a, 1991b). The main requirements of the policy included the necessity of obtaining fully informed permission or consent from the parent or other legal guardian for a child's participation in research; obtaining assent, when possible, from the child; and ensuring that the risk/benefit ratio is favorable to the child.

In evaluating the concept of risk, several variants are described in the CFR. Minimal risk is defined as risk that is not greater than that ordinarily encountered in daily life or during routine physical or psychological assessments (DHHS, 1991a, § 46.102(i)). Minimal risk is not equivalent to no risk, and the ways in which it is calibrated and defined differ considerably from one investigation to another and from one IRB to another. Research that involves greater than minimal risk but also includes the prospect of direct benefit is justified if the potential benefit outweighs the potential harm (DHHS, 1991b, §46.405). According to 45 CFR 46, a benefit must be reasonably expected if a study is to be considered to have the prospect of direct benefit. Risks, however, must be presented if they are foreseeable. This formulation is much broader and could include possible but unlikely problems. Treatment studies tend to fall into this category. Deliberation of the risks and benefits involves careful consideration of the severity of the child's illness, the availability of alternative treatments, and the estimates of the safety and efficacy of the experimental treatment that the child may receive if enrolled in the study. Table 4.1 lists the kinds of research by level of risk and the decisional elements to weigh when considering the involvement of children.

Research that does not contain direct benefit to the participant is among the most controversial. Examples of these kinds of studies include invasive medical procedures, exposure to situations that may provoke anxious or upsetting responses, and administration of agents that are potentially toxic. Federal regulations stipulate that this kind of research may be conducted only if, in addition to the other requirements, the following conditions are also met:

1. The study involves only a minor increase over minimal risk;
2. The procedure involves "experiences to the subjects that are commensurate with those inherent in their actual or expected medical, dental, psychological, social or educational situations";
3. The study has the potential to provide knowledge that is of "vital importance" to understanding or treating the pediatric illness; and
4. Parental permission and child assent are obtained (DHHS, 1991b, §46.406)

The final category of risk involves projects that present greater than a minor increase over minimal risk. These studies are rarely proposed and are considered only if

TABLE 4.1. Elements to Consider in Evaluating the Ethics of Research in Children

Type of research	Critical elements
Research that has potential benefit to research subject	Risk/benefit must be favorable to the research subject
Research that has no potential benefit to the research subject	No greater than minimal risk is allowed
Research that has no potential benefit but relevant knowledge can be gained	No more than a minor increase over minimal risk is allowed
	Subjects are exposed to experiences reasonably commensurate with those inherent in their lives
	Research is likely to yield knowledge that is of vital importance for amelioration of the condition
Research that is not otherwise approvable under the foregoing criteria	Secretary of HHS can determine that proposed research presents a reasonable opportunity to further understanding, prevention, or alleviation of a serious problem affecting health/welfare of children

they have the potential to increase scientific knowledge about a serious public health problem affecting children. They require special review and approval by the DHHS.

OBTAINING INFORMED CONSENT

Informed consent is in some sense the ethical cornerstone on which rests human subjects' protections. It requires that individuals understand and are free to choose their participation. Ethical dilemmas concerning consent may arise in any type of treatment or intervention study, including pharmacological, psychosocial, preventive, or service trials. As Levine (1981) indicates, the consent process should include specific elements: an invitation to participate; statements of the purpose of the study and the basis of participant selection; measures for ensuring that a person's decision to participate is voluntary; and explanations of procedures, benefits, risks, and discomforts; of how untoward consequences will be handled; of alternatives to participation; and of financial considerations, confidentiality, and opportunities for continuing disclosure.

Applebaum and Grisso (1988) identified four central criteria to consider when assessing the adequacy of informed consent procedures, listed in Table 4.2. These issues are capacity, understanding, reasoning, and ability to express a choice. Capacity involves the ability of the individual to provide consent. Although it is not the same as competence, which is a legal term, it refers to a basic capacity for understanding language, linguistic convention, and the meaning attached to words. Understanding refers to the ability of the individual to comprehend the terms of the agreement involved in consent. Understanding is sometimes believed to have occurred if the individual can repeat back what he or she has heard, but new methods of ensuring understanding are being developed by L. Roberts (1998) for consent involving adult patients with potential limitations (e.g., patients with schizophrenia). Reasoning refers to the ability of the individual to balance risks and benefits and to foresee or anticipate both. Finally, the ability of the individual to express a choice is essential to the concept of informed consent. It is distinct from understanding in a receptive sense, as it entails the active ability to weigh options and select according to one's preferences. It is probably a key aspect of the consent process yet has rarely been studied.

Obtaining consent can become complex in research with adolescents because it generally must involve both the adolescent and the parent or guardian. In research involving minimal risk, it has sometimes been sufficient to obtain the informed consent of one parent. However, in research with greater than minimal risk, obtaining permission of both parents (if available) is generally advisable.

Children, by virtue of their limited legal status and because they cannot legally consent to research participation, are often considered to be a vulnerable population. In addition, children with psychiatric disorders may have (but do not necessarily have) limita-

TABLE 4.2. Criteria for Assessing the Adequacy of Informed Consent

Appreciating the situation	Ability to evaluate the options realistically
Understanding	Ability to comprehend terms of agreement
Reasoning	Ability to balance risks and benefits
Communicating choices	Ability to maintain and communicate stable choices

Note. Data from Appelbaum and Grisso (1988).

tions with respect to understanding the conditions by which their participation is being solicited. Therefore, special efforts must be made to ensure that children's assent to participate is voluntary and that they understand fully the risks and benefits of participation. It is often prudent to ask whether a particular study's aims could be directed toward a less vulnerable population first. A clear rationale should be provided as to why children with psychiatric disorders, as opposed to children or adolescents without these conditions, are the population of interest for a particular study.

There are variations from state to state in the laws authorizing minors to consent to either treatment or participation in research. Adolescents who are 18 or older are legally adults in all but three states, in which the age is 19 (Hoagwood, Jensen, & Leshner, 1997). There are circumstances under which children can give their own consent, based on their status, the specific services sought, or the type of study (e.g., high-risk populations) (English, 1991). Some states allow minors who are living apart from their parents (e.g., homeless, emancipated, or married minors) to consent to receive healthcare or mental healthcare (English, 1991). Laws relating to consent for minors are changing in many states and thus are subject to variation. As a consequence, it is advisable for the researcher to become well acquainted with the laws governing minor status and consent in the state in which the research is to be conducted.

Impairments in decisional capacity, as may occur with children whose cognitive capacities are developing or among psychiatrically impaired individuals, have implications for informed consent procedures. These impairments may be transient, intermittent, or permanent (Roberts, 1998). Clinical syndromes may create distortions of thought, impaired attention or memory, ambivalence, emotional lability, lack of motivation, distractibility, or impulsivity (Bonnie, 1997; Dresser, 1996; Elliott, 1997; Expert Panel Report, 1998; Roberts, 1998). In studies involving persons with mental illnesses that may impair their judgment, an investigator should strongly consider using an independent qualified professional to assess the potential participants' capacity to provide informed consent. Children, whose cognitive, affective, and physiological development is emerging, do not possess full decisional capacity and thus are usually dependent on others for providing such (Munir & Earls, 1992); generally it is the parents who are placed in this role. However, among adolescents there are cases in which independent professionals have been engaged in research projects, and paid as independent consultants, to assess adolescents' understanding of the informed consent protocol and to ensure that participation is entirely voluntary (Fisher, 1996).

A variety of features may be included in protocols to improve the process of obtaining informed consent. These include repeated exposure to the information in the protocol; multiple avenues of communication (verbal, written, etc.); language use that is simple, in small units, and comprehensible; use of "patient educators" who can review relevant information with the potential subject, explain the study's purpose and process, and answer any questions; and specific attention to particular aspects of consent, including motivation, culture, and personal history of previous involvement in research projects (Applebaum & Grisso, 1995; Bonnie, 1997; Roberts, 1998; Sutherland, Meslin, & Till, 1994).

WEIGHING RISKS AND BENEFITS

Analysis of the risks and benefits of participation in research is made by the investigator, and the appropriateness of the balance is ascertained by the IRB. The purpose of the study must include demonstration of its potential benefits as well as an explicit discussion as to how the investigator intends to minimize risk. In assessing risks, investigators occasionally overlook some of the distinct advantages to participation in research. For example, in addition to the increased access to treatment that is available from participation in treatment trials, participation in research can also provide youth with information about the effectiveness of treatments, the availability of community services, and the perceptions of their peers (Hoagwood, Jensen, & Fisher, 1996).

However, the weighing of risks and benefits in research on child and adolescent mental health can be among the most complex to address. The primary premise is that risks and benefits should be viewed from the standpoint of the research participant, not the investigator or institution. No risk is considered acceptable if the research does not have the potential to benefit the participant or will not strengthen knowledge about the condition or its treatment. The scientific validity of the design is one important factor for evaluating the potential benefit of a study. The design should reduce risks to the maximum extent possible while preserving the scientific integrity of the design. For example, active treatment comparison arms are desirable, as opposed to wait-list controls or placebo conditions. Whenever feasible, the design should also maximize benefits to increase the likelihood that advantages to individual participants or to other populations will be accrued. For example, a study of the comparative effectiveness of two empirically validated treatments would confer benefit and reduce risk for all subjects enrolled in the study. Finally, a careful assessment of the range of potential positive outcomes—both direct and indirect—should be taken into account when determining the likely impact of a treatment (Fisher, 1996).

Just as there are both direct and indirect benefits which must be considered, there are also direct and indirect risks. The notion of what constitutes a risk needs to be assessed broadly to encompass physical risks, psychological risks, and the social dimensions of risk (Levine, 1981; Roberts, 1998). The latter could include risks such as stigma, labeling, or community distrust. For example, some studies of service interventions have been viewed as "hit and runs," with services put into place temporarily for the purpose of studying them, but with no provision being made from the outset to try to ensure their continuation if they are found to be effective after the study is completed (Hoagwood et al., 1996). In some ways, risks from medication trials may be easier to identify than risks from psychosocial treatments or service interventions. For example, the risks from medication treatment trials may include dizziness, sleeplessness, tics, heart palpitations, and so on, whereas most often the risks from participation in psychosocial treatment trials are harder to quantify or predict. Nevertheless, they must be considered and included in the informed consent protocol. Such things as the possibility of memory flashbacks, transient discomforts, increased restlessness, or anxiety through exposure to memories or events may be among the risks associated with participation in psychosocial treatment trials.

The other side of the risk coin, however, is that the lack of a scientifically valid and useful knowledge base about effective psychosocial treatments for children and adolescents has created a situation wherein millions of children are exposed to treatments or interventions everyday in schools, mental health clinics, or other service venues for which there is no evidence whatsoever of their impact. In fact, most studies of programs for youth who receive public mental health services through either the mental health, welfare, education, or justice systems indicate that upwards of 90% of such programs have no evidence to support their impact, and some, in fact, are known to be harmful (Burns, Hoagwood, & Mrazek, 2000; Dishion, McCord, & Poulin, 1999; Rones & Hoagwood,

2000; U.S. Department of Health and Human Services, 1999; U.S. Public Health Service, 2000). The ethics of a public mental health system that delivers untested clinical services and treatments should certainly be called into question.

Concerns about the use of placebos have been voiced for decades. Foremost among these concerns is the argument that the ethical duty of clinical investigators is to avoid harm and that placebo arms, by definition, promote risk by providing no treatment at all for a period of time. This argument is at the core of the World Medical Association's revision of the Declaration of Helsinki (World Medical Association [WMA], 2000), which argues that clinical research involves an ethical obligation of the investigator to conduct research based on the therapeutic value for the participant.

The WMA first developed the Declaration of Helsinki in 1964 as a statement to guide physicians in research involving human subjects. The Declaration contains a series of statements about what ought or ought not to occur in medical research (WMA, 2000). In 2000, the WMA issued a revision tightening its stance against the use of placebos by stating that in any medical trial all patients, including those in control conditions, must be assured of receiving an active treatment. In essence, this statement precluded the use of placebos in research. However, the statement aroused considerable controversy and discussion, including a major conference by the NIH in November 2000. In the fall of 2001, the WMA stated that under certain circumstances, placebo-controlled trials could be ethically acceptable, if sound methodological reasons were provided. The interpretation of this statement has yet to achieve any consensus internationally, and some countries (e.g., Brazil) continue to ban all placebo-controlled studies.

Questions about the ethics involved in the use of placebos might be more usefully thought of as issues involving the role of expectancy values (generally transient expectations) versus the role of conditioned responses. Expectancies are generally considered transient responses, whereas conditioned responses may involve synaptic remodeling. The scientific questions thus become those related to the psychological expectancies that lead to placebo responses, the time course of placebo responses, and the mechanisms that underlie these responses.

While questions about the ethical appropriateness of placebos arise more often in pharmacological treatment trials than in studies of psychosocial treatments, the principle is the same: withholding treatments for children who have clear treatment needs and for whom an effective treatment exists creates an ethical problematic. However, use of placebo treatment arms is also one of the strongest scientific strategies for demonstrating treatment impact vis-à-vis nonspecific factors (e.g., attention). The issues investigators must weigh in deciding in favor of or against inclusion of a placebo arm include the appropriateness of comparison treatments for the population to be studied (e.g., have they only been used with adults?), the status of the scientific evidence supporting alternative treatments (e.g., is the support for alternative treatments that are reasonably commensurate with one another?), and the nature of the research questions being examined (Roberts, Lauriello, Geppert, & Keith, 2001). Improvements in design can also provide additional protections, as described by Charney (2000).

It is also important to note that high-risk protocols that involve placebo arms may require special preparation to incorporate into consent forms or other research materials the perspectives of families or other stakeholders. Further discussion of the models for establishing formal means of enlisting community stakeholder perspectives is provided later.

ENGAGING FAMILIES, YOUTH, AND COMMUNITY STAKEHOLDERS

Because the issues about the weighing of relative risks and benefits depend in large measure on community norms, and because federally funded studies must demonstrate adequate representation of the population diversity which exists within the communities being examined, there are now a growing number of studies that are establishing formal means of incorporating community perspectives into the research protocol. In fact, some researchers have called such inclusion the only means of ensuring that an ethical compact exists (Jensen, Hoagwood, & Trickett, 1999). There are a variety of ways in which community or stakeholder perspectives can be incorporated into research studies, and many of the more robust models have arisen from work within the HIV/AIDS community. For example, Lynn and McKay (in press) have adapted an advisory board model from an HIV prevention program to their work with families of youth with mental illnesses, and Ireys, Devet, and Sakwa (2002) have adapted a model from a family support program for families of chronically ill children to families of children with severe emotional disturbances. Both of these models involve the establishment of a community advisory board whose membership includes parents or caretakers of youth with mental illnesses, and community stakeholders, case managers, or policymakers. These boards are actively engaged in every phase of the research project from its inception (including design, selection of measures, recruitment, implementation) to the final dissemination of the results.

Another model for enlisting community collaboration in research studies entails the involvement of special consultants with knowledge of the values, attitudes, or perspectives of the community in which the project will be carried out. These expert consultants may be involved at any phase of the project to provide advice and guidance about the suitability or acceptability of designs, measures, or recruitment of vulnerable populations. Often they are included on a scientific advisory board and meet once or twice a year to provide input on these issues as the study is designed and conducted. This model is less intense and elicits far less substantive guidance about the perspectives of stakeholders but is more commonly selected by investigators, in part because it seems to be less time-consuming and intrusive to the overall objectives of the scientific enterprise. However, those perceptions may well be false. There have been a number of recently launched large clinical trials that have encountered serious obstacles to recruitment and acceptance of the study in a range of communities because the investigators failed to include, in a substantive way, community input on the design and conduct of the study from the beginning. In addition, there is no evidence to suggest that the involvement of community perspectives will undermine the scientific validity of the study; to the contrary, some have argued that this is the only way to create an ethically valid and grounded science base (Jensen, Hoagwood, & Trickett, 1999).

One problem that often arises in either of these models, however, is the extent to which any individual person or group of persons can realistically "speak" for a "community." In fact, the notion of what constitutes a community is itself controversial (Fisher et al., 2002). However, it behooves the would-be investigator to attempt to understand the context in which the study is to occur, and often this understanding entails special attention to the perspectives of those who will be the ultimate beneficiaries of the outcomes of the study (i.e., the families, caseworkers, providers, administrators, or policymakers in the community in which the treatment will or can be provided).

Beyond consideration of community perspectives in the design and conduct of treatment studies, there are those who have argued that research subjects themselves are best seen as active collaborators in the research process (Atkisson, Rosenblatt, & Hoagwood, 1996). The relationship between investigator and research participant is most respectful when it is structured as a collaborative partnership. This stance requires that participants be fully informed about the risks and benefits of the study, that they understand that the partnership is voluntary, and that they can discontinue participation at any time. This role of the research participant as collaborator actively engaged in the study contrasts with the passive stance that has typically described much medical research in the past. As Atkisson et al. (1996) point out, the role of research participant as collaborator is an ideal that is never fully realized in any study—there are numerous obstacles to it.

The principles of collaboration—whether directed at community stakeholders or at research participants themselves—are especially important in studies involving psychosocial treatments for children and adolescents, in part because profound misunderstandings of what constitutes mental illnesses and misperceptions about the need for and consequences of treatments have created a climate wherein distrust and suspicion about research and researchers abound. These misperceptions are compounded by widespread ignorance about the goals of science, about what evidence-based practice is, and about the reasons why the application of research findings to practice is needed. Direct and open communication among stakeholders and researchers will not be a panacea, but it is probably an essential element for accomplishing the goals of creating an ethical and valid science base on psychosocial treatments for youth.

PROVIDING CLINICAL FEEDBACK: THE THERAPEUTIC DILEMMA

The blueprint report of the National Advisory Mental Health Council (NIMH, 2001) called for an increase in the number of studies of treatment efficacy, effectiveness, and process for children and adolescents with mental disorders. In the past 5 years, the number of pediatric trials of treatments—both pharmacological and psychological—has quadrupled. The number of child and adolescent treatment trials is expected to continue to rise, in large part because of the urgency of the public health need for scientific knowledge about effective interventions. In addition, however, there is an increasing interest in studies that attend to issues of treatment process, not only outcome. Such studies are essential if the active ingredients that lead to therapeutic change are to be discovered.

For psychosocial treatment researchers, especially those involved in long-term treatment studies, issues can arise about the extent of an investigator's responsibility to inform subjects about their progress or about comorbid conditions. The appropriateness of providing feedback is generally thought to depend on the research goal and on the definition of "clinical" services. For example, one IRB ruled that because information about a participant was obtained by nonclinicians (i.e., graduate students) it was not clinical and thus no obligation existed to inform the participant about treatment needs or to refer the participant for treatment. But some standards of clinical responsibility suggest that any investigator undertaking a treatment research project is simultaneously agreeing to either provide appropriate intervention when needed or to refer the participant to another resource (Fisher, 1996).

USING INCENTIVES

Recruitment for participation involves consideration of several questions in advance. How significant are the study's aims? Why are particular populations, especially if they are vulnerable populations, needed for answering the questions of interest? Can the study be conducted on less vulnerable populations first? In addition, for studies supported by public health funds, there is a public health responsibility to ensure that the highest quality of science is supported and that only issues of genuine importance are targeted for such studies (Hyman, 1999).

Incentives offered for research participation need to be considered with respect to two issues: respect for participants' time and compensation for such, and lack of coercion (Macklin, 1981; Roberts, 1998). Investigators working with populations that are socioeconomically disadvantaged have special responsibilities to ensure that both research benefits and risks are not unfairly distributed. Once again, the establishment of community advisory boards can be helpful in ascertaining the community's perceptions of risks associated with recruitment and the types of recruitment strategies that may be viewed as coercive. Perceptions of risk and coercion vary enormously according to cultural norms, previous experiences that members of a community may have had with research, and attitudes toward different kinds of treatments or services (e.g., concerns about medications and their risks, and concerns about custody and how disclosure of a child's behavior might affect one's rights as a parent).

In cases in which monetary incentives are provided to research participants, such incentives may be viewed as inducements that are fair compensation for one's time. On the other hand, such compensation may also be viewed in some communities as coercive, that is, as offering inducements that are outside the bounds of convention and that will be used to manipulate rather than compensate. The perceptions of the ways in which monetary inducements may be viewed within particular community contexts need to be carefully considered by investigators prior to designing a study. Community advisory boards can be helpful in reflecting back to investigators the community values, expectations, and beliefs about incentives.

ENSURING CONFIDENTIALITY

Research on psychosocial treatments for children and adolescents may involve the divulgence of sensitive information about a child or family that may not have been previously revealed to others or that could produce harm if discovered. Ethical considerations about recruitment and consent can provide important safeguards against the revelation of confidential information, but additional protections are needed to ensure that information remains confidential. Investigators are obligated to ensure that information collected during a research protocol is not divulged to others in a manner inconsistent with the participant's understanding. Procedures for protecting confidentiality must ensure that a participant retains control over what is shared and with whom (Fisher, 1996).

Routine procedures for maintaining confidentiality of data include the use of subject codes rather than identifiers, secure storage, limited access to data, disposal of unnecessary identifying information, and appropriate supervision of research personnel. With newer technologies available for protecting electronic information, but with the additional risks that electronic transmission poses, investigators must be especially cautious to ensure that identifiable information collected during research projects is safeguarded.

The Certificate of Confidentiality is a federally sponsored document that provides immunity to investigators from any governmental or civil order to disclose identifying information from research records. The Certificate is granted under section 301(d) of the Public Health Service Act. The Certificate provides additional protection against disclosure of confidential information to outside parties. When a Certificate of Confidentiality is granted, both its protections and limitations should be explained to the child and the caregiver. The application for the Certificate can be obtained by most federal research institutions.

OTHER SPECIAL CONSIDERATIONS AND STRATEGIES

Roberts (1998) has developed a process for helping investigators develop protocols to ensure that ethically important research elements—design, informed consent, and assurances of confidentiality, for example—explicitly deal with human subjects' protection. The Research Protocol Ethics Assessment Tool is an evaluative checklist for use with participants who may have mental health problems. Although not designed for child and adolescent populations, it can be useful as an assessment tool by investigators who wish to ensure that key aspects of the research project are adhering to the highest ethical standards.

Other resources exist for investigators seeking guidance about obtaining informed consent. In 1998, the NIH convened a conference to provide practical advice to IRBs on issues related to involving individuals with a questionable capacity to consent. A summary of the conference is available in a document issued by the NIH (Expert Panel Report, 1998). Finally, the NIH now requires all investigators seeking funding for research to obtain continuing education in the protection of human subjects. The requirement for such is described in the NIH Guide (NIH, 2000).

SUMMARY AND CONCLUSION

It is as unethical to conduct studies that have not ensured adequate human subjects' protection as it is to withhold examination of treatments from children who need them. Creating an ethically grounded science base requires more than attending to the jots and tittles within legally grounded regulations or guidelines. It requires principled commitment to the intrinsic value of science and to the belief that no harm must ensue from participation in research. It requires attention to the values, histories, and beliefs of the culture or the community the researcher enters. These are principles that need thoughtful consideration at the beginning of investigations, not at the end.

As noted in the Surgeon General's Report on Mental Health (U.S. Department of Health and Human Services, 1999), research on the efficacy and effectiveness of treatments and other mental health services for children and adolescents lags far behind the adult field and remains one of the most significant public health arenas in which to advance the health of the nation's children. However, the task of constructing designs that will provide adequate safeguards against potential harm is complex and requires deliberate attention to a range of issues. As has been described in this chapter, these issues include ensuring that truly informed consent has been obtained from the participants. What constitutes "understanding of a study" has yet to be fully examined scientifically, but the elements involved in consent include capacity, understanding, reasoning, and ability to express choices. If children or adolescents with limited cognitive abilities are part of a research population, then procedures must be in place to ensure that a guardian, caretaker, or independent professional with the best interests of the child in mind can make that decision.

Striking a balance between the benefits that can accrue to individuals or to society as a whole through research and the potential harm from participating in a particular study requires that the investigator carefully consider the varieties of harm—both direct or indirect—that may ensue, as well as the varieties of potential benefit. The primary standpoint from which such decisions are made must be that of the research participant, not the investigator or institution. Designs can often be constructed that will maximize benefit and minimize harm (e.g., the use of active treatment comparisons).

Consideration of issues such as the use of monetary incentives often rests on the values implicit within the particular community, neighborhood, or setting in which the study is to be carried out. Such consideration can often benefit from guidance provided by community leaders, families of children with mental health problems, or stakeholders. Models of ways to establish formal means of enlisting such guidance are being used in a variety of studies involving HIV/AIDS, chronic physical illnesses, and, more recently, childhood mental illnesses. Beyond obtaining consultation from community stakeholders, however, the active participation of persons who represent the perspectives of the ultimate beneficiaries of science augments the validity and generalizability of the findings and, most important, provides the ethical grounding that either makes the research ultimately meaningful or relegates it to dusty academic shelves.

Although the challenges to conducting research on psychosocial treatments for youth may appear daunting, the alternative—which unfortunately is the status quo for the majority of children in the public mental health system, namely, providing untested or even harmful treatments or services to children and adolescents with mental health needs—is simply untenable. Knowledge about the impact of treatments and their application within the mental health system must be generated and the pace accelerated. The ethical principles by which these advances can be made extend beyond those described in the Belmont Report. In addition to ensuring that research participants experience no harm (beneficence), are treated respectfully (respect), and are treated equitably (justice), one can add a higher-order principle that the rational generation of knowledge must be ceaseless. It is through constant examination, analysis, and reanalysis that the self-correcting process of science, as a method for generating knowledge as well as uncertainty, can be sustained.

REFERENCES

Applebaum, P. S., & Grisso, T. (1988). Assessing patients' capacities to consent to treatment. *New England Journal of Medicine, 319,* 1635–1638.

Applebaum, P. S., & Grisso, T. (1995). The MacArthur Treatment Competence Study I, II, III. *Law and Human Behavior, 19,* 105–174.

Arnold, L. E., Stoff, D. M., Cook, E., Cohen, D. J., Kruesi, M., Wright, C., Hattab, J., Graham, P., Zametkin, A., Castellanos, F. X., McMahon, W., & Lechman, J. F. (1995). Ethical issues in biological psychiatric research with children and adolescents. *Journal of the American Academy of Child and Adolescent Psychiatry, 34,* 929–939.

Attkisson, C. C., Rosenblatt, A., & Hoagwood, K. (1996). Research ethics and human subjects protection in child mental health services research and community studies. In K. Hoagwood, P. S. Jensen, & C. B. Fisher (Eds.), *Ethical issues in mental health research with children and adolescents* (pp. 43–58) . Mahwah, NJ: Erlbaum.

Bhatara, V., Feil, M., Hoagwood, K., Vitiello, B., & Zima, B. (2002). Trends in combined pharmacotherapy with stimulants for children. *Psychiatric Services, 53*, 244–245.

Bonnie, R. J. (1997). Research with cognitively impaired subjects. *Archives of General Psychiatry, 54*, 105–111.

Burns, B. J., Hoagwood, K., & Mrazek, P. (2000). Effective treatment for mental disorders in children and adolescents. *Clinical Child and Family Psychology Review, 2*, 199–254.

Charney, D. S. (2000). The use of placebos in randomized clinical trials of mood disorders: Well justified, but improvements in design are indicated. *Biological Psychiatry, 47*, 687–688.

Dishion, T. J., McCord, J., & Poulin, F. (1999). When interventions harm: Peer groups and problem behavior. *American Psychologist, 54*, 755–765.

Dresser, R. (1996). Mentally disabled research subjects: The enduring policy issues. *Journal of the American Medical Association, 276*, 67–72.

Elliott, C. (1997). Caring about risks: Are severely depressed patients competent to consent to research? *Archives of General Psychiatry, 54*, 113–116.

English, A. (1991). Runaway and street youth at risk for HIV infections: Legal and ethical issues in access to care. Special issue: Homeless youth. *Journal of Adolescent Health, 12*, 504–510.

Expert Panel Report to the National Institutes of Health. (1998, February). *Research involving individuals with questionable capacity to consent: Ethical issues and practical considerations for institutional review boards (IRBs)* Bethesda, MD: National Institutes of Health.

Fisher, C. (1996). Casebook on ethical issues in research on child and adolescent mental disorders. In K. Hoagwood, P. Jensen, & C. Fisher (Eds.), *Ethical issues in child and adolescent mental health research* (pp. 135–166). Mahwah, NJ: Erlbaum.

Fisher, C., Hoagwood, K., Boyce, C., Duster, R., Frank, D. A., Grisso, T., Levine, R. J., Macklin, R., Spencer, M. B., Takanishi, R., Trimble, J. E., & Zayas, L. H. (2002). Research ethics for mental health science involving ethnic minority children and youth. *American Psychologist, 57*(12), 1024–1040.

Hoagwood, K., Jensen, P. S., & Fisher, C. (Eds.). (1996). *Ethical issues in child and adolescent mental health research*. Mahwah, NJ: Erlbaum.

Hoagwood, K., Jensen, P. S., & Leshner, A. I. (1997). Ethical issues in research on child and adolescent mental disorders: Implications for a science of scientific ethics. In S. W. Henggeler & A. B. Santos (Eds.), *Innovative approaches for difficult–to-treat populations* (pp. 459–476). Washington, DC: American Psychiatric Press.

Hyman, S. E. (1999). Protecting patients, preserving progress: Ethics in mental health research. *Academic Medicine, 74*, 258–259.

Ireys, H., Devet, K. A., & Sakwa, D. (2002). Family support and education. In B. J. Burns & K. Hoagwood (Eds.), *Community treatment for youth: Evidence-based interventions for severe emotional and behavioral disorders* (pp.154–175). New York: Oxford University Press.

Jensen, P. S. (1998). Ethical and pragmatic issues in the use of psychotropic agents in young children. *Canadian Journal of Psychiatry, 43*, 585–588.

Jensen, P. S., Bhatara, V., Vitiello, B., Hoagwood, K., Feil, M., & Burke, L. B. (1999). Psychoactive medication prescribing practices for U.S. children: Gaps between research and clinical practice. *Journal of the American Academy of Child and Adolescent Psychiatry, 38*(5), 557–565.

Jensen, P. S., Hoagwood, K., & Trickett, E. (1999). Ivory tower or earthen trenches? Community collaborations to foster real-world research. *Journal of Applied Developmental Science, 3*, 206–212.

Levine, R. J. (1981). *Ethics and regulation of clinical research*. Baltimore: Urban & Schwartzenberg.

Lynn, C., & McKay, M. (in press). School social work: Promoting parent–school involvement through collaborative practice models. *Social Work in Education*.

Macklin, R. (1981). "Due" and "undue" inducements: On paying money to research subjects. *IRB: Review of Human Subjects Research, 3*, 1–6.

Munir, K., & Earls, F. (1992). Ethical principles governing research in child and adolescent psychiatry. *Journal of the American Academy of Child and Adolescent Psychiatry, 31*, 408–414.

National Advisory Mental Health Council Workgroup Report. (2001). *Blueprint for change: Research on child and adolescent mental health.* Washington, DC: National Institute of Mental Health.

National Bioethics Advisory Commission. (1998). Research involving persons with mental disorders that may affect decisionmaking capacity [On-line]. Available: *http://www.bioethics.gov*

National Commission for the Protection of Human Subjects of Biomedical and Behavioral Research. (1979). *The Belmont Report: Ethical principles and guidelines for the protection of human subjects of research.* Washington, DC: U.S. Government Printing Office.

National Institutes of Health. (1999, March 31). Research on ethical issues in human subjects (PA-99-079, NIH Guide) [On-line]. Available: *http://grants.nih.gov/grants/guide/notice-files/PA-99-079.html*

National Institutes of Health (2000, June 5). Required education in the protection of human research participants (OD-00-039, NIH Guide) [On-line]. Available: *http://grants.nih.gov/grants/guide/notice-files/NOT-OD-00-039.html*

Roberts, L. W. (1998). Ethics of psychiatric research: Conceptual issues and empirical findings. *Comprehensive Psychiatry, 39,* 99–110.

Roberts, L. W., Lauriello, J., Geppert, C., & Keith, S. J. (2001). Placebos and paradoxes in psychiatric research: An ethics perspective. *Biological Psychiatry, 49,* 887–893.

Roberts, R. E., Attkisson, C. C., & Rosenblatt, A. (1998). Prevalence of psychopathology among children and adolescents. *American Journal of Psychiatry, 155,* 715–725.

Rones, M., & Hoagwood K. (2000). School-based mental health services: A research review. *Clinical Child and Family Psychology Review, 3,* 223–241.

Shore, D. &, Hyman, S. E. (1999). NIMH symptom challenge and medication discontinuation. *Biological Psychiatry, 46,* 1009–1010.

Sutherland, H. J., Meslin, E. M., & Till, J. E. (1994). What's missing from current clinical trial guidelines? A framework for integrating science, ethics, and the community context. *Journal of Clinical Ethics, 7,* 297–303.

U.S. Department of Health and Human Services. (1991a). Protection of human subjects. Basic HHS policy for protection of human research subjects. Code of Federal Regulations, Title 45, Public Welfare: Part 46, Subpart A: 46.101–46.124, Revised June 18, 1991, Effective August 19, 1991, Office of the Federal Register, National Archives and Records Administration, Washington, DC, October 1, 1994 (45 CFR Subtitle A), pp. 116–127.

U.S. Department of Health and Human Services. (1991b). Protection of human subjects, Subpart D: Additional protections for children involved as subjects in research, Code of Federal Regulations, Title 45, Public Welfare: Part 46, Subpart D: 46.401 – 46.409, Revised June 18, 1991, Effective August 19, 1991, Office of the Federal Register, National Archives and Records Administration, Washington, DC, October 1, 1994 (45 CFR Subtitle A), pp. 132–135.

U.S. Department of Health and Human Services. (1999). *Mental health: A report of the Surgeon General.* Rockville, MD: U.S. Department of Health and Human Services, Substance Abuse, and Mental Health Services Administration.

U.S. Public Health Service. (2000). *Report of the Surgeon General's Conference on Children's Mental Health: A national action agenda.* Washington, DC: U.S. Department of Health and Human Services.

Vitiello, B. (2002) Ethical issues in pediatric psychopharmacology research. In D. Rosenberg, S. Gershon, & P. Davanzo (Eds.), *Pharmacotherapy for child and adolescent psychiatric disorders* (pp. 7–22). New York: Marcel Dekker.

Vitiello, B., Jensen, P. S., & Hoagwood, K. (1999). Integrating science and ethics in child and adolescent psychiatry research. *Biological Psychiatry, 46,* 1044–1049.

World Medical Association. (2000). *Declaration of Helsinki. Ethical principles for medical research involving human subjects* [On-line]. Available: *www.wma.net/e/policy*

Zito, J. M., Safer, D. J., DosReis, S., Gardner, J. F., Boles, M., & Lunch, F. (2000). Trends in the prescribing of psychotropic medications to preschoolers. *Journal of the American Medical Association, 283,* 1025–1030.

II

PROGRAMS OF RESEARCH

A

Internalizing Disorders
and Problems

5

Child-Focused Treatment of Anxiety

PHILIP C. KENDALL, SASHA G. ASCHENBRAND,
AND JENNIFER L. HUDSON

OVERVIEW

Anxiety disorders are among the most common forms of psychopathology in children and adolescents (Anderson, Williams, McGee, & Silva, 1987; Fergusson, Horwood, & Lynskey, 1993), and they are associated with a negative impact in multiple domains (e.g., social, familial, and academic). Evidence suggesting that levels of anxiety worsen over time (Strauss, Lease, Last, & Francis, 1988) highlights the importance of addressing these problems in children. Data also suggest that the majority of anxiety disorders do not remit with the simple passage of time (e.g., Keller et al., 1992) and that anxious (social phobic) youth are at increased risk for subsequent depression and/or substance use/abuse disorders. Given the prevalence of and interference caused by anxiety disorders in children, the development and evaluation of efficacious and effective treatments is warranted.

The treatment program the *Coping Cat* (Kendall, 1990; Kendall, Choudhury, Hudson, & Webb, 2002a, 2002b)[1] was developed at the Child and Adolescent Anxiety Disorders Clinic (CAADC) at Temple University and is for anxiety-disordered children between the ages of 7 and 13 years. The *C.A.T. Project*, a teen program, is also available. The program consists of (1) a treatment manual to guide the therapist and (2) a workbook for use by each child client. Both are specifically tailored for children with a principal diagnosis of separation anxiety disorder (SAD), generalized anxiety disorder (GAD), and social phobia (SoP). Although the strategies outlined in the treatment manual could also benefit children with other anxiety disorders (specific phobias, obsessive–compulsive problems, posttraumatic stress) the program has been designed more specifically for the basic similarities within SAD, GAD, and SoP. These disorders do not occur alone: Comorbidity is the "norm" and provides a challenge for the therapist (Hudson, Krain, & Kendall, 2001; Kendall, Kortlander, Chansky, & Brady, 1992). The treatment employed at CAADC accepts comorbid conditions (we exclude psychosis and IQ < 80 but include children with various other disorders and Asperger's) provided that the target anxiety disorder is a principal/primary diagnosis. For example, the program is appropriate for a child with GAD and comorbid dysthymia. In a case in which dysthymia/depression is assessed as more severe and impairing than anxiety, treatment for depression would be recommended. We use a thorough process to determine whether anxiety is the child's primary problem. First, an initial phone screen reduces the probability of inappropriate referrals. Once the family comes in for an evaluation, intensive structured interviews conducted separately with parents and children are used to assign diagnoses. We rely on clinician severity ratings of interference and distress to determine which diagnoses are principal/primary if a child has multiple conditions. Although we can never be 100% certain that we have teased apart which diagnoses are principal/primary, we make a definitive decision in tough cases and proceed with appropriate treatment. During treatment, the focus is on the child's anxiety diagnoses and not the comorbid diagnoses. Interestingly, the treatment has been found to have beneficial effects on some comorbid conditions in addition to the targeted principal diagnoses (Kendall, Brady, & Verduin, 2001).

Guiding Theory and Main Treatment Themes

Potential historical causes of anxiety are not the focus of treatment. Similarly, pointing fingers of causal blame does not occur in the treatment. Rather, the treatment accepts the child where he or she is at the beginning of treatment and looks forward and works to accomplish new goals. Prior events and explanations are considered only to the extent that the therapist needs them to arrange the most effective activities and experiments to help alter the child's threat-focused interpretations of situations and events.

Our treatment of anxiety in youth is guided by an integrationist perspective often labeled cognitive-behavioral, which includes considerations of the child's internal and external environments. The cognitive-behavioral model incorporates and emphasizes behavior, cognition, affect, and social factors. Therefore, cognitive-behavioral treatment strategies with children and adolescents use enactive, performance-based procedures and structured sessions as well as cognitive and affective interventions to effect change in thoughts, feelings, and behavior. The model places an emphasis on the learning process and the influence of contingencies and models in the child's environment, simultaneously highlighting the centrality of the individual's information-processing and emotional experiencing style in the development and reduction of psychological difficulties. The cognitive-behavioral model represents a hybrid of cognitive, behavioral, emotion-focused, and social strategies for change. As such, the model abandons reliance on any single/simple model and supports an integrative understanding of the relationships of cognition and behavior to emotional functioning, within the larger social context of the individual. Social and interpersonal contexts, including peers and the family, are important to consider in the design and outcomes of therapy, and must therefore be a part of treatment and the guiding cognitive-behavioral model.

Combining/integrating treatment strategies is consistent with the multicomponent conceptualization of anxiety as having cognitive, behavioral, and physiological features. First, anxious affect is associated with physiological arousal manifested, for example, by gastrointestinal distress and muscle tension. Thus, the treatment program teaches the child to identify physiological responses and employ relaxation strategies and diaphragmatic breathing in response to the physiological cues. Second, research has shown that anxious children display cognitive bias toward threat: anxious children demonstrate cognitive distortions, overestimating the likelihood of negative events (e.g., negative evaluation from peers and developing an illness) and the impact of the negative event (e.g., certain social rejection and certain death). Hence, the program provides opportunities for the child to consider alternative interpretations of situations and to develop/learn coping thoughts to replace anxious thoughts. Finally, anxious children avoid rather than approach stressful or potentially threatening situations. In avoiding feared situations, the child prevents him- or herself from learning that (1) a negative event is not as likely as predicted, (2) a feared consequence is less likely and less negative than anticipated, and, most important, the child never learns that (3) he or she can actually cope with the situation. The program provides opportunities for exposure to the feared situations, teaches the child to problem-solve and consider alternate behavioral responses, and offers multiple chances to practice actively coping in the formerly distressing situations.

The treatment protocol (therapist manual) follows a structured and organized set of sessions and emphasizes a "coping model." That is, the goal of therapy is not to forever remove all anxiety but, instead, to "build a cognitive template" (Kendall, 1993, p. 236) to be useful in the management of (coping with) anxiety in the future. Identifying the cognitive processes associated with excessive anxious arousal, training in cognitive strategies for anxiety management, and behavioral relaxation and performance-based practice opportunities are sequenced within the manual to build skill on skill. The child is given opportunities to learn that that he or she can enter anxiety-provoking situations using the skills acquired and, ultimately, cope successfully with the situation. The treatment guides the child to approach anxiety-provoking situations in a gradual fashion to maximize the child's experience of mastery. To help build the child's coping template, the therapist frequently uses coping modeling. That is, the therapist demonstrates the desired coping behaviors in the feared situation so that the child can imitate the therapist's behavior. Importantly, the therapist models the process of coping and not solely the end product of mastery. The therapist not only models the coping behavior but may also disclose personal examples of stressful situations similar to the child's difficulties. The therapist describes to the child the strategies that were useful in dealing with situation. Again, the aim is to demonstrate that having some distress is reasonable, that a strategy can be used to address the distress, and that the distress can be met head on (avoidance is not needed). The therapist models coping with anxiety, not total mastery. Related to this, the therapist demonstrates that successful task completion does not require perfection.

Practice and skill rehearsals are essential to ensure that the child develops the coping strategies. The program relies on both in-session (with the therapist in and out of the office) and out-of-session (without the therapist) practice. Role-plays and imaginal and *in vivo* exposure tasks provide excellent opportunities to practice coping skills. As noted, the child's social environment is considered crucial to the cognitive-behavioral model, and hence the therapist encourages the child each week to complete homework tasks—"Show That I Can" (STIC) tasks. In addition to building the child's confidence, these STIC tasks are designed to allow the child to use the skills taught and practiced in sessions in real-life situations. The child will practice within a therapy session how to deal with a situation at school, but STIC tasks are used to encourage the child to practice the skills with peers/family during the week. To help the child with this transition, the therapist creates real-life-like situations for practice within therapy and may invite siblings or age-matched peers who are further along in their treatment to assist with the practice.

In the individual treatment (Kendall, 1994), the therapist meets/works primarily with the anxious child (e.g., once a week for 16 weeks) and meets with the parents on two occasions (i.e., to address issues regarding the parent's response to the child's anxiety and to inform parents of upcoming features of the treatment). Meeting with the child individually provides an opportunity for the child to trust and build a relationship with the therapist. The trusting relationship may help the child to be more willing to participate in the challenging practice and exposure parts of the program. Without trust, a hesitant child may refuse to approach anxiety-provoking situations. An important component of the program is building rapport with the child. The therapist spends time to get

to know the likes and dislikes of the child and uses some time at the end of more structured parts of the sessions to play a game or activity chosen by the child. Does working
with the child in the sessions (not including parents) facilitate the child's gaining autonomy from parents? There are data showing a relationship between anxiety and overinvolved parenting (Hudson & Rapee, 2001; Siqueland, Kendall, & Steinberg, 1996), and
it may be that not involving parents in each session gives the child the needed opportunity to develop skills independently of his or her parents. It may also be the case that direct
involvement of parents in the child's sessions provides an opportunity to directly address
parenting behavior that may be maintaining the child's anxiety. Whether or not the child
or the child and parents are best seen in sessions may be differentially related to the
child's diagnosis: Younger separation-anxious youth may benefit more from including
parents, whereas socially anxious teens may benefit more from private, parents-not-
included sessions. We are currently evaluating the potential differential effects of child
and family versions of the treatment.

   Although the treatment manual offers a structured session-by-session approach, an
important emphasis within the manual-based treatment is therapist flexibility (Hudson et
al., 2001; Kendall, 2001; Kendall, Chu, Gifford, Hayes, & Nauta, 1998). The therapist,
being mindful of the goals of each session and features of the child, adapts the protocol
to the individual needs of the child, tailoring the program to an optimal "fit." Although
the manual provides solid guidelines from which to work, the therapist is nevertheless required to be flexible and creative in applying the guiding manual as treatment (see
Kendall et al., 1998).

CHARACTERISTICS OF THE TREATMENT PROGRAM

The following discussion highlights features of the Coping Cat program, our integrated
cognitive-behavioral treatment for youth with anxiety disorders. The typical program
consists of 16–18 individual sessions and integrates the demonstrated efficiencies of the
behavioral approach (e.g., exposure, relaxation, and role plays) with an added emphasis
on the social-cognitive information-processing factors associated with each individual's
anxiety. The overall objective is for the client to recognize signs of unwanted anxious
arousal and to let these signs serve as cues for the use of the strategies the child has
learned. In this progressive skill-building approach, identifying the cognitive processes
associated with excessive anxious arousal, training in cognitive strategies for anxiety
management, and behavioral relaxation and performance-based practice opportunities
are sequenced within the treatment manual and within the child client's *Coping Cat
Workbook* (see the order form on the web page at *www.childanxiety.org*). The treatment program places the greatest emphasis on the following general strategies:

   • Coping modeling
   • Identification and modification of anxious self-talk
   • Exposure to anxiety-provoking situations
   • Role-play activities
   • Contingent rewards for effort
   • Homework assignments (STIC tasks)
   • Affective education
   • Awareness of bodily reactions and cognitive activities when anxious
   • Relaxation procedures

- Graduated sequence of training tasks and assignments
- Application and practice of newly acquired skills in increasingly anxiety-provoking situations
- Design and completion of a "child-developed" commercial

TABLE 5.1. An Overview of the Sequence and Content of the Sessions of the Coping Cat (and C.A.T. Project) for Anxiety in Youth

Session	Purpose of session
1	Build rapport: provide orientation and overview of the program; encourage the child's participation and verbalizations during sessions; introduce STIC tasks and rewards; play a "Personal Facts" game; have some *fun*!
2	Talk about treatment goals; identify different feelings and somatic responses to anxiety; normalize fear/anxiety; develop hierarchy of anxiety-provoking situations; play "Feelings Charades"; create a "Feelings Dictionary."
3	Review distinguishing anxious feelings from other feelings; learn more about somatic responses to anxiety; identify individual somatic responses to anxiety.
4 (Parent session)	Provide information about treatment to the parent(s); give parents opportunity to discuss concerns; learn more about the situations in which the child becomes anxious; provide ways in which parents may be involved.
5	Introduce relaxation training; review recognition of somatic cues; make and decorate a relaxation tape; let child show skills to a parent.
6	Review relaxation training; help child recognize anxious self-talk; help child generate less anxiety-provoking self-talk; use cartoons to identify self talk.
7	Review anxious self-talk and reinforce changing anxious self-talk into coping self-talk; introduce cognitive strategies to manage anxiety; review relaxation training.
8	Introduce self-evaluation and reward; review skills by introducing the FEAR plan; make a FEAR plan poster and a wallet-size card with the FEAR acronym.
9 (Parent session)	Explain second half of treatment; acknowledge that this portion of treatment will provoke greater anxiety; encourage parents to discuss concerns with the therapist.
10	Practice the four-step coping (FEAR) plan under low-anxiety-provoking conditions, both imaginal and *in vivo* (out-of-office).
11	Continue practicing skills for coping with anxiety in low-level imaginal and *in vivo* situations.
12	Practice skills for coping with anxiety in imaginal and *in vivo* scenarios that provoke moderate anxiety.
13	Practice skills for coping with anxiety in *in vivo* situations that produce moderate levels of anxiety.
14	Practice skills for coping with anxiety in imaginal and *in vivo* situations that produce high anxiety; begin planning "commercial."
15	Practice skills for coping with anxiety in real challenging situations that produce high levels of anxiety; continue planning the "commercial."
16	Continue practicing coping with anxiety in *in vivo* situations that produce high levels of anxiety; review and summarize the program; make plans with parents to help the child maintain and generalize newly acquired skills; bring closure to the therapeutic relationship; tape the "commercial"; award the certificate.

The entire treatment is divided into two segments. The first eight sessions focus on skills training, whereas the second eight sessions focus on skills practice. For a summary of the sequence and content of specific sessions, see Table 5.1. Throughout, the therapist introduces concepts in order from basic to more difficult, gradually building the child's skills. This sequencing is perhaps most easily seen in the second half of treatment where the clinician and child collaborate to develop and refine a hierarchy of exposure tasks. The exposure tasks provide the child with increasingly challenging opportunities to demonstrate and practice his or her skills in real-life situations, thereby increasing the child's sense of competence. With multiple opportunities for rehearsal and practice built into the treatment, the child gains a sense of self-reliance and eventually decreases his or her dependence on others for reassurance. The focus on cognitive processing guides the child to internalize concepts and generalize his or her skills to settings outside those directly addressed during treatment. Increasing competence is attributed to the child, with the help of the therapist, who serves as a collaborative and supportive coach.

Throughout treatment, the therapist serves as a coping model as new skills and concepts are introduced. Before asking the child to do or try something, the therapist goes first. The therapist demonstrates not only each new skill for the child but also the obstacles that might be experienced and strategies that may be used to overcome these obstacles. The therapist then invites the child to participate in role playing, perhaps role playing the situation first with the child tagging along to make role-plays less intimidating. Eventually, the child does role-play scenes, practicing the newly acquired skills. Role-plays are varied according to the child's skill level and understanding of concepts (e.g., it is often unnecessary for a therapist to model the role-play first when working with an adolescent). The therapist derives role-plays from the child's fear hierarchy or from other events that are known to provoke anxiety. During each session and throughout the treatment, the level of anxiety is gradually increased, beginning with nonstressful situations and progressing to anxious situations. The mantra—"practice in private, perform in public"—guides the therapist's creation of role-plays and selection of exposure situations.

The first half of treatment (educational phase) introduces several basic concepts to the child, concepts that are later integrated into a "plan." The concepts/skills begin with an awareness of bodily reactions and feelings in general to feelings and recognition of physical symptoms that are specific to anxiety. The child comes to recognize physical reactions as a cue to the presence of anxiety. Each child also learns to recognize and focus on "self-talk"—what the child thinks and says to him- or herself when anxious. This self-talk concerns both the child's expectations and fears about what might happen and the role the child sees for him- or herself in the situation. Related to this situation, the child learns problem-solving skills as a way to generate actions that need to be taken, including the modification of anxious self-talk into coping self-talk and the tactic of trying out different ideas as a way to cope more effectively with anxiety. The child is given experience with self-evaluation and reward. As described in the next section of this chapter, these parts combine to make the FEAR plan.

To facilitate the child's involvement in (ownership of) the program, to provide some fun activities, and to ensure effective communication and learning of the various concepts, chapters in the *Coping Cat Workbook* parallel the treatment sessions provided by the therapist. The child and therapist work with the session content and homework assignments (STIC tasks)—the therapist privately guided by the manual, the child and therapist using the workbook in sessions.

The First Half: Building the FEAR Plan

The four concepts taught in the program are summarized by the acronym, FEAR: a useful mnemonic to help children remember the steps to deploy when anxious. FEAR stands for the following:

F—Feeling frightened? (awareness of physical symptoms of anxiety)
E—Expecting bad things to happen? (recognition of anxious self-talk)
A—Attitudes and Actions that will help (behavior and coping self-talk to use when anxious)
R—Results and rewards (self-evaluation and administration of self-reward for effort)

For fun, and to increase learning, the child makes a poster (and/or wallet-size card) summarizing the FEAR plan.

Feeling Frightened?

As children learn the FEAR plan, they also learn to use several strategies to cope with their anxiety. Are you "Feeling frightened?" An awareness of physical symptoms related to anxiety cues the child to do something to address the arousal. For instance, taking a deep breath or using muscle relaxation techniques. Relaxation training helps the child recognize that he or she does have control over his or her physical reactions. In typical fashion for relaxation training, the body's major muscle groups are sequentially relaxed through tension-releasing exercises designed to inform the child of states of tension and to use perceived muscle tension as a cue to initiate relaxation procedures. The particular muscle groups and somatic sensations that accompany anxiety are specific to each child, so greater awareness of the child's unique responses permit targeting specific muscle groups when anxious. Pictures in the workbook, with guidance from the therapist, assist the child in learning about symptoms of "feeling frightened."

Relaxation techniques are practiced via coping modeling and role-plays. The therapist describes anxiety-provoking scenarios and models recognition of anxious feelings and accompanying tension and somatic responses. The therapist demonstrates coping by taking deep breaths and relaxing specific muscle groups, describing what is being done step by step. The child tags along with the therapist during a similar sequence. Once the child has learned some relaxation skills, parents are invited into the session and the child teaches the parents.

Expecting Bad Things to Happen?

E stands for Expecting bad things to happen. Cognitive strategies identify and challenge the child's faulty expectations. The child learns to identify and then "test out" and eventually reduce negative expectations. To modify maladaptive expectations (self-talk), the therapist helps to identify unfairly negative self-statements for the child. Together, the child and therapist try out new ways of viewing situations, using different expectations and coping self-talk as a framework. Anxiety-producing misinterpretations of events and situations are questioned and tested out, with strategies for coping being used to replace them.

Children are not known for their willingness to tell adults what they are thinking. Any experienced therapist will confirm that when a child is asked, "What are you thinking," the likely answer is "Nothing" or "I dunno." With content in the *Coping Cat Workbook*, the therapist introduces the idea of self-talk using cartoons with empty thought bubbles. The therapist describes nonstressful situations and asks the child to provide examples of thoughts that might accompany the events. The child is then asked to develop different sets of possible thoughts for more ambiguous situations. The concept of self-talk is expanded to anxiety-provoking situations, beginning with low anxiety-provoking situations and progressing to higher degrees of anxiety. The child and therapist fill in the possible thoughts for the different cartoon situations before the child is asked about his own thoughts and before the thoughts are targeted for change.

Modeling and role-play are used to help the child practice the skill of identifying and challenging negative self-talk (unfounded and unwanted expectations). Accurate assessment and understanding of the child's characteristic dysfunctional thoughts are crucial to effective building of a coping template. It is worth noting that the goal is not to completely eradicate perceptions of stress. Rather, the goal is to teach the child to recognize and change unfounded perceptions of stress and to use realistic perceptions of stress as cues to initiate coping strategies. The emphasis is not on teaching positive self-talk but on "checking out" and reducing negative self-talk.

Attitudes and *Actions* That Might Help

The third step in the FEAR plan, Attitudes and Actions that might help, is taught as problem solving. The goal is to develop the child's confidence in his or her ability to meet daily challenges. Problem solving begins with the therapist helping the child to understand that problems are a part of everyday life and encouraging the child not to rely on initial reactions that might be maladaptive. The child is asked to reconsider a problem in clearly defined problem ways and with clearly defined goals. Next, the child (and therapist) generates alternative solutions for the problem. These ideas may not all be the best, but judgment is withheld until the next step, when the dialogue turns to an evaluation of each proposed solution and a selection of the one (best one) to put into effect. The child and therapist can then anticipate several related aspects of the chosen solution.

The therapist introduces problem solving to the child by suggesting that when anxious or worried, it will be easier to manage anxiety if there are steps to follow. After reviewing the topic of an awareness of bodily cues and anxious self-talk, the therapist points out that it might be helpful to take some action that will help change the situation or the reaction to it. The therapist and child discuss the suggested alternatives, determine which may be the most feasible alternative, and make a plan to put the solution into action. Throughout, the therapist models problem solving and asks the child to tag along. Skills are practiced in session under conditions involving gradually increasing degrees of anxiety and the therapist has the child try out and record (in the workbook) problem solving in situations outside session.

Results and *Rewards*

The last step of the FEAR plan, Results and Rewards, is based on self-monitoring and contingent reinforcement. Approach behavior is strengthened through appropriate reward and reinforcement. To reduce anxious behavior, shaping and positive reinforcement are frequently used. Some children diagnosed with anxiety disorders have self-doubting thoughts and low self-confidence. Other anxious children hold themselves to exceptionally high standards of achievement and are unforgiving if they fail to meet these standards. The therapist addresses these maladaptive expectations by rewarding the child for minor achievements and for partial successes, as well as for all forward-moving effort. Perfection is not an option and is never expected.

For young children, the therapist may introduce the concept of self-rating and reward by describing a reward as something that is given when someone is pleased with work that was done. For the older child, the therapist and child may discuss parental evaluation and rewards and gradually introduce the idea of self-rating by describing how a child can decide whether he or she is satisfied with his or her own work. Once the child understands self-monitoring/self-rating, the therapist provides opportunities for the child to practice making self-ratings and rewarding him- or herself for effort. The therapist uses coping modeling and role-play techniques to demonstrate self-rating and self-reward.

The Second Half: Exposure and Practice

The second segment of the program is largely devoted to the application and practice of the newly acquired FEAR plan within exposure to increasingly anxiety-provoking situations. The main strategy used is exposure, both imaginal and *in vivo*. Exposure tasks involve placing the child in situations that are fear-evoking, having the child experience distress, and having the child become accustomed to the situation and practicing using coping strategies. The program follows a gradual exposure model, in which the child moves up a hierarchy of anxiety-provoking situations, as determined by the child's anxiety level. The child experiences anxiety during exposure tasks, but it is important that the child's anxiety level not be so high as to result in the child's perception of the need for even greater avoidance. For all exposure tasks, the therapist collaborates with the child to make sure that the child understands the situation, ways to handle the situation, and the intended goal of the experience.

The therapist employs the following strategies when guiding the training and practice of the new skills. The process begins with an imaginal, in-office exposure to a non-stressful situation. Situations presented to each child are individually designed based on the child's particular fears and worries (as assessed during the initial evaluation, the ongoing sessions, and the collaborative development of the hierarchy). Future sessions also involve imaginal, in-office exposure, but the situations are designed to produce low levels of anxiety and are followed by actual, *in vivo* experiences (out-of-office) in low-stress situations. Subsequent sessions involve exposure to situations that cause gradually increasing levels of stress in the child, again first in imaginal settings and, once these are mastered, then in *in vivo* situations. For example, a child may initially have to ask a secretary for a key to a room, whereas a later task may require that the child purchase a chosen snack from a streetside food vendor. Exposure tasks need not be of long duration and several can be arranged for one session; it should be kept in mind that the clients are children and what is an exposure task for them may not be seen as distressing to adults. Exposure tasks are eventually designed to be in situations that are even more stressful for the child—it is an impressive event for a child who was once avoidant of speaking to peers to meet a peer and have a conversation. Typically the child may express surprise that the interaction went so well and be boosted to try future peer interactions.

Part of the practice segment of the program includes giving the child the chance to practice telling others about how to manage anxiety. While nearing the completion of the program, the child creates and produces a "commercial" summarizing his or her experiences. The child, with the therapist's help, puts together a product—a video, a booklet, or an audiotape that help can inform other children about how to manage anxiety. The production of a "commercial" gives the child a chance to be the expert, gives the therapist a chance to see what the child has learned, and provides an opportunity for the child and therapist to share what has been accomplished with others. In addition, making a tape gives the child clear evidence of our support, provides tangible documentation of success, offers a final reward at the end of the program, and helps to bolster treatment-produced gains.

A Role for Parents

Parental involvement in our program is integral to helping the child to overcome clinically significant anxiety. Although the program focuses on helping the individual child to learn to think and behave differently, parents participate in a supportive role—they are consultants and collaborators, not co-clients. Accordingly, the child-focused treatment program does not provide family therapy but does involve parents as consultants. Parents are important in determining the accurate child diagnoses and in ensuring the child's acceptance and participation in the program. Therapists also meet with the parents during sessions 4 and 9 to collaborate with them on treatment plans and to maintain their cooperation and support. Parents are given opportunities to discuss their concerns about their child and to provide further information that might be helpful. It is not uncommon for unstructured conversations to include comments about the parents' impressions of the child's anxiety and the therapist's offering specific ways that parents might help in the achieving of positive outcomes.

Given the role parents play in their child's treatment, even when not in a family-oriented treatment, therapists should be aware of the particular problems that families of anxious children may experience. These problems may include increased anxiety among family members, the presence of other types of psychopathlogy, and particular problems in parenting styles such as overprotectiveness, restriction, intolerance for negative emotions, and guilt about the child's problems. Given that parents play a role in the success of child-focused treatment and that there is a hypothesized role for parents in the development and/or maintenance of childhood anxiety, we have developed a family Coping Cat program. The same strategies are employed, but the sessions include parental participation. A manual describing this program is available (Howard, Chu, Krain, Marrs-Garcia, & Kendall, 2000).

Flexibility within Fidelity

Critics of manual-based treatment offer potentially reasonable objections, many of which rest on the assumption that manuals involve a prearranged and rigid approach to treatment. Critics often assume that manuals are designed to implement specific procedures using a steadfast, linear approach. Given this level of assumed rigidity, critics complain that manual-based treatment precludes any individuality of the therapist. Clearly, such assumptions are unwarranted and there is a rational middle ground between the complete freedom of an unstructured treatment and the rigid adherence to a manual. This middle ground consists of using the manual as a guide and with integrity yet allowing it to become vibrant and alive when put into practice. Practitioners are best prepared to achieve flexible applications of manual-based treatments when there is an understanding of the treatment on multiple levels, including the model on which the treatment is based and the elements involved in the process of treatment.

The Coping Cat program can be used with both necessary fidelity and desired flexibility. The model behind the program drives the treatment, not specific sentences or exact applications of techniques. As stated earlier, the treatment model includes cognitive change and behavioral exposure tasks. However, affective and educational factors affect this relationship. Moreover, the child's involvement in treatment, a variable that is likely influenced by a lively, flexible manual and an engaging therapist, influences both the exposure and the cognitive and educational components. Our model for understanding the impact of the Coping Cat program assigns a key role to child involvement, a factor that is facilitated by a living, breathing manual. For example, in each session the therapist has the freedom to adapt the treatment goals to the needs/interests of the child. There are many opportunities for such flexibility within fidelity. A child may modify the acronym FEAR to his or her own liking. One child completing the program transformed the FEAR plan into a military-inspired "Scouting, Intelligence, Battle, and Recon" plan. Flexibility can also include adjustments of the sessions to real-world events, while keeping to role-plays and exposure tasks, cognitive processing of the events, and problem-solving discussions. For example, the therapist might have to adjust a planned session to accommodate current events in the child's life, such as an upcoming, anxiety-provoking birthday party or a recent argument with a parent. The emphasis is on adapting and tailoring the treatment (not changing the treatment) to the individual needs of the child.

EVIDENCE FOR THE EFFECTS OF TREATMENT

In this section, we summarize the results of outcome research using applications of the Coping Cat program with anxious children. Drawing on the foundations provided by the American Psychological Association (APA) Task Force on Psychological Intervention Guidelines, Chambless and Hollon (1998) proposed a scheme for determining when a psychological treatment for a specific problem or disorder may be considered to be established in efficacy or to be possibly efficacious. According to their system, a treatment may be considered efficacious (i.e., established) or possibly efficacious (i.e., promising but in need of replication) if it has been shown to be more effective than no treatment, a placebo, or an alternate treatment across multiple trials conducted by different investigative teams. Treatments that meet these criteria, except for replication or independent replication, are designated as probably efficacious. According to two recent reviews, the Coping Cat program of cognitive-behavioral therapy (CBT) for childhood anxiety is probably efficacious (Kazdin & Weisz, 1998; Ollendick & King, 2000). It can be argued that CBT for child anxiety warrants designation as an established efficacious treatment, but this classification depends in part on whether the Coping Cat program and the Australian adaptation (Coping Koala) are judged to constitute the same treatment as a conceptual replication.

Randomized Clinical Trials

Building on a promising initial evaluation of the Coping Cat program using a multiple baseline design (Kane & Kendall, 1989), several randomized clinical trials have been conducted by at least two different research teams (Barrett, Dadds, & Rapee, 1996; Kendall, 1994; Kendall et al., 1997). The first published randomized clinical trial (Kendall, 1994) evaluating the Coping Cat program employed 47 children, ages 9–13 years, who were referred from multiple community sources. Participants received a primary anxiety disorder diagnosis of SAD, overanxious disorder (OAD), or avoidant disorder (AD)—Kendall and Warman (1996) found that children meeting DSM-III criteria for OAD/AD were not dissimilar to children diagnosed by DSM-IV criteria as GAD/SoP. The results indicated that, compared to wait-list control children, children who received the treatment evidenced a significant positive change from pre- to posttreatment on self-report, parent report, and behavioral observation measures. The central measure of outcome was the independent diagnostic evaluation: Both children's and parents' diagnostic interview data indicated that 64% of the treated children no longer met diagnostic criteria for their primary diagnosis at posttreatment, whereas only 5% of the wait-list control children no longer met diagnostic criteria at this time. Treatment-produced gains were maintained at 1-year follow-up. In a longer follow-up study, Kendall and Southam-Gerow (1996) reassessed 36 of the 47 children treated in the 1994 clinical trial. The length of time from completion of the treatment program to long-term assessment ranged from 2 to 5 years, with an average of 3.35 years. On both self-report and parent-report measures, and in terms of diagnostic status, treatment-produced gains were maintained at 3.35-year follow-up.

A second randomized clinical trial of the treatment (Kendall et al., 1997) involved 94 children, ages 9–13 years. Using the Anxiety Disorders Interview Schedule—Child/Parent (ADIS C/P; Silverman & Albano, 1997), participants received a primary diagnosis of one of the target anxiety disorders. The outcomes of the study supported the efficacy of the treatment for childhood anxiety, with 50% of treated cases being free from the primary anxiety disorder at posttreatment. For those cases in which the primary anxiety diagnosis remained at posttreatment, analyses showed significant reductions on severity scores. Children who received the Coping Cat treatment demonstrated significant positive change on self-report, parent report, and some behavioral observation measures. Clinically significant gains were evident in the returning of the average scores of the treated children to within the normative range for scores on these measures. Also, the gains were maintained at a 1-year follow-up. It is also worth noting that a 7.4-year follow-up of 90% of the cases treated in the 1997 study revealed evidence of the long-term maintenance of gains—and some positive impact on the sequelae of anxiety, such as on indicators of substance abuse (Kendall, Safford, Flannery-Schroeder, & Webb, 2003).

Given the criteria for establishing treatment efficacy, and given the overall worthiness of replications in general, the project conducted in Australia and reported by Barrett et al. (1996) merits mention. These authors evaluated the efficacy of an Australian adaptation of the Coping Cat program, the Coping Koala, against a program of combined CBT plus family anxiety management training. Among the reported results, it was found that 72% of children (ages 7–14) with primary diagnoses of SAD, OAD, or SoP no longer met diagnostic criteria a year after child-focused treatment. An average of 6 years after treatment, 52 of the 79 original clients (ages 14–21) were reassessed with diagnostic interviews, clinician ratings, and self- and parent report measures (Barrett, Duffy, Dadds, & Rapee, 2001). Analyses of diagnostic status revealed that 86% of participants no longer met criteria for an anxiety disorder.

To examine the efficacy of the Coping Cat program in group format, Flannery-Schroeder and Kendall (2000) compared group treatment, individual treatment, and a wait-list control condition providing services for 37 children ages 8–14 years. All the children were diagnosed with primary anxiety disorders, as assessed by the ADIS C/P. When diagnostic status was considered at posttreatment, significantly more of the treated youth (73% individual, 50% group) than the wait-list youth (8%) were free of the primary anxiety disorder diagnosis they had received at pretreatment. Other measures supported the superiority of the treatment conditions over the wait-list, but only children receiving individual treatment showed significant improvements on self-report measures of anxious distress. The three conditions did not differ with regard to measures of social functioning. At a 3-month follow-up assessment, treatment gains were maintained.

Variables Affecting Treatment Outcome

In addition to research evaluating the effectiveness of the Coping Cat program for childhood anxiety, studies have examined potential factors that might moderate treatment outcome. Researchers have considered potential moderating factors such as gender, ethnicity, comorbidity, symptom severity, and cognition. Few of these factors have been found to significantly predict treatment outcome. Treadwell, Flannery-Schroeder, and Kendall (1995) examined gender and ethnic differences in the levels of anxious symptomatology reported by 178 children (ages 9–13) who sought treatment at the CAADC. This study also investigated differences in treatment sensitivity by gender and ethnicity in 81 children diagnosed with a childhood anxiety disorder. No differences in the prevalence or intensity of fears as a function of gender or ethnicity were found among child, parent, teacher, and diagnostic ratings of the anxious youth. Moreover, reductions in anxious symptomatology and the absence of anxiety disorder diagnoses due to treatment were comparable across gender and ethnicity.

Kendall et al. (2001) examined comorbidity as a potential moderator of treatment outcome for 173 children (ages 9–13) who had been treated for a DSM-III-R/DSM-IV primary anxiety disorder diagnosis at the CAADC. The incidence of comorbidity among cases treated and evaluated at CAADC was high: 79% of the 173 participants received at least one comorbid diagnosis at pretreatment. At posttreatment, comorbid and noncomorbid cases were compared: 68% of noncomorbid children were free of their primary diagnosis, as compared with 71% of the comorbid children. Both groups showed significant reductions in pretreatment diagnosis and on parent and child self-report measures. These results suggest that treatment was equally effective with comorbid and noncomorbid anxious children.

Southam-Gerow, Kendall, and Weersing (2001) investigated the correlates of good versus poor treatment response in 135 children and adolescents (ages 7–15) who had received CBT for a primary anxiety disorder. Although, as reported in earlier publications, participants had generally improved, the results of analyses of the combined data set indicated a few factors that were correlated with a less favorable treatment response. These factors included higher levels of maternal- and teacher-reported child-internalizing psychopathology reported at pretreatment, higher levels of maternal self-reported depressive symptoms, and older child age. However, factors such as ethnicity, gender, family income, family composition (i.e., dual- vs. single-parent household), child-reported symptomatology, and maternal-reported level of child externalizing problems did not moderate treatment response.

To examine a mediator of treatment response, Treadwell and Kendall (1996) investigated the relationship between childhood anxiety disorders, the valence and content of self-statements (positive or negative), and the impact of treatment on children's internal dialogues. Participants were 151 children (ages 8–13); 71 had anxiety disorders and 80 were control participants. Positive and negative self-statements and a states-of-mind (SOM) ratio were examined. The SOM model proposes five categories of self-talk, including positive dialogue (considered optimal for psychological adaptation), negative dialogue (associated with moderate anxiety or depression), internal dialogues of conflict (associated with self-doubt, worry, and mild anxiety or depression), positive monologue (positive self-statements possibly indicating mania, grandiosity, and impulsiveness), and negative monologue (a decreased rate of positive self-statements associated with severe depression or acute stages of panic). Results indicated that the negative self-statements and SOM ratio (but not positive self-statements) of children with anxiety disorders significantly predicted anxiety. Results also indicated that negative (but not positive cognition) and SOM ratio predicted improvement in anxiety after treatment and mediated treatment gains. The treatment-produced gains were mediated by reductions in the children's negative self-talk; the power of nonnegative thinking!

Although few variables differentiate good treatment responders from less favorable treatment responders, one study did identify differences between treatment completers and treatment noncompleters. Kendall and Sugarman (1997) examined the differences between treatment completers ($n = 146$) and terminators ($n = 44$, including both refusers and dropouts). They found that treatment terminators were more likely to live in a single-parent household, be ethnic minorities, and report less anxious symptomatology than treatment completers. Follow-up interviews indicated that these factors were influential in the terminators' decisions to discontinue treatment. Socioeconomic status and level of parental education, however, were not predictors of early treatment termination.

Transporting Treatment from the Research Clinic to the Practice Clinic

Evidence from research clinic outcomes supports the efficacy of the treatment program for childhood anxiety. A question remains—will the effectiveness will be comparable in non-research-oriented clinic settings? At present, there is a noted absence of data. The dearth of data on the "transportability" of research-clinic treatments to service clinic settings may be explained by the difficulties inherent in this process—difficulties that fall into research, therapist/clinic, and client categories (Kendall & Southam-Gerow, 1995).

Does the conduct of research affect the transportability of treatment? To conduct clinical trials, researchers seek relatively homogeneous samples and set certain inclusion/exclusionary criteria. At CAADC, the main inclusion criterion is the presence of a principal anxiety disorder diagnosis, and exclusionary criteria are few (current psychoactive medication use for anxiety or depression, psychosis, IQ below 80). Does this create a highly select sample of cases? One set of comparisons (Southam-Gerow, Weisz, & Kendall, in press) indicates that whereas research clinic cases are more severe in terms of anxiety, clinical setting cases are more comorbid with externalizing problems. Currently, at CAADC, a child who meets criteria for a comorbid internalizing or externalizing diagnosis is included in the research sample. The treatment manual and other publications (e.g., Hudson et al., 2001) outline specific flexible adaptations of the manual for the case when comorbid conditions are present. For example, when treating an anxious child with attention-deficit/hyperactivity disorder, the therapist may need to make several modifications to the sessions such as shortening the length of the session or providing frequent breaks in order to maintain the child's attention. Behavior management strategies may also be useful in helping the child to remain seated and focused during his or her therapy session. The therapist may reward the child for on-task behavior or remove privileges for disruptive or impulsive behavior. A recent study (Kendall et al., 2001) found that comorbid anxiety and behavior disorders did not detrimentally influence treatment outcome.

Therapist/clinic factors, including clinic procedures, theoretical orientation, and supervision practices, may influence transportability. In research clinics, projects are often subsidized such that clients do not have to pay for treatment. The economics of therapy may have implications for outcomes: child clients may be more likely to complete treatment if cost is not a concern for their parents. If cost is an issue, clients may terminate early, making evaluations of success difficult to complete. To prevent premature termination, community-based therapists can address financial issues openly with parents in the early stages of the treatment program and discuss alternative treatment and payment options (e.g., fortnightly sessions). Current research is examining the efficacy of bibliotherapy in the treatment of childhood anxiety disorders (Rapee, Abbott, & Gaston, 2002). Therapist-assisted self-help may reduce the number of required therapy sessions, reduce cost, and potentially be a viable alternative for families where cost is an issue.

The fact that the Coping Cat treatment is manual-based helps to guide therapy and ensure that clinicians are providing the prescribed treatment. Manuals can facilitate transportability, because critical components of the treatment are specified and explained. Although manuals help in the dissemination of empirically validated treatments, they do not by themselves guarantee accurate implementation. Treatment integrity checks are conducted at research clinics, but these checks are not a priority in nonresearch settings. Moreover, focused group supervision, which is conducted weekly at the CAADC, can be a powerful force in buttressing therapist involvement and fostering positive child outcomes. Such supervision can include discussion of the flexible administration of the protocol and strategies for solving various therapeutic problems. In almost all service settings, group supervision among colleagues trained in the same disorder-specific treatment is a luxury that is not feasible. Theoretical differences among staff members may also pose an obstacle to focused supervision and thereby to transportability. Thus, it would be important for therapists in service settings to find a supervisor with adequate training in the manual or at least whose theoretical framework matches that of the treatment. Additional supervisor and therapist training may be required for this to be a workable option.

Client characteristics may have an impact on the transportability of the treatment. Clients seeking help at the CAADC may have expectations about "specialized" treatments for anxiety, as they are seeking treatment at an anxiety disorders clinic. Such expectations may enhance treatment, as clients may be more compliant. Community clinics are not typically perceived as specialty centers, so their services might be less likely to be influenced by positive expectancies. Nevertheless, therapists using the manual within community settings can promote themselves as coaches who specialize in coping skills to deal with anxiety. The aim of therapy then, is to transfer these "special" skills to the child and family. This approach may increase the positive expectancies of the family and increase their commitment and compliance with the program. Although speed bumps may influence the transporting of the Coping Cat (and C.A.T. Project) program from the research clinic to the practice setting, an accurate picture of the nature of the transportability of treatments requires specific studies of the outcomes of treatments as implemented within fidelity in service settings. Systematic study of the factors that impede or facilitate the process of transportability is needed.

DIRECTIONS FOR FUTURE RESEARCH

The development and evaluation of the treatment reported herein began in 1984. It can be said that much has been accomplished over the nearly two decades of work, but several important questions remain for the next decade of research: questions involving components analyses, comparisons to alternate treatments, examinations of the optimal role of parents, studies of the processes (and other potential mediators) of treatment response, and investigations of the role of medications in the overall treatment of anxiety disorders in youth. Each question merits discussion.

Which of the several components of the integrative intervention can be considered an active treatment component? The Coping Cat program is multifaceted, integrating educational, cognitive, affective, social, parent/family, and behavioral elements. Although it is not likely that one component will rise over all others as the sole active force in favorable gains, components analyses should help clarify where best to place one's therapeutic emphasis.

Future research would benefit from inclusion of comparisons to conditions other than wait-list. A randomized clinical trial is currently under way at the CAADC to evaluate relative outcomes among two active conditions (family CBT, child-focused CBT) and a family treatment involving education about anxiety, support for dealing with an anxious child, and therapeutic attention. Not unlike the comparison of individual to group treatment (Flannery-Schroeder & Kendall, 2000), the results of this study will provide valuable information about outcomes relative to conditions that offer more than a wait list.

In general, the literature supports the belief that including parents in treatment of child psychopathology has a beneficial effect on the outcomes. For instance, including parents in the treatment of oppositionality in youth is preferred over child-focused treatment. However, we do not yet have compelling data on the preferred role for parents in the treatment of anxiety disorders in youth. Parents of anxious youth may be too involved in their child's lives, and the preferred intervention may be to have the parent less involved (and not in sessions). With the parent out of the session, the child can develop a relationship with the therapist and begin to have favorable experiences with new ways of behaving. In contrast, it may be preferred that parents are in the sessions such that the therapist can directly address the need for greater granting of autonomy to the child, the need for more tolerance of negative emotions, and the need to permit the child to have experiences from which to learn (as opposed to avoiding experience to be safe). Not to complicate matters unnecessarily, but the role of parents may also be different for older and younger children and for children with different types of anxiety diagnoses.

Given evaluations of the role of parents in the treatment of a child with an anxiety disorder, it would be interesting and informative to examine whether treatment for the child has any beneficial (spillover) effects for the parents. Many children with anxiety disorders have parents with anxiety difficulties, and reductions in parental anxiety may come about concurrently with treatment for the child's anxiety. We are currently using structured interviews at pre- and post-treatment to assess parental psychopathology and to evaluate any changes in symptomatology that might be related to treatment.

Another interesting area for future research concerns the process of therapy and its relationship to therapeutic outcomes. Now that the intervention has been found to have promise with regard to outcomes, it would be fruitful to examine further the processes and therapeutic mechanisms that contribute to psychological change (Kazdin & Kendall, 1998). Some data suggest that reduction in negative thinking mediates positive outcomes, but what other factors are involved? Process variables within our manual-based treatment, such as the therapeutic alliance, therapist flexibility, and child involvement, are currently being examined.

For adults, medications are often a part of a combined psychological and pharmacological approach. There are some data suggesting that select medications may be useful for obsessive–compulsive disorder in children, but there are notably few studies of medications for the anxiety disorders discussed in this chapter. Currently under way, a four-condition study will compare the Coping Cat treatment (CBT), medication (Sertraline), the combination of the two, and a pill placebo. This study will combine data from six sites (Temple, Duke, Johns Hopkins, NYU/Columbia, UCLA, and the Western Psychiatric Institute and Clinic) and should be useful to inform practitioners of the potential role of medications. Also of interest, what are the effects of medications on the contribution of the exposure tasks to treatment outcomes? If exposure tasks are active ingredients and if they require that the participant child experience anxious arousal, will these psychological forces be undermined because the medicated child may not experience the anxious arousal (and thereby not have the benefits of the habituation) that is provided as part of the exposure task? On the other hand, might the medications facilitate the child's initial comfort with treatment and similarly facilitate an active and involved approach to treatment?

One cannot forgot the 25–35% of cases for whom the outcomes are not optimal. True, it seems reasonable to conclude that the treatment is reasonably effective given the reported results, but the results are not uniformly positive. Advances are likely to be found in (1) the addition of booster sessions and further contacts for those cases not reaching preferred level of improvement at the end of the time-limited treatment, (2) investigations of developmental factors (cognitive, social emotional, or physical) that may help to individually tailor treatments and improve the percentage of improved cases, and (3) getting to know more about how nonanxious youth manage their unwanted distress. Some of the processes involved in normal adjustment to anxious arousal may contribute meaningfully to the further refining of our current program.

SUMMARY AND CONCLUSIONS

Anxiety disorders in youth are a significant and prevalent form of psychological distress. Using appropriate methodologies for evaluations, cognitive-behavioral youth-focused treatment has a favorable record of success in treating disturbingly anxious 8–13-year-olds who have a high incidence of comorbid conditions. The treatment integrates an understanding of cognition, behavior, and emotional functioning within a larger social context.

The cognitive-behavioral treatment methods, including a therapist manual and a child workbook, build on a child–therapist relationship, but importantly also provide education into the physiological signs of anxiety, the normality of anxiety, the self-talk associated with anxiety, the use of relaxation to reduce anxiety, and behavioral skills to address the management of anxiety. A central component of the treatment is the hierarchical use of exposure tasks to provide real experiences with the arousal and management of anxious distress. Generally, the first half of treatment is the educational (preparation) phase, whereas the second half is the exposure (practice) phase. The main features of the educational phase are summarized with a four-step FEAR plan and the plan is implemented and practiced in the second half of the program. The CBT therapist is active and serves as a coping model who appropriately self-discloses and who arranges the challenging *in vivo* exposure tasks for the child. Roughly two-thirds of those treated, including both genders, various ethnicities, and several primary anxiety disorders, have been found to benefit meaningfully. Initial evidence suggests that older children with more severe psychopathology may be more often among those who do less well after treatment.

Additional scientific investigation is needed (1) using comparison conditions that are potentially more potent than wait lists, (2) into the forces that are a part of the process of the effective intervention, and (3) toward the improvement of the treatment for those who, to date, have not been positive treatment responders. Also, there is a need for a greater understanding of the role of developmental factors in the nature and treatment of anxiety disorders in children and adolescents.

ACKNOWLEDGMENTS

The research reported in this chapter was supported by grants from the National Institutes of Health (e.g., MH44042; MH60653, MH59087) awarded to Philip C. Kendall.

NOTES

1. Contact the publisher at (610) 896-9797 or via e-mail at *info@workbookpublishing.com,* or visit the website at *www.workbookpublishing.com*

REFERENCES

Anderson, J. C., Williams, S., McGee, R., & Silva, P. A. (1987). DSM-III disorders in preadolescent children: Prevalence in a large sample from a general population. *Archives of General Psychiatry, 44,* 69–76.

Barrett, P. M., Dadds, M. R., & Rapee, R. M. (1996). Family treatment of childhood anxiety: A controlled trial. *Journal of Consulting and Clinical Psychology, 64,* 333–342.

Barrett, P. M., Duffy, A. L., Dadds, M. R., & Rapee, R. M. (2001). Cognitive-behavioral treatment of anxiety disorders in children: Long-term (6 year) follow-up. *Journal of Consulting and Clinical Psychology, 69,* 1–7.

Chambless, D., & Hollon, S. (1998). Defining empirically supported treatments. *Journal of Consulting and Clinical Psychology, 66,* 5–17.

Fergusson, D. M., Horwood, L. J., & Lynskey, M. T. (1993). Prevalence and comorbidity of DSM-III-R diagnoses in a birth cohort of 15 year olds. *Journal of the American Academy of Child and Adolescent Psychiatry, 32,* 1127–1134.

Flannery-Schroeder, E. C., & Kendall, P. C. (2000). Group and individual cognitive-behavioral treatments for youth with anxiety disorders: A randomized clinical trial. *Cognitive Therapy and Research, 24*(3), 251–278.

Howard, B. L., Chu, B., Krain, A., Marrs-Garcia, A., & Kendall, P. C. (2000). *Cognitive-behavioral family therapy for anxious children: Therapist manual* (2nd ed.). Ardmore, PA: Workbook Publishing. Available: *www.workbookpublishing.com*

Hudson, J. L., Krain, A., & Kendall, P. C. (2001). Expanding horizons: Adapting manual-based treatments for anxious children with comorbid diagnoses. *Cognitive and Behavioral Practice, 8,* 338–346.

Hudson, J. L., & Rapee, R. M. (2001). Parent–child interactions and the anxiety disorders: An observational analysis. *Behaviour Research and Therapy, 39,* 1411–1427.

Kane, M., & Kendall, P. C. (1989). Anxiety disorders in children: A multiple-baseline evaluation of a cognitive-behavioral therapy. *Behavior Therapy, 20,* 499–508.

Kazdin, A. E., & Kendall, P. C. (1998). Current progress and future plans for developing effective treatments: Comments and perspectives. *Journal of Clinical Child Psychology, 27,* 217–226.

Kazdin, A. E., & Weisz, J. (1998). Identifying and developing empirically supported child and adolescent treatments. *Journal of Consulting and Clinical Psychology, 66,* 18–35.

Keller, M. B., Lavori, P. W., Wunder, J., Beardslee, W. R., Schwartz, G., & Roth, B. (1992). Chronic course of anxiety disorders in children and adolescents. *Journal of the American Academy of Child and Adolescent Psychiatry, 31*, 595–599.

Kendall, P. C. (1990). *Coping Cat Workbook*. Ardmore, PA: Workbook Publishing.

Kendall, P. C. (1993). Cognitive-behavioral therapies with youth: Guiding theory, current status, and emerging developments. *Journal of Consulting and Clinical Psychology, 61*, 235–247.

Kendall, P. C. (1994). Treating anxiety disorders in children: Results of a randomized clinical trial. *Journal of Consulting and Clinical Psychology, 62*, 100–110.

Kendall, P. C. (2001). Flexibility within fidelity. *Clinical Child and Adolescent Psychology Newsletter, 16*(2), 1–5.

Kendall, P. C., Brady, E., & Verduin, T. (2001). Comorbidity in childhood anxiety disorders and treatment outcome. *Journal of the American Academy of Child and Adolescent Psychiatry, 40*, 787–794.

Kendall, P. C., Choudhury, M., Hudson, J., & Webb, A. (2002a). *The C.A.T. project therapist manual*. Ardmore, PA: Workbook Publishing.

Kendall, P. C., Choudhury, M., Hudson, J., & Webb, A. (2002b). *The C.A.T. project workbook for the cognitive-behavioral treatment of anxious adolescents*. Ardmore, PA: Workbook Publishing.

Kendall, P. C., Chu, B., Gifford, A., Hayes, C., & Nauta, M. (1998). Breathing life into a manual. *Cognitive and Behavioral Practice, 5*, 177–198.

Kendall, P. C., Flannery-Schroeder, E., Panichelli-Mindel, S., Southam-Gerow, M., Henin, A., & Warman, M. (1997). Therapy for youth with anxiety disorders: A second randomized clinical trial. *Journal of Consulting and Clinical Psychology, 65*, 366–380.

Kendall, P. C., Kortlander, E., Chansky, T. E., & Brady, E. U. (1992). Comorbidity of anxiety and depression in youth: Treatment implications. *Journal of Consulting and Clinical Psychology, 60*, 869–880.

Kendall, P. C., Safford, S., Flannery-Schroeder, E., & Webb, A. (2003). *Child anxiety treatment: Maintenance of outcomes in adolescence and impact on substance use and depression at 7.4 year follow-up*. Manuscript submitted for publication, Temple University.

Kendall, P. C., & Southam-Gerow, M. (1995). Issues in the transportability of treatment: The case of anxiety disorders in youths. *Journal of Consulting and Clinical Psychology, 63*, 702–708.

Kendall, P. C., & Southam-Gerow, M. (1996). Long-term follow-up of a cognitive-behavioral therapy for anxiety-disordered youth. *Journal of Consulting and Clinical Psychology, 64*, 724–730.

Kendall, P. C., & Sugarman, A. (1997). Attrition in the treatment of childhood anxiety disorders. *Journal of Consulting and Clinical Psychology, 65*, 883–888.

Kendall, P. C., & Warman, M. (1996). Anxiety disorders in youth: Diagnostic consistency across DSM-III-R and DSM-IV. *Journal of Anxiety Disorders, 10*, 453–463.

Ollendick, T. H., & King, N. J. (2000). Empirically supported treatments for children and adolescents. In P. C. Kendall (Ed.), *Child and adolescent therapy: Cognitive-behavioral procedures* (2nd ed., pp. 386–425). New York: Guilford Press.

Rapee, R. M., Abbott, M. J., & Gaston, J. (2002, March). *Bibliotherapy in the treatment of childhood anxiety disorders*. Paper presented at the Anxiety Disorders Association of America National Conference, Austin, TX.

Silverman, W., & Albano, A. M. (1997). *The Anxiety Disorders Inverview Schedule for Children (DSM-IV)*. San Antonio: Psychological Corporation.

Siqueland, L., Kendall, P. C., & Steinberg, L. (1996). Anxiety in children: Perceived family environments and observed family interaction style. *Journal of Clinical Child Psychology, 25*, 225–237.

Southam-Gerow, M. A., Kendall, P. C., & Weersing, V. R. (2001). Examining outcome variability: Correlates of treatment response in a child and adolescent anxiety clinic. *Journal of Clinical Child Psychology, 30*, 422–436.

Southam-Gerow, M. A., Weisz, J., & Kendall, P. C. (in press). Anxiety-disordered youth in research and service clinics: Examining client differences and similarities. *Journal of Clinical Child and Adolescent Psychology.*

Strauss, C., Lease, C., Last, C., & Francis, G. (1988). Overanxious disorder: An examination of developmental differences. *Journal of Abnormal Child Psychology, 11,* 433–443.

Treadwell, K. R. H., Flannery-Schroeder, E. C., & Kendall, P. C. (1995). Ethnicity and gender in relation to adaptive functioning, diagnostic status, and treatment outcome in children from an anxiety clinic. *Journal of Anxiety Disorders, 9,* 373–384.

Treadwell, K. R. H., & Kendall, P. C. (1996). Self-talk in youth with anxiety disorders: States of mind, content specificity, and treatment outcome. *Journal of Consulting and Clinical Psychology, 64,* 941–950.

6

Parental Involvement in the Treatment of Anxious Children

PAULA M. BARRETT AND ALISON L. SHORTT

OVERVIEW

Anxiety disorders in children and adolescents (hereafter the term "children" includes adolescents) are characterized by anxiety that is excessive in frequency, intensity, duration, or their combination. To be considered clinically significant, the anxiety must interfere with the child's functioning in family, school, or peer settings or cause the child distress. Persistent anxiety is broadly recognized to have a negative impact on interpersonal relationships, social competence, peer relations, and school adjustment (Barrett, 1999). Estimated prevalence rates for childhood anxiety disorders vary but are typically found to range between 8 and 12% (Anderson, Williams, McGee, & Silva, 1987; Costello & Angold, 1995). Contemporary findings indicate the prevalence of adolescent anxiety in Australia to be as high as 15% (Boyd, Kostanski, Gullone, Ollendick, & Shek, 2000).

In the majority of cases, it is the parent or caregiver who makes the decision to seek treatment; children rarely refer themselves for treatment. Parents seeking treatment for their child want an intervention that is effective, time-limited, and acceptable. Parents seek treatment that will improve their child's functioning and minimize the disruption to family life that arises as a result of the child's anxiety. This disruption may take the form of a child making persistent requests for reassurance. In addition, anxious children frequently enlist their parents' help in avoiding difficult situations such as attending social events, going to camp, or sleeping in a room by themselves. Many parents find it difficult to know how to parent their anxious child in such situations. Consequently, parents seeking treatment for their child's anxiety frequently request guidance about what they can do to help their child to overcome his or her worries or fears.

In working with children we recognize that children function in a context that influences their behavior (Bronfenbrenner, 1979; Lerner, 1991). That context includes children's relationships with their parents, siblings, other family members, peers, and other systems such as their school and neighborhood community. Children's dependence on their parents or caregivers, and evidence that parental influences are involved in children's anxiety, raise questions about the appropriate focus of treatment (Kazdin, 2000). Should treatment focus on a child directly, on the parents, or on a combination of the two? To answer this question, clinicians need to gather information about whether the forces that promote or sustain the child's anxiety could be within the family context, and whether changing contextual influences could be a valuable way to alter child functioning.

The decision whether treatment should involve parents, and if so what role parents should play, is based on knowledge of the child's anxiety as well as parental and family factors that may moderate treatment outcome. To this end, during the assessment, information should be gathered from the child and from significant people in the child's life (e.g., mothers, fathers, and teachers). Multiple instruments, including interviews, self-reports, and measures of anxiety and avoidance behavior in day-to-day life (e.g., monitoring and behavioral avoidance tests), can be used. Information about the child and the parents' motivation for treatment, the patterns of reinforcement relating to avoidance behaviors, and the extent to which the child is seeking and receiving reassurance may be obtained. Children may be observed interacting with their parents, and parents and children may be asked to complete self-report measures of perceived parenting behaviors. Information about family history of anxiety, mood, or other disorders should also be obtained, as it will help to guide the choice of treatment strategy. In some cases child-only treatment may be sufficient; in others, parent involvement in treatment may seem most likely to optimize treatment effectiveness. The empirical literature on parent involvement in child anxiety treatment is sparse; however, some evidence is emerging which indicates that a cognitive-behavioral treatment targeting the child and parents may be the treatment of choice for some anxious children.

This chapter focuses on family-based treatment for anxiety disorders in children, with a central focus on treatment outcome research conducted by our research team. This research has pursued answers to questions arising from our clinical work—questions about the role and involvement of parents in the treatment of anxious children. The majority of this chapter focuses on describing a family-based cognitive-behavioral treatment for anxious children and their parents called FRIENDS (Barrett, Lowry-Webster, & Turner, 2000a, 2000b, 2000c, 2000d, 2000e, 2000f). The program name, "FRIENDS," is an acronym for the strategies taught:

F—Feeling worried?
R—Relax and feel good.
I—Inner thoughts.
E—Explore plans.
N—Nice work so reward yourself.
D—Don't forget to practice.
S—Stay calm, you know how to cope now.

The idea of using an acronym to help children remember the strategies taught came from the Coping Cat program, which uses the FEAR acronym (Kendall, 1990; see Chapter 5, this volume). To this end, the model underlying this treatment program and research examining its efficacy are discussed in turn.

Conceptual Model Underlying Treatment

Individual cognitive-behavioral treatment (ICBT) focuses on dysfunctional cognitions and how these affect the child's subsequent emotions and behavior (Kendall et al., 1992, 1997). Cognitive distortions are considered to play a central role in childhood anxiety because they lead to misperceptions of the child's coping abilities, environmental threats, or both. Treatment aims to help children to develop new skills, facilitate new experiences for children to test dysfunctional as well as adaptive beliefs, and assist children in processing new experiences. Modeling and direct reinforcement are used to facilitate the child's learning of new approach behaviors and cognitive strategies believed to address processes such as information processing style, attributions, and self-talk (Kazdin, 2000). The basic techniques used in ICBT are *in vivo* exposure, relaxation training, role playing, modeling, and contingency management.

Family-based cognitive-behavioral treatment (FCBT) shares a similar rationale to ICBT. Cognitive distortions are seen as central to the maintenance of anxiety symptoms; however, the family is seen as the optimal environment for effecting change in the child's dysfunctional cognition. Parents are in a unique position to facilitate new experiences in which children can test dysfunctional beliefs, and parents living with the child can assist the processing of new experiences on a daily basis. Also, parents are influential role models in children's lives—a parent modeling adaptive beliefs and cognitive processing of day-to-day events and rewarding a child for approaching situations in an optimistic manner can be especially helpful for anxiety reduction. In summary, treatment effectiveness is seen as maximized by treating children directly, and by involving parents in complementary and ancillary roles.

CHARACTERISTICS OF THE TREATMENT PROGRAM

The FRIENDS Program

The child component of the FRIENDS program (Barrett et al., 2000a, 2000b, 2000c, 2000d, 2000e, 2000f) originated with the development of the *Coping Koala Group Workbook* (Barrett, 1995), an Australian adaptation of Kendall's *Coping Cat Workbook* (Kendall, 1990). The FRIENDS program encourages children to (1) think of *their body as their friend* because it tells them when they are feeling worried or nervous by giving them clues; (2) *be their own friend*, and reward themselves when they try hard; (3) *make friends*, so that they can build their social support networks; and finally (4) *talk to their friends* when they are in difficult or worrying situations.

The FRIENDS program targets parents as well as anxious children. The case for involving parents in the treatment of anxious children is supported by research findings implicating parental factors in the genesis and maintenance of anxiety. Parental factors, including high parental control, parental anxiety, and parental reinforcement of avoidant coping strategies, have been associated with children's anxiety symptoms (Barrett, Rapee, Dadds, & Ryan, 1996; Rapee, 1997; Shortt, Barrett, Dadds, & Fox, 2001; Siqueland, Kendall, & Steinberg, 1996). Moreover, parental anxiety may moderate treatment outcome. Cobham, Dadds, and Spence (1998) found that children with one or more parent with an anxiety disorder responded less well to treatment. More recently, Southam-Gerow, Kendall, and Weersing (2001) reported that higher levels of maternal self-reported depressive symptoms were associated with less favorable outcomes following cognitive-behavioral treatment for anxious youth. Our clinical experience suggests that even when parenting factors do not appear to play a significant role in the development or maintenance of the child's anxiety, enlisting the parents help to change aspects of the child's environment is an excellent way to reduce the child's anxiety and effect positive change.

The FRIENDS program is founded on three specific models: peer learning, experiential learning, and family-directed problem solving. Each is discussed in turn. The

FRIENDS program is designed for implementation with groups of participants of similar age. We believe that peer group training is effective because children learn best by observing and helping others. Furthermore, learning in a peer context provides a safe and familiar environment in which participants can practice newly learned skills. Most of the activities outlined in the FRIENDS program are based on experiential learning. This means that participants are encouraged to learn from their own experiences. The FRIENDS program encourages group participants to play an active role in learning by brainstorming ideas, learning from new experiences, and building on past experiences. In each session there is a mix of pairs work and small and large group activities. This mix facilitates relationship building and helps to improve group cohesion and affiliation. These experiential activities also appear to increase children's enjoyment. The acceptability of the treatment from the child's perspective is important. As mentioned previously, it is usually the parent or caregiver who seeks treatment for his or her child—however, the child's comfort with attending treatment seems to be an important factor in ensuring that the family remains in treatment. In sum, ensuring a pleasant affective environment during treatment helps to maintain the child's motivation and willingness to participate.

The underlying philosophy of the FRIENDS program is that therapists, parents, and children possess valuable knowledge and experiences that they bring to the group. Family members are encouraged to work together to find solutions to their problems. A collaborative "team" approach is emphasized in which the therapist, parent(s), and the child work together with a shared goal of increasing both the child's and parent's confidence. The parent component of the FRIENDS program is also conducted in a group format. It is aimed at empowering parents by helping them to recognize the skills they already have as parents and using these skills to help their children overcome anxiety problems. Parents are taught to recognize and deal appropriately with their own anxiety. Parents are also trained in reinforcement strategies, including specific praise (e.g., "I'm so glad you went to the school sports carnival and cheered for your team"; "Staying at your friends house all afternoon was a great achievement") and tangible rewards (e.g., staying up an extra half hour) for their child's gradually facing feared situations. Planned ignoring is used as a method for dealing with excessive complaining. Parents role-play contingency management strategies with examples of their child's fearful behaviors, and participants are encouraged to learn from each other's role-plays and home experiences. Group processes include the normalization of anxiety and parenting difficulties, role-playing difficult situations with their children, and peer learning through discussion of successes and difficulties. In addition, parents are taught cognitive techniques to challenge unhelpful thoughts. Parents also receive brief training in communication, partner support, and problem-solving skills. Finally, we encourage the development of a support maintenance network among parents.

Main Themes of the Treatment Program

It is generally accepted that anxiety is a multidimensional construct that consists of physiological, cognitive, and emotional elements. The FRIENDS program addresses child and youth anxiety by focusing on the physiological, cognitive processes, and learning processes that are believed to interact in the development, maintenance, and experience of anxiety. Figure 6.1 displays a model identifying these processes and how the skills taught in the FRIENDS program target each. Physiological skills taught include increasing children's awareness of somatic cues to let them know they are feeling worried or scared (e.g., butterflies in the stomach and heart beating fast). Children then learn deep breathing and progressive muscle relaxation. They are encouraged to practice these skills regularly so that they can learn to identify when they are feeling tense and they can use this cue to relax their

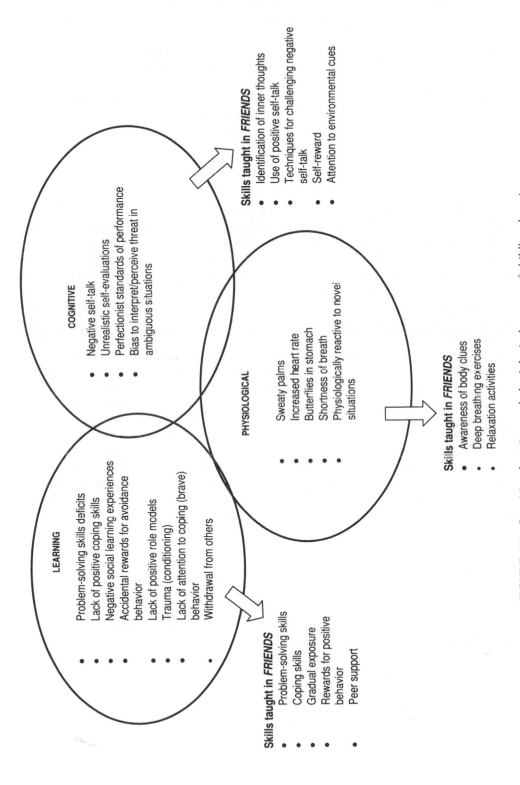

FIGURE 6.1. Cognitive, learning, and physiological aspects of childhood anxiety.

muscles. Cognitive skills include recognition of how one's thinking affects how one feels and what one does. Children and youth experiencing anxiety tend to engage frequently in negative self-talk. The FRIENDS program teaches participants to recognize negative self-talk and to cope with worrying situations by learning to challenge unhelpful thoughts. Anxious children often have perfectionist standards. To help children make more realistic self-evaluations, participants learn to view situations in terms of partial success. Partial success involves teaching children to concentrate on the positive aspects of a situation and on what they did well. Behavioral skills taught in FRIENDS include problem solving and graded exposure to difficult situations. Furthermore, children are encouraged to reward themselves for using coping skills as they try to approach difficult situations.

Participants

The FRIENDS program targets primary and high school–age children with persistent or severe anxiety that causes significant distress and/or interference in their lives. While the FRIENDS program is also widely used among nonclinic class members to promote emotional resilience (Barrett & Turner, 2001), children with diagnoses of generalized anxiety disorder (GAD), separation anxiety disorder (SAD), or social phobia (SoP) are likely to benefit from this integrated CBT program, regardless of age, gender, or ethnicity (Barrett, Sonderegger, & Xenos, in press). Unlike other available programs which target children ages 7 to 14 years in the same program, FRIENDS recognizes the developmental needs of children at different ages with two parallel forms: FRIENDS for Children (7–11 years) and FRIENDS for Youth (12–16 years). We believe that it is vital that treatment programs cater to developmental differences in children's abilities to understand self and other's emotional states, to regulate their own behavior, and to engage in metacognition (i.e., the ability to think about their own thinking). The developmental literature tells us that these abilities are usually fully developed only in late childhood (Hergenhahn & Olson, 1999). Having two different forms of the FRIENDS programs also ensures that the content and activities are age appropriate. A recent study by Southam-Gerow et al. (2001) reported that older children responded less favorably to CBT for anxiety. They suggested that CBT programs might be less palatable to older youth, who may view exercises and assignments as somewhat "childish." To combat this view, A FRIENDS for Youth program has been designed to be specifically "teen friendly." There is more opportunity for group discussion rather than didactic interaction during the treatment sessions.

Program Format

The FRIENDS treatment program is designed for implementation in a group format (GCBT). Treating anxious children in groups offers several advantages. First, it enhances cost-effectiveness because it allows more efficient use of the therapist's time. Second, social withdrawal and social reservedness is often associated with anxiety, and the group setting exposes children to peer interaction and provides them with opportunities to learn social skills (Flannery-Schroeder & Kendall, 2000). Finally, group format increases opportunities for positive modeling and normalization of worries and fears.

Content of Treatment

The child and adolescent components of the FRIENDS for Children and FRIENDS for Youth programs each comprise 10 sessions and 2 booster sessions. Each session is designed to run for approximately 1 hour. The initial 10 sessions are conducted weekly for optimal effectiveness, and the booster sessions are conducted 1 month and 3 months following completion of treatment. The booster sessions provide additional opportunities for children to practice the skills learned in the previous sessions and to facilitate the generalization of these skills to help them cope with situations encountered in everyday life. Table 6.1 presents an overview of the FRIENDS for Children program and Table 6.2 shows an overview of the FRIENDS for Youth program. These tables illustrate how each strategy represented by a letter in the FRIENDS anagram is covered in the sequence of therapy. Table 6.3 outlines the content of the four parent sessions of the FRIENDS program.

The family skills component of FRIENDS is designed to run in a group format for approximately 6 hours. The format of the parent sessions is flexible. It is presented as four 1½ hour sessions; however, session content can be broken into more or fewer sessions depending on the individual needs of the group. This flexibility allows the program to be adapted for clinic or community settings. In a clinic setting it may be desirable to see the parents after each child session to monitor the child's progress, to gather additional information on child functioning, and to ensure effective implementation of the parenting strategies. In this case the sessions could be broken down to 10 35- to 40-minute sessions. In contrast, in a school setting it might be better to run a full-day parenting workshop. With regard to the content of the parent sessions, like other parent training programs (Barrett, 1998; Silverman et al., 1999) parents are taught how to use appropriate reinforcement strategies. In addition, FRIENDS incorporates cognitive re-

TABLE 6.1. Outline of FRIENDS for Children Sessions

Session	Content
1	Rapport building and introduction of group participants Establishing group guidelines Normalization of anxiety and individual differences in anxiety reactions
2	Affective education and identification of various emotions
3	Introduce the relationship between thoughts and feelings
4	F: Feeling worried? (identifying physiological symptoms of worry) R: Relax and feel good (relaxation activities and identification of pleasant activities to do when feeling worried or sad)
5	I: Inner thoughts (identifying self-talk, thinking helpful thoughts)
6	Challenging negative self-talk E: Explore plans (identifying a positive role model and people the child can turn to for support)
7	Problem-solving skills (six-stage problem-solving plan) Introduce the concept of graded exposure (the step plan)
8	Designing a step plan for feared objects/ situations (graded exposure) N: Nice work, reward yourself (rewards for partial success)
9	D: Don't forget to practice (practicing the FRIENDS skills) S: Stay calm (reflect on ways to cope in difficult situations)
10	Generalization and maintenance of the FRIENDS strategies
Booster 1	Review of FRIENDS strategies
Booster 2	Review of FRIENDS strategies

TABLE 6.2. Outline of FRIENDS for Youth Sessions

Session	Content
1	Introduction of group participants and rationale for the group Establishing group guidelines and confidentiality contracting Personal goal setting
2	Building self-esteem
3	Increase awareness of communication styles: verbal and non-verbal Introduce the relationship between thoughts and feelings Developing friendship skills
4	F: Feeling worried? (identifying physiological symptoms of worry) R: Relax and feel good (relaxation activities and visualization)
5	I: Inner thoughts (identifying self-talk, challenging negative self-talk, thinking more positively, attention training)
6	E: Explore plans (identifying social support network, conflict resolution strategies)
7	Problem-solving skills
8	Graded exposure (the step plan) N: Nice work, reward yourself (rewards for partial success)
9	D: Don't forget to practice (practicing the FRIENDS skills) S: Stay calm (reflect on ways to cope in difficult situations)
10	Generalization and maintenance of the FRIENDS strategies
Booster 1	Review of FRIENDS strategies
Booster 2	Review of FRIENDS strategies

structuring for parents and partner support training and encourages families to build supportive social networks. Parents are also encouraged to practice the skills learned in FRIENDS as a family, on a daily basis.

Skills Emphasized in Treatment: The FRIENDS Anagram

F—Feeling Worried?

This is the first skill taught in the treatment program. It involves affective education and teaching children to identify physiological and behavioral indicators of anxiety. Some young people have difficulty making the connection between the physical symptoms of anxiety and the situations that make them feel scared or worried. For example, a child who feels sick just before going to school each Friday is unlikely to be feeling sick from an illness. It is more likely that the child is feeling worried about something that is going to happen at school that day, such as a Friday afternoon test.

R—Relax and Feel Good

The second strategy covered in the program builds on the first. Children are taught that we can feel better and improve our performance by learning relaxation exercises. Children are encouraged to think of relaxation as a skill like riding a bike that needs to be practiced regularly. Engaging in enjoyable activities when feeling worried or sad is another way to help children cope with their worries.

TABLE 6.3. Content and Activities from the Parent Sessions of the FRIENDS Program

Session	Content
1	• Rapport building and introduction of participants. • Psychoeducation about physiological, cognitive, and learned aspects of anxiety and how strategies taught in the FRIENDS program target each of these. • Explanation of FRIENDS acronym and ideas behind the FRIENDS program (the importance of making friends, being your own friend, etc.). • Parents practice deep breathing, progressive muscle relaxation and discuss ways of creating calm time for themselves.
2	• Parents identify their own thoughts in different situations and learn to challenge unhelpful thoughts. • Parents learn to use questioning to help their child combat unhelpful thoughts. • Parents learn problem-solving skills and discuss ideas for their child's graded exposure hierarchy for a feared object/situation
3	• The concepts of observational learning, reinforcement, praise and planned ignoring are discussed. • The importance of (1) rewarding children for approaching difficult situations, and (2) learning to evaluate performance in terms of partial success and to set reasonable achievable goals, are emphasized. • Parents are encouraged to think about their own approaches to difficult situations. (Do they approach or avoid?) Parents are encouraged to think through the consequences of this behavior for themselves and their child.
4	• Strategies for promoting positive family skills are discussed. Parents reflect on their strengths as people and parents. The importance of spending quality time with partners and children, and building social networks is emphasized. • Parents discuss ways of presenting a "united front" when dealing with children. This included ideas for supporting other adults (e.g., partners and teachers) to manage the child's anxiety more effectively. • Parents identify strategies for maintaining gains, discuss potential difficulties, and make plans for continued practice of the FRIENDS strategies learned.

I—Inner Thoughts

This step introduces the cognitive strategies of the treatment program. The FRIENDS program teaches children how the way they talk to themselves influences what they do and how they feel. Children are encouraged to identify negative-self talk and to challenge it.

E—Explore Plans

The fourth step looks for ways to solve problems in difficult or worrying situations and teaches two specific plans of action. First, the Six Block Problem Solving Plan involves thinking through (1) what is the problem—define it!, (2) list all possible solutions, (3) list what might happen for each solution, (4) select the best solution based on the consequences, (5) make a plan for putting this solution into practice and Do It!, and finally (6) evaluate the outcome in terms of strengths and weaknesses, and if it did not work return to block (2) and try again. The second plan for dealing with anxiety-provoking situations is the step plan. The step plan involves children constructing a graded exposure hierarchy that they will implement during the remainder of the program. In implementing the step plan, children are encouraged to use the strategies covered in previous sessions (e.g., relaxation, deep breathing, and challenging unhelpful thoughts) as they climb each step.

N—Nice Work so Reward Yourself

The fifth step teaches children to evaluate their performance in terms of partial success and to set reasonable, achievable goals. In the parent program, parents are encouraged to reward their child's approach behavior. On this step, children are encouraged to reward themselves whenever they try their hardest. Simply studying for an examination or entering a singing competition may deserve a reward if these situations require courage and effort. Learning to self-reward facilitates children's independence, and they are also taught to evaluate their performance in terms of partial success.

D—Don't Forget to Practice

The sixth step reminds the child that the skills and strategies learned in FRIENDS need to be practiced on a regular basis. Children are encouraged to role-play difficult situations with family and/or peers. For example, if a child has a class talk to do, then role playing in front of members of her family will allow her to practice her presentation skills and her FRIENDS skills to help her cope in this situation.

S—Stay Calm

Finally, this last step reminds children that they can stay calm because they know how to cope with their worries.

Therapist Manuals and Workbooks

One of the goals in designing FRIENDS was to ensure that the program was user-friendly and able to be used in research and community settings. To this end, the FRIENDS for Children and FRIENDS for Youth programs are manualized and consist of three parts:

1. A group leader's manual that clearly describes the activities the therapist needs to implement in each session;
2. A workbook for each child or youth to complete as they work through the program; and
3. A parent information booklet detailing strategies to help overcome anxiety problems and to deal with common parenting difficulties.

The manuals permit flexible implementation to allow for family individuality and the needs of specific groups (the manuals are published by Australian Academic Press and can be ordered from the FRIENDS website: *http://www.friendsinfo.net*).

Evaluation of Treatment

A multiple informant and multimethod approach to the assessment of anxiety is recommended. As mentioned earlier, clinical interviews with the child and his or her parent, self-reports, and parent and teacher behavior ratings should be included as a matter of course at the beginning, middle, and end of treatment. Follow-ups at 6 months and 12 months after treatment, and longer term, should also be included whenever possible. Measures of cognition and behavioral avoidance may also yield information about the cognitive and behavioral changes associated with treatment. When evaluating family-based treatments, there is a clear need to include measures of family functioning, parental psychopathology, and observations of parent–child interaction. Also, although treatments are routinely evaluated in terms of efficacy, the assessment of treatment acceptability has not been consistent. We believe that it is important to evaluate the acceptability of treatment programs as programs with high acceptability are more likely to be transported from research to community settings and this will help to ensure the long-term viability of anxiety treatment programs.

EVIDENCE FOR THE EFFECTS OF TREATMENT

For many years, researchers have espoused the importance of parental involvement in helping anxious children; however, empirical investigations of the effectiveness of including parents in treatment are relatively scarce. Howard and Kendall (1996) were the first to evaluate the effectiveness of CBT plus parent involvement using a multiple baseline design. Six clinically anxious children ages 9 to 13 years participated, and four of these children showed positive changes in diagnostic status, standardized parent and teacher report measures, and parent and child reports of coping at posttreatment.

Barrett, Dadds, and Rapee (1996) conducted the first randomized, controlled trial of CBT plus family anxiety management training (FAM). The FAM component formed the basis for the parenting sessions in the FRIENDS program. It involved (1) training parents in contingency management, (2) giving parents skills to better manage their own anxiety, and (3) training parents in problem solving and communication skills. Barrett et al. randomly assigned 79 children (ages 7–14 years) to either child-only CBT, CBT + FAM, or a wait-list condition. At posttreatment, 61% of children in the child-only CBT group were diagnosis free compared to 88% of children in the combined treatment and less than 30% in the wait-list condition. At 12-month follow up, the relative superiority of CBT + FAM was maintained. However at a long-term follow-up conducted 5–7 years after completion of treatment, child-only CBT and CBT + FAM were equally effective, with 87% and 86% of participants in these respective groups diagnosis free.

Interestingly, age and gender appeared to moderate the effectiveness of the additional parent component. Specifically, younger children (ages 7–10 years) and girls who completed the CBT + FAM condition were more likely to be diagnosis free than were their peers in the child-only CBT condition. For boys and children ages 11 to 14 years, the child-alone CBT was as effective as CBT + FAM at posttreatment and at follow-up. Barrett et al. suggested that enhancing parenting skills may be important for younger children, but for older children individual work may be sufficient to reduce anxiety. A recent study by Cobham et al. (1998) identified parental anxiety as another potential moderator of treatment effectiveness. In their study of 67 children, children with an anxious parent were found to be more likely to be free of their anxiety diagnosis if they received child CBT plus parental anxiety management (PAM) (CBT + PAM). Children without an anxious parent responded positively regardless of whether they were assigned to child-only CBT or CBT + PAM.

In 1998, Barrett reported the results of a study evaluating a GCBT family-based intervention for childhood anxiety disorders. Sixty children ranging from 7 to 14 years old were randomly allocated to three treatment conditions: GCBT, GCBT plus family management (GCBT + FAM), and wait list. At posttreatment, 56% of children in the GCBT, 71% of children in the GCBT + FAM, and 25% of children in the wait-list group no longer met criteria for any anxiety disorder diagnosis. At 12-month follow-up, 65% of children in the GCBT group and 85% of children in the GCBT + FAM were diagnosis free. At posttreatment and follow-up, comparison of the GCBT and GCBT + FAM conditions revealed that children in the GCBT + FAM condition showed significant improvements on measures of diagnostic status, parents' perception of their ability to deal with the child's behavior, and change in family disruption by child's behavior. These results suggest that CBT family interventions for childhood anxiety disorders can be effectively administered in a group format. In support of the findings from Barrett et al.'s (1996) earlier study, the addition of a family management component led to more favorable outcomes.

In summary, research by our team provides preliminary support for using CBT plus parent involvement over child-only CBT for some children. However, there is a clear need for these findings to be replicated by different groups of investigators. To date, research by others comparing child-alone CBT to CBT plus parent involvement in the treatment of anxious children has yielded contrary results that challenge the assumption that a combined treatment approach leads to better outcomes. For example, Spence, Donovan, and Brechman-Toussaint (2000) randomly allocated 50 socially phobic children (ages 7 to 14 years) to either a child-alone CBT group, a CBT-plus-parent-involvement group, or a wait-list control. At posttreatment, significantly fewer children in the treatment conditions retained a clinical diagnosis of social phobia compared to the wait-list condition. Children in the CBT conditions, with and without parent involvement, showed comparable improvements at posttreatment. At 12-month follow-up, there was a trend toward superior results when parents were involved in treatment; however, this effect was not statistically significant. Similarly, in a recent study by Heyne et al. (2002), 61 school-refusing children (ages 7 to 14 years) were randomized to a child therapy program, a parent and teacher training program, or a combination of the two. Although all groups showed significant improvement from pretreatment to posttreatment, there was some evidence that the combined program produced better immediate outcomes. Children in the child-only therapy group showed the least improvement in school attendance compared to the other groups, and children in the combined condition displayed significantly fewer internalizing behaviors than children in the child-alone group. However, by follow-up, the attendance and adjustment of those in the child therapy group equaled that of children whose parents and teachers were involved in treatment, whether on their own (parent/teacher training) or together with their children (combined child therapy and parent/teacher training). It appeared that working with the child alone or caregivers alone may be just as effective as a combined treatment approach. The results of these two studies suggest that for some children, a less time-consuming child-alone CBT approach may be sufficient to reduce anxiety. The challenge for future researchers is to be able to identify child and family characteristics that will enable clinicians to match anxious children to either child-alone or child-plus-parents intervention. There is preliminary evidence (Barrett et al., 1996; Cobham et al., 1998) to suggest that younger age and high parental anxiety are characteristics that may lead a clinician to select a combined parent and child treatment over CBT for the child alone.

A number of recent trials of CBT for anxious children have included some parent involvement (e.g., Flannery-Schroeder & Kendall, 2000; Mendlowitz et al., 1999; Silverman et al., 1999). Integration of these research findings is complicated by a lack of definition about what constitutes parent involvement in treatment. More work is needed to identify the specific strategies that need to be included in parent sessions and the role parents should play in treatment. Our reading of this literature leads us to question the extent to which parent involvement in all these studies is comparable to each other. We wonder whether these studies represent trials of the same treatment or whether they report on trials of qualitatively different treatments. One of the most important tasks for researchers is to manualize the parent components of treatment and to clearly describe the content of the parent sessions in research articles.

Recent research suggests that CBT for anxious youth can be effectively delivered in a group format. In addition to the Barrett (1998) trial discussed earlier, our research team recently completed a randomized controlled trial of the FRIENDS for Children program for young children ages 6 to 10 years (Shortt, Barrett, & Fox, 2001). Seventy-one children were randomly allocated to FRIENDS for Children treatment or a 10-week wait-list control. At posttreatment, 69% of children who completed treatment were diagnosis free, compared to 6% in the wait-list condition. Studies by research teams in the United States comparing GCBT to wait-list control groups have yielded similarly positive results (see Flannery-Schroeder & Kendall, 2000; Silverman et al., 1999). GCBT for childhood anxiety disorders is now regarded as a "probably efficacious" treatment.

In recent years our research interests have expanded. We have adopted a joint focus on both treatments for children already suffering from anxiety and prevention and early intervention programs which intervene prior to the development of significant anxiety symptomatology (see Barrett & Turner, 2001). This decision to adopt a joint focus is based on our belief that treating children who are already experiencing significant anxiety problems may not be the most effective or efficient means of reducing the incidence of childhood anxiety in the general population.

Strengths and Weaknesses of the Treatment Approach

An important issue for family intervention is the *type* of family intervention. Family treatment is not a uniform entity, because every family is different. Many families need some type of intervention; consequently, the parent component of FRIENDS is integrated and targets a number of areas of parent functioning and parenting behavior. Programs such as FRIENDS, which teach strategies for parents to better manage their own anxiety symptoms and include some cognitive therapy with parents, appear to go some way in minimizing the negative effect that parental psychopathology has on treatment outcome. However, there is a clear need for future studies to examine how family interventions can be tailored to the needs of individual families.

A limitation of our research to date is that characteristics of the participants may limit generalization to clinical practice. To get large numbers of participants, we have used community advertisements (e.g., newspapers and school newsletters) to notify parents about the treatment. Even though all participants are screened to ensure that they meet diagnostic criteria for an anxiety disorder, it has been argued that participants who volunteer for treatment research are different from those families who typically are seen in clinical work (Kazdin, 2000). Children recruited for research may be less severely disturbed, may show less impairment across multiple domains (e.g., school and peer relations), and typically do not have comorbid externalizing disorders. The families of these children may be less disturbed than families that present at a clinic setting. Families usually have to function at a reasonable level in order to comply with the higher demands of the research setting (e.g., repeated interviews, questionnaires, and other assessment tasks). Given that families presenting in clinical practice may be more disturbed, there may be a greater need for a treatment program which targets parents and family functioning, as well as child anxiety and coping. In a similar vein, if parents of clinically referred samples have higher rates of disorders than do parents of nonreferred children with milder forms of the problem, there may be a greater need for adjunctive individual therapy with the parent to target the parent's own anxiety or other problems. In summary, future examination of the efficacy of FRIENDS in the clinic setting would be welcomed.

It is our view that one of the most important future developments in the childhood anxiety area will be to ensure satisfactory dissemination of effective treatments into the community. Evidence-based approaches are commonly used in research and university clinic settings but are less common among practitioners in the community. When this is considered with the fact that many anxious children and adolescents are still not presented at mental health settings, the need for interventions that are user-friendly and able to be implemented in community settings such as schools is clear. One of the key strengths of the FRIENDS treatment program is that both the parent and child components are manualized, and the manuals and associated materials for children and parents are easily accessed from the publisher.

Recommendations Regarding Implementation in Practice

Parental involvement in treatment is a complex issue. Therapists need to be able to engage parents and work with them as they interact with their children. In working with parents, it is important for therapists to express their interest in and concern about the parents as individual people as well as parents. In the FRIENDS program this expression is achieved by activities in which parents share information about themselves and their achievements as people. In our experience, one of the best ways to build an alliance with parents is to demonstrate empathy and understanding for the impact that having an anxious child has on them and their family. As mentioned earlier, anxious children often make persistent requests for reassurance from parents. Generally anxious children frequently bombard parents with "what if?" questions about future events, while children with separation fears ask parents for reassurance about the parents' whereabouts when the child is not with them. An anxious child's hesitancy to participate in activities can inhibit the family's social life and limit spontaneity (Siqueland & Diamond, 1998). We have worked with families that go to the same holiday destination year after year to avoid their child's fear of the unknown, as well as families that find day-to-day life marked by their child's inability to make decisions about simple tasks such as which breakfast cereal to have or what to take to school.

Working with parents is made easier by recognizing some of the common patterns of parent–child interaction in families with anxious children. Of course, it is equally important to remember that no one pattern characterizes all families with an anxious child. Clinicians should also consider that the processes by which parents and children influence each other are likely to be reciprocal in nature (Dadds & Roth, 2001). This means that the patterns of parent–child interaction observed may reflect a parent's own anxiety affecting the child or the anxious child's attempts to coerce his or her parents into maintaining a reassuring closeness, but most likely these patterns reflect both parent and child factors. There is accumulating research that suggests parents can and do influence their children's behavior. Our own research suggests that parent–child interactions can maintain the children's anxiety symptoms (e.g., Barrett et al., 1996; Dadds, Spence, Holland,

Barrett, & Laurens, 1997). Parents may influence their child to engage in more avoidant behavior by questioning their child's ability to perform the task successfully ("Do you really think you'd be able to go up to a group of kids you didn't know?", "Do you really think you'd be able to stay home by yourself with a sitter?") and by reminding them of previous experiences which did not turn out well. Rather than rewarding the child's courageous attempts, parents can ignore approach behaviors and pay attention to the child's concerns about the situation and his or her ability to cope with it. Another common pattern is that the parents' attempts to soothe their child become "protection traps" (Ginsburg, Silverman, & Kurtines, 1995). In this cycle, parents' love for their child accompanied by recognition that their child is sensitive to challenge leads parents to "protect" their child from distress by encouraging them to avoid a feared object or situation.

The FRIENDS treatment program attempts to capitalize on these reciprocal parent–child interactions so that treatment gains are maintained in the long term. During treatment, children learn skills to better manage their anxiety, and parents learn strategies to encourage their child to engage in approach behaviors that they may not have felt confident enough to do previously. The parent may begin to behave differently—encouraging the child to relax, challenge negative thinking, and approach difficult situations one step at a time. This new approach behavior is rewarded and is self-rewarding. As the child successfully manages new challenges, his or her confidence will increase and he or she will seek more independence. The child has the experience to challenge catastrophic cognitions concerning anxiety-provoking situations. The child develops increasing confidence in his or her ability to cope with challenging situations.

DIRECTIONS FOR FUTURE RESEARCH

There is clearly a need for more research examining the processes of change in therapy. Silverman and Kurtines (1996) have proposed a transfer of control model that is helpful for conceptualizing the process of effective therapeutic change in children. They suggest that therapy involves a gradual "transfer of control" where the sequence is generally from therapist to parent to child. The therapist is viewed as an expert consultant who possesses the knowledge of the skills and methods necessary to produce therapeutic change, and who then transfers the use of these skills and methods to the parent, and subsequently from parent to child. This model for the process of change needs to be investigated empirically.

As evidenced by the research reviewed previously, most treatment outcome studies to date have examined the efficacy of integrated programs that combine a number of CBT strategies to target anxious symptomatology. A consequence of this combination is that the relative efficacy of each strategy is unknown. The identification of the key change-producing procedure or procedures might allow briefer or more effective programs to be developed. Barrett has recently begun work on a controlled trial examining the relative efficacy of the different components of integrated CBT programs (e.g., exposure vs. cognitive strategies vs. psychoeducation and support). This trial will also examine whether the helpfulness of each strategy depends on the age of the child. Similar trials by other research groups are encouraged.

The findings from the Shortt, Barrett, Dadds, and Fox (2001) study provide supportive evidence for the use of the FRIENDS for Children program with anxious children ages 7 to 10 years. A controlled trial evaluating the FRIENDS for Youth program in a sample of clinically anxious adolescents is currently under way. An important area for further research is to investigate specific group processes in both child and parent sessions, which may help or hinder treatment outcome. Studies could examine whether positive processes such as therapeutic alliance, therapist empathy, group cohesion, and identification with the group have a positive relationship with treatment effectiveness.

Finally, there is a need for more studies to include measures of the social validity of their intervention programs. Although treatments are routinely evaluated in terms of efficacy, the assessment of treatment acceptability has not been consistent. Interventions need to be evaluated in terms of the willingness of practitioners to use them and of clients to accept them (Foster & Marsh, 1999). Therapeutic manuals have the advantage of allowing for a high degree of standardization. The precise outline of activities provided is easily translated into criteria for treatment integrity. However, a disadvantage of manuals in a clinic setting is that therapists are concerned that using a manual may limit their flexibility in addressing issues relevant to treatment but not covered in the manual. The need for programs to be perceived as flexible is magnified for group treatment when therapists try to cater to the individual needs of many children. In designing FRIENDS, effort was made to make the manuals flexible. The extent to which we have been successful awaits further research. Further research examining the relationship between treatment integrity, therapist flexibility, and treatment outcome is also needed.

A second issue in terms of social validity concerns the degree of treatment acceptability. Researchers need to question multiple sources (e.g., children, parents, and teachers) about their experience of treatment and treatment effectiveness. When assessing the acceptability of integrated treatment programs, a combination of global satisfaction measures and measures of satisfaction with each element in the treatment package (e.g., exposure, peer learning, and homework activities) are desirable. Our research suggests that children and parents participating in the FRIENDS program are satisfied with the treatment (Shortt et al., 2001). This is an important finding, as programs with high acceptability are more likely to be transported from research to community settings.

A weakness of previous research in the childhood anxiety area is that most participants have been Caucasian and English speaking. Few studies have examined the efficacy of cognitive-behavioral treatment programs for children from culturally diverse backgrounds. Young people of non-English speaking backgrounds (NESB) frequently experience anxiety and stress as a direct consequence of migration and cultural adjustment. Having identified a lack of culturally appropriate interventions for use with ethnic minority groups, members of our research team have adapted the FRIENDS program for culturally diverse primary and high school–age students, with ethnically sensitive appendices for Chinese and former Yugoslavian migrants/refugees (Barrett, Sonderegger, & Sonderegger, 2001a, 2001b). Preliminary findings suggest that NESB children who completed the FRIENDS program showed improved coping skills and were better able to combat the anxieties associated with living in a different culture (Barrett, Moore, & Sonderegger, 2000; Barrett, Sonderegger, & Sonderegger, 2001c; Barrett et al., in press).

SUMMARY AND CONCLUSIONS

Childhood anxiety problems that interfere with family, peer relation, or school functioning have an alarming prevalence rate. However, clinically validated interventions that deal with pervasive anxiety concerns are becoming increasingly sophisticated. In understanding the variables that influence children's behavior (e.g., children's relationships with their parents, siblings, other family members, peers, school, and neighborhood community), researchers in recent years have enquired whether treatments should focus directly on children or be broadened to include family and school functioning contexts. Although there is a relative dearth of empirical literature on the involvement of families and community in child anxiety treatment programs, this chapter presents emerging evidence for one family-directed peer and experiential learning program (FRIENDS), which demonstrates the efficacy of using cognitive-behavioral strategies with primary and high school–age children. This program uses the acronym FRIENDS to help participants remember successful coping strategies, as well as encouraging children to both think of themselves and their bodies as friends and understand the value of making and taking to friends. Complex multiphasic concerns are addressed by focusing on the physiological, cognitive processes, and learning processes linked with the development, maintenance, and experience of anxiety. In this regard, the program may also be used as a prevention to develop resilience against anxiety among nonclinic populations.

Although many evidence-based approaches are commonly used in research and university clinic settings, empirically validated intervention programs are only as good as their satisfactory dissemination into the community. Because many anxious children and adolescents fail to present at mental health clinics, the administration of the FRIENDS program has been largely adopted by school and community groups. Moreover, to ensure that emotional resilience and treatment gains are sustained overtime, the FRIENDS program incorporates parents into the treatment regime and capitalizes on reciprocal parent–child interactions. At the same time that children are learning skills to better manage their anxiety, parents learn strategies to encourage their children to engage exposure, coping, and problem-solving behaviors.

With regard to treatment of anxious children, several published studies provide support for the use of GCBT. In this chapter, the FRIENDS program has been described in detail and is offered as a group CBT program for anxious children and their parents. The use of the FRIENDS program over other group programs may be indicated when the client is an adolescent (as FRIENDS for Youth was developed specifically to meet the developmental needs of adolescents), or when case formulation suggests that a child's parents and/or peer relationships may be maintaining the anxiety symptoms. Although empirical investigations using the FRIENDS program have yielded positive results among diverse ages and ethnic groups, in order to delineate the most successful components of the intervention, future studies need to examine specific group processes in both child and parent sessions, including therapeutic alliance, therapist empathy, group cohesion, and group identification. Continued social validity studies will only further enhance the intervention over time. It is our hope that therapists find the FRIENDS program a useful intervention for their anxious clients. Furthermore, we hope that the recognition and treatment of anxiety disorders in non-mental health settings become a higher research priority.

REFERENCES

Anderson, J. C., Williams, S., McGee, R., & Silva, W. (1987). DSM-III disorders in preadolescent children. *Archives of General Psychiatry, 44*, 69–76.

Barrett, P. M. (1995). *Group Coping Koala Workbook*. Unpublished manuscript, School of Applied Psychology, Griffith University, Brisbane, Australia.

Barrett, P. M. (1998). Evaluation of cognitive-behavioral group treatments for childhood anxiety disorders. *Journal of Clinical Child Psychology, 27*, 459–468.

Barrett, P. M. (1999). Interventions for child and youth anxiety disorders: Involving parents, teachers, and peers. *The Australian Educational and Developmental Psychologist, 16,* 5–25.

Barrett, P. M., Dadds, M. R., & Rapee, R. M. (1996). Family treatment of childhood anxiety: A controlled trial. *Journal of Consulting and Clinical Psychology, 64*(2), 333–342.

Barrett, P. M., Lowry-Webster, H., & Turner, C. (2000a). *FRIENDS program for children: Participants workbook.* Brisbane: Australian Academic Press.

Barrett, P. M., Lowry-Webster, H., & Turner, C. (2000b). *FRIENDS program for children: Parents' supplement.* Brisbane: Australian Academic Press.

Barrett, P. M., Lowry-Webster, H., & Turner, C. (2000c). *FRIENDS program for children: Group leaders manual.* Brisbane: Australian Academic Press.

Barrett, P. M., Lowry-Webster, H., & Turner, C. (2000d). *FRIENDS program for youth: Participants workbook.* Brisbane: Australian Academic Press.

Barrett, P. M., Lowry-Webster, H., & Turner, C. (2000e). *FRIENDS program for youth: Parents' supplement.* Brisbane: Australian Academic Press.

Barrett, P. M., Lowry-Webster, H., & Turner, C. (2000f). *FRIENDS program for youth: Group leaders manual.* Brisbane: Australian Academic Press.

Barrett, P. M., Moore, A. F., & Sonderegger, R. (2000). The FRIENDS Program for young former-Yugoslavian refugees in Australia: A pilot study. *Behaviour Change, 17,* 12–21.

Barrett, P. M., Rapee, R. M., Dadds, M. R., & Ryan, S. M. (1996). Family enhancement of cognitive style in anxious and aggressive children. *Journal of Abnormal Child Psychology, 37,* 187–203.

Barrett, P. M., Sonderegger, R., & Sonderegger, N. L. (2001a). *Universal supplement to FRIENDS for Children: Group leaders manual for participants from non-English speaking backgrounds.* Bowen Hills, Queensland: Australian Academic Press.

Barrett, P. M., Sonderegger, R., & Sonderegger, N. L. (2001b). *Universal supplement to FRIENDS for Youth: Group leaders manual for participants from non-English speaking backgrounds.* Bowen Hills, Queensland: Australian Academic Press.

Barrett, P. M., Sonderegger, R., & Sonderegger, N. L. (2001c). Evaluation of an anxiety prevention and positive-coping program (FRIENDS) for children and adolescents of non-English speaking background. *Behaviour Change, 18,* 78–91.

Barrett, P. M., Sonderegger, R., & Xenos, S. (in press). Using FRIENDS to combat anxiety and adjustment problems among young migrants to Australia: A national trial. *Clinical Child Psychology and Psychiatry.*

Barrett, P. M., & Turner, C. (2001). Prevention of anxiety symptoms in primary school children: Preliminary results from a universal school-based trial. *British Journal of Clinical Psychology, 40,* 399–410.

Boyd, C. P., Kostanski, M., Gullone, E., Ollendick, T. H., & Shek, D. T. (2000). Prevalence of anxiety and depression in Australian adolescents: Comparisons with worldwide data. *Journal of Genetic Psychology, 161,* 479–492.

Bronfenbrenner, U. (1979). *The ecology of human development: Experiments by nature and design.* Cambridge, MA: Harvard University Press.

Cobham, V. E, Dadds, R., & Spence, S. H. (1998). The role of parental anxiety in the treatment of childhood anxiety. *Journal of Consulting and Clinical Psychology, 66,* 893–905.

Costello, E. J., & Angold, A. (1995). Epidemiology. In J. S. March (Ed.), *Anxiety disorders in children and adolescents* (pp. 109–124). New York: Guilford Press.

Dadds, M. R., & Roth, J. H. (2001). Family processes in the development of anxiety problems. In M. W. Vasey & M. R. Dadds (Eds.), *The developmental psychopathology of anxiety disorders in children* (pp. 278–303). New York: Oxford University Press.

Dadds, M. R., Spence, S. H., Holland, D. E., Barrett, P. M., & Laurens, K. R. (1997) Prevention and early intervention for anxiety disorders: A controlled trial. *Journal of Consulting and Clinical Psychology, 65,* 627–635.

Flannery-Schroeder, E. C., & Kendall, P. C. (2000). Group and individual cognitive-behavioral treatments for youth with anxiety disorders: A randomized clinical trial. *Cognitive Therapy and Research, 24,* 251–278.

Foster, S. L., & Marsh, E. J. (1999). Assessing social validity in clinical treatment research: Issues and procedures. *Journal of Consulting and Clinical Psychology, 67,* 308–319.

Ginsburg, G. S., Silverman, W. K., & Kurtines, W. K. (1995). Family involvement in treating children with phobic and anxiety disorders: A look ahead. *Clinical Psychology Review, 15*(5), 457–473.

Hergenhahn, B. R., & Olson, M. H. (1999). *An introduction to theories of personality* (5th ed.). Upper Saddle River, NJ: Prentice-Hall.

Heyne, D., King, N. J., Tonge, B. J., Rollings, S., Young, D., Pritchard, M., & Ollendick, T. H. (2002). Evaluation of child therapy and caregiver training in the treatment of school refusal. *Journal of the American Academy of Child and Adolescent Psychiatry, 41,* 687–695.

Howard, B., & Kendall, P. C. (1996). Cognitive-behavioral family therapy for anxiety disordered children: A multiple baseline evaluation. *Cognitive Therapy and Research, 20,* 423–443.

Kazdin, A. E. (2000). *Psychotherapy for children and adolescents: Directions for research and practice.* New York: Oxford University Press.

Kendall, P. C. (1990). *The Coping Cat Workbook.* Ardmore, PA: Workbook Publishing.

Kendall, P. C., Chansky, T. E., Kane, M. T., Kim, R., Kortlander, E., Ronan, K. R., Sessa, F. M., & Siqueland, L. (1992). *Anxiety disorder in youth: Cognitive-behavioral interventions.* Needham Heights, MA: Allyn & Bacon.

Kendall, P. C., Flannery-Schroeder, E., Panichelli-Mindel, S. M., Southam-Gerown, M., Henin, A., & Warman, M. (1997). Treatment of anxiety disorders in youth: A second randomized clinical trial. *Journal of Consulting and Clinical Psychology, 65,* 366–380.

Lerner, R. M. (1991). Changing organism-context relations as the basic process of development: A developmental contextual perspective. *Developmental Psychology, 27,* 27–32.

Mendlowitz, S. L., Manassis, K., Bradley, S., Scapillato, D., Miezitis, S., & Shaw, B. F. (1999). Cognitive-behavioral group treatments in childhood anxiety disorders: The role of parental involvement. *Journal of the American Academy of Child and Adolescent Psychiatry, 38,* 1223–1229.

Rapee, R. M. (1997). Potential role of childrearing practices in the development of anxiety and depression. *Clinical Psychology Review, 17,* 47–68.

Shortt, A. L., Barrett, P. M., Dadds, M. R., & Fox, T. L. (2001). The influence of family and experimental context on cognition in anxious children. *Journal of Abnormal Child Psychology, 29,* 585–596.

Shortt, A. L., Barrett, P. M., & Fox, T. (2001). Evaluating the FRIENDS program: A cognitive behavioral group treatment for anxious children and their parents. *Journal of Clinical Child Psychology, 30,* 525–535.

Silverman, W. K., & Kurtines, W. M. (1996). *Anxiety and phobic disorders: A pragmatic approach.* New York: Plenum Press.

Silverman, W. K., Kurtines, W. M., Ginsburg, G. S., Weems, C. G., Lumpkin, P. W., & Carmichael, D. H. (1999). Treating anxiety disorders in children with group cognitive behavior therapy: A randomized clinical trial. *Journal of Consulting and Clinical Psychology, 67,* 995–1003.

Siqueland, L., & Diamond, G. S. (1998). Engaging parents in cognitive behavioral treatment for children with anxiety disorders. *Cognitive and Behavioral Practice, 5,* 81–102.

Siqueland, L., Kendall, P. C., & Steinberg, L. (1996). Anxiety in children: Perceived family environment and observed family interaction. *Journal of Clinical Child Psychology, 25,* 225–237.

Southam-Gerow, M. A., Kendall, P. C., & Weersing, V. R. (2001). Examining outcome variability: Correlates of treatment response in a child and adolescent anxiety clinic. *Journal of Clinical Child Psychology, 30,* 422–436.

Spence, S. H., Donovan, C., & Brechman-Toussaint, M. (2000). The treatment of childhood social phobia: The effectiveness of a social skills training-based, cognitive-behavioral intervention, with and without parental involvement. *Journal of Child Psychology and Psychiatry and Allied Disciplines, 41,* 713–726.

7

Cognitive-Behavioral Group Treatment for Adolescent Depression

GREGORY N. CLARKE, LYNN L. DEBAR,
AND PETER M. LEWINSOHN

OVERVIEW

The Clinical Problem

Recent epidemiological research has confirmed that adolescent depression is a significant public mental health problem. Adolescent major depression has an estimated point prevalence ranging from 3% to 5%, and a lifetime rate of 20% by age 18 (Birmaher et al., 1996; Lewinsohn, Hops, Roberts, Seeley, & Andrews, 1993). Major depression prevalence among younger, prepubertal children is estimated to be much lower, about 1% (Birmaher et al., 1996). Among prepubertal children, the ratio of depressed boys to girls is roughly equal. However, by early adolescence girls are two to three times more likely to be depressed than boys (Birmaher et al., 1996; Lewinsohn et al., 1993), similar to adult gender ratios. Cohort data also suggest increasing depression prevalence in children born in the latter half of this century, and the initial onset age of depression appears to be dropping as well (Lewinsohn et al., 1993).

Youth who have had an episode of depression have a high probability of recurrence, ranging from 12% relapse within 1 year to 33% within 4 years (Lewinsohn, Clarke, Seeley, & Rohde, 1994). This often chronic and recurrent illness is associated with significant impairment in family, social, and academic functioning. Depressed youth have an increased risk of suicide, other psychiatric difficulties, and substance abuse (Rohde, Lewinsohn, & Seeley, 1991). Rates of youth depression and the most common comorbidities have been well documented by community epidemiology studies (Lewinsohn et al., 1993).

Conceptual Model and Assumptions Underlying Treatment

Underlying this treatment program is the fundamental assumption that depression results from learned maladaptive behaviors and responses, interacting with a biological or inherited risk for depression. Therefore, we hypothesize that learning new, presumably more adaptive behaviors can be curative or at least palliative. This treatment model focuses on specific learned behaviors, particularly social behaviors which involve interpersonal skills such as assertiveness, listening to and communicating with others, and addressing conflict. This is often referred to as the social learning model of depression (Lewinsohn, Hoberman, Teri, & Hautzinger, 1985). This model is closely tied to what has been called the behavioral theory, in which depression is hypothesized to arise from low rates of rewards (response-contingent positive reinforcement) and high rates of negative reinforcement (punishment or withdrawal of reinforcement) (summarized by Lewinsohn et al., 1985). The behavioral theory of depression implies that depression will be decreased by modifying social behaviors so that they lead to more reward and less punishment.

Another construct thought to underlie depression is internal and highly negative or irrational thinking, perhaps best described in the cognitive model of depression of Beck, Rush, Shaw, and Emery (1979). This theory hypothesizes that depression results from highly negative and irrational (unrealistic) beliefs or schemas that are largely automatic and that lead the depression-prone person to interpret ambiguous situations in a highly negative and pessimistic way ("Those people must be laughing at me, because they know I am a failure"). This theory implies that changing underlying beliefs in the more positive and realistic direction will lead to a decrease in depression.

One overall model unifies these various contributing theories and underlies our intervention, the Adolescent Coping With Depression (CWDA) program. This unifying theory is the multifactorial model of depression proposed by Lewinsohn et al. (1985). Briefly, increased dysphoria/depression is presumed to be the result of multiple etiological elements acting in combination. These factors include negative cognition; high rates of negative reinforcement, low rates of positive reinforcement, stressful events, predisposing vulnerabilities or risk factors (e.g., being female, a previous history of depression, and having depressed parents), and the absence of protective factors that help the person avoid becoming depressed (e.g., high self-esteem and coping skills). This model recognizes that there may be multiple pathways into depression; each person experiences a unique and idiosyncratic combination of these factors. Conversely, this model implies that people can recover from depression in multiple ways, through the amelioration of one or more of these etiological factors. Interestingly, the model does not necessarily require that the curative methods address the same etiological factor that led to the onset of depression. That is, it may not be necessary to know the specific "cause" in order to match the treatment to this factor. Many interventions, possibly unrelated to the causal factors, may be curative alone or in combination. The CWDA intervention is guided by the hypothesis that teaching individuals new cognitive and behavioral skills strengthens their repertoire of coping techniques and helps them overcome their depression. Furthermore, the skills acquired in the CWDA course provide youth with some "immunity" against the development of later affective episodes, even if the youth may have a putatively inherited biological risk.

Goals and Main Themes of the Treatment Program

The CWDA course (Clarke, Lewinsohn, & Hops, 2001) employs a psychoeducational approach to treating youth depression in a group or class-like setting. Our rationale for this approach was severalfold. First, we hypothesized that teenagers would be comfortable with the group learning model, given its similarity to school. We hoped that the psychoeducational approach might make the group, and depression, less stigmatizing and increase youth comfort. Of course, we try to avoid those aspects of school that might alienate some of the participants. We do not judge or grade their answers, participation and attendance are encouraged but voluntary, and all the topics are highly personal and relevant (their own feelings and behavior) rather than abstract and of little obvious relevance to the teens' lives (these are common complaints about math and history classes). The second reason for employing a psychoeducational approach was ease of use for therapists. Few community- and school-based mental health professionals have extensive training in cognitive-behavioral therapy (CBT), which is a barrier to more widespread use of this evidence-tested treatment. Our detailed manual and the psychoeducational approach make the implementation of the CWDA course easier for novice therapists or those experienced therapists who are new to CBT. In general, our CBT treatment and prevention trials (discussed later) have been staffed by community therapists with several years of general adolescent therapy experience but only minimal CBT training prior to our studies. Nonetheless, with a moderate amount of experiential training these individuals are able to deliver the group prevention and treatment programs based on the CWDA program and obtain sizable clinical benefit. At a minimum, we do expect therapists to have at least a master's degree in one of several disciplines with a mental health background (psychology, psychiatry, social work, nursing), and several years of prior experience working with groups of adolescents. Therapists should also be comfortable assessing depression and other comorbidities and formulating and acting on a crisis plan to address any of the many problems that may arise (e.g., suicidal behavior, substance abuse, or emergent bipolar disorder).

The CWDA program directly focuses on symptom relief, a treatment aim it shares with most other CBT interventions. The course is divided into specific modules, or component skills training sections of several sessions each. Each module targets a particular depression symptom or deficit, such as depressive thinking, poor social skills, low rates of pleasant activities, and so on. Each module provides training in a skill or technique specifically designed to reduce or eliminate that domain of dysfunction. For example, the behavioral therapy module is meant to address low rates of pleasurable activities. For anyone familiar with CBT this seems obvious. However, this approach to treating depression is in direct contrast to historical treatments such as psychodynamic therapy, which focus on more distal and presumed root causes such as childhood experiences. Table 7.1 lists the specific CWDA therapy components and their intended targets.

Table 7.1 makes it immediately obvious that the CWDA intervention is multimodal.

TABLE 7.1. CWDA Therapy Components and Their Intended Targets

CWDA skill modules	Targets
Cognitive restructuring	Irrational or highly negative beliefs, guilt, hopelessness, worthlessness
Behavioral therapy	Social withdrawal, impaired interpersonal interactions, anhedonia
Problem solving, communication, negotiation	Impaired interpersonal interactions, conflict, anger, marital/family problems, poor problem solving
Relaxation training	Tension/anxiety, social anxiety
Goal setting	Identifying short and long-term life goals, and potential barriers to achieving these

The program consists of several component skills or techniques, each of which could be considered an entire, comprehensive treatment for depression in its own right. The rationale for such treatment clearly arises out of the multidimensional theoretical background for the CWDA program, reviewed earlier. We believe that there are many possible approaches to recovering from depression, any one or more of which might be effective for any given individual. Because the present state of research cannot currently support optimal matching of persons to specific treatments, we have opted to offer several treatments with the hope that group participants will find that at least one of these techniques works for them. Further, because this is a group program, each of the participants may find that a different skill works for him or her—and thus we must present all skills to all participants.

We tell group participants in advance that not every skill or technique will be equally useful for all adolescents but that we expect at least some of the group members will find each new skill helpful. We ask that all group participants try each new skill and not reject any one out of hand before trying it. In practice, of course, this can be a problem. When a new skill is presented, some youth will claim that they have tried it before and it did not do anything for them. In these cases, we ask that they try the skill again. But if a teen is adamant that he or she will not benefit from a given skill, we ask the teen to respect that other youth in the group may want to learn and benefit from this technique.

The CWDA course therapist is expected to be active and directive. A portion of each session is didactic, in which the therapist presents the basics of new skills. There is the risk that didactic presentations will be dry and boring, so therapists are encouraged to provide frequent opportunities for adolescent participation: asking questions, soliciting youth examples, and so on. Even after the didactic presentation, during practice and individual problem solving, the therapist is expected to be actively assisting participants through coaching, hints, and so on. The only significant exception are those group exercises during which the therapist may wish to withhold comments because group members are providing feedback and advice to one another. With teenagers this peer feedback seems to be especially valued by group members. Even if teens trust and like the group therapist they nonetheless may discount the therapist's feedback because she or he is an adult. Feedback from the other adolescent group members may be more palatable as it comes from a peer "who understands my life."

Homework is also a regular component of the CWDA program, and it is encouraged but voluntary. Early in each session the therapist and group members review the previous session and the assigned homework. Youth who did not complete their homework between sessions often use this period to fill out the forms. Homework is meant to increase adolescent generalization of these new skills to their life outside the therapy session. If homework is not possible or acceptable, therapists should find other methods of promoting skill generalization. One example would be to encourage skills practice immediately before and after sessions, such as engaging in problem solving with parents in the waiting room right after sessions.

CHARACTERISTICS OF THE TREATMENT PROGRAM

The original version of the CWDA program (Clarke, Lewinsohn, & Hops, 2001) is a mixed-gender group consisting of 16 2-hour sessions, typically delivered twice a week over 8 weeks. Group membership is between 6 and 10 depressed adolescents, ages 13 to 18. In our research studies we most often conduct groups with a single therapist, but for training purposes we sometimes include a second, trainee therapist who coleads the group before eventually leading a later group him- or herself. The course is described in a therapist manual with scripted sessions and explanatory narrative. A companion youth workbook is provided to each participating teenager, and it contains relevant exercises and worksheets for acquiring and practicing the CWDA skills.

The adolescent CWDA program is a developmentally appropriate adaptation of the adult Coping With Depression course, developed by Lewinsohn, Steinmetz, Antonuccio, & Teri (1984). We changed the adult program to make it more appropriate for teenagers by simplifying the homework and lectures; using cartoons to illustrate cognitive distortions; adding more participatory exercises; and adding problem-solving, communication, and negotiation skills training to address conflict issues with family, peers, and other adults such as teachers.

Another developmentally relevant change was to create a parallel parent course (Lewinsohn, Rohde, Hops, & Clarke, 1991), meant to be offered to the parents or guardians of youth enrolled in the CWDA treatment program. This parent course consists of eight 1-hour sessions offered once a week on one of the same nights as the teen group. A separate parent group therapist leads these sessions, although for some later sessions the adolescent and parent groups meet together to practice family problem-solving techniques. However, research summarized later (Clarke, Rohde, Lewinsohn, Hops, & Seeley, 1999; Lewinsohn, Clarke, Hops, & Andrews, 1990) suggests that there is little incremental benefit from this parent group over that achieved by the adolescent group alone. Part of the reason for this may be the relatively lackluster parent participation we have experienced, despite several attempts to schedule the parent group at the most convenient times. The parents who seem to attend are those who need it least, whereas those who have clear family conflict are often unavailable.

Who Is Treated?

In all of our treatment outcome trials the target patients are depressed youth, with or without other comorbidities. Major depression and/or dysthymia was a requirement for the CWDA randomized trials (Clarke et al., 1999; Clarke et al., 2002; Lewinsohn et al., 1990; Rohde et al., 2001). However, our impression is that youth with subdiagnostic levels of depression would also benefit. This conclusion is supported by the findings of our two depression prevention randomized trials, which used a prevention program that is a subset of the CWDA program (Clarke, Hawkins, Murphy, & Sheeber, 1995; Clarke et al., 2002). In our earlier, highly controlled CWDA treatment *efficacy* studies (Clarke et al., 1999; Lewinsohn et al., 1990), we excluded a greater number of comorbid conditions than was the case in our prevention studies (Clarke et al., 1995; Clarke, Hornbrook, et al., 2001) and our later, more "real-world" CWDA *effectiveness* trial (Clarke et al., 2002). In general, however, we always excluded youth with active psychotic disorders and bipolar disorder. We often permitted active substance abuse or dependence, as long as youth were not intoxicated while attending sessions. Infrequently we excluded a youth with significant and imminent risk of suicide. However, we included most youth with active suicidal ideation and behavior, as long as the risk was not judged to be extremely high or imminent.

Content of Treatment

As indicated earlier, the original CWDA program is multimodal, consisting of several distinct skills training modules spread throughout the intervention. Figure 7.1 provides a

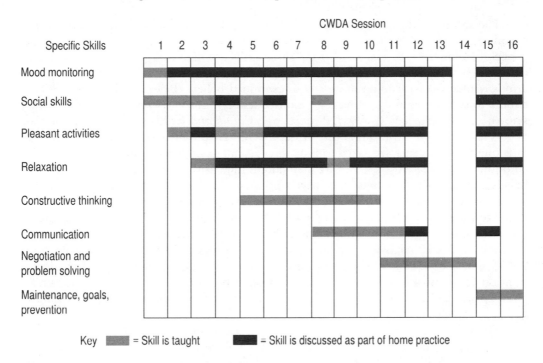

FIGURE 7.1. Timeline of CWDA skills and sessions. From Clarke, Lewinsohn, and Hops (2001). Copyright 2001 by Gregory N. Clarke. Reprinted by permission.

schematic of the skill modules and indicates the sessions in which those skills are addressed. The first session orients teenagers to the course features and presents the general social learning model of depression as justification for the skills training that will come later. We also establish course "ground rules" during the first session; these include confidentiality about what is said in the group, what they can expect of each other, and our expectation that they support each other.

The CWDA intervention has at its core two main intervention components. The first of these is behavioral therapy, also referred to as behavioral activation. This approach involves working with youth to increase their rates of age-appropriate and individually tailored pleasant activities and is primarily addressed in CWDA sessions 2 through 5. Group leaders help youth select a personalized list of 10 to 20 fun activities that they would like to do more often, and collect baseline information on their rates of these activities and their daily moods. In most cases, youth find a positive correlation between their mood and ratings of fun activities, further supporting the rationale for increasing the number of fun activities they do each day. A minority of teens will argue that the causal direction of any association between mood and activities is in the other direction: They only do fun things when they feel good, rather than the other (and more therapeutic) way around. We agree that this may be the case for these teens, but challenge them to test their interpretation by consciously increasing their rate of fun activities and seeing what impact it has (or does not have) on their mood. The later sessions focus on setting small but achievable goals for increasing their activity level, making a written contract with themselves with small rewards for meeting their goals, and problem-solving solutions to barriers to doing more fun activities, such as chores and homework obligations.

The second main component is cognitive therapy and is an adolescent-appropriate modification of Beck's therapy (Beck et al., 1979) and the rational emotive therapy approach of Ellis (Ellis & Harper, 1961). These skills are delivered primarily in sessions 5 through 10. The group therapist initially introduces the basic concepts of triggering situations (Antecedents) leading to mostly unexamined beliefs (Beliefs), which in turn contribute to the development of feelings (Consequences). The early sessions employ widely known cartoons such as *Garfield, Peanuts,* and *Calvin and Hobbes* to illustrate common beliefs leading to frustration, anger, or depression. By the later sessions, these cartoons fade out as adolescents are asked to provide personal examples of situations, beliefs, and emotional reactions. Adolescents are then taught the basics of determining whether these beliefs are irrational, unrealistic, or overly negative and judgmental. In those cases, they are coached through the creation of more realistic positive counterthoughts and then asked to rate how their mood changes with this new belief. Some time may be spent examining family origins of unrealistic thoughts, especially in those circumstances in which we have conducted trials with offspring of depressed parents (Clarke, Hornbrook, et al., 2001). One nice feature of the group versions of the CWDA program is that challenges to negative or unrealistic thoughts can come from other adolescents, rather than from the adult group leader. As previously mentioned, this peer feedback is often more palatable and believable to teenagers.

The CWDA program also includes several subsidiary components, including relaxation training (addressed in sessions 3 and 8) to cope with tension and social anxiety often associated with depression. Teens are taught progressive muscular relaxation methods, and a shorter, more "portable" deep-breathing technique. Successful relaxation is valuable for reducing tension, but it is also helpful in later sessions of the CWDA program to overcome social anxiety that may sabotage other therapy goals such as increasing the frequency of social activities in the pleasant activities section. Another subsidiary component is problem solving, negotiation, and communication skills, addressed in sessions 9 through 14. Adolescents and parents each learn and practice the basics of these skills in their separate groups, with a focus on parent–child conflict. In session 14, teens and patents come together in a single, combined group to employ their recently acquired skills to problem-solve some relatively low-intensity family problems (this explains why few activities are shown in Figure 7.1 for session 14). We do not start with the higher-intensity problems immediately, because feelings about these problems are often so intense that they increase the chances of failure—before the family can lean how to apply the problem-solving skills. Once a family can competently use these skills to address low-intensity conflicts, they are encouraged to gradually address more serious and contentious problems. Finally, because some depressed adolescents have difficulty making and retaining social connections, rudimentary social skills are taught in group sessions 1 through 3 and revisited in sessions 5 and 8. These skills include approaching people and starting conversations, making and maintaining friendships, and practicing positive nonverbal behaviors such as appropriate smiling and eye contact.

Toward the end of the course, the emphasis shifts from specific skills addressing domains of dysfunction to more general topics. These include reviewing long- and short-term goals in several areas (social, academic, family, employment, etc.), identifying barriers to achieving these goals and problem-solving solutions to address these barriers, discussing how to maintain gains by continuing to use the skills they have learned, developing plans to recognize if they become depressed again, and creating a personal depression prevention plan, including what to do in an emergency. Unlike traditional, individual psychotherapy, the end of the CWDA course has only a cursory focus on termination issues. Some time in the final session is spent reviewing individual progress since the beginning of the group, identifying areas of competence and areas still to work on, feelings about the group ending, and a discussion of what each adolescent might do to replace the support that the group may have provided.

Throughout the group, youth are asked to monitor their daily mood on a 7-point scale, which is meant to provide them with an ongoing measure of their progress but is also important for specific exercises related to increasing pleasant activities, described earlier. In general, we find that orienting adolescents to ongoing self-evaluation contributes to the overall self-change, self-improvement approach of the CWDA group.

Although the specific content and skills training varies by session, the structure and within-session sequencing of activities is similar across most group meetings. The typical group session follows this sequence: (1) review of the agenda for that day's session; (2) review of homework from the previous session, including catch-up for those who did not complete homework; (3) didactic presentation of the new skills, emphasizing adolescent examples and participation; (4) practice of the new skills (peer and therapist feedback are both important); (5) problem-solve solutions to barriers to implementing the new skills; and (6) complete homework assignment.

Although we would ideally like all teens to acquire and generalize all the skills taught in the CWDA course, we acknowledge that not every skill will be equally useful for each teen. This is meant to relieve perfectionistic pressure for those teens who believe they must master each module, as well as forestall pessimism among youth who find the first few modules to be either too difficult or not pertinent for them ("Let's see if the next section will be more helpful for you").

How to Determine When Treatment Is "Finished"

The original CWDA program is a group intervention with a fixed duration of 16 2-hour sessions. The "acute phase" course ends at the same time for all participants, regardless of degree of recovery. Therefore, the issue of when treatment is finished is moot. However, recognizing that approximately one third of youth entering the group may not be fully recovered at the end of the course, we developed and tested a continuation component for the CWDA program, consisting of monthly group booster sessions (Clarke et al., 1999). Youth are offered clinically relevant refresher courses in the various skills taught in the acute CWDA program—most often to address new or ongoing problems for one or more of the group members (e.g., a youth still bothered by unrealistic thoughts of guilt and worthlessness would prompt a review of the cognitive restructuring module). We found that youth who were partially recovered at the end of acute treatment and were assigned to this continuation program continued to improve at higher rates (Clarke et al., 1999; summarized later).

The original CWDA program also is a fixed membership group. That is, all youth in a given group are enrolled at the beginning, and no additional youth are added at any later point. Because participating youth need to learn the overall model of depression and the intervention in the early sessions, they may not benefit if they miss this fundamental information by entering the group in later sessions. This restriction sometimes creates difficulty in settings such as inpatient units where census is highly fluid and youth presence may be brief. To address this issue, Rohde[1] and colleagues have created a variation of the CWDA program for use with delinquent adolescents with comorbid depression held for an average of 30 days in a county juvenile detention facility. This version of the program is designed to be used in a circular (endlessly repeating) fashion and permits the entry of new group members between each new skill module. The 16 original CWDA sessions have been divided into three six-session modules consisting of the following skills: (1) first module: social skills, pleasant activities; (2) second module: relaxation, cognitive restructuring; and (3) third module: communication, problem solving, and life goals/maintenance. Because new members are entered into the group at the junction between modules, each new module begins with a reintroduction of the premise of the group, a review of group norms and guidelines, and instructions on how to monitor mood. Group members typically stay in the group for three modules to learn the entire skill repertoire but do not stay in the group indefinitely. Although this variant of the CWDA program has not yet been tested in rigorous outcome studies, our impression is that it seems to work much better than just entering youth at each individual session.

Variants of the CWDA Program

Other, recent modifications of the CWDA program include variations to prevent depression, treating depression in delinquent youth, providing group or individual treatment in managed care settings, and providing adjunct CBT for individual depressed youth (rather than groups) started on selective serotonin reuptake inhibitor medications. All these variants are described later. Robinson[2] (personal communication, November 2001) is developing a culturally relevant version for African American youth, but this version is not yet available and we cannot describe it in detail at this time.

We shortened the CWDA program and focused on a single-skill training module (cognitive restructuring) to develop a group prevention program called the Coping with Stress course. This program consists of 15 1-hour sessions, typically delivered over 5 weeks to groups of 6 to 10 adolescents ages 13 to 18. We have conducted two randomized trials using this intervention with at-risk offspring of depressed parents (Clarke, Hornbrook, et al., 2001) and with youth with subdiagnostic depressive symptoms (Clarke et al., 1995), with positive preventive effects in both studies.

Rohde and colleagues (2001) recently conducted a randomized trial evaluating a slightly modified version of the original CWDA program (not the endlessly repeating variant described above) with depressed youth with comorbid conduct disorder; the results of this study are summarized later. Rohde and colleagues are now in the process of creating a variant of the CWDA program that includes modules to address anger management, impulse control, and other skills relevant to disruptive behavior control (personal communication, November 2001). This new program will focus on prosocial coping to negative emotions, as opposed to the treatment of clinical depression.

Asarnow and Jaycox blended elements of the CWDA program with aspects of the Penn Depression Prevention Program intervention (Jaycox, Reivich, Gillham, & Seligman, 1994). They created brief group and individual versions of a CBT program for use in a quality-improvement randomized trial they are conducting in several private and public mental health settings (Asarnow, Jaycox, & Tompson, 2001).

Our group (Clarke, DeBar, Ludman, Asarnow, & Jaycox, 2001) recently modified the Asarnow and Jaycox CBT program to create a shorter, individual version for depressed youth also receiving antidepressant medication. This "adjunct CBT" variant, currently being evaluated in a randomized effectiveness trial, permits variable duration (from five to nine sessions) depending on the degree of youth recovery/response at the halfway point. The program consists of an initial introductory session, a four-session cognitive restructuring module, and a four-session behavioral activation module. Youth and therapists jointly decide which module to employ first, based on the youth's prior therapy and life experiences and a match with each youth's natural coping strategies. In this "stepped intensity" approach, youth who are still depressed after the first half of the program are continued for an additional four sessions (for a total of nine sessions), whereas youth who are recovered at the fifth session are given the option of continuing with the remaining skill module (to consolidate gains) or discontinuing with an option to restart therapy if depression recurs. In either case, youth receive brief (10-minute) continuation telephone calls on a monthly and then bimonthly basis during the year after acute treatment. These calls check for depression recurrence, provide support, and provide any needed referrals or case management to address other life events that may emerge (pregnancy, family conflict, substance abuse). Finally, because all these youth are being treated with antidepressant medication prescribed by their usual health care physician, the CBT therapist also acts to monitor medication compliance, side effects, benefit from medication (or lack of thereof), and any signs of planning to discontinue medication. Depending on the medication issues, the CBT therapist consults with the prescribing physician and/or youth or family and helps to encourage (and even schedule) follow-up medication visits when necessitated by medication-related issues. The CWDA program has also served as one of the main source materials for the individual CBT intervention currently being employed in a large, multisite, national randomized trial for adolescent depression called the Treatment of Adolescent Depression Study (TADS; March & Vitiello, 2001). Results are not expected for several years.

Finally, we are in the process of creating an Internet-based, self-help variation of the CWDA program for youth who are depressed. This web site is still in development but will ultimately provide on-line, self-guided training and practice of cognitive and behavioral therapy techniques for adolescents with low-grade depression. Our ultimate intent is to conduct randomized trials of this program, perhaps compared to live CWDA therapy groups or to other Internet resources.

How to Obtain Manuals and Supporting Materials

We had originally published the CWDA manual in the traditional manner, through a publisher (Clarke, Lewinsohn, & Hops, 2001). However, we have recently opted for another way to distribute these materials. The therapist manual and adolescent workbook for CWDA are now available only on the Internet at *www.kpchr.org/public/acwd/acwd.html*. Other therapy materials related to the CWDA program, such as the spin-off prevention program (Clarke et al., 1995), are also available there. All these materials are available free of charge and may be photocopied and employed by anyone in any setting. Although we retain copyright, we are also open to modification of these materials by other researchers or clinicians to better serve other audiences or target groups, as long as these modifications are also made freely available. We no longer distribute paper copies of these programs; the Internet site is the only method for obtaining copies of these interventions.

EVIDENCE FOR THE EFFECTS OF TREATMENT

To date, the CWDA course has been evaluated in four randomized trials. In all cases, we have used a structured psychiatric interview, the Children's Schedule for Affective Disorders and Schizophrenia (K-SADS), to diagnose major depression, dysthymia, and other comorbid disorders. Other self- and parent report measures were also administered in these studies but are not reported here.

The first two of these studies (Clarke et al., 1999; Lewinsohn et al., 1990) shared the same basic design. Youth diagnosed with major depression and/or dysthymia according to the third edition of the *Diagnostic and Statistical Manual of Mental Disorders* (DSM-III; American Psychiatric Association, 1980) were randomly assigned to one of three conditions: (1) youth enrolled in the group CWDA course, but no parent involvement; (2) youth enrolled in the CWDA course and parents enrolled in the parallel parent group; or (3) a wait-list control condition. In the first trial, 59 depressed youth were randomized (Lewinsohn et al., 1990); in the second trial 123 depressed youth were randomized (Clarke et al., 1999). The principal outcome was recovery from major depression and/or dysthymia at posttreatment and through a 2-year follow-up period. Compared to the wait-list condition, the active treatment conditions resulted in significantly more depression recovery in both studies. The posttreatment depression recovery rate in this first study was 46% for the treatment groups versus 5% for the control condition. The second study found higher depression recovery rates in the treatment groups (67%) than in the wait-list condition (48%). However, contrary to expectations there were few or no significant advantages for parent involvement in either study.

The second CWDA study (Clarke et al., 1999) also included a linked but separate trial of a continuation treatment following the end of the acute treatment phase (the 8-week CWDA course). The continuation program (described earlier) aimed to improve ongoing recovery from depression and minimize relapse. Youth who had completed the acute phase CWDA groups were randomly reassigned to one of three conditions for the remaining 24-month follow-up period: (1) assessments every 4 months with monthly booster sessions, (2) assessments only every 4 months, or (3) assessments only every 12 months. The booster sessions did not reduce the rate of depression recurrence in the follow-up period but did accelerate recovery among depressed youth who were still depressed at the end of the acute phase CWDA groups.

More recently, Rohde et al. (2001) completed a randomized trial of the CWDA program for depressed, delinquent youth recruited through local juvenile justice departments. Ninety-six youth ages 13 through 17 meeting DSM-IV (American Psychiatric Association, 1994) criteria for major depression or dysthymia and conduct disorder were randomized to either the CWDA course, or to a life-skills tutoring course (an attention–placebo control condition). Depression recovery at posttreatment was 26% in the CWDA condition versus 14% in the life-skills condition (odds ratio = 3.4, 95% confidence interval = 1.3–9.3). However, by 12 months posttreatment there were no differences between conditions for depression outcomes. There were also no differences for overall conduct disorder diagnoses at any time point, although youth in the CWDA condition had lower levels of aggression/rule violation symptoms immediately following acute treatment (this advantage disappeared by the final, 12-month follow-up). Overall, we detected a modest acute treatment advantage for the CWDA program for depression but not conduct disorder, but this advantage did not persist over the yearlong follow-up.

Finally, we recently completed a randomized, effectiveness trial of the CWDA course for depressed adolescent offspring of depressed patents (Clarke et al., 2002). Potentially depressed adults were found by reviewing antidepressant medication dispenses, mental health appointments, and medical charts in the health maintenance organization (HMO) where this trial was conducted. Informational letters signed by each parent's treating physician were mailed to the appropriate adults. Eligible offspring ages 13 to 18 who met current DSM-III-R (American Psychiatric Association, 1987) criteria for major depression and/or dysthymia were randomized to either usual HMO care (*n* = 47) or usual care plus the CWDA program ($n = 41$). We were unable to detect any significant advantage for the CBT program over usual care at posttreatment, or over the 24-month follow-up, for any depression or other outcomes. This study failed to find significant benefit for the CWDA program, in contrast to the other three randomized trials that did find an effect (Clarke et al., 1999; Lewinsohn et al., 1990; Rohde et al., 2001). The reasons are not clear, but it may be because the comparison condition in the Clarke et al. (2002) study was another active depression treatment: usual care in this HMO consisting primarily of brief psychotherapy and/or antidepressant medication. This was not the case in the other three trials, where the comparison condition was either wait-list or an attention placebo condition with no focus on depression.

Although this chapter is primarily about the CWDA treatment program, we have also conducted several studies of a depression prevention program, the Coping with Stress (CWS) course, that is derived from and closely related to the CWDA intervention. In both these randomized trials with high-risk youth (Clarke et al., 1995; Clarke, Hornbrook, et al., 2001) we found significant preventive effects for the CWS program, with significantly fewer prospective cases of major depression among youth participating in the prevention program compared to youth in the usual care control condition.

We have examined the effects of mediators and moderators on outcomes for the first randomized trial of the CWDA treatment program (Clarke, Hops, Lewinsohn, & Andrews, 1992). We found that improved depression diagnostic outcomes were associated with greater number of past psychiatric diagnoses, parent involvement in treatment, and younger age at onset of first depressive episode. Improved depression self-report scores were associated with lower intake depression and anxiety, higher enjoyment and frequency of pleasant activities, and more rational thoughts. Interestingly, we failed to find any association between degree of "between-session" homework completion and improved outcome (Clarke et al., 1992). It may be that homework completed between sessions plays no role in improving depression. However, the fact that noncompliant youth have a chance to "make up" their homework at the beginning of each session may diminish the statistical association between homework completion and outcome

In each of our outcome studies we have measured therapist fidelity to the CWDA manual, using a scale developed for this purpose (Clarke, 1998). Fidelity is typically high, with mean ratings ranging between 78 and 94% compliance with the defined program. However, therapist fidelity is rated for one therapist treating many youth in a group, and outcome is recorded for individual youth. All these youth in a given group have highly variable depression recovery but are exposed to the same level of therapist treatment fidelity. Because of this "data mismatch" between a group therapist and individual youth outcomes, we have not been able to analytically examine the relationship between the two (see Clarke, 1998, for more details).

We have also examined the importance of youth participant adherence with the program. One aspect of adherence is homework completion, discussed earlier. Another aspect is attendance, which might be seen as a proxy for "dose." In two studies (Clarke et al., 1992, 1999) we failed to find an association between number of sessions attended and depression outcomes. In child psychotherapy in general, there have been mixed findings regarding the relationship between psychotherapy dose and outcomes. Two problems are that treatment attendance may be at least partly dependent on rapidity of recovery (those that recover quickly are more likely to drop out prematurely, having reached a personal level of satisfactory recovery) and on depression severity (those that are more disordered may be more inclined to stay in treatment longer). Both of these factors would lead to a pattern of lower doses associated with better outcomes and higher doses associated with poorer outcomes, contrary to the expected dose relationship.

A final treatment process issue is the degree to which teenagers acquire new knowledge and skills as a function of attending group sessions, the degree to which this knowledge translates to new "antidepressant" behaviors skills that generalize beyond therapy sessions, and then finally the degree to which these skills lead to recovery from depression. We have not yet tested this entire causal pathway in a single study, but various elements are being examined in separate studies currently under way. For example, working with data from a randomized trial of the CWDA program with delinquent and depressed youth described later in this chapter (Rohde et al., 2001), Kaufman and Rohde (personal communication, November 2001) have found that depression improvement is partially mediated by change on social skills and fully mediated by change on constructive thinking.

DIRECTIONS FOR FUTURE RESEARCH

Despite the progress we have made, there are still several unanswered questions about the CWDA course. One principal remaining hurdle is a randomized trial of the CWDA program conducted by researchers other than ourselves, in order to get beyond the "founders effect." Another limitation of the extant CWDA studies is our reliance on white, mostly middle-class participants. Three of the CWDA trials were conducted with fairly homogeneous samples of white, middle-class depressed youth with only limited comorbidity. One CWDA study has been conducted with depressed youth with comorbid conduct disorder (Rohde et al., 2001), but these were still predominantly white youth. However, Robinson has recently received funding to modify the CWDA program for use with inner-city African American youth, with outcome studies to follow.

Similar modifications and studies need to be conducted with many other special populations. For example, we have given some thought to variations of the CWDA program for single-gender groups, on the assumption that the dynamics of these groups might enhance outcomes as well as to take advantage of what is emerging about differences in depression among teenage girls and boys. Wisdom[3] has created a version of the CWDA program for girl-only groups (personal communication, December 2001). The revised group includes both discussing the real-world stressors the girls experience within the context of the cognitive and behavioral modules and teaching skills to help girls analyze messages about stereotypes, communicate clearly and assertively, and maintain healthy relationships. This variation has been piloted but has not yet been tested in a randomized trial. Conducting more rigorous evaluations of this and related variations is a high priority.

SUMMARY AND CONCLUSIONS

In the decade since the publication of both the CWDA manual (Clarke et al., 1990) and our first randomized trial (Lewinsohn et al., 1990), we have conducted three other randomized trials of this program. We have also broadened the target population to include depressed teenagers with comorbid conduct disorder as well as children of depressed parents. Several special purpose variations of the CWDA program have been created by ourselves and others for prevention, individual CBT, and use with special populations. With one exception (Clarke, Hornbrook, et al., 2001), all the studies of the CWDA program or its spin-off programs have yielded significant, positive treatment or prevention results. Somewhat surprising, the addition of a companion parent group does not significantly improve outcomes. In general, we conclude that the CWDA course has been moderately well tested and is certainly well along the continuum toward becoming an evidence-based treatment. However, we still need to test the benefit of the CWDA program with special populations, particularly minority adolescents, teenagers with greater psychiatric comorbidity, and same-gender groups.

Dissemination and adoption of the CWDA program in practice settings remains a challenge. We developed the original CWDA course as a psychoeducational program in part to facilitate its adoption in practice settings, particularly where groups of adolescents would be easy to form—such as schools and day treatment facilities. The highly scripted therapist manual and youth workbook were meant to provide clear direction for therapists new to CBT. Despite these features, we have heard that it is practically difficult for providers in many traditional settings to bring together a sufficient number of depressed youth at the same time in order to start a fixed-membership, fixed-duration group of any kind. This feedback has led us to develop the circular (endlessly repeating) modification of the CWDA course and the individual brief (five- to nine-session) variation. We believe that both of these adaptations of the CWDA program will ease adoption in practice settings.

NOTES

1. Paul Rohde, PhD, can be reached at the Oregon Research Institute, 1715 Franklin Boulevard, Eugene, OR 97403.
2. LaVome Robinson, PhD, can be reached at the Department of Psychology, DePaul University, 2219 North Kenmor, Chicago, IL 60614.
3. Jennifer Wisdom, PhD, can be reached at the Kaiser Permanente Center for Health Research, 3800 North Interstate Avenue, Portland, OR 97227.

REFERENCES

Asarnow, J. R, Jaycox, L. H., & Tompson, M. C. (2001). Depression in youth: Psychosocial interventions. *Journal of Clinical Child Psychology, 30,* 33–47.

Beck, A. T., Rush, A. J., Shaw, B. F., & Emory, G. (1979). *Cognitive therapy of depression.* New York: Guilford Press.

Birmaher, B., Ryan, N. D., Williamson, D. E., Brent D. A., Kaufman, J., Dahl, R. E., Perel, J., & Nelson, B. (1996). Childhood and adolescent depression: A review of the past 10 years. Part I. *Journal of the American Academy of Child and Adolescent Psychiatry, 35,* 1427–1439.

Clarke, G. N. (1998). Intervention fidelity in adolescent depression prevention and treatment. *Journal of Prevention and Intervention in the Community, 17,* 19–33.

Clarke, G. N., DeBar, L. L., Ludman, E., Asarnow, J. R., & Jaycox, L. H. (2001). *Collaborative care, cognitive-behavioral program for depressed youth in a primary care setting.* Retrieved February 17, 2003, from the Kaiser Permanente Center for Health Research website: *http://www.kpchr.org/public/acwd/acwd.html*

Clarke, G. N., Hawkins, W., Murphy, M., & Sheeber, L. B. (1995). Targeted prevention of unipolar depressive disorder in an at-risk sample of high school adolescents: A randomized trial of group cognitive intervention. *Journal of the American Academy of Child and Adolescent Psychiatry, 34,* 312–321.

Clarke, G. N., Hops, H., Lewinsohn, P. M., & Andrews, J. (1992). Cognitive-behavioral group treatment of adolescent depression: Prediction of outcome. *Behavior Therapy, 23,* 341–354.

Clarke, G. N., Hornbrook, M. C., Lynch, F. L., Polen, M., Gale, J., Beardslee, W. R., O'Connor, E., & Seeley, J. R. (2001). A randomized trial of a group cognitive intervention for preventing depression in adolescent offspring of depressed parents. *Archives of General Psychiatry, 58,* 1127–1134.

Clarke, G. N., Hornbrook, M. C., Lynch, F. L., Polen, M., Gale, J., O'Connor, E. A., Seeley, J., & DeBar, L. L. (2002). Group cognitive behavioral treatment for depressed adolescent offspring of depressed parents in an HMO. *Journal of the American Academy of Child and Adolescent Psychiatry, 41,* 305–313.

Clarke, G. N., Lewinsohn, P. M., & Hops. H. (2001). *Instructor's manual for the Adolescent Coping with Depression course.* Retrieved April 5, 2002, from Kaiser Permanente Center for Health Research website: *www.kpchr.org/public/acwd/acwd.html*

Clarke, G. N., Rohde, P., Lewinsohn, P. M., Hops, H., & Seeley, J. R. (1999). Cognitive-behavioral treatment of adolescent depression: Efficacy of acute group treatment and booster sessions. *Journal of the American Academy of Child and Adolescent Psychiatry, 38,* 272–279.

Ellis, A., & Harper, R. A. (1961). *A guide to rational living.* Hollywood, CA: Wilshire Books.

Jaycox, L. H., Reivich, K. J., Gillham, J., & Seligman, M. E. (1994). Prevention of depressive symptoms in school children. *Behaviour Research and Therapy, 32,* 801–816.

Lewinsohn, P. M., Clarke, G. N., Hops, H., & Andrews, J. A. (1990). Cognitive-behavioral treatment for depressed adolescents. *Behavior Therapy, 21,* 385–401.

Lewinsohn, P. M., Clarke, G. N., Seeley, J. R., & Rohde, P. (1994). Major depression in community adolescents: Age at onset, episode duration, and time to recurrence. *Journal of the American Academy of Child and Adolescent Psychiatry, 33,* 809–818.

Lewinsohn, P. M., Hoberman, H. M., Teri, L., & Hautzinger, M. (1985). An integrative theory of unipolar depression. In S. Reiss & R. R. Bootzin (Eds.), *Theoretical issues in behavioral therapy* (pp. 313–359). New York: Academic Press.

Lewinsohn, P. M., Hops, H., Roberts, R. E., Seeley, J. R., & Andrews, J. A. (1993). Adolescent psychopathology: I. Prevalence and incidence of depression and other DSM-III-R disorders in high school students. *Journal of Abnormal Psychology, 102,* 133–144.

Lewinsohn, P. M., Rohde, P., Hops, H., & Clarke, G. N. (1991). *The Coping With Depression Course—Adolescent version: Instructor's manual for the parent course.* Retrieved April 5, 2002, from Kaiser Permanente Center for Health Research website: *www.kpchr.org/public/acwd/acwd.html*

Lewinsohn, P. M., Steinmetz, J. L., Antonuccio, D. O., & Teri, L. (1984). A behavioral group therapy approach to the treatment of depression. In D. Upper & S. M. Ross (Eds.), *Handbook of behavioral group therapy* (pp. 303–329). New York: Plenum Press.

March, J. S., & Vitiello, B. (2001). Advances in paediatric neuropsychopharmacology: An overview. *International Journal of Neuropsychopharmacology, 4,* 141–147.

Rohde, P., Clarke, G. N., Mace, D. E., Jorgensen, J., Seeley, J. R., & Gau, J. (2001, October). *Cognitive-behavioral treatment for depressed adolescents with comorbid conduct disorder.* Paper presented at the annual conference of the American Academy of Child and Adolescent Psychiatry, Honolulu.

Rohde, P., Lewinsohn, P. M., & Seeley, J. R. (1991). Comorbidity of unipolor depression: II. Comorbidity with other mental disorders in adolescents and adults. *Journal of Abnormal Psychology, 100,* 214–222.

8

Cognitive-Behavioral Therapy for Adolescent Depression

Comparative Efficacy, Mediation, Moderation, and Effectiveness

V. Robin Weersing and David A. Brent

OVERVIEW

A growing body of naturalistic studies has documented that depression in youth, particularly during adolescence, is common, of relatively long duration, and recurrent. Specifically, depression has a point prevalence among adolescents of approximately 5%, may produce long-lasting impairments in social and occupational functioning (e.g., Rohde, Lewinsohn, & Seeley, 1994), and substantially increases the risk of early mortality by suicide (e.g., Brent et al., 1993).

This chapter provides an overview of our laboratory's program of research on the treatment of depression and suicidality in adolescents. Many of the findings we report are drawn from the Brent et al. (1997) clinical trial, which tested the effects of cognitive-behavioral therapy (CBT), systemic-behavioral family treatment (SBFT), and nondirective supportive therapy (NST). Data from this investigation have been used to evaluate the efficacy of CBT relative to alternate treatments, probe possible mechanisms of CBT action, and delineate moderators of treatment effects. In addition to these core clinical trial findings, we present preliminary results from three recent projects: (1) investigating the efficacy of CBT with seriously suicidal youth (Barbe, Bridge, Birmaher, Kolko, & Brent, 2002); (2) testing the effects of CBT with "treatment resistant" youth who have already failed a medication protocol for depression; and (3) probing the effectiveness of CBT for adolescent depression under conditions approximating real-world clinical practice (Weersing, Weisz, & Brent, 2002).

Conceptual Models Underlying Treatment

Factors implicated in the onset and maintenance of depression in youth fall into two broad, conceptual categories: (1) intraindividual cognitive and biological vulnerabilities (e.g., depressogenic information processing; Gladstone & Kaslow, 1995); and (2) interpersonal and environmental factors (e.g., family expressed emotion; Asarnow, Goldstein, Tompson, & Guthrie, 1993). In the Brent et al. (1997) clinical trial, CBT and SBFT were chosen as representatives of these two plausible and conceptually distinct approaches to treating depression. CBT attempts to alleviate the symptoms of depression by changing youths' cognitive distortions, encouraging activities that promote positive mood, and teaching teens problem-solving skills to promote better coping with negative life events. In contrast, SBFT focuses on interpersonal antecedents of depression by working to reduce family conflict, improve intrafamilial support, and improve family communication patterns. Next, we provide a brief overview of the relevant theories and empirical findings related to these treatment models.

Cognitive Vulnerability Model

Several theories of depression fall under the umbrella of the cognitive vulnerability model. The most well-known of these is the cognitive theory of depression developed by Beck and colleagues (see Beck, Rush, Shaw, & Emery, 1979). In brief, Beck et al. noted that depressed individuals have inaccurate, overly negative views of themselves, the world, and possibilities for the future—a negative cognitive triad of depressogenic beliefs. This cognitive triad is hypothesized to be resistant to disconfirmation by contradictory positive information, in part because of systematic errors in depressed individuals' information processing (e.g., selective abstraction of negative information). At a deeper level, both the cognitive triad and errors in information processing are thought to derive from more stable cognitive structures, or schemas. Schemas are core beliefs and recollections that organize past experience and, when activated by internal or external stimuli, bring that past experience to bear on the current situation. Depressogenic schemas are thought to develop from early negative experiences, to become activated during analogous stressful circumstances in the present, and to predispose the individual to dysfunctional beliefs and errors in processing information and, thus, symptoms of depression.

The Beck model was developed to describe and explain adult depression; however, there is evidence to suggest that depressed adolescents display similar patterns of negative beliefs and errors in information processing (see Gladstone & Kaslow, 1995, for review). Data also indicate that a depressogenic cognitive style may precede actual symptoms of depression in adolescents and may serve as a risk factor for future depressive episodes (Lewinsohn et al., 1994; Lewinsohn, Allen, Seeley, & Gotlib, 1999). Given this evidence, a cognition-focused intervention was included in the Brent et al. (1997) clinical trial, based in large part on the adult treatment program developed by Beck.

Negative Life Events and Family Conflict

Experiencing negative, uncontrollable events has been linked to helplessness and apathy in both humans and animals (see Abramson, Seligman, & Teasdale, 1978). In adolescents, first onset and recurrence of depression are often preceded by negative psychosocial events, including family conflict, physical illness, breakup of romantic relationships, and loss of friendships (Lewinsohn et al., 1999). Of these, familial stress may play a particularly important role; parental depression, parent–child conflict, parental divorce, low family cohesion, and high levels of "expressed emotion" have all been found to increase the risk of depression in adolescents (e.g., Asarnow et al., 1993; Lewinsohn et al., 1994).

In CBT, treatment addresses these environmental factors by targeting irrational, overly negative thoughts about these events and by teaching general problem-solving and hypothesis-testing skills to enable patients to better cope with and solve life problems. Given the strength of evidence linking familial factors to the onset, maintenance, and recurrence of depression in adolescents, an explicitly family-based intervention (SBFT) also was included in the clinical trial design. The SBFT intervention was crafted to directly address the negative family context that may produce depression in youth.

CHARACTERISTICS OF THE TREATMENT PROGRAMS

The Brent et al. (1997) clinical trial investigated the efficacy of psychosocial interventions for adolescent depression. Youths, ages 13 to 18, with major depressive disorder were randomly assigned to one of three treatments: CBT, SBFT, and NST. The sample of depressed youths was predominantly Caucasian and female and suffered from moderate rates of comorbidity. Study design and sample characteristics are provided in greater detail in the section on treatment evidence and efficacy.

As described previously, CBT and SBFT were designed to address specific etiological factors thought to underlie the onset and maintenance of depression in teens. NST was included in the clinical trial design to control for nonspecific aspects of treatment, such as therapist attention and warmth. All interventions met for the same number of sessions (12 to 16, plus boosters) and on a similar schedule (weekly in the active phase, plus two to four monthly booster sessions). Parents of youth in all three cells also were provided psychoeducation about the nature and seriousness of depressive illness (Brent, Poling, McKain, & Baugher, 1993). We next describe the specific aspects of each treatment, providing the greatest detail about the CBT intervention and briefer coverage of the comparison treatment conditions.

Cognitive-Behavioral Treatment

Format and Duration

CBT was delivered individually to depressed adolescents on a weekly schedule. Youth received between 12 and 16 sessions of the active intervention and were eligible to receive up to four additional booster treatment sessions over a 4-month follow-up period. Therapists presented themselves as collaborators and coaches and encouraged teens to take an active role in their own recovery. Occasionally, therapists would be in contact with parents to provide general information about the progress of treatment; however, as CBT was to be compared against an explicitly family-based model (SBFT), these sessions were kept to a minimum.

Content of Treatment and Skills Taught

CBT sessions focused primarily on altering the irrational, overly negative cognitions viewed to be at the root of depressive symptomatology. Youth were taught to identify their automatic thoughts, accurately label thoughts as distorted or overly pessimistic, and challenge their depressive thinking about themselves and the world.

In addition to focusing on depressogenic cognitions, CBT therapists targeted difficulties in affect regulation and impulsivity, particularly as related to self-injurious, risky, and suicidal behaviors. Youth were taught how to identify their feelings, use behavioral activities and distraction to regulate mood, and solve problems in a calm and logical manner. These general problem-solving skills were viewed as an important both for alleviating symptoms in the current depressive episode and for their ability to aid in relapse prevention by helping adolescents to effectively cope with future negative life events and interpersonal difficulties.

Developmental Adaptation of the Beck Model

This CBT treatment protocol represents a developmental adaptation of the classic Beck CBT approach. As adolescents are not autonomous agents, despite their desires to be so, a family psychoeducation component (Brent, Poling, et al., 1993) was added to gain parent support for treatment attendance, goals, and completion of homework assignments. The collaborative empiricism of Beck et al. (1979) was articulated to adolescents, often seeking independence from adult authorities, as "I'm going to teach you how to be your own therapist." As teens frequently do not complete homework, *in vivo* experiences, such as monitoring cognitions associated with in-session affective shifts, were used to illustrate and socialize the adolescent to the cognitive model.

Because adolescents present with a wide range of cognitive abilities and prior experience with treatment, it may be necessary to educate adolescent clients to the "language" and process of psychotherapy. To accomplish this goal, the CBT therapists summarized, or had the adolescent summarize, frequently in session to be sure that the therapist and young client were indeed speaking the same language. Throughout treatment, the level of abstraction was kept to a minimum and concrete examples, linked to youths' personal experience, were used whenever possible.

Comparison Treatments

The family-based intervention included in the trial, SBFT, was a combination of two treatments that have been used effectively with dysfunctional families of adolescents. The first phase of SBFT employed the methods of functional family therapy (Alexander & Parsons, 1982). The therapist attempted to clarify the concerns that brought the family to treatment and to redefine the adolescent patient's problem as a problem both for and of the entire family system. In this process, the therapist worked to engage the entire family in solving this problem. Dysfunctional patterns of interaction and inappropriate alliances were identified, and the relationship between these family problems and the patient's symptoms were elucidated. Following this problem definition stage, the second phase of SBFT was more behavioral in focus and was based on the model articulated by Robin and Foster (1989). Family members were encouraged to try out new patterns of interaction and were given positive practice assignments within session and for homework. Family members also were coached to improve their communication skills more generally in order to better solve family problems in the future.

In addition, NST was included in the clinical trial to control for nonspecific aspects of the therapeutic experience such as therapist time and attention, the provision of a warm trusting relationship, and the passage of time. These elements of treatment are common to all forms of therapy, and although they may be necessary for treatment success, they may not be sufficient. In NST, youth were encouraged to explore and express their feelings. Therapists adopted a warm, nonjudgmental, and nondirective stance, offering general support, reflection and clarifications, and messages of hope. Therapists did not provide specific instructions for changing life circumstances or feelings and did not interpret teens' statements or encourage them to adopt a different perspective when evaluating their lives.

Treatment Manuals and Therapist Training

Detailed manuals were created for CBT, SBFT, and NST.[1] Readers are referred to Brent et al. (1996) for additional discussion of the CBT, SBFT and NST manual content and for sample case illustrations.

Therapists in the clinical trial were master's-level clinicians, with a median of 10 years of professional experience treating distressed adolescents. Before participating in the treatment study, each therapist received 6 months of intensive treatment-specific training. To be certified for participation in the study, therapists were required to treat two cases with the appropriate treatment manual to criterion. During the clinical trial, therapists were provided with ongoing supervision, and therapy tapes were rated for adherence. As a check on treatment integrity, a random 25% of session tapes from each therapy condition were rated by external consultants expert in each of the three treatment models. Analyses of these ratings indicated that the three types of treatment were readily discernable from each other and that sessions within each modality were of "acceptable" quality or better (over 90% of sessions rated, across all cells).

EVIDENCE FOR THE EFFECTS OF TREATMENT

Design of the 1997 Clinical Trial

Depressed adolescents were recruited from two sources: (1) the Child and Adolescent Mood and Anxiety Disorder Clinic at Western Psychiatric Institute and Clinic (two-thirds), and (2) newspaper advertisements (one-third). Youth were screened for presence of DSM-III-R major depressive disorder (MDD) and were required to evidence Beck Depression Inventory (BDI; Beck, Steer, & Garbin, 1988) scores in at least the borderline clinical range (greater than or equal to 13). Youth were excluded from the study if they met criteria for psychosis, bipolar disorder, obsessive–compulsive disorder, eating disorder, recent substance abuse, current physical or sexual abuse, pregnancy, or chronic physical illness. Youth were between the ages of 13 and 18 and of normal intelligence. The sample was predominantly Caucasian (85%) and female (75%) and had moderate rates of comorbid anxiety disorder (32%) and dysthymia (22%).

One hundred and seven youth met entry criteria and were randomly assigned to CBT, SBFT, or NST. As described previously, youth were seen for 12 to 16 sessions of active treatment and were eligible for up to four follow-up booster appointments. Assessments were conducted at intake, the sixth treatment session, treatment termination, every 3 months in the first year following termination, and 2 years after termination. Primary outcome measures were diagnostic status, self-rated depression symptoms on the BDI, interviewer-rated depression, and functional status. In addition, information was collected on youths' feelings of hopelessness, cognitive distortions, and suicidality. Parents' current and lifetime psychopathology was assessed, as were family environment variables.

Status of the Evidence

Comparative Efficacy of CBT, SBFT, and NST

At posttreatment assessment, CBT appeared to be most efficacious intervention for depression. Significantly more of the depressed teens receiving CBT (83%) no longer met diagnostic criteria for MDD, compared to youth who received NST (58%). Full clinical remission[2] of depression symptoms also was more common in the CBT cell (60%) than in either NST (39%) or SBFT (38%). In addition, CBT youth experienced improvement in their BDI scores more quickly than did youth in SBFT, and they improved on interviewer-rated depression symptoms more quickly than youth in SBFT or in NST. Treatments did not differ in their effects on functioning or suicidality, although serious suicidality moderated depression treatment efficacy (discussed further later).

Despite the results favoring CBT at posttreatment, there were no differences in depression between treatment groups at 2-year follow-up (Birmaher et al., 2000). In terms of current MDD, descriptive data did favor CBT (6%) over SBFT (23%) and NST (26%), although these rates were not significantly different.

Treatment Expectancy and Credibility

At intake, parents and youth viewed all three treatments as equally credible and expected positive improvement. Over the course of treatment, parents' positive views of CBT were maintained, whereas parents' views of treatment credibility deteriorated for adolescents in both SBFT and NST.

Predictors of Treatment Effects and Moderators

Across treatment cells, poorer posttreatment response was predicted by greater cognitive distortion, higher levels of hopelessness, more severe depression at intake, older youth age, and referral from clinical sources rather than newspaper advertisement. For the sample as a whole, intake depression severity predicted failure to recover from depression, a chronic course, and recurrences over the follow-up period (Birmaher et al., 2000). Parent–child conflict, both at intake and over follow-up, similarly predicted lack of recovery, chronicity, and recurrence. Across cells, youth with "double depression" (comorbid depression and dysthymia) were more likely to withdraw from the study due to failure to respond to treatment.

In terms of treatment moderators, CBT appeared to be the best treatment for youth with serious suicidality (attempt and/or ideation with plan; Barbe et al., 2002). CBT was equally efficacious for treating depression in those with current or lifetime suicidality as in those without such a history. In contrast, NST did particularly poorly in treating depression in those with current or lifetime suicidality, compared to those without such a history (response rate of 26% vs. 64%). This finding was mediated by the differential impact of CBT versus NST on decreasing feelings of hopelessness. In addition, CBT was particularly more efficacious than the other interventions when youth met criteria for a comorbid anxiety disorder. Finally, maternal depressive symptoms also moderated treatment efficacy, insofar as the presence of maternal depression eliminated the generally superior effect of CBT.

In sum, youths with severe and chronic depressions (e.g., double depression, greater cognitive distortions) experienced worse outcomes across a variety of domains. There also was evidence to suggest that negative family environment (e.g., maternal depression, family conflict) boded poorly for treatment outcome. Perhaps most important, CBT continued to be superior to SBFT and to NST when controlling for all these adverse predictors, and, moreover, the efficacy of CBT did not significantly deteriorate with increasing numbers of adverse predictors (Brent et al., 1998).

Predictors of Additional Service Use

Over the course of the follow-up assessment period, more than half of the clinical trial participants sought additional treatment (Brent, Kolko, Birmaher, Baugher, & Bridge, 1999). Although CBT was the most efficacious intervention in the short term, youth who received CBT were no less likely to seek additional services than youth in the comparison treatment conditions. Treatment was most often sought for additional difficulties with depression (62%), but therapy was also obtained for general family problems (33%) and for youth acting-out behavioral problems (31%). Given these target complaints, it is not surprising that intake depression severity, comorbid disruptive behavior problems, and family difficulties predicted additional service use across treatment cells.

Mechanisms of Action

Our research group has conducted three studies to evaluate the mechanisms of action in CBT. In the first, Kolko, Brent, Baugher, Bridge, and Birmaher (2000) investigated the mediating role of cognitive and family process variables in producing the 1997 clinical trial outcomes. As hypothesized, CBT did produce significant, specific changes on a measure of cognitive distortions compared to SBFT and NST. However, CBT was not superior to the comparison treatments in changing feelings of hopelessness.[3] In addition, contrary to hypotheses, CBT was as effective as SBFT in changing general family functioning and was more effective than SBFT in improving marital satisfaction and parents' feelings of behavioral control. Thus, although CBT affected one theoretically specific mechanism of cognitive change, it also produced nonspecific changes in "mediators" belonging to another theoretical model of intervention (SBFT). Furthermore, these specific changes in cognitive distortions did not statistically mediate the effects of CBT on self-rated depression symptoms.[4]

Two additional studies examined the shape of change in depression symptoms over the course of treatment for clues to mechanisms of therapeutic action (Gaynor et al., in press; Renaud et al., 1998). In the first investigation, youth were identified who showed a "rapid response" to treatment, namely, an improvement of 50% or more in BDI scores between pretreatment and the second session of therapy. These rapid responders had received little "active intervention" by the second session of treatment, and the three treatment groups—CBT, SBFT, and NST—did not differ in the number of rapid responders (31% of sample, overall). Taken together, these results suggest that rapid response to treatment was likely due to nonspecific intervention factors, such as therapist warmth. Of note, the relationship between nonspecific, rapid response and treatment outcome varied by intervention. Pairwise comparisons revealed that youth in NST were much less likely to achieve clinical remission of depression, if they failed to experience a rapid response to intervention by the second treatment session. This was true for NST youth at posttreatment (21% vs. 100%) and follow-up assessment (55% vs. 88%). Although these data did not shed immediate light on the mechanism of action in CBT, they did imply that our placebo-control intervention, NST, most likely did operate through nonspecific mechanisms of action, such as remoralization. The data also suggested that the overall effects CBT and SBFT were not dependent on an early placebo response to treatment.

In Gaynor et al. (in press), we sought to build on the Renauld study by investigating the effects of large, sudden improvements occurring during the course of treatment. It has been hypothesized that "sudden gains" *during* depression treatment are a CBT-specific mechanism of action. Sudden gains are thought to result from the cognitive consolidation of CBT lessons—an "aha!" experience, after which patients experience rapid relief from depression. Our study was the first to investigate sudden gains in an adolescent population, and we were among the first to compare rates and effects of sudden gains across different types of treatment.

Results of the study did not support the hypothesis that sudden gains are a CBT-specific mechanism of action. There was a similar rate of sudden gains across CBT, SBFT, and NST (39% overall). Moreover, sudden gains were associated with positive outcome across all three types of treatment. There was a marginally significant interaction indicating that youth who failed to achieve a sudden improvement during treatment fared better in CBT than in the comparison conditions. Taken together with the equivalent rates of sudden gains across cells, these data may indicate that (1) sudden gains are a nonspecific treatment phenomenon, and (2) the superior effects of CBT at posttreatment may be a result of gradual acquisition of cognitive restructuring and problem-solving skills over the course of treatment.

DIRECTIONS FOR FUTURE RESEARCH

Interventions for Treatment-Resistant Depression

There appears to be a need to boost the acute treatment efficacy of CBT for a subset of treatment-resistant youth. Adolescents with dysthymia comorbid with major depression were significantly more likely to drop out of the Brent et al. (1997) clinical trial, and global severity of depression at intake predicted a poor course over the 2-year follow-up period. Data with adult samples support the value of combination treatments—CBT plus medication—for chronically and severely depressed individuals (Keller et al., 2000). In our own work, we are currently testing the efficacy of a combination CBT + SSRI treatment for adolescents who have failed a previous community trial of antidepressant medication.[5]

For this investigation, the 1997 CBT treatment protocol was modified in a number of respects. It seemed likely that a sample of treatment-resistant youth would (1) present with severe and clinically complicated depression, (2) meet criteria for a number of comorbid diagnoses, and (3) have significant mood lability and high levels of suicidality. Accordingly, crisis-intervention modules were built into the revised CBT treatment as well as greater emphasis on teaching problem-solving and affect regulation skills. The structure of the original treatment manual also was substantially deconstructed. All the manual components were repackaged as modules, rather than sessions. Therapists thus were given greater flexibility to spend multiple sessions on critical skills and customize treatment for youths' personalities and life circumstances. Families also have been afforded a greater role in treatment than in the original 1997 CBT clinical trial. Given the central role of parent–child conflict in referral, recovery, and treatment of adolescent depression, a CBT approach to family problem solving was included as an explicit part of the treatment package.

This project is still in its earliest stages, and efficacy data on the modified intervention are not yet available. Pending empirical data on the treatment of chronic and severely depressed teens, combination therapy may be warranted in practice to prevent premature therapy termination and boost treatment response.

Continuation Treatment

As an additional area for treatment development and research, the long-term efficacy of CBT may be able to be improved through continuation treatment. The 1997 clinical trial treatment protocol did include a small number of monthly booster sessions, and CBT effects were maintained during the booster period. However, by 2-year follow-up, rates of depression recurrence were not significantly different between CBT, SBFT, and NST (although descriptive data did favor CBT). One investigation with depressed teens has found that the addition of 6 months (median) of CBT continuation treatment produced a significantly lower relapse rate than CBT alone (20% vs. 50%; Kroll, Harrington, Jayson, Fraser, & Gowers, 1996). These results are promising and additional work investigating models of continuation treatment would be a welcome addition to the treatment literature.

Effectiveness of CBT in Practice

Data from the Brent et al. (1997) clinical trial suggest that CBT may have the promise of effectiveness in real-world clinical contexts. CBT was the most efficacious intervention at posttreatment both on dimensional symptom measures and in terms of clinical remission of MDD. In addition, CBT was the most "robust" intervention in the face of adverse treatment indicators, such as high levels of hopelessness and comorbid anxiety.

To measure the effectiveness of CBT more directly, we recently completed a project in which we assessed the outcomes of adolescents treated in a depression specialty clinic. The Services for Teens at Risk (STAR) Center is an outpatient clinic, run by our research group, that serves depressed and suicidal adolescents and their families. The STAR Center is housed in the general child outpatient service at Western Psychiatric Institute and Clinic and draws youth from that service as well as youth referred after inpatient care for a suicide attempt. Teens seen at the STAR Center receive a combination of CBT and medication management. These services are free to families, as in most clinical trials, but STAR therapy is open-ended, and the content of therapy sessions is unmonitored. Youth seen at the STAR Center meet criteria for significant mood disorder; however, they also often meet criteria for comorbid diagnoses, such as substance abuse. The STAR Center, thus, shares many features with CBT clinical trials but has a patient base and setting similar to outpatient clinical practice. Given this blend of research and practice characteristics, we viewed the STAR Center as a natural laboratory in which to begin assessing the effectiveness of CBT under clinically representative conditions. To accomplish this task, we reviewed the medical records of youth treated in STAR between 1995 and 2002. In this time span, 80 youths who met criteria for MDD and self-reported significant depression symptoms (BDI greater than 12) received a course of CBT in STAR. All 80 youths were between the ages of 13 and 18 and were predominantly Caucasian (85%) and female (77%). These teens evidenced a broader range of comorbid diagnoses than did youth in the Brent et al. (1997) clinical trial, and 20% of the STAR sample would have been excluded from the clinical trial on the basis of comorbid diagnoses (e.g., substance abuse). In terms of treatment, the content of the CBT intervention in the clinical trial and STAR was similar, but the number of sessions in STAR was much more variable, and 75% of STAR youths received concurrent medication treatment.

As part of their routine clinical care, youths in STAR completed the BDI each session, and we were able to examine BDI symptom trajectories as an index of treatment effectiveness. Preliminary results indicate that CBT in the STAR Center produced significant improvement in depression symptoms approximately 6 months after intake (i.e., BDI trajectory falling within the normal range). This time to recovery is almost twice as long as in the 1997 CBT clinical trial (Brent et al., 1997). However, results of STAR Center CBT may compare quite favorably to outcomes achieved by eclectic community therapy. In sample of 67 depressed youths treated in community mental health centers, a similar level of symptom reduction did not occur until 12 months after intake (for details, see Weersing & Weisz, 2002; Weersing et al., 2002).

Whereas our preliminary data from STAR suggest that CBT for depressed adolescents may prove to be effective in real-world clinical practice, formal dissemination trials of CBT have yet to be conducted. There are reasons to suspect that clinical trial effects for CBT may be reduced in the context of clinical practice. In addition to differences in youth characteristics, the staff and settings of community practice are likely quite different from clinical trials, and even from the STAR Center. To be feasible for use in general clinical practice, CBT protocols may need to be shorter, simpler, and more focused than current clinical trial manuals. Of course, these "feasibility" modifications will need to be balanced against possible decrements in efficacy, especially given data that longer-term continuation CBT may be indicated for a substantial portion of youth. In short, we see a good deal of work to done in order to successfully develop and disseminate a CBT protocol optimized for community practice settings.

Treatment Mechanisms

Finally, we see value in additional studies attempting to uncover the mechanisms of action and critical components of CBT. Work in this area has suggested that a percentage of youth, across all treatment modalities, may respond quickly to depression psychoeducation and warm therapeutic contact (i.e., demonstrate a rapid response to treatment; Renaud et al., 1998). For youth who do not show sudden improvements in symptoms, CBT may "work" through the gradual acquisition of emotional regulation, cognitive restructuring, and problem-solving skills. Our data supporting these hypotheses are somewhat indirect (Gaynor et al., in press), and results have not been consistent across all measures (Kolko et al., 2000). Stronger evidence on the mediators of treatment effects may help to guide the design of future interventions and provide the most efficient and effective care for depressed adolescents.

SUMMARY AND CONCLUSIONS

In sum, CBT appears to be an efficacious intervention for the treatment of depression in adolescents. In the Brent et al. (1997) clinical trial, 60% of teens treated with CBT experienced clinical remission[6] of depression by posttreatment, a significantly higher percentage than in SBFT (38%) or NST (39%). Outcomes on dimensional measures of depression symptoms, both youth-report and interviewer-rated, also supported the superiority of CBT. In addition, youth treated with CBT experienced relief from depression more quickly than youth in either of the comparison treatments.

There also is evidence to suggest that CBT may work well outside of clinical trial contexts, under the conditions of real-world clinical care. Data for this conclusion come from two sources. In the clinical trial dataset, CBT was more "robust" to adverse treatment indicators, such as hopelessness, suicidality, and comorbid anxiety, than either SBFT or NST (Brent et al., 1998). Furthermore, the efficacy of CBT did not change appreciably as the number of adverse treatment indicators increased. Additional support for the effectiveness of CBT in practice comes from our investigation of CBT in the STAR Center. In the STAR Center, depressed teens provided with CBT experienced substantial improvement in their depression symptoms in approximately 6 months—twice as long as in the 1997 clinical trial sample but twice as quickly as youth treated with traditional psychotherapy in community clinics (Weersing et al., 2002).

Despite this evidence of short-term efficacy, and the promise of effectiveness in practice, the news on CBT effects is not all good. A substantial portion of adolescents treated with CBT remain symptomatic at posttreatment (40%), and the superior effects of CBT relative to SBFT and NST appear to dissipate over long term follow-up. In addition, although CBT produced substantial changes in depression, CBT was no more efficacious than alternate treatments in improving teens' functioning or feelings of suicidality. Findings such as these highlight the need for additional research on treatment-refractory depressed youth and the efficacy of longer-term, continuing-care treatment models.

ACKNOWLEDGMENTS

Preparation of this chapter was facilitated by National Institute of Mental Health (NIMH) Institutional Research Training Grant MH18269 supporting V. Robin Weersing. Data collection for Brent et al. (1997) was supported by NIMH MH46500 and MH18269.

NOTES

1. Manuals for the three treatments are available from David Brent at Western Psychiatric Institute and Clinic, University of Pittsburgh Medical School, 3811 O'Hara Street, Pittsburgh, Pennsylvania 15213.
2. Remission was defined as the absence of diagnosable MDD and at least three consecutive Beck Depression Inventory (BDI) scores of less than nine. See Birmaher et al. (2000) for a discussion of issues surrounding the definition of remission, recovery, and recurrence of depression.
3. These results held for the sample, and all treatment cells, as a whole. Among youth with data on suicidality, CBT did produce better effects on hopelessness than NST, and these changes in hopelessness mediated the superior efficacy of CBT in treating seriously suicidal youth (Barbe et al., 2002).
4. This may be due, in part, to missing data. Some youths were missing data on cognitive distortions, and these participants could not be included in the mediational analyses. When these youths were excluded, the previously significant effect of CBT on BDI scores, reported for the sample as a whole, lapsed into marginal significance (see Kolko et al., 2000, for details). As there was no effect of treatment on outcome (BDI scores), the attempt to search for mediated effects was cut short.
5. This investigation also includes cells testing the effects of medication-switch and medication-switch-plus-CBT. These design features are less critical for our current discussion. Details of the full multisite study design are available from the authors.
6. Remission was defined as the absence of diagnosable MDD and at least three consecutive BDI scores in the normal range (< 9).

REFERENCES

Abramson, L. Y., Seligman, M. E. P., & Teasdale, J. (1978). Learned helplessness in humans: Critique and reformulation. *Journal of Abnormal Psychology, 87,* 49–74.

Alexander, J., & Parsons, B. V. (1982). *Functional family therapy.* Pacific Grove, CA: Brooks-Cole.

Asarnow, J. R., Goldstein, M. J., Tompson, M., & Guthrie, D. (1993). One-year outcomes of depressive disorders in child psychiatric in-patients: Evaluation of the prognostic power of a brief measure of expressed emotion. *Journal of Child Psychology and Psychiatry, 34,* 129–137.

Barbe, R. P., Bridge, J., Birmaher, B., Kolko, D. J., & Brent, D. A. (2002). Suicidality and its relationship to treatment outcome in depressed adolescents. Manuscript submitted for publication.

Beck, A. T., Rush, A. J., Shaw, B. F., & Emery, G. (1979). *Cognitive therapy of depression.* New York: Guilford Press.

Beck, A. T., Steer, R. A., & Garbin, M. G. (1988). Psychometric properties of the Beck Depression Inventory: Twenty-five years of evaluation. *Clinical Psychology Review, 8,* 77–100.

Birmaher, B., Brent, D. A., Kolko, D., Baugher, M., Bridge, J., Iyengar, S., & Ulloa, R. E. (2000). Clinical outcome after short-term psychotherapy for adolescents with major depressive disorder. *Archives of General Psychiatry, 57,* 29–36.

Brent, D. A., Holder, D., Kolko, D., Birmaher, B., Baugher, M., Roth, C., & Johnson, B. (1997). A clinical psychotherapy trial for adolescent depression comparing cognitive, family, and supportive treatments. *Archives of General Psychiatry 54,* 877–885.

Brent, D. A., Kolko, D., Birmaher, B., Baugher, M., & Bridge, J. (1999). A clinical trial for adolescent depression: Predictors of additional treatment in the acute and follow-up phase of the trial. *Journal of the American Academy of Child and Adolescent Psychiatry, 38,* 263–271.

Brent, D. A., Kolko, D., Birmaher, B., Baugher, M., Bridge, J., Roth C., & Holder, D. (1998). Predictors of treatment efficacy in a clinical trial of three psychosocial treatments for adolescent depression. *Journal of the American Academy of Child and Adolescent Psychiatry, 37,* 906–914.

Brent, D. A., Perper, J. A., Moritz, G., Allman, C., Roth, C., Schweers, J., Balach, L., & Baugher, M. (1993). Psychiatric risk factors of adolescent suicide: A case control study. *Journal of the American Academy of Child and Adolescent Psychiatry, 32,* 521–529.

Brent, D. A., Poling, K., McKain, B., & Baugher, M. (1993). A psychoeducational program for families of affectively ill children and adolescents. *Journal of the American Academy of Child and Adolescent Psychiatry, 32,* 770–774.

Brent, D. A., Roth, C. M., Holder, D. P., Kolko, D. J., Birmaher, B., Johnson, B. A., & Schweers, J. A. (1996). Psychosocial interventions for treating adolescent suicidal depression: A comparison of three psychosocial interventions. In E. D. Hibbs & P. S. Jensen (Eds.), *Psychosocial treatments for child and adolescent disorders: Empirically based strategies for clinical practice* (pp. 187–206). Washington, DC: American Psychological Association.

Gaynor, S. T., Weersing, V. R., Kolko, D. J., Birmaher, B., Heo, J., & Brent, D. A. (in press). The prevalence and impact of large sudden improvements during adolescent psychotherapy for depression: A comparison across cognitive-behavioral, family, and supportive therapy. *Journal of Consulting and Clinical Psychology.*

Gladstone, T. R. G., & Kaslow, N. J. (1995). Depression and attributions in children and adolescents: A meta-analytic review. *Journal of Abnormal Child Psychology, 23,* 597–606.

Keller, M. B., McCullough, J. P., Klein, D. N., Arnow, B., Dunner, D. L., Gelenberg, A. J., Markowitz, J. C., Nemeroff, C. B., Russell, J. M., Thase, M. E., Trivedi, M. H., & Zajecka, J. (2000). A comparison of nefazodone, the cognitive behavioral-analysis system of psychotherapy, and their combination for the treatment of chronic depression. *New England Journal of Medicine, 342,* 1462–1470.

Kolko, D., Brent, D., Baugher, M., Bridge, J., & Birmaher, B. (2000). Cognitive and family therapies for adolescent depression: Treatment specificity, mediation and moderation. *Journal of Consulting and Clinical Psychology, 68,* 603–614.

Kroll, L., Harrington, R., Jayson, D., Fraser, J., & Gowers, S. (1996). Pilot study of continuation cognitive-behavioral therapy for major depression in adolescent psychiatric patients. *Journal of the American Academy of Child and Adolescent Psychiatry, 35,* 1156–1161.

Lewinsohn, P. M., Allen, N. B., Seeley, J. R., & Gotlib, I. H. (1999). First onset versus recurrence of depression: Differential processes of psychosocial risk. *Journal of Abnormal Psychology, 108,* 483–489.

Lewinsohn, P. M., Roberts, R. E., Seeley, J. R., Rohde, P., Gotlib, I. H., & Hops, H. (1994). Adolescent psychopathology: II. Psychosocial risk factors for depression. *Journal of Abnormal Psychology, 103,* 302–315.

Renaud, J., Brent, D. A., Baugher, M., Birmaher, B., Kolko, D. J., & Bridge, J. (1998). Rapid response to psychosocial treatment for adolescent depression: A two-year follow-up. *Journal of the American Academy of Child and Adolescent Psychiatry, 37,* 1184–1190.

Robin, A. L., & Foster S. L. (1989). *Negotiating parent–adolescent conflict: A behavioral–family systems approach.* New York: Guilford Press.

Rohde, P., Lewinsohn, P. M., & Seeley, J. R. (1994). Are adolescents changed by an episode of major depression? *Journal of the American Academy of Child and Adolescent Psychiatry, 33,* 1289–1298.

Weersing, V. R., & Weisz, J. R. (2002). Community clinic treatment of depressed youth: Benchmarking usual care against CBT clinical trials. *Journal of Consulting and Clinical Psychology, 70,* 299–310.

Weersing, V. R., Weisz, J. R., & Brent, D. A. (2002, April). *Treatment of youth depression: Benchmarking community TAU and open-clinic CBT against clinical trials.* Paper presented at the International Conference on Mental Health Services Research, Washington, DC.

9

Interpersonal Psychotherapy for Depressed Adolescents

Laura Mufson and Kristen Pollack Dorta

OVERVIEW

Over the past two decades, there has been increased recognition of the public health importance of addressing the growing rates of adolescent depression in both clinical and research settings. Epidemiological research has demonstrated that the prevalence of depression symptoms and depressive disorders in children and adolescents ranges from 1.6% to 8.9% (Angold & Costello, 2001). Research also has demonstrated that within the adolescent population, the rates of depression are significantly higher for girls than for boys (Angold & Costello, 2001). Adolescent depression often runs a chronic and relapsing clinical course, and it has a high morbidity and cost to society due to the accompanying rates of school dropout, teenage pregnancy, suicide, and substance abuse.

Depressed adolescents, however, are a largely underserved population (Wu et al., 1999). Wu et al. found that these adolescents are underidentified and/or underreferred. The undertreatment of adolescents can be explained by a combination of their limited access to and underutilization of mental health care.

Treating Adolescent Depression

Researchers and clinicians in the field of adolescent depression turned to their adult counterparts as a model for embarking on a program of psychotherapy research in an effort to create a body of evidence-based treatment for adolescent depression. Manualized and, therefore, standardized treatments are the only ones feasible to assess in controlled clinical trials. The focus on short-term or time-limited psychotherapies is more consistent with current trends in managed health care. Developing treatments that are brief and manageable must be an objective for anyone aiming to better meet the needs of the multitude of depressed adolescents.

Given the substantial rates of depressed mood and depressive disorders within the adolescent population and the negative developmental trajectories associated with adolescent depression, this area deserves considerable attention with respect to clinical intervention. Although a number of psychosocial and medication interventions for adolescent depression exist, relatively little research has been done to assess the efficacy of these interventions in comparison to the field of adult depression. Interpersonal psychotherapy for depressed adolescents (IPT-A) is one psychosocial treatment that has been shown to be efficacious.

Origins and Conceptual Model of IPT-A

IPT-A is an adaptation of interpersonal psychotherapy (IPT). IPT is a brief treatment that was developed and tested for depressed adults (Klerman, Weissman, Rounsaville, & Chevron, 1984). The focus of IPT treatment is on the patients' depressive symptoms and their current interpersonal context regardless of the etiology of the disorder. The theoretical roots of this treatment can be found in the interpersonal schools of thought and, more specifically, in the teachings of Harry Stack Sullivan and Adolf Meyer, who moved the focus of psychiatry away from the individual by arguing that one's personality is the culmination of recurrent patterns of interpersonal interactions (Sullivan, 1953). Diagnosis and intervention, therefore, must focus on not only the symptoms and behaviors that comprise the disorder but also the individual's interpersonal interactions and the communications involved in these interactions. Diagnosis includes the identification of maladaptive interpersonal patterns that are seemingly related to one's depression and the intervention involves the disruption of these patterns (Kiesler, 1991).

Research Support for an Interpersonal Conceptualization of Depression

An interpersonal approach to the conceptualization and treatment of depression is well supported by research (Hammen, 1999; Joiner, Coyne, & Blalock, 1999). Research has demonstrated that depression, even at subclinical levels, is related to significant interpersonal problems and interpersonal stress (Puig-Antich et al., 1993; Stader & Hokason, 1998). In addition, research has documented that interpersonal experiences are often precipitants of the onset of depression (Hammen, 1999).

Rationale for the Adaptation for Adolescents

The rationale for the adaptation of IPT for adolescents lies in research evidence, the developmental relevance of the treatment, and the clinical need in the community. Clinical research conducted in the 1970s and 1980s clearly established the efficacy of IPT for the treatment of depression in adults (DiMascio et al., 1979; Elkin et al., 1989; Weissman et al., 1979). Research also has demonstrated the similarities between adolescent and adult depressive symptoms (Ryan et al., 1987). Finally, research has clearly documented the critical role that interpersonal events and interpersonal skills can play in the development and sequelae of adolescent depression (Hammen, 1999; Marx & Schulze, 1991; Stader & Hokason, 1998).

IPT also was selected for use with adolescents due to its developmental relevance to the adolescent population. IPT-A focuses largely on current interpersonal issues that are likely to be areas of most concern and importance to adolescents. Discussing interpersonal events is something adolescents can relate to and are accustomed to doing in their daily lives. IPT-A is an active treatment with a large psychoeducational component aimed at building competencies and skills in the adolescent. It is structured and organized in such a way that the adolescent can take increasingly more control of and play an increasingly more active role in the treatment as it progresses. Research has shown that depressed individuals develop less effective problem-solving strategies than do nondepressed individuals (Marx & Schulze, 1991). Specifically, Marx and Schulze demonstrated that depressed individuals displayed a "passive, resigned orientation" (p. 365) to problem solving that can lead to a sense of helplessness further exacerbating their depression. This would suggest that depressed individuals may need to develop more active, action-oriented approaches to problem solving to give them a sense of being an agent of change and empowerment. As such, the increasingly active role of adolescents in IPT-A treatment serves as a model for the changes that many depressed adolescents need to pursue in aspects of their lives.

Finally, IPT-A is a treatment approach that may be easily disseminated to a variety of settings because it is manualized and brief. Therapist training is facilitated by standardized guidelines for treatment that may be used for teaching as well as for monitoring continued adherence to the evidence-based treatment. These factors ensure both quality of care and comparability of care across settings. Given the critical need to reach depressed adolescents, IPT-A could prove helpful in increasing access to care, specifically evidence-based care.

How IPT-A Differs from IPT

Several alterations were made to the IPT manual to increase the model's appropriateness for the treatment of adolescent depression. Although the overall goals and problem areas of IPT are employed in IPT-A, the latter also includes a fifth problem area, "single-parent family." This area was included given the frequency with which it occurs for adolescents, its empirically demonstrated connection to depressive symptoms, and the interpersonal challenges and difficulties associated with this situation.

A second adaptation is the addition of a parent component to the treatment protocol. Although IPT-A is an individual treatment, for many adolescents some degree of involvement on the part of the parent or guardian is often advisable and critical in promoting the well-being of the adolescent and encouraging the success of the treatment. Parent involvement in IPT-A is flexible and can range from no involvement to attendance at several sessions. Recommendations typically include at least involvement in the initial phase in order to be educated about the disorder and the treatment. The role of the parent/ guardian in treatment is presented for each phase of the treatment as described later in this chapter.

Another difference is that the objectives of IPT-A and related techniques have been adapted to be more developmentally relevant to the adolescent population. The objectives have been altered slightly to take into account developmental tasks including individuation, establishing autonomy, developing interpersonal relations with members of the opposite sex and with potential romantic partners, coping with initial experiences with death and loss, and managing peer pressures.

The techniques employed in the treatment for working toward the goals of decreasing depressive symptoms and improving interpersonal functioning have been geared toward adolescents. Techniques employed specifically with adolescents include giving them a rating scale from 1 to 10 to rate their symptoms so it is easier for them to monitor improvement; doing more basic social skills work; conducting explicit work on perspective-taking skills to counteract adolescent black-and-white thinking about solutions to problems; and learning how to negotiate, specifically, parent–child tensions. Finally, strategies were developed for dealing with specific issues that may arise in the course of treating adolescents, including school refusal, physical or sexual abuse, involvement of child protective agencies, and dealing with suicidality.

CHARACTERISTICS OF THE TREATMENT PROGRAM

The general goals of IPT-A are to decrease depressive symptoms and to improve interpersonal functioning. Neither these goals nor the techniques employed to attain these goals are novel in the treatment of depression. What is unique is the overall way in which these techniques and goals are combined in a treatment program for adolescent depression.

Patient Selection

Based on clinical experience, the patients who are best suited for IPT-A are those who are motivated to be in treatment or, at least, to "feel better" or function better in one or more interpersonal areas related to their depression. In addition, patients should be able to establish a therapeutic alliance, be willing to receive time-limited treatment, and be able to agree with the therapist that at least one interpersonal problem exists. Adolescents whose families are supportive of treatment and are willing to participate in treatment are more likely to have a positive outcome to the treatment.

IPT-A is not recommended for patients who have a long-standing history of severe interpersonal problems; rather, it is most suited to those who have an identifiable interpersonal event that served as a precipitant or clear exacerbating factor in the patient's depression. IPT-A is not appropriate for treating adolescents who are mentally retarded or currently in crisis, suicidal or homicidal, psychotic, bipolar, or substance abusing.

Course of Treatment

Attaining the goals of reducing depressive symptoms and improving interpersonal functioning involves four primary objectives in IPT-A: (1) identify the problem area, (2) relate depressive symptoms to problem areas, (3) focus on current relationships, and (4) help the patient master the interpersonal context of his or her depression. These objectives are further delineated and addressed to varying degrees throughout the three phases of IPT-A treatment: the initial phase, the middle phase, and the termination phase. Descriptions of the three phases of treatment are presented next.

Initial Phase

The initial phase of IPT-A typically includes sessions one through four. There are seven objectives for this phase of treatment:

1. Diagnose the depression.
2. Explain the theory and goals of IPT-A.
3. Explain the patient's and parents' roles in treatment.
4. Assess patient suitability for IPT-A.
5. Conduct the interpersonal inventory in order to relate the depression to the interpersonal context.

   6. Identify the interpersonal problem area(s).
   7. Make a treatment contract.

Diagnose the Depression

For the most part, the diagnostic assessment is conducted prior to beginning the treatment; however, it is important to reconfirm the diagnosis through a thorough assessment during the initial session. During ensuing sessions, the therapist conducts somewhat briefer assessments to evaluate any change in symptoms. Using a variety of sources, preferably including both the parent and the patient, the patient's current symptoms and history of depressive symptoms are assessed using a clinical interview. At this time, other symptoms, such as mania, psychosis, substance abuse, or suicidality, which might make IPT-A an inappropriate treatment for that patient, are also reviewed. The adolescent's general psychosocial functioning should be assessed using multiple informants whenever possible. A variety of assessment tools including interviews and self-report or clinician-report rating scales may be employed.

   Another important component of the assessment is education. Both the adolescent and the parent(s) should be educated about depression. The therapist should review the symptoms, discuss what is known about the illness, discuss treatment options, and provide a realistic explanation of potential outcomes of treatment.

Explain the Theory and Goals of IPT-A

As with most treatments, the first sessions of IPT-A involve establishing the therapeutic alliance and defining the structure and context of the treatment. These steps help to ensure that the course of treatment will be as predictable as possible and to decrease the possibility of dropout. For IPT-A, defining the structure and context involves describing the assessment and treatment process, which includes explaining the brief, time-limited nature of IPT-A and clearly defining the roles of the therapist and patient from the beginning. With respect to the former, IPT-A is a once-weekly, 12-week treatment. The therapist is encouraged, particularly in the first few weeks of treatment, also to make brief, weekly phone contact with the patient and family between sessions to further foster the therapeutic relationship and establish treatment adherence.

Explain the Patient's and Parents' Roles in Treatment

It is recommended that the patient's parent(s) participate in at least one session during the initial phase of treatment. This session may or may not be the first one. During the session with the parent(s), the therapist can obtain valuable information that will aid in establishing the patient's diagnosis and determining the patient's level of interpersonal functioning. In addition, the parent(s) should be provided with key information regarding the approach to and course of treatment. The goal is to enlist the parent(s) as collaborative therapists in treating the adolescent's depression given that they have more frequent contact with the adolescent.

Conduct Interpersonal Inventory to Relate the Depression to the Interpersonal Context

The next focus of IPT-A is on interpersonal diagnostics. The therapist conducts the interpersonal inventory, an interpersonal assessment of the patient's most important relationships. The goal is to identify those interpersonal issues that are most closely related to the onset and/or persistence of the patient's depression. The inventory consists of a series of discussions aimed at gathering information about the adolescent's relationships with significant others. Although the primary informant for the inventory is the adolescent, other significant people in the adolescent's life, including parents and teachers, may also serve as informants if their involvement is acceptable to the adolescent.

The information gathered about each significant relationship includes the frequency, content, and context of contacts with this person; the terms and/or expectations of the relationship and whether it has met these; the positive and negative aspects of the relationship; the changes the patient would like to see in the relationship; any ideas on how to initiate and carry out those changes; the impact of the adolescent's depression on the relationship and vice versa; and the impact of that relationship on other relationships and vice versa. While conducting the interpersonal inventory, the therapist should also probe for any significant life events that may be related to the depression.

Identify Interpersonal Problem Area(s) and Make a Treatment Contract

Following the interpersonal assessment, the therapist illustrates for the patient the association between key interpersonal issues and the onset, persistence, and/or exacerbation of the depression. Using this information, the therapist helps the adolescent identify an interpersonal problem area that will be the focus of treatment. The five potential problem areas, all of which are discussed in more detail later in this chapter, include grief due to death, separation, or illness; interpersonal disputes; role transitions; interpersonal deficits; and single-parent family situations. Once the problem area is defined, the patient and therapist establish a verbal treatment contract. In this contract, adolescent's and family's roles in treatment are specified, treatment goals are identified, expectations for treatment are clarified, and practical details regarding the treatment are reviewed. An excerpt of a verbal treatment contract would be as follows:

> "As we discussed, it seems as though your depression is very related to the conflict you and your mom are having about expectations for you around the house and at school. We will be further clarifying the specific areas where you disagree and trying to identify new strategies that may help you get along better. You will help this process by bringing in information each week about your mood and anything that has happened in your relationship that week. Together we will work on identifying better ways to deal with the situations. In order for treatment to work best, you need to come every week on time. If you are unable to make it, it is important to call and cancel. We have met four times and have eight more weeks left. In the next few weeks, if it seems like it may be helpful, we might invite your mother into the session so I can help you work directly on the communication. Don't worry, we will discuss this together first. Do you have any questions about the treatment so far?"

In addition to being helpful to treatment, this contract serves as a model for all interpersonal relations in that it reflects clarity in communication and expectations.

Middle Phase

The primary focus of the middle phase of IPT-A, which consists of sessions five through eight, is on further exploration and clarification of the problem area, developing new strategies for managing the issues related to the problem, and implementing those strategies. The specific objectives for this phase are as follows:

1. Monitor depressive symptoms.
2. Consider adjunctive therapy (medication).
3. Aid patient in discussing topics related to identified problem area.
4. Relate patient's feelings to interpersonal events and relationships.
5. Conduct communication analysis.
6. Develop and adapt interpersonal problem-solving strategies.

Although the techniques employed and strategies recommended are specific to each problem area, the general strategies include exploration, encouragement of affect expression, linking affect to interpersonal events, clarification of conflicts, communication analysis, decision analysis, and behavior-change techniques, including role-plays. The treatment approach for each problem area is discussed later in this chapter.

The role that family and key school personnel play in this phase of treatment is specific to each case. As a rule, however, the more collaboration, the more likely the adolescent will generalize any treatment gains to settings outside treatment. For those children not attending school regularly, the therapist should work closely with the school and family to facilitate reentry as soon as possible.

Termination Phase

In many ways, the termination phase of IPT-A, which includes sessions nine through twelve, is similar to the termination process of other treatments. The objectives for this phase of treatment include the following:

1. Review warning symptoms of depression.
2. Review identified problem area.
3. Review strategies for improving relationships.
4. Review changes in adolescent and/or family.
5. Anticipate potential future situations and review strategies for managing those situations.
6. Discuss feelings about ending treatment/relationship with therapist.
7. Discuss possibility of recurrence of depression and strategies for managing such a recurrence.

The therapist should review the course of the patient's depressive symptoms as well as his or her current symptoms, the associations between depressive symptoms and the identified interpersonal problem area(s), and the strategies that have proved most helpful to the patient. The potential recurrence of depression and the warning signs of symptoms for that particular adolescent should be highlighted and strategies for managing these reviewed. The therapist should have a similar meeting with the patient's parent in order to review progress made toward the treatment goals, warning signs for recurrence of symptoms, plans to manage future stressors, and further treatment options or referrals if these are needed.

Interpersonal Problem Areas

The primary area of interpersonal functioning to be targeted for an individual adolescent is defined by the identified interpersonal problem area. In IPT-A there are five interpersonal problem areas (see Table 9.1). Each problem area has an array of strategies that can be employed to accomplish the goals associated with the specific problem area as well as the more general treatment goals of IPT-A. IPT-A makes no assumptions regarding the temporal associations between the interpersonal problem areas and depression. The interpersonal problem area may have preceded the depression or occurred in response to the depression, or, in the most likely scenario, the two may have reciprocal exacerbating effects. In the sections that follow we briefly discuss each problem area. For a more detailed discussion of each area, see the IPT-A manual (Mufson, Moreau, Weissman, & Klerman, 1993).

Problem Area 1: Grief

Many bereaved adolescents experience some depressive symptoms, including dysphoria, anhedonia, and appetite disturbance. Not every adolescent who experiences a death, however, develops depression. Therefore, grief is considered a problem only if it is prolonged or becomes abnormal. IPT-A is particularly useful for adolescents who have previously experienced depression; whose support network is particularly limited; who have a lack of understanding of death; who have experiences involving multiple or sudden deaths; who had a conflicted relationship with a deceased person; who have an overly dependent surviving parent; or who experienced a death by suicide or homicide. These situations have all been identified as risk factors for more complicated bereavement and the potential onset of depression (Clark, Pynoos, & Goebel, 1994).

According to IPT-A, the first step in treating the grief reaction is to help the adolescent discuss the loss in significant detail, including his or her relationship with the deceased and the events surrounding the loss. The therapist encourages the adolescent to monitor, identify, and express feelings associated with the relationship and the loss. Over the course of the grief work, the therapist encourages the adolescent to begin to create a

TABLE 9.1. Interpersonal Problem Areas in Interpersonal Psychotherapy for Depressed Adolescents

Problem areas	Treatment goals
Grief	1. Help adolescent mourn effectively 2. Reestablish interests and relationships
Interpersonal disputes	1. Identify the dispute 2. Develop a plan of action 3. Modify communication and expectations
Role transitions	1. Understand what transition means to teen 2. Identify the demands of new situation 3. Understand what has been gained/lost 4. Learn new skills
Interpersonal deficits	1. Reduce social isolation 2. Improve social skills 3. Increase self-confidence 4. Improve and expand relationships
Single-parent families	1. Understand feeling related to situation 2. Understand feelings related to parents 3. Alleviate guilt about situation 4. Define roles and expectations in relationships

more realistic memory of the deceased individual and of their relationship and its associated feelings. Eventually, the therapist encourages the adolescent to look for ways to develop new relationships or further develop established relationships to substitute for the
support and roles that were lost. The therapist and adolescent must both explore the
adolescent's fears about new relationships and actively rehearse skills needed to develop
relationships or engage in new activities.

Problem Area 2: Interpersonal Disputes

A dispute involving interpersonal roles exists when one individual and a significant other
(or others) have nonreciprocal expectations about their relationship (Klerman et al.,
1984). Such disputes occur frequently between adolescents and their parents or
guardians and often center on issues such as sexuality, authority, money, and life values.
Such disputes do not inherently result in adolescent depression. In fact, they are a fundamental part of many adolescents' struggles to attain autonomy and a reflection of the
process of individuation. However, when these disputes become chronic and the adolescent and parents are unable to manage the dispute, it can become more problematic and
can place considerable stress on the adolescent and parents. In these cases, interpersonal
disputes can serve as a precipitant of adolescent depression. Some adolescents who are
depressed may be particularly ill equipped to manage these disputes. In such cases, the
disputes may exacerbate the adolescent's depression.

In treating this problem area, it is important first to clearly identify and define the
dispute. A dispute may be in one of three possible stages (Klerman et al., 1984): renegotiation, impasse, and dissolution. During renegotiation, the adolescent and significant other are communicating with each other and are attempting to resolve the dispute. During
the second stage, impasse, the adolescent and significant other have stopped communicating and have stopped trying to discuss or resolve the conflict but still have a desire to
mend the relationship. During the final stage, dissolution, the adolescent and significant
other have decided that the dispute cannot be resolved and have chosen to end their relationship. This latter stage is infrequently encountered among adolescents except for situations in which the adolescent wants to end a romantic relationship. Otherwise, attempts
are made to preserve workable family relationships.

The work involves clarifying the expectations that both the adolescent and the parent have for themselves, for each other, and for the relationship. The therapist should
then work with the adolescent and parent to modify their communication and expectations for each other and their relationship. If a resolution seems impossible, the therapist
works with the adolescent to develop strategies for coping with parental expectations
that cannot be changed and perhaps seeking out other adaptive relationships that may
address the same emotional needs more effectively. Although it is ideal in most cases for
the parent to participate in some treatment sessions, this problem area can be addressed
with an adolescent alone when necessary.

Problem Area 3: Role Transitions

Role transitions are changes that occur due to a person's progression from one social role
to another. They can be more predictable changes, which are associated with normal developmental shifts that occur at different stages in adolescence, or they can be more unexpected and associated with both adolescence and some additional change or stressor in
the life of the adolescent. Some of the determinants of how successfully a role transition

is managed include the adolescent and family members' flexibility, the adolescent's psychological functioning, and the adolescent's perceived social support. Transitions are often associated with increased pressures and responsibilities and thus can place high demands on the adolescent who may feel that he or she is unable to meet self-expectations or the expectations of others. The adolescent may experience a loss of self-esteem as he or she struggles to gain confidence in his or her new role. The transition may result in some impairment in interpersonal functioning and in depression when it occurs too rapidly, is experienced as a loss by the individual, is associated with secondary changes or stressors, or is met by the inflexibility of either the adolescent or significant others in the adolescent's life.

Treatment of this problem area involves identifying and defining the role transition and then clarifying what this transition means to the adolescent, what demands are associated with the new role, and what has been gained and lost in the transition. Encouraging the adolescent to explore his or her feelings related to each of these areas is critical. The therapist aids the adolescent in learning new skills that will facilitate acceptance of the new role by the adolescent or the family and increase the adolescent's confidence in managing the role.

If the role transition in any way involves the adolescent's family, family members should be involved in some of the treatment sessions whenever possible. If the family members have difficulty with the transition (e.g., parents are inhibiting their adolescent's movement toward increased autonomy), treatment can address the difficulty. In such a case, the therapist can act as a coach to the parents by helping them learn ways to support the adolescent outside treatment sessions. Ideally, support will increase the chance that the adolescent will generalize the gains made and the skills acquired to his or her daily life.

Problem Area 4: Interpersonal Deficits

An adolescent is considered for this problem area when he or she appears to lack the social skills needed to establish and maintain appropriate relationships with family, peers, or other significant people. IPT-A and this problem area are relevant only to the treatment of adolescents who are depressed and whose interpersonal deficits are less pervasive and/or a consequence of either their depression or a specific stressor.

Interpersonal deficits can impede an adolescent's achievement of developmental tasks, particularly those in social domains. These adolescents can experience social isolation and decreased self-confidence and self-esteem, which can lead to or exacerbate feelings of depression. The depression can lead to further social withdrawal and isolation, which often results in a significant lag in interpersonal skills even after the adolescent's depression has resolved.

IPT-A employs a number of strategies for addressing this problem area, including reviewing past significant relationships and interpersonal experiences and exploring repetitive and parallel interpersonal problems. The therapist helps the adolescent recognize the association between the impact of his or her deficits on relationships and depressive symptoms. New strategies, including communication skills, for approaching situations are identified and practiced using role-plays. The adolescent is encouraged to apply these strategies to maintain existing relationships and form new ones.

Family members may be involved in treatment, particularly when the adolescent's interpersonal deficits affect family relationships. It is important that the interpersonal skills learned in treatment be practiced outside the therapy session. The family can play a critical role in supporting and encouraging the adolescent as he or she develops and practices these skills.

Problem Area 5: Single-Parent Families

Single-parent family status can be the result of parental absence or abandonment, parental divorce or separation, or the death of a parent. Each situation presents unique emotional conflicts for the adolescent and the custodial parent, and each family and adolescent bring to the situation a different history of skills, stressors, and strengths for managing the situation. Research has demonstrated that transitions in family structure as well as, more specifically, parental divorce and single-parent family structures, are associated with an increased risk for negative outcomes, including decreased well-being, depression, and relational problems (Aseltine, 1996; Cornwell, Eggebeen, & Meschke, 1996; Spruijt & de Goede, 1997), which does not suggest that adolescents in single-parent homes are inevitably going to evidence more negative outcomes or, even more specifically, depression. Rather, they simply seem to be at greater risk for such outcomes as compared to peers who reside in two-parent homes in which no such transitions in family structure have occurred. This problem area is intended for those adolescents who are experiencing depressive symptoms and whose symptoms seem to be closely associated either temporally or conceptually with their single-parent family status.

In addressing this problem area, the therapist encourages the adolescent to recognize the feelings related to the single-parent family status and any associations between the situation and the depressive symptoms. The therapist helps the adolescent to clarify expectations of current relationships and define roles in the new family structure. In many cases, involvement of the custodial parent, and sometimes involvement of the noncustodial parent if available, is extremely helpful to the treatment process.

EVIDENCE FOR THE EFFECTS OF TREATMENT

Initial IPT-A Project

The initial IPT-A project was focused on adapting IPT to the treatment of adolescents, developing a detailed training program for therapists interested in conducting IPT-A, and conducting an open clinical trial. Once the open trial was completed, a randomized controlled clinical trial was conducted in an outpatient hospital setting. The development and empirical testing of IPT-A were designed to follow similar phases that characterize the development of pharmacological agents (Rush, 1984). Initial goals are to assess feasibility and acceptability with a subsequent shift to the goal of demonstrating efficacy.

Training

Mufson, the first author, was trained as an IPT therapist by one of the original developers of IPT, Gerald Klerman. The training program for IPT-A, used in the controlled clinical trial, includes reading the treatment manual, attending a 2-day course on the treatment (which includes viewing videotapes and participating in role-plays), using IPT-A to treat at least two patients (and videotaping these sessions), and attending weekly supervision with an expert in IPT-A. In addition, to certify competence, three randomly selected videotapes per training case are reviewed and rated for competence by two additional experts in IPT-A.

Empirical Support for IPT-A

To date, Mufson has conducted both an open clinical trial and a controlled clinical trial of IPT-A. The open trial provided preliminary support for the use of IPT-A. The purpose of the open trial was to gain experience in IPT-A and to determine whether the treatment was feasible and acceptable to the adolescent population. The sample consisted of 14 12- to 18-year-olds who were referred to a hospital outpatient clinic due to depressive symptoms or who responded to an advertisement for the treatment of adolescent depression. The results of this study indicated a significant decrease in adolescents' depressive symptomatology and in symptoms of psychological and physical distress. Adolescents also demonstrated significant improvement in their general functioning at home and at school. Finally, none of the adolescents qualified for a diagnosis of depression (according to the revised third edition of the *Diagnostic and Statistical Manual of Mental Disorders* [DSM-III-R]; American Psychiatric Association, 1987) at the end of treatment (Mufson et al., 1994).

Although these results were promising, their significance is difficult to determine in the absence of randomization and a comparison group. In addition, because the only therapist was the developer of the adaptation, treatment effects could be attributed to the specific therapist's skill rather than to the treatment techniques themselves. To test that premise, Mufson needed to train other therapists and assess treatment efficacy as delivered by other trained therapists.

The next study was a randomized controlled clinical trial comparing IPT-A to clinical monitoring in a sample of clinic-referred depressed adolescents (Mufson, Weissman, Moreau, & Garfinkel, 1999). Adolescents were identified using a clinician-rated scale, the Hamilton Rating Scale for Depression (HRSD; Williams, 1988), and a self-report measure, the Beck Depression Inventory (BDI; Beck, Steer, & Garbin, 1988; Strober, Gree, & Carlson, 1981), as well as two clinical interviews, the Schedule for Affective Disorders and Schizophrenia for School-Age Children (K-SADS-PL; Kaufman et al., 1997), and the NIMH Diagnostic Interview Schedule for Children, Version 4 (DISC IV; Shaffer, Fisher, Lucas, Dulcan, & Schwab-Stone, 2000). Adolescents with a diagnosis of major depressive disorder who were not currently suicidal or psychotic and were not diagnosed with a chronic medical illness, bipolar I or II, conduct disorder, substance abuse disorder, eating disorder, or obsessive–compulsive disorder were included in the study. Of the 57 adolescents who were determined to be eligible for the study, 48 agreed to be randomized.

Adolescents were randomized to IPT-A or clinical monitoring. Clinical monitoring was originally designed to be the closest approximation to a wait-list condition and was to be considered an "ethical wait list." Patients were assigned a therapist, had one session a month but could call if they needed another session. If they needed more than one session, it would be seen as a failure to be maintained in the condition and they would be removed from the study and referred for more treatment. Although funded in this form, institutional review board (IRB) review required significant modifications to the condition. Adolescents in the clinical monitoring condition would receive once-monthly 30-minute sessions with a therapist with the option for a second session each month. They would also be seen bimonthly by the independent evaluator. During the 1 week of the month without a face-to-face meeting, the therapists needed to have a phone contact with the adolescent to assess clinical status and safety. Thus the adolescents in the clinical monitoring condition received a therapeutic check-in at least 3 out of 4 weeks of the month. Treatment in both conditions was provided for 12 weeks.

Therapists received training in IPT-A consistent with the training program discussed earlier. Adolescents in IPT-A had weekly 45-minute therapy sessions with additional parent sessions during the initial and termination phase and when needed in the middle phase of treatment. Adolescents enrolled in the study, in either treatment condition, were assessed at weeks 0, 2, 4, 6, 8, 10, and 12. The outcomes assessed included diagnosis and symptoms levels (HRSD, BDI, Clinical Global Impression Form [CGI]) as well as global and social functioning (Children's Global Assessment Scale and Social Adjustment Scale—Self Report Version, respectively), parent–child relationship (Parental Bonding Instrument), life events, and social problem-solving skills (Social Problem-Solving Inventory—Revised).

The results of this controlled trial were promising with respect to the efficacy of IPT-A in comparison to clinical monitoring. Treatment outcome was assessed in several ways. First, with respect to rates of treatment completion, significantly more IPT-A patients (88%) completed treatment than did the control patients (46%). Given the rates of noncompletion, particularly in the control group, all subsequent analyses were conducted using both a completer sample (n = 32 adolescents) and an intent-to-treat sample (n = 48 adolescents). In addition, all analyses were conducted on outcome measures at termination while controlling for the baseline assessment of the measures.

For both the completer and the intent-to-treat samples, IPT-A patients reported significantly fewer depressive symptoms. Using standards for recovery set forth by the National Collaborative Study for the Treatment of Depression (Elkin et al., 1989), significantly more IPT-A patients as compared to control patients met the recovery criteria for major depression. The results of this study revealed that treatment with IPT-A also resulted in improved overall social functioning as compared to treatment in the control condition as well as improved functioning in the domains of peer and dating relationships. Though treatment for many teens focused on family issues, there was a nonsignificant trend toward improvement with IPT-A. This may be due to the likelihood of greater difficulty or longer period of time needed to affect changes in the more entrenched relationship patterns with family. In addition, it may be the perceived high rates of depression in the parents of these teens that hampered their ability to change in response to the adolescents' efforts for changing their interactions.

Finally, although these results were somewhat tentative due to some missing data, IPT-A patients demonstrated better skills than control patients in certain areas of social problem-solving skills, including positive problem-solving orientation and rational problem solving. With respect to the latter, IPT-A patients exhibited better performance in the generation of alternatives and solution implementation and verification. Although further research with different comparison groups and across different adolescent populations is needed, the results of this randomized controlled trial suggest that IPT-A is an efficacious treatment for adolescent depression.

A second research group has also been conducting studies of IPT for depressed Puerto Rican adolescents using a different modification of the adult manual tailored to the Puerto Rican culture. Rosselló and Bernal (1999) conducted a study of IPT versus CBT versus wait list for depressed teens. They found that IPT and CBT resulted in a greater reduction in depressive symptoms than did the wait-list condition. Also, IPT was significantly better than the wait-list condition at increasing self-esteem and improving social adaptation. This study provided additional support for the efficacy of the interpersonal approach to depression in adolescents.

CURRENT AND FUTURE DIRECTIONS

Currently, we are conducting an effectiveness study of IPT-A in school-based health clinics in the New York metropolitan area. This investigation is guided by a public health model of clinical intervention and intervention research (Leibowitz, 2000). Studies conducted according to a public health model occur in actual practice settings and face all the realities and complexities of those settings and the people served by them. Such research aims to address some of the potential limitations of more traditional efficacy trials, including a lack of generalizability and practicality. Using a public health model seems particularly important for evaluating treatments to be provided to more impoverished communities and to adolescents in general, as both of these populations are highly likely to receive services outside hospitals or research clinics.

Our current effectiveness study is a randomized, controlled trial comparing the outcome of IPT-A to that of mental health treatment as it is usually provided at the school-based health clinics. We selected school-based health clinics as the setting for the study because they provide an alternative and uniquely available community-based setting for providing care to adolescents, particularly in the current health care climate in which services can be difficult to access and are increasingly costly. Through this study, we hope to gain further support for the effectiveness, generalizability, feasibility, and cost-effectiveness of IPT-A.

Currently, we also are conducting a small-scale, randomized trial comparing a group model of IPT-A (IPT-AG) to individual IPT-A. The feasibility and acceptability of IPT-AG have been tested in two open trials. It appears that based on adolescent reports, our clinical impressions, and limited data, adolescents find IPT-AG interesting and helpful. Also, adolescents reported improvement in depressive symptomatology. The current investigation will provide preliminary efficacy data. If the treatment is efficacious, we hope to conduct a more extensive clinical trial.

With respect to research, in the near future we hope to pursue a controlled trial comparing IPT-A to medication and/or to combined IPT-A and medication. In addition, more long-term follow-up studies are needed to establish the long-term impact of IPT-A, particularly given the documented patterns of recurrence and persistence of depression in adolescents. Related to this area of research, an important area of clinical application of IPT-A is as a continuation and/or maintenance treatment. There is increased demand for continuation treatments that can be used with more short-term treatment models.

SUMMARY AND CONCLUSIONS

Interpersonal psychotherapy for depressed adolescents (IPT-A) is a short-term, manualized, individual treatment for adolescent depression. The focus of the treatment is on alleviating depressive symptoms and improving interpersonal functioning. The treatment consists of three phases (initial, middle, and termination) each of which takes approximately four sessions. By the conclusion of the initial phase the therapist identifies one or two interpersonal problem areas where there are difficulties in relationships related to the adolescent's depression. This serves as the focus of treatment and determines the treatment goals and relevant strategies the therapist employs to attain these goals. The therapist plays an active and directive role in the treatment. The adolescent also is expected to be increasingly active over the course of the treatment.

Whenever possible, parents or guardians are involved in the treatment periodically in order to receive psychoeducation about depression, to learn and practice effective communication skills, and to support the adolescents gains in treatment. The therapist also maintains collateral contact with other individuals and agencies (e.g., school personnel) involved with the adolescent whenever this is appropriate and deemed helpful to the treatment.

The efficacy of IPT-A has been demonstrated in two randomized controlled clinical trials (Mufson et al., 1999; Rosselló & Bernal, 1999). In the clinical trial conducted by Mufson and colleagues, IPT-A was superior to clinical monitoring with respect to decreasing depressive symptoms, rates of recovery from depression, and rates of retention in treatment. In addition, adolescents who received IPT-A demonstrated significant improvement in certain areas of social functioning and interpersonal problem-solving skills as compared to adolescents who received clinical monitoring. These findings, together with the results of Rosselló and Bernal (1999), demonstrate the effectiveness of IPT with depressed adolescents.

Current empirical investigations of IPT-A aim to reach a broader range of depressed adolescents by providing treatment in community-based practice settings and/or with adaptations to make treatment delivery more cost-effective and accessible to more teens. Specifically, an effectiveness trial of IPT-A delivered in school-based health clinics and a small-scale randomized trial of the group version of IPT-A are currently under way. If effective, the group version of IPT-A could be a more cost-effective treatment. Results from these studies are not yet available, but preliminary feedback suggests that both models are at least acceptable and feasible. Findings from these studies will, ideally, be part of the solution to the public health need to provide more empirically based efficacious and cost-effective treatments to depressed adolescents while decreasing the barriers to their access to care.

ACKNOWLEDGMENTS

Excerpts of this chapter have been reprinted from Mufson and Pollack Dorta (2000). Copyright 2000 by the Analytic Press. Reprinted by permission.

REFERENCES

American Psychiatric Association. (1987). *Diagnostic and statistical manual of mental disorders* (3rd ed., rev.). Washington, DC: Author.

Angold, A., & Costello, E. J. (2001). The epidemiology of depression in children and adolescents. In I. M. Goodyer (Ed.), *The depressed child and adolescent* (2nd ed., pp. 143–178). New York: Cambridge University Press.

Aseltine, R. (1996). Pathways linking parental divorce with adolescent depression. *Journal of Health and Social Behavior, 37,* 133–148.

Beck, A. T., Steer, R. A., & Garbin, M. G. (1988). Psychometric properties of the Beck Depression Inventory: Twenty-five years of evaluation. *Clinical Psychology Review, 8,* 77–100.

Clark, D., Pynoos, R., & Goebel, A. (1994). Mechanisms and processes of adolescent bereavement. In R. Haggerty (Ed.), *Stress, risk, and resilience in children and adolescents: Processes, mechanisms, and interventions* (pp. 100–145). Cambridge, UK: Cambridge University Press.

Cornwell, G., Eggebeen, D., & Meschke, L. (1996). The changing family context of early adolescence. *Journal of Early Adolescence, 16,* 141–488.

DiMascio, A., Klerman, G. L., Weissman, M. M., Prusoff, B. A., Neu, C., & Moore, P. (1979). A control group for psychotherapy research in acute depression: One solution to ethical and methodological issues. *Journal of Psychiatric Research, 15,* 189–197.

Elkin, I., Shea, M. T., Watkins, J. T., Imber, S. D., Sotsky, S. M., Collins, J. F., Glass, D. R., Pilkonis, P. A., Leber, W. R., Docherty, J. P., Fiester, S. J., & Parloff, M. B. (1989). National Institute of Mental Health Treatment of Depression Collaborative Research Program: General effectiveness of treatments. *Archives of General Psychiatry, 46,* 971–983.

Hammen, C. (1999). The emergence of an interpersonal approach to depression. In T. Joiner & J. Coyne (Eds.), *The interactional nature of depression: Advances in interpersonal approaches* (pp. 22–36). Washington, DC: American Psychological Association.

Joiner, T., Coyne, J., & Blalock, J. (1999). On the interpersonal nature of depression: Overview and synthesis. In T. Joiner & J. Coyne (Eds.), *The interactional nature of depression: Advances in interpersonal approaches* (pp. 3–20). Washington, DC: American Psychological Association.

Kaufman, J., Birmaher, B., Brent, D., Rao, U., Flynn, C., Moreci, P., Williamson, D. & Ryan, N. (1997). Schedule for Affective Disorders and Schizophrenia for School-age Children—Present and Lifetime Version (K-SADS-PL): Initial reliability and validity data. *Journal of the American Academy of Child and Adolescent Psychiatry, 36*(7), 980–988.

Kiesler, D. (1991). Interpersonal methods of assessment and diagnosis. In C. R. Snyder & D. R. Forsyth (Eds.), *Handbook of social and clinical psychology: The health perspective* (pp. 438–468). Elmsford, NY: Pergamon Press.

Klerman, G. L., Weissman, M. M., Rounsaville, B. J., & Chevron, E. S. (1984). *Interpersonal psychotherapy of depression.* New York: Basic Books.

Leibowitz, B. D. (2000). A public health approach to clinical therapeutics in psychiatry: Directions for new research. *Dialogues of Clinical Neuroscience, 2*(3), 309–313.

Marx, E., & Schulze, C. (1991). Interpersonal problem-solving in depressed students. *Journal of Clinical Psychology, 47,* 361–367.

Mufson, L., Moreau, D., Weissman, M. M., & Klerman, G. L. (1993). *Interpersonal psychotherapy for depressed adolescents.* New York: Guilford Press.

Mufson, L., Moreau, D., Weissman, M. M., Wickramaratne, P., Martin J., & Samoilov, A. (1994). The modification of interpersonal psychotherapy with depressed adolescents (IPT-A): Phase I and Phase II studies. *Journal of the American Academy of Child and Adolescent Psychiatry, 33,* 695–705.

Mufson, L., & Pollack Dorta, K. (2000). Interpersonal psychotherapy for depressed adolescents: Theory, practice, and research. In A. E. Esman (Ed.), *Adolescent psychiatry: The annals of the American Society for Adolescent Psychiatry* (Vol. 25, pp. 139–168). Hillsdale, NJ: Analytic Press.

Mufson, L., Weissman, M. M., Moreau, D., & Garfinkel, R. (1999). Efficacy of interpersonal psychotherapy for depressed adolescents. *Archives of General Psychiatry, 56,* 573–579.

Puig-Antich, J., Kaufman, J., Ryan, N. D., Williamson, D. E., Dahl, R. E., Lukens, E., Todak, G., Ambrosini, P., Rabinovich, H., & Nelson, B. (1993). The psychosocial functioning and family environment of depressed adolescents. *Journal of the American Academy of Child and Adolescent Psychiatry, 32,* 244–253.

Rosselló, J., & Bernal, G. (1999). The efficacy of cognitive-behavioral and interpersonal treatments for depression in Puerto Rican adolescents. *Journal of Consulting and Clinical Psychology, 67*(5), 734–745.

Rush, A. J. (1984). A phase II study of cognitive therapy of depression. In J. B. Williams & R. L Spitzer (Eds.), *Psychotherapy research: Where are we and where should we go?* (pp. 216–235). New York: Guilford Press.

Ryan, N. D., Puig-Antich, J., Ambrosini, P., Rabinovich, H., Robinson, D., Nelson, B., Iyengar, S., & Twomey, J. (1987). The clinical picture of major depression in children and adolescents. *Archives of General Psychiatry, 44,* 854–861.

Shaffer, D., Fisher, P., Lucas, C. P., Dulcan, M. K., & Schwab-Stone, M. E. (2000). NIMH Diagnostic Interview Schedule for Children Version IV (NIMH DISC IV): Description, differences from previous versions and reliability of some common diagnoses. *Journal of the American Academy of Child and Adolescent Psychiatry, 39*(1), 28–38.

Spruijt, E., & de Goede, M. (1997). Transitions in family structure and adolescent well-being. *Adolescence, 32,* 898–911.

Stader, S., & Hokanson, J. (1998). Psychosocial antecedents of depressive symptoms: An evaluation using daily experiences methodology. *Journal of Abnormal Psychology, 107,* 17–26.

Strober, M., Gree, J., & Carlson, C. (1981). Utility of the Beck Depression Inventory with psychiatrically hospitalized adolescents. *Journal of Consulting and Clinical Psychology, 48,* 482–483.

Sullivan, H. S. (1953). *The interpersonal theory of psychiatry.* New York: Norton.

Weissman, M. M., Prusoff, B. A., DiMascio, A., Neu, C., Goklaney, M., & Klerman, G. L. (1979). The efficacy of drug and psychotherapy in the treatment of acute depressive episodes. *American Journal of Psychiatry, 136,* 555–558.

Williams, J. B. W. (1988). A structured interview guide for the Hamilton Depression Rating Scale. *Archives of General Psychiatry, 45,* 742–747.

Wu, P., Hoven, C., Bird, H., Cohen, P., Alegria, M., Dulcan, M., Goodman, S., Horwitz, S., Lichtman, J., Narrow, W., Rae, D., Reiger, D., & Roper, M. (1999). Depressive and disruptive disorders and mental health service utilization in children and adolescents. *Journal of the American Academy of Child and Adolescent Psychiatry, 38,* 1081–1092.

10

Primary and Secondary Control Enhancement Training for Youth Depression

Applying the Deployment-Focused Model of Treatment Development and Testing

JOHN R. WEISZ, MICHAEL A. SOUTHAM-GEROW,
ELANA B. GORDIS, AND JENNIFER CONNOR-SMITH

OVERVIEW

Most children and adolescents have felt sad or down. But youngsters who meet criteria for depressive *disorders* in the fourth, most recent, edition of the *Diagnostic and Statistical Manual of Mental Disorders* (DSM-IV; American Psychiatric Association, 1994), have serious and debilitating problems. *Major depressive disorder,* for example, involves one or more episodes in which at least five depressive symptoms have been present for at least 2 weeks. One of these five must be either an increase in depressed or irritable mood (in adults, this must be *depressed* mood) or greatly diminished interest or pleasure. The other symptoms may include significant changes in weight (loss or gain), sleep (insomnia or hypersomnia), or psychomotor activity (slowing or agitation); increased fatigue, increased feelings of worthlessness or guilt; diminished concentration or decisiveness; or recurrent thoughts of death or suicidal thoughts or actions. A second relevant condition, *dysthymic disorder,* entails sad or irritable mood (in adults, this must be *depressed* mood) most of the day, for more days than not, for at least 1 year (2 years in adults), and the presence, while depressed, of at least two of the following: poor appetite or overeating, insomnia or hypersomnia, low energy or fatigue, low self-esteem, poor concentration or decisiveness, and feelings of hopelessness. Less studied but potentially relevant is a third category, *minor depressive disorder,* which is similar to major depressive disorder except that fewer symptoms are required. At any one point in time, about 2–5% of all youths meet criteria for a depressive disorder, but by the end of adolescence, as many as 20% may have met criteria at some time in their young life (see, e.g., Lewinsohn, Hops, Roberts, Seeley, & Andrews, 1993).

The emphasis on diagnosis has increased in recent years, but a large proportion of the research literature on youth depression has focused on youngsters who show elevated levels of depressive symptoms, often assessed via self-report questionnaires or interviews, without formal diagnostic assessment. From this literature on symptomatic youth, together with research focused squarely on diagnostic groupings, some general trends are evident:

- Rates of depression increase with age, with a modest increase from preschool to elementary school ages, and a substantial leap in adolescence.
- Gender differences are nonexistent or modest up until puberty, but rates of depression grow markedly higher in girls than boys thereafter, especially in late adolescence.
- Youth depression is often comorbid with other dysfunction, particularly anxiety disorders and disruptive behavior disorders. In one review (Angold & Costello, 1993), the presence of youth depression increased the probability of another disorder by at least 20 times.
- Youth depression is associated with serious functional problems, including poor academic achievement, disturbed interpersonal relationships, and markedly depressed scores on measures of global adjustment and functioning (see Hammen & Rudolph, 1996).
- Youth depression predicts later depression as well as increased long-term risk of substance use, employment problems, and marital difficulties (see, e.g., Gotlib, Lewinsohn, & Seeley, 1998; Rao, Daley, & Hammen, 2000).

This overall picture highlights the need to develop interventions that can help young people combat depression. Our work on this front has focused on psychosocial, behavioral, and cognitive processes. But before we describe this work, we would like to comment on the role of biological factors and the potential of biological interventions.

Although antidepressants are now the second most frequently prescribed class of psychotropics for pediatric populations in the United States (Weisz & Jensen, 1999), guidelines for child and adolescent use are not as well developed as for adult use, and there are puzzling differences between preadolescent and adolescent response (see, e.g., Ryan et al., 1986). In fact, recently published practice parameters by the American Academy of Child and Adolescent Psychiatry for the treatment and assessment of children and adolescents with depressive disorders recommended psychosocial therapy as the first treatment for most depressed youth (American Academy of Child and Adolescent Psychiatry, 1998). At present, the evidence base on tricyclic antidepressants shows weak effects with children, and only a few studies to date have tested the effects of selective serotonin reuptake inhibitors (SSRIs). As the evidence base on SSRIs and other antidepressants grows, it seems likely that a subset of youths will remain who do not respond well, and that most who do respond will not recover completely from all signs of depression. Logically, we know that cause and cure are not inextricably linked; thus even a depressed state that is heavily influenced by biological factors may, in principle, be treated effectively by a psychosocial intervention. And, of course, some parents would rather have their child try "talk therapy" before considering psychotropic medication. What appears to be happening in the field is that psychosocial intervention and medication are viewed increasingly as complementary interventions, partners in the treatment armamentarium. In this emerging partnership, our role has been to build primarily on a psychosocial model of depression and a psychological model of change, to which we now turn.

The Skills-and-Thoughts Depression Framework

The *skills-and-thoughts depression framework* focuses on skill deficits and habits of thought that set the stage for, and may prolong, depression in young people. The conceptual framework draws heavily from the theoretical and empirical work of numerous pioneers in the field (see References). The skills-and-thoughts perspective holds, in part, that characteristic skill deficits and cognitive habits can generate sad affect *and* make the child vulnerable to depressive symptoms in response to adverse, stressful, or ambiguous life events. Moreover, these deficits and habits may actually generate their own stressful events (e.g., unsuccessful interactions and social rejection), which then stimulate further depression, in cyclic fashion (see Hammen & Goodman-Brown, 1990).

Among the *skill deficits* documented in the literature on child depression (see reviews by Hammen & Rudolph, 1996; Weisz, Rudolph, Granger, & Sweeney, 1992) are (1) *poor problem-solving skills, with deficits in the generation, evaluation, and enactment of solutions*; (2) *maladaptive activity selection* (i.e., generally low activity level, failure to seek out pleasant activities, and tendency to engage in solitary and self-focused activities); (3) *tension and poorly developed self-soothing ability*, which leads to worry and avoidance of novel or potentially challenging situations; (4) *a diffident or otherwise unengaging social style*, which prevents satisfying interactions and impedes development of close relationships; and (5) *inferior performance in specific school- and/or peer-valued skill domains* (e.g., sports), which generates unfavorable social comparisons by self and others and undermines both peer status and self-esteem.

Among the *habits of thought* documented in the literature (see reviews by Gladstone & Kaslow, 1995; Weisz et al., 1992) are (1) *negative cognitions* (e.g., inappropriate self-blaming, catastrophizing, and failure to find the "silver lining"), which lead to unduly depressive interpretations of events, (2) *solitary cognition*—failure to bring others' perspectives into the picture, which leaves the individual's negative cognitions unchallenged; (3) *rumination* over unhappy events and cognitions, which magnifies their impact through repeated exposure; and (4) *perceived helplessness–hopelessness–lack of control*, which can lead to low level persistence in coping with stress and challenge.

Individual Differences

A key element in the skills-and-thoughts model is the notion that individuals can differ markedly from one another in the extent to which particular skill deficits or habits of thought play a role in their depression. For some, specific skill deficits and resulting low self-esteem may be central, whereas for others, there may be few skill deficits but a pervasive tendency to apply negative, depressogenic cognitions to daily events. There is no assumption that all, or even most, depressed youth show *all* the difficulties listed in the preceding two paragraphs. Noting such marked individual differences has led us to emphasize case formulations and the importance of tailoring treatment procedures to fit characteristics and contexts of the individual youngsters in treatment.

Reciprocal, Cyclic Process and Self-Generation of Stress

The skills-and-thoughts model construes the various skill deficits and habits of thought as operating in reciprocal, cyclic fashion, with each factor potentially exacerbating the effects of the other. For example, an unengaging social style may prevent the development of close relationships, increasing the likelihood of solitary cognition and thus leaving a child's depressogenic cognitions unchallenged and unaltered. The various processes may also cause depressed individuals to generate their own stressful events, as when lack of skill in a sport leads to poor performance and social rejection. A central task in treatment is to break this cycle of reciprocal influence and self-generated stress by providing clients with a collection of solution-relevant tools.

Role of Sociocultural and Familial Context

Finally, the model recognizes that each individual's depression occurs within a unique familial and sociocultural context. To understand fully each individual's depression, and to intervene effectively, requires an understanding of the relation between the symptoms and their context.

The Primary–Secondary Control Model of Change

The change model that drives the Primary and Secondary Control Enhancement Training (PASCET) program is the *two-process model* of control and coping (Rothbaum, Weisz, & Snyder, 1982; Weisz, McCabe, & Dennig, 1994; Weisz, Rothbaum, & Blackburn, 1984a, 1984b). In this model, *primary control* involves efforts to cope by making objective conditions (e.g., the activities one engages in, the outcome of a sports event, and one's acceptance by others) conform to one's wishes. In contrast, *secondary control* involves efforts to cope by adjusting oneself (e.g., one's beliefs, expectations, or interpretations of events) to fit objective conditions, to influence their subjective impact without altering the events themselves. The model holds that depression may be addressed, in part, by learning to apply primary control to distressing conditions that are modifiable, and secondary control to those conditions that are not.

This change model meshes well with the skills-and-thoughts depression model described earlier. In general, the skill deficits are addressed by primary control coping strategies taught in the PASCET program, and the habits of thought are addressed by secondary-control coping strategies taught in the PASCET program. Reduction in depression is construed as coming about gradually, through a growing working knowledge, and implementation (via in-session exercises and practice assignments) of the various primary and secondary coping strategies that may be used to combat depressive symptoms and the conditions that trigger them.

The model recognizes that change is most likely to occur if the coping skills are taught and practiced, in ways that fit into the individual's particular style and manner of expressing depression, and into the sociocultural and family context of the individual's life. Thus, the change agent (i.e., therapist) is expected to learn as much as possible about the distinctive character of the individual's depression, and about the family, school, and peer social situation in relation to the individual's symptoms, and then to make the learning exercises and practice activities relevant to the individual and his or her context. In this theme and others, we owe much to such insightful leaders as Henggeler, Schoenwald, Borduin, Rowland, and Cunningham (1998) and Persons (1993).

Finally, the model recognizes that individual change ultimately involves a personal decision to select certain change mechanisms over others. Intervention is thus construed as teaching young clients about an array of primary and secondary control coping skills and strategies for change and helping each youth select those for emphasis that seem most relevant personally and most likely to be helpful. This notion connects with the "toolbox concept," discussed later as we describe the treatment program itself.

CHARACTERISTICS OF THE TREATMENT PROGRAM

The PASCET program is a structured intervention for depression, designed for use with youngsters ages 8–15. Treatment sessions, take-home practice assignments, and parent handouts are built on research findings concerning cognitive and behavioral features of depression in children and adolescents, and on the two-process model of perceived control and coping, discussed previously. As suggested by that model, youngsters are trained to gain control of their mood by developing skills that will help them cultivate primary and secondary control. The treatment procedures used are derived primarily from the rich cognitive-behavioral tradition.

In its current form, the program involves individual child sessions complemented by parent, family, and school contact, with therapists guided through all these steps by a treatment manual. Youngsters take part in about 10 structured, manualized sessions, followed by about 5 individually tailored sessions, involving (1) applications of the most personally relevant PASCET coping skills to important situations or problems in the youth's life and (2) planning for future applications of the PASCET skills after the treatment has ended. Within-session exercises and take-home practice (i.e., homework) assignments are guided by an *ACT & THINK Practice Book*, which the youngsters use during treatment and keep thereafter. Individual youth sessions are complemented by contact with parents in three forms. First, each individual youth session ends with a *summary conference* in which the youth and therapist are joined by one or both parents or other family members to review the main points of the day's session, go over the youth's practice assignment for the upcoming week, and make plans for family members to collaborate in the practice assignment. In each summary conference, the therapist provides family members with a handout summarizing information about the session and the practice assignment. Second, separate *parent sessions* are held, at the beginning, middle, and end of the youth's treatment, to discuss the treatment program, solicit parent perspectives on the youth's mood and behavior at home, and help parents find resources to improve their parenting skills, address marital difficulties, or treat their own mental health problems. And third, the therapist makes one *home visit*, to meet the youth's family and learn about the living environment. In addition, the therapist makes at least one *school visit*, to learn about the youth from relevant school personnel and to observe the school environment.

Skills Emphasized in the Program

An ACT & THINK Chart, provided to parents and youths, summarizes the skills emphasized in the treatment program. In identifying ways to convey the skills to young people, we learned a great deal from an array of excellent youth treatment researchers (e.g., Clarke, Lewinsohn, & Hops, 1990; Kazdin, Seigel, & Bass, 1992; Lewinsohn & Rohde, 1993; Stark, 1990; reviewed in Weisz, Valeri, McCarty, & Moore, 1999). The first set of skills (listed in Table 10.1) fits within the ACT acronym; these skills emphasize primary control.

- *Activities that solve problems.* To counter resignation in the face of difficulties, we encourage youngsters to tackle daily problems by applying systematic problem solving (see Kazdin, Chapter 14, this volume; Kazdin et al., 1992; Spivack, Platt, & Shure, 1976). We teach and practice STEPS ("*Say what the problem is. Think of solutions. Examine each one. Pick one and try it out. See if it worked.*").
- *Activities I enjoy.* To counter maladaptive activity selection, therapists work with the youth to create a menu of specific activities that are reliable mood enhancers *and* that are readily accessible without adult help (Disneyland and Magic Mountain are out; music and phoning a friend are in). We try to include some activities with others and some altruistic activities, to counter the self-focus that can exacerbate sad feelings. Youngsters select and practice activities from the menu and record and discuss the impact of those activities on their mood.
- *Calm* . . . To address the tension and anxiety that often accompany depression, we teach both progressive muscle relaxation with mental imagery and diaphragmatic breathing exercises that we label "secret calming," for use in public situations.
- . . . *and Confident.* To deal with the unengaging social style that can sometimes accompany depression, therapists and youth identify behaviors that show a "positive self" and "negative self"; they do role-plays involving both styles. *In vivo* exercises (i.e., in-session exercises in real-world situations, such as approaching the clinic secretary using the positive self skills) and take-home practice assignments provide opportunities to try out the "positive self" skills and observe their impact on self and others.
- *Talents.* To address specific skill gaps that can undermine both social standing and self-esteem, youth identify skills they want to enhance (academic, athletic, artistic, social, etc.), then work with therapists to break the skill down into steps and implement a practice schedule.

As the initial sessions focusing on the ACT skills are completed, therapists focus discussion on the fact that some of the difficult situations they confront may be hard for youth to change through their own actions. For these more intractable problems, young-

---

TABLE 10.1. Coping Skills Emphasized in the PASCET Program

ACT (primary control) skills
- Activities that solve problems [Use systematic steps to find solutions to everyday problems.]
- Activities I enjoy [Create a menu of pleasant activities, schedule them, record impact on mood.]
- Calm [Learn and practice two methods of achieving relaxation and self-soothing.]
- Confident [Identify and practice ways to show a positive self; observe effects on self and others.]
- Talents [Break desired skills into steps and implement a practice schedule.]

THINK (secondary control) skills
- Think positive [Identify and alter cognitions that are unrealistically negative.]
- Help from a friend [Call on others who can offer helpful views on troubling situations.]
- Identify the "silver lining" [Learn to find the benefits embedded in adverse situations.]
- No replaying bad thoughts [Use distraction to cut short rumination over bad experiences.]
- Keep thinking—Don't give up [Plan multiple coping steps until emotional state improves.]

sters may only be able to feel better by changing how they think about their situation. This discussion launches a second phase of treatment, focused on the THINK skills:

- *Think positive.* Here the focus is on identifying and altering cognitions that are unrealistically negative. Therapists use multiple approaches (e.g., self-disclosure, vignettes, role-plays, and video clips) to build their young clients' skills in recognizing and reshaping distorted thinking.
- *Help from a friend.* Together, therapist and youth create a list of people with whom to "think things over"—people who can offer helpful perspectives on troubling situations. Practice focuses partly on forming the habit of reaching out when troubled, and evaluating the impact.
- *Identify the "silver lining."* Therapist and youth work to cultivate the skill of finding benefit made possible by situations that seem otherwise adverse.
- *No replaying bad thoughts.* Here the goal is to combat tendencies to ruminate about bad experiences and thus spiral toward depression by identifying and practicing highly distracting activities—activities so engaging they prevent unproductive rumination.
- *Keep thinking—Don't give up.* To combat passivity and helplessness, we encourage youngsters to persevere in thinking of ways to cope. Therapists work to instill the idea that first attempts often fail, and that sequential coping—Plan A, B, C, etc.—is often required for success. Youngsters develop and practice their own multistep coping plans.

Selecting "Best-Fit" Coping Skills, Designing Sequential Coping Plans

After initial exposure and practice has focused on each of the skills noted previously (which requires about 10 sessions), therapist and youth identify a few of the skills that seem most useful. The remainder of the treatment (usually about five sessions) is devoted to individually tailored role-plays, in-session *in vivo* exercise, and between-session practice assignments, focused on the use of those few skills that are most personally relevant and helpful, in response to the conditions and events that are the most common sources of distress. Typically, the skills are strung together in the form of stepwise coping plans (à la the last of the aforementioned THINK skills). For example, one youngster who was troubled at night over thoughts of his parents' separation and divorce developed the following coping plan: His Plan A (i.e., first coping strategy) was to call a friend who had faced the same problem and who really knew how to make him feel better. If that strategy was unavailable (e.g., his friend couldn't talk on the phone then) or if it failed to dispel the sad feelings, Plan B was to distract himself through reading and listening to music. If those two strategies failed to help, or only helped somewhat, Plan C was to listen to his relaxation tape (made in the session with his therapist), so he could get calm, put a pleasant image in his mind, and go to sleep. Ideally, parents who have been involved through collaborative practice sessions with their children continue to prompt and praise the use of coping skills while therapy is ongoing, and afterward when the therapist is no longer in the picture.

Case Formulation and the Toolbox Concept

The individualizing process is guided by case formulations (see Persons, 1993). The therapist's experience in individual youth sessions, parent sessions, home visit, and school visit is used to create, then continually revise and update, an individual formulation—a coherent, integrated description of the youth and his or her life situation, emphasizing the antecedents and behavioral expression of his or her depression, the coping strategies from the PASCET protocol that are most likely to be helpful to this particular youth, and how these coping strategies may best be applied given the conditions and constraints of this youngster's life. This therapist formulation is used, together with input from the youth and parent(s), to plan the best ways to introduce and apply core coping skills during the structured sessions, and to design the individually tailored sessions that occur in roughly the last third of the treatment protocol. We view the initial phase of treatment as providing youngsters with a *toolbox* containing a variety of skills. The full course of treatment involves identifying those few tools that appear most useful to the individual youth, and then practicing their use to proficiency. When proficiency is demonstrated in the *in vivo* exercises and practice assignments, and when parents or other family members appear ready to support continued use of the skills, it is time for termination.

In a later section, we review our research on effects of the PASCET program. But first we discuss the model of treatment development and testing that guides this research.

STRATEGY FOR TREATMENT DEVELOPMENT AND TESTING: THE DEPLOYMENT-FOCUSED MODEL

Our work with the PASCET program has been guided by a deployment-focused model (DFM) of treatment development and testing (Weisz, in press-a, in press-b). The model is intended in part to promote the movement of clinical trials into service settings, and thus to promote the development of tested treatments that are ready for use in clinical practice. It certainly is the case that despite a strong body of clinical trials research on child and adolescent treatments, most of the interventions studied have not actually made their way into routine use in clinical practice settings or become part of the usual standard of care for practitioners. Indeed, even mature evidence-based treatments that have undergone rather extensive efficacy testing have, for the most part, not been subject to "effectiveness tests" (i.e., trials testing the treatments as provided to naturally referred individuals treated by practitioners in the settings and under the conditions of everyday practice).

The proposed DFM is explicitly geared to ensuring that tests in practice settings do occur, and thus to producing treatments that are designed to work well in those settings. The model is guided by three primary aims: (1) developing treatments that can fit smoothly into everyday practice and work well with clinic-referred individuals treated in clinic settings by practicing clinicians; (2) generating evidence on treatment outcome in actual clinical practice, the kind of evidence clinicians and clinic administrators most need to assess the likely utility of the treatments for their settings; and (3) producing a body of evidence on the nature, necessary and sufficient components, boundary conditions (i.e., moderators), and change processes (i.e., mediators) associated with treatment impact that will have a high level of external validity because it is derived from research in the practice context. The model entails six steps of treatment development and testing, as shown in Figure 10.1.

- *Step 1: Theoretically and clinically guided construction of the treatment protocol.* The initial step is development, refinement, pilot testing, and manualizing of the treatment protocol. Theory and evidence on the nature and treatment of the target condition, the clinical literature (e.g., published case studies), and input from experienced clinicians

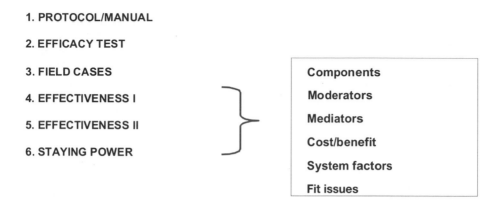

1. PROTOCOL/MANUAL

2. EFFICACY TEST

3. FIELD CASES

4. EFFECTIVENESS I

5. EFFECTIVENESS II

6. STAYING POWER

Components

Moderators

Mediators

Cost/benefit

System factors

Fit issues

FIGURE 10.1. Steps in the deployment-focused model of treatment development and testing. Copyright 2002 by J. R. Weisz. Reprinted by permission.

are used to guide the design of treatment components. The goal is the production of a well-grounded (i.e., theoretically and empirically), manualized treatment program that possesses a high degree of adaptability across a variety of clinical situations. The treatment protocol should grow out of a clearly articulated model of the condition being treated, and of the mechanism(s) by which change in that condition is brought about.

• *Step 2: Initial efficacy trial under controlled conditions, to establish potential for benefit.* Next, an initial *efficacy* trial is used to assess whether the treatment (compared to a control group) can produce beneficial effects with youth treated under controlled laboratory conditions. The focus is the systematic study of volunteers, not clinically referred cases, to avoid the risk of exposing severely disordered individuals to an untested intervention.

• *Step 3: Single-case applications in practice settings, with progressive adaptations to the protocol.* Next comes a series of single-case tests with clinic-referred individuals, treated in clinical settings representative of those for which the treatment is ultimately intended. Ideally, there is dual supervision (i.e., one supervisor from the research team who is expert in the treatment protocol to ensure faithfulness to the core treatment principles, plus a second who is an experienced clinic staff member) to monitor the appropriateness of the treatment for the family and the clinical setting. Successive modifications are made to the treatment protocol to ensure goodness of fit while also adhering to the model of change. The process of Stage 3 guides decisions as to the *type* of manual best suited to the clinical context, with choices ranging from highly structured, session-by-session instructions (see, e.g., Clarke et al., 1990) to broad treatment principles with illustrations of how to apply them (see, e.g., Henggeler et al., 1998).

• *Step 4: Initial effectiveness test.* The fourth step involves an initial group-design effectiveness trial in which the newly adapted treatment protocol is tested in a practice setting, with clinically referred youngsters who meet criteria for the target condition, and with treatment provided by practitioners who work in the setting. Outcomes are compared for youth randomly assigned to either the manualized treatment or the usual treatment procedures in the setting. In this initial effort to move from a series of individual cases and successive modifications in the protocol to more uniform applications of the protocol across clients and therapists, two goals are paramount. One is to provide initial evidence on whether introducing the target treatment improves outcomes relative to the intervention clients in the setting would have otherwise received. Another is to begin what is likely to be a lengthy process of investigator education. That is, efforts to apply the protocol effectively within a group-design trial will likely teach treatment developers a great deal about setting conditions, characteristics of referred youth and their families, therapist responses to training and supervision, and numerous other factors that need to be addressed to deploy the intervention effectively across groups of clinicians and youth in the practice context. Lessons learned in this process can inform the design of subsequent effectiveness tests.

• *Step 5: Further tests of effectiveness and dissemination.* These subsequent tests are additional group-design clinical trials, with the target treatment provided to referred clients, in practice settings, by staff practitioners. As in Step 4, clients are randomly assigned to either the target treatment or usual care. Each subsequent effectiveness test builds on lessons learned in previous trials regarding ways to fit the treatment into the setting, ways to engage the kinds of clients who seek care there, ways to build therapist proficiency in the protocol, and ways to address a variety of problems that may arise with attempts to change current practices via dissemination of new procedures. The individual studies are intended to assess the disseminability and effectiveness of the treatment program under the most representative clinic conditions possible. The series of studies is intended to refine procedures for deploying the protocol to the point that it fits so well into the setting and works so well with referred clients that it can continue to be used effectively after the treatment researchers are gone.

• *Step 6: Tests of goodness of fit and sustainability in practice contexts.* The final step focuses on the fit of the treatment program to the practice context in which it is employed. The aim is to identify factors that predict (a) the likelihood that practitioners will use the treatment, (b) the degree to which those who do use it will adhere to the protocol, and (c) the extent to which use of the protocol improves youth outcomes. An overarching focus will be assessment of staying power (i.e., continued use, with treatment integrity and youth outcomes maintained) over time in various practice settings.

• *Additional foci throughout Steps 4, 5, and 6: Components, moderators, mediators, cost–benefit, system factors, and fit issues.* There is much additional learning that can be done within Steps 4–6. As shown in Figure 10.1, a goal in these studies is to use variations in design and measurement to (a) ascertain the necessary and sufficient components of our complex treatment packages, (b) identify moderators of outcome that set boundaries around treatment impact, (c) assess whether proposed change processes in treatment do in fact mediate outcomes, (d) assess treatment costs in relation to benefits, (e) investigate which organizational factors in the systems and settings where the treatments are used (e.g., community mental health clinics, inpatient psychiatric units, primary care clinics, schools, and social service agencies) relate to how effectively the treatments are used, and (f) test variations in treatment procedures, packaging, training, and delivery designed to improve fit to various settings in which the treatment is deployed. The aim is to generate a mosaic of information about the target treatment, its most essential ingredients, the factors that enhance or undermine its success, the boundary conditions that define the effective range of the treatment, the change processes that account for its effects, and procedural modifications that can magnify treatment effects or extend their duration.

Of course, the large body of published *efficacy* research with children and adolescents already includes numerous dismantling studies, and moderator and mediator tests are more and more evident in recent years (see Weersing & Weisz, 2002). It might be argued that the control and precision of efficacy designs make them particularly appropriate for such work. Our concern is that what we learn through dismantling studies, moderator assessment, and mediator tests in efficacy trials may not apply so well to a treatment when it is used in clinical service settings. Because the clients, therapists, and conditions of treatment in those settings can differ in so many ways from those of efficacy tests (see, e.g., Southam-Gerow, Kendall, & Weisz, in press), the degree to which separate components of the treatment package can produce effects in practice may be quite different from what was found in those tests (see also Strosahl, Hayes, Bergan, & Romano, 1998). Similarly, the impact of various moderators and the processes that mediate treatment effects may be different for real-world clinical cases and settings than in an experimental sample tested in a university research clinic. For example, we might find that our treatment works well across the range of socioeconomic status (SES) tested in our university research clinic, in which clients are all study volunteers who are paid or treated free of charge, but that when we test the treatment in community clinics, where clients are neither paid nor given free treatment, SES has a substantial effect on both attendance and outcome (see Kazdin & Wassell, 1999, for discussion of other barriers to participation). In general, it seems possible that the most externally valid and practically useful answers to questions about treatment outcome, necessary and sufficient ingredients, moderators, and mediators may come from research with referred samples seen under genuine clinical practice conditions.

APPLYING THE DEPLOYMENT-FOCUSED MODEL TO THE PASCET PROGRAM

We are following the DFM rather closely in our efforts to develop and test the PASCET program.

Developing a Manual for the Protocol

In developing the initial manual and treatment materials for the PASCET protocol, we drew from a variety of empirical, theoretical, and clinical sources, as have many treatment developers before us. Fortunately, there is a rich empirical literature on the characteristics of depressed youth (see, e.g., Hammen & Rudolph, 1996) and a rich treatment literature packed with interventions for addressing those characteristics (see, e.g., Lewinsohn, Clarke, Hops, & Andrews, 1990; Starke, Reynolds, & Kaslow, 1987). And clinician colleagues were generous in sharing ideas and feedback as the manual and materials were being developed.

Initial Efficacy Test of the PASCET Program

In our initial efficacy test of the manualized program (Weisz, Thurber, Sweeney, Proffit, & Legagnoux, 1997), we focused on elementary school youngsters who showed elevated levels of depressive symptomatology, assessed via the self-report Children's Depression Inventory (CDI; Kovacs, 1992) and the Children's Depression Rating Scale—Revised (CDRS-R; Poznanski & Mokros, 1996), a standardized clinical interview. The 48 children from grades 3–6 included 26 boys and 22 girls, with a mean age of 9.6 years; 30 were Caucasian and 18 were ethnic minority youngsters (primarily African American). Participants were randomly assigned to the PASCET program (an abbreviated version of the one described earlier) or to a no-treatment control group. Those in the PASCET con-

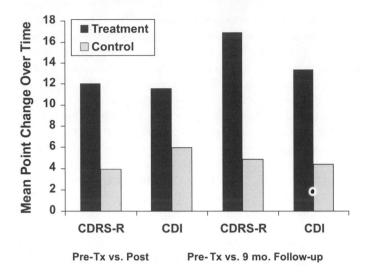

FIGURE 10.2. Treatment group and control group change in Children's Depression Rating Scale—Revised (CDRS-R) and Children's Depression Inventory (CDI) scores from pretreatment (Pre-Tx) to posttreatment (Post) and from pretreatment to follow-up assessment 9 months after the end of treatment (9-mo. follow-up). From Weisz, Thurber, Sweeney, Proffitt, and LeGagnoux (1997). Copyright 1997 by the American Psychological Association. Reprinted by permission.

dition were formed into small groups (three to five), meeting once weekly, each with two cotherapists. The therapists included one licensed doctoral-level clinical psychologist and five graduate students in a clinical psychology doctoral program; study-related training and supervision included pretreatment reading, review, and discussion of the treatment manual, with weekly meetings (60–90 minutes each) to review previous sessions and role play upcoming sessions.

Outcomes were assessed posttreatment, and again after 9 months. At both assessment points, the treatment group showed significantly greater reductions than did the control group in depressive symptomatology on the CDI and CDRS-R (see Figure 10.2). Posttreatment and follow-up between-group comparisons both showed significantly less depression on the self-report questionnaire for the treated children than the untreated children; mean differences ran in the same direction but were not significant on the clinical interview measure. The clinical significance of group differences was supported by the fact that treated children, more than controls, shifted from above to within the normal range on both measures. These group differences were significant at posttreatment for the questionnaire measure (50% vs. 16%) and at follow-up for both the questionnaire measure (62% vs. 31%) and the interview measure (69% vs. 24%).

In the context of the DFM, a primary function of the initial efficacy trial was to assess whether the treatment program has the potential for benefit. With the findings supporting potential benefit, we moved to the next step in the DFM—field cases.

Trying PASCET with Referred Community Clinic Cases, and Adapting the Protocol to Fit

Following the DFM approach, we next took the PASCET protocol into one of the primary settings for which it is ultimately intended: the community mental health clinic. We used the program with clinic-referred youth, adapting it as needed to make it work in the new setting and with these youth who were markedly more disturbed and distressed than the ones we had seen in schools in the initial trial. Therapists were advanced clinical trainees, individually supervised jointly by (1) senior clinic staff therapists, suggesting adjustments to fit client and clinic characteristics, and (2) the first author (JRW), encouraging adherence to the core principles of the PASCET model. As a result of these field trials of the program, we made a number of changes designed to make the protocol fit smoothly into the clinic setting and work effectively with referred youth. Following are a few examples:

- We changed from a group format to an individually administered format because the sensitivity of personal and family issues (e.g., sexual abuse and parental infidelity) made group discussion clinically inappropriate, and the logistical challenge of scheduling multiple depressed youth at common meeting times proved too formidable to manage.
- We added problem-solving training, as reports of new problems were a near-weekly occurrence in our clinic youth, and positive self-presentation skills, as ineffective social style was so often an issue for the clinic youth.
- The complexity of our youngsters' family and school situations, and our need to understand these to fashion appropriate interventions, led us to expand parent involvement and to add home and school visits.
- We lengthened the treatment, devoting more time to introducing the various skills, practicing them in session and at home, discerning each youth's few "best fit" skills, and individualizing their application to each youth's real-life situations.
- We improved the organization of the therapist manual and youth practice book, based on feedback from therapists, clinic supervisors, and youth themselves, as to what was needed to make these aids most useful.

With these and other clinic-experience-inspired refinements, the PASCET program took the form detailed previously in the section "Characteristics of the Treatment Program," leaving us positioned for Step 4 in the model.

Design of the Initial Effectiveness Trial

The first PASCET effectiveness trial is currently under way, with children and adolescents referred to community mental health clinics. One goal is to provide an initial test of whether the protocol can produce greater relief from youth depression than the usual treatment procedures in the clinics. A broader goal is to begin identifying the challenges that will need to be addressed to deploy the intervention effectively across groups of clinicians and youth in the practice context.

All study therapists are regular staff and trainees of the five Los Angeles area clinics participating in the project. To ensure that any group differences in outcome (i.e., between PASCET and usual care) reflect differences in treatment method, not therapist characteristics, all therapists have been randomized to continue providing treatment in their usual manner or to receive training and supervision in the PASCET program. PASCET training is done in one 6-hour program, and group supervision typically involves about a half hour per week for each client.

We work with youth ages 8–15 who have been referred through normal channels to any of our five participating clinics. (We do not run ads or otherwise recruit participants, because we want findings to generalize to youth who are normally referred to community clinics.) Youngsters and their parents are administered standardized diagnostic interviews, and youth are invited to participate if they meet criteria for major depressive disorder, minor depressive disorder, or dysthymic disorder. When youth and families agree to take part, they are randomized to usual care or to PASCET. The usual care condition is a particularly strong comparison against which to pit PASCET because each therapist's usual care procedures tend to involve the intervention methods in which the therapist is most experienced and believes most strongly. By contrast, therapists in the PASCET condition use procedures that are less familiar to them, procedures they are still learning while doing treatment. This state of affairs provides a test of how clinician therapists, employed in service clinics, fare when using PASCET, supported by a level of training and supervision that is actually feasible for them in normal practice. After all, it is these kinds of therapists, working in normal practice conditions, to whom we ultimately want to disseminate the treatment program if it is found to be effective.

Outcome assessments for the project take place when treatment ends and at later follow-ups. We expect to learn from the results regardless of the outcome. But even before we reach that point, we have learned a good deal from the study that helps us understand the challenge of spanning the gap between treatment research and clinical care in service settings. Among the lessons we have learned:

• Depression is not easy to identify among youngsters referred to community mental health clinics. The most common reason for referral to such clinics tends to be externalizing, disruptive behavior. Few youth appear to be referred because they are quietly depressed. One important consequence may be that many quietly depressed youngsters remain unreferred and untreated. This fits with previous studies suggesting that a majority of depressed youth do not receive treatment, even in samples of insured youth with access to services.

• Comorbidity is rampant among depressed youth in our community clinics. Perhaps in part because externalizing, disruptive behavior is the most common ticket of admission to such clinics, most (> 80%) of our depressed youth also meet criteria for one or more disruptive behavior disorders (conduct disorder, oppositional defiant disorder, attention-deficit/hyperactivity disorder); additional comorbidities, such as anxiety disorders, are also common.

• We have often broadened the treatment focus to respect parent and youth concerns and to keep families engaged in treatment. This is true in part because so many of our youngsters were initially referred in whole or in part because of their externalizing problems. In each study case, further assessment has identified depression warranting treatment, but a failure by the therapist to also address initial referral concerns can understandably reduce parents' motivation to keep their children in treatment (see Garcia & Weisz, 2002). The need to expand our scope of treatment has generated a more flexible use of the manual than we had originally envisioned.

• Generating skilled use of a manual-guided treatment is a difficult task with therapists who were trained in different approaches to therapy. The great majority of our therapists are idealistic, highly professional, and strongly committed to helping children. But few have ever used a treatment manual before. The structured, sequential approach embodied in the manual often clashes with therapists' previous experience and training, particularly when the previous orientation emphasized listening and reflecting rather than bringing an agenda to the session. There are marked individual differences among therapists in the degree of success experienced in making the transition to a structured, manualized approach. But most therapists seem to find the challenge intriguing, and several have indicated that it actually made them feel more confident to approach each session with a specific plan. This enthusiasm is tempered by the fact that therapist turnover in the clinics often hampers acquisition of polished expertise in the protocol.

• Youngsters in community clinic care tend to come from highly stressed families in which crises are common. Indeed, many of our youth bring a *crisis of the week* to most sessions, and these crises can derail a therapist's session plan. Part of the art of using a manualized treatment, we believe, is turning such crises into skill-building opportunities. That is, whenever possible, we try to have therapists convey the skills covered in treatment by applying them to real-world problems or crises the youth has brought to the session. The ideal is genuinely to address the concern the youth has brought to the therapist while also conveying a useful skill for coping with that concern.

• Testing a new treatment in clinical practice settings can be challenging, logistically and otherwise. Indeed, doing this study has helped us understand why so many other investigators have not. To make the project feasible for full-time clinic therapists, we must send mobile supervision teams to the various clinics each week. To make the project feasible for youth and their families (to ensure a truly representative sample), we must send mobile assessment teams to locations the families can reach easily, at all assessment points in the study (and often to find no family there). To identify relevant cases, we must find our way within each clinic's distinctive and often evolving procedures for referral, intake, and case assignment. This, together with the need to balance research requirements against the clinics' ultimate responsibility for clinical care, has created complicated questions, which are typically addressed differently by the seven human subjects committees monitoring the study. This has led to an ongoing state of affairs best described as *dueling internal review boards* (IRBs). At present, it appears that neither the research establishment nor the clinical care establishment (outside universities, at least) seems ideally suited to the kind of collaboration needed in effectiveness research. Changes may be needed if research of this type is to proliferate.

DIRECTIONS FOR FUTURE RESEARCH

The treatment approach described in this chapter is a work in progress. We have begun the process of testing it, but a great deal remains to be done. In this chapter we have used research on the PASCET program to illustrate a generic model of treatment development and testing. This DFM is designed to produce treatments that fit well into practice contexts and work well with individuals treated in those contexts. It is also designed to produce externally valid evidence on treatment effects and on such related topics as the boundary conditions of treatment impact (moderators), the necessary and sufficient components of the program, and the change processes through which the treatment works when it does (mediation). In general, for many treatments, we suspect that these objectives can be well served by carrying out much of the treatment development and testing process in the practice settings for which the treatment programs are ultimately intended.

That said, we must emphasize that at present neither the world of research nor the world of clinical practice seems well-suited to work that brings the two worlds together. As we illustrated in the chapter, our effectiveness study has presented significant challenges, logistically and clinically. These are quite understandable, given the substantial gulf between research and practice in objectives, constraints, and even daily work requirements. To make research that spans this gulf a viable and attractive option for both investigators and clinicians may well require a more comprehensive effort than is feasible for any one research team. The effort may need to encompass multiple fronts including personnel (clinicians with productivity requirements stand to lose by participating in research), funding (effectiveness research is costly), ethics (dueling IRBs make for inefficient human subjects review), and many others. For effectiveness research to prosper, changes may be needed to ensure that the benefits outweigh the costs, for both investigators and practicing clinicians.

We have one final thought on future research in the area. One possible explanation we have considered for the slow pace of dissemination research is that treatments with a good evidence base are *disorder focused* (i.e., focused on the amelioration of a single mental disorder). However, as noted previously, a large body of evidence indicates that many youngsters in clinical samples meet criteria for multiple disorders. Moreover, many youth have multiple problems requiring clinical attention yet do not qualify for a formal diagnosis. Furthermore, the perception among some influential clinicians is that evidence-based treatments are not applicable in their settings because their cases are more complex than those in research settings (e.g., Fensterheim & Raw, 1996), and there is emerging evidence that clinical cases may indeed be more complex, on average, than research cases (e.g., Hammen, Rudolph, Weisz, Burge, & Rao, 1999; Southam-Gerow et al., in press). Thus, as we described in our experience with PASCET in community clinics, one way to improve mental health care for children and families in clinical practice may be to nudge treatment programs toward increased capacity to focus on multiple problems, even when they do not fall neatly within the same diagnostic category.

SUMMARY AND CONCLUSIONS

The PASCET program focuses on treatment of depressed youngsters ages 8–15. The program grows out of the cognitive-behavioral tradition and builds on the primary–secondary control model of change. In treatment sessions and in take-home assignments, youngsters learn and practice coping skills of two types: primary control skills for altering objective events in their lives and secondary control skills for altering the subjective impact of stressors (i.e., the thoughts and feelings they provoke). Over the course of the program, youth are encouraged to identify a small number of the coping skills that work particularly well for them and to practice applying those skills sequentially in response to distressing events or conditions. Parents are taught the skills as well, and encouraged to support their children's use of them.

Our research group has focused not only on development of this particular depression treatment program but also on a more general strategy for treatment development. Our DFM is intended to support the development of treatments that are ready for dissemination to and effective use in clinical practice contexts. Toward that end, the model calls for steps of development and testing that move expeditiously from an initial efficacy trial to adaptations and tests of the treatment with referred youth, treated by practicing clinicians, and in clinical practice contexts.

We have begun applying the DFM to the PASCET program. An initial efficacy trial of the program with youngsters recruited from schools showed evidence that PASCET has the potential to alleviate depressive symptoms, producing markedly more movement from the clinical range to the normal range on depression measures in comparison to a randomly assigned control group. This trial was followed by a series of cases treated in the community mental health clinic setting, with progressive adaptations to the protocol made in response to the treatment challenges we encountered there. With the protocol thus adapted, we have begun a trial of the PASCET program in multiple community mental health clinics, targeting depressed children who have been referred to the clinics through normal channels, and with treatment administered by community clinic therapists. The therapists have been randomly assigned to learn and apply the PASCET program or to continue doing their own preferred usual treatment procedures for working with depressed youth.

We are midway into this community clinic trial at present. But we have already learned a good deal about the challenge of bringing structured, manual-guided treatment into a clinical practice context. Our experience underscores numerous differences between the conditions that have traditionally been created to test treatments and the conditions in which most treatments are employed in clinical practice. We hope our work can contribute to bridging some of those differences. The bridging task seems an important one, particularly if we want the treatments tested in research to make their way into the world of clinical practice.

ACKNOWLEDGMENTS

The work described in this chapter was supported by research grants (RO1 MH49522, R01 MH57347) and a Research Scientist Award (K05 MH01161) from the National Institute of Mental Health, which we gratefully acknowledge. We also offer sincere thanks to the colleagues on our research team who have played such important roles in supporting the research and enhancing the intellectual climate. These include Trilby Cox, Alanna Gelbwasser, Kristin Hawley, Mandy Jensen, Anna Lau, Cari McCarty, Bryce McLeod, Phoebe Moore, Antonio Polo, Tamara Sharpe, Lynne Sweeney, Chris Thurber, Sylvia Valeri, and Robin Weersing,

REFERENCES

American Academy of Child and Adolescent Psychiatry. (1998). Practice parameters for the assessment and treatment of children and adolescents with depressive disorders. *Journal of the American Academy of Child and Adolescent Psychiatry, 37*(10, Suppl.).

American Psychiatric Association (1994). *Diagnostic and statistical manual of mental disorders* (4th ed.). Washington, DC: Author.

Angold, A., & Costello, E. J. (1993). Depressive comorbidity in children and adolescents: Empirical, theoretical, and methodological issues. *American Journal of Psychiatry, 150,* 1779–1791.

Clarke, G., Lewinsohn, P., & Hops, H. (1990). *Leader's manual for adolescent groups: Adolescent coping with depression course.* Eugene, OR: Castalia.

Fensterheim, H., & Raw, S. D. (1996). Psychotherapy research is not psychotherapy practice. *Clinical Psychology: Science and Practice, 3,* 168–171.

Garcia, J. A., & Weisz, J. R. (2002). When youth mental health care stops: Therapeutic relationship problems and other reasons for ending youth outpatient treatment. *Journal of Consulting and Clinical Psychology, 70,* 439–443.

Gladstone, T. R. G., & Kaslow, N. J. (1995). Depression and attributions in children and adolescents: A meta-analytic review. *Journal of Abnormal Child Psychology, 23,* 597–606.

Gotlib, I. H., Lewinsohn, P. M., & Seeley, J. R. (1998). Consequences of depression during adolescence: Marital status and marital functioning in early adulthood. *Journal of Abnormal Psychology, 107,* 686–690.

Hammen, C., & Goodman-Brown, T. (1990). Self-schemas and vulnerability to specific life stress in children at risk for depression. *Cognitive Therapy and Research, 14,* 215–227.

Hammen, C., & Rudolph, K. D. (1996). Childhood depression. In E. J. Mash & R. A. Barkley (Eds.), *Child psychopathology* (pp. 153–195). New York: Guilford Press.

Hammen, C., Rudolph, K., Weisz, J. R., Burge, D., & Rao, U. (1999). The context of depression in clinic-referred youth: Neglected areas in treatment. *Journal of the American Academy of Child and Adolescent Psychiatry, 38,* 64–71.

Henggeler, S. W., Schoenwald, S. K., Borduin, C. M., Rowland, M. D., & Cunningham, P. B. (1998). *Multisystemic treatment of antisocial behavior in children and adolescents.* New York: Guilford Press.

Kazdin, A. E., Seigel, T., & Bass, D. (1992). Cognitive problem-solving skills training and parent management training in the treatment of antisocial behavior in children. *Journal of Consulting and Clinical Psychology, 60,* 733–747.

Kazdin, A. E., & Wassell, G. (1999). Barriers to treatment participation and therapeutic change among children referred for conduct disorder. *Journal of Clinical Child Psychology, 28,* 160–172.

Kovacs, M. (1992). *Children's Depression Inventory Manual.* North Tonowanda, NY: Multi-Health Systems.

Lewinsohn, P. M., Clarke, G. N., Hops, H., & Andrews, J. (1990). Cognitive-behavioral treatment for depressed adolescents. *Behavior Therapy, 21,* 385–401.

Lewinsohn, P. M., Hops, H., Roberts, R. E., Seeley, J. R., & Andrews, J. A. (1993). Adolescent psychopathology: I. Prevalence and incidence of depression and other DSM-III-R disorders in high school students. *Journal of Abnormal Psychology, 102,* 133–144.

Lewinsohn, P. M., & Rohde, P. (1993). The cognitive-behavioral treatment of depression in adolescents: Research and suggestions. *The Clinical Psychologist, 46,* 177–184.

Persons, J. B. (1993). Case conceptualization in cognitive-behavior therapy. In K. T. Kuehlwein & H. Rosen (Eds.), *Cognitive therapies in action: Evolving clinical practice* (pp. 33–53). San Francisco: Jossey-Bass.

Poznanski, E. O., & Mokros, H. B. (1996). *Children's Depression Rating Scale—Revised (CDRS-R) Manual.* Los Angeles: Western Psychological Services.

Rao, U., Daley, S. E., & Hammen, C. (2000). Relationship between depression and substance use disorders in adolescent women during the transition to adulthood. *Journal of the American Academy of Child and Adolescent Psychiatry, 39,* 215–222.

Rothbaum, F., Weisz, J. R., & Snyder, S. (1982). Changing the world and changing the self: A two-process model of perceived control. *Journal of Personality and Social Psychology, 42,* 5–37.

Ryan, N. D., Puig-Antich, J., Cooper, T., Rabinovich, H., Ambrosini, P., Davies, M., King, J., Torrer, D., & Fried, J. (1986). Imipramine in adolescent major depression: Plasma level and clinical response. *Acta Psychiatrica Scandinavica, 73,* 275–288.

Southam-Gerow, M. A., Weisz, J. R., & Kendall, P. C. (in press). Youth with anxiety disorders in research and service clinics: Examining client differences and similarities. *Journal of Clinical Child and Adolescent Psychology.*

Spivack, G., Platt, J. J., & Shure, M. B. (1976). Youth with anxiety disorders in research and service clinics: Examining client differences and similarities. *Journal of Clinical Child and Adolescent Psychology.*

Stark, K. (1990). *Childhood depression: School-based intervention.* New York: Guilford Press.

Stark, K. D., Reynolds, W. R., & Kaslow, N. J. (1987). A comparison of the relative efficacy of self-control therapy and a behavioral problem-solving therapy for depression in children. *Journal of Abnormal Child Psychology, 15,* 91–113.

Strosahl, K. D., Hayes, S. C., Bergan, J., & Romano, P. (1998). Assessing the field effectiveness of Acceptance and Commitment Therapy: An example of the manipulated training research method. *Behavior Therapy, 29,* 35–64.

Weersing, V. R., & Weisz, J. R. (2002). Mechanisms of action in youth psychotherapy. *Journal of Child Psychology and Psychiatry, 43,* 3–29.

Weisz, J. R. (in press-a). Milestones and methods in the development and dissemination of child and adolescent psychotherapies: Review, commentary, and a new deployment-focused model.

In E. D. Hibbs & P. S. Jensen (Eds.), *Psychosocial treatments for child and adolescent disorders: Empirically based strategies for clinical practice* (2nd ed.). Washington, DC: American Psychological Association.

Weisz, J. R. (in press-b). *Psychotherapy for children and adolescents: Evidence-based treatments and case examples.* Cambridge, UK: Cambridge University Press.

Weisz, J. R., & Jensen, P. S. (1999). Efficacy and effectiveness of child and adolescent psychotherapy and pharmacotherapy. *Mental Health Services Research, 1,* 125–157.

Weisz, J. R., McCabe, M. A., & Dennig, M. D. (1994). Primary and secondary control among children undergoing medical procedures: Adjustment as a function of coping style. *Journal of Consulting and Clinical Psychology, 62,* 324–332.

Weisz, J. R., Rothbaum, F. M., & Blackburn, T. F. (1984a). Standing out and standing in: The psychology of control in America and Japan. *American Psychologist, 39,* 955–969.

Weisz, J. R., Rothbaum, F. M., & Blackburn, T. F. (1984b). Swapping recipes for control. *American Psychologist, 39,* 974–975.

Weisz, J. R., Rudolph, K. D., Granger, D. A., & Sweeney, L. (1992). Cognition, competence, and coping in child and adolescent depression: Research findings, developmental concerns, therapeutic implications. *Development and Psychopathology, 4,* 627–653.

Weisz, J. R., Thurber, C., Sweeney, L., Proffitt, V. D., & LeGagnoux, G. L. (1997). Brief treatment of mild-to-moderate child depression using primary and secondary control enhancement training. *Journal of Consulting and Clinical Psychology, 65,* 703–707.

Weisz, J. R., Valeri, S. M., McCarty, C. A., & Moore, P. S. (1999). Interventions for child and adolescent depression: Features, effects, and future directions. In C. A. Essau & F. P. Petermann (Eds.), *Depressive disorders in children and adolescents* (pp. 383–436). Northvale, NJ: Harwood.

B

Externalizing Disorders
and Problems

11

A Cognitive-Behavioral Training Program for Parents of Children with Attention-Deficit/Hyperactivity Disorder

Arthur D. Anastopoulos and Suzanne E. Farley

OVERVIEW

Attention-deficit/hyperactivity disorder (AD/HD[1]; American Psychiatric Association, 1994) is a chronic and pervasive condition characterized by developmentally inappropriate levels of inattention, impulsivity, and/or hyperactivity. Occurring in as many as 5–7% of the general child population, AD/HD is one of the most frequently cited reasons for referral to mental health professionals, pediatricians, and school personnel (Barkley, 1998).

Because AD/HD appears so often in clinical settings, it is of paramount importance for practitioners to be well versed in its assessment (Anastopoulos & Shelton, 2001) and treatment (Barkley, 1998). Consistent with the treatment emphasis of this text, this chapter provides an in-depth discussion of one of the more commonly employed interventions for AD/HD—namely, parent training (PT). It begins with a brief overview of those aspects of AD/HD that have direct bearing on the use of PT with this population. This overview is followed by a discussion of the rationale for using this form of treatment. Next, we present a detailed description of the PT program that we have used both clinically and in our research. After reviewing some of the evidence addressing the efficacy of this intervention, this chapter concludes with a brief discussion of the advantages and limitations of PT and gives suggestions for future research.

Clinical Presentation

Having AD/HD places individuals at risk for a multitude of psychosocial difficulties across their lifespan (Anastopoulos & Shelton, 2001). For example, preschoolers with AD/HD place enormous caretaking demands on their parents and frequently display aggressive behavior when interacting with siblings or peers. Difficulties acquiring academic-readiness skills may be evident as well, but these tend to be of less clinical concern than the family or peer problems that preschoolers present. As children with AD/HD move into their elementary school years, academic problems take on increasing importance. Together with their ongoing family and peer relationship problems, such school-based difficulties set the stage for the development of low self-esteem and other emotional concerns. Similar problems persist into adolescence but on a much more intense level. New problems may develop as well (e.g., traffic violations and experimentation with alcohol and drugs), stemming from the increased demands for independence, self-regulation, and self-control that teenagers with AD/HD face.

In addition to being affected by its primary symptoms, individuals with AD/HD are at increased risk for having secondary or comorbid diagnoses (Jensen, Martin, & Cantwell, 1997). Oppositional defiant disorder (ODD) is especially common early on, affecting approximately 40% of the preschoolers and elementary school–age children who have AD/HD. As many as 20–30% of these children eventually display secondary features of conduct disorder (CD). When AD/HD is accompanied by either ODD or CD, there is also an increased risk for depression and anxiety disorders to be present, especially during adolescence. Antisocial personality disorder, major depression, and substance abuse are just a few of the many comorbid problems that may be found among adults with AD/HD. In combination with AD/HD, such comorbid conditions increase the severity of an individual's overall psychosocial impairment, thereby making the prognosis for such individuals less favorable.

Whether alone or in combination with various comorbid conditions, AD/HD can also have a significant impact on the psychosocial functioning of parents and siblings (Barkley, 1998). Research has shown, for example, that parents of children with AD/HD often become overly directive and negative in their parenting style. In addition to viewing themselves as less skilled and less knowledgeable in their parenting roles, they may also experience considerable stress in their parenting roles, especially when comorbid oppositional defiant features are present. Parental depression and marital discord may arise as well. Whether these parent and family complications result directly from the child's AD/HD is not entirely clear at present. Clinical experience suggests that they probably do, at least in part, given the increased caretaking demands that children with AD/HD impose on their parents. These demands include more frequent displays of noncompliance, related to the child's difficulties in following through on parental instructions. In addition, parents of these children often find themselves involved in resolving various school, peer, and sibling difficulties, which occur throughout childhood and into adolescence as well.

Approach to Treatment

In view of its chronicity, pervasiveness, and comorbidity, AD/HD is not a condition that lends itself to one-dimensional treatment approaches. To address all the problems that children and adolescents with AD/HD so often present, clinicians must employ multiple treatment strategies in combination, each of which addresses a different aspect of the child's or adolescent's psychosocial difficulties. Among those treatments that have received adequate, or at the very least preliminary, empirical support are pharmacotherapy, PT in contingency management methods, parent counseling, classroom applications of contingency management techniques, and cognitive-behavioral training (Pelham, Wheeler, & Chronis, 1998). Despite such support, these interventions should not be viewed as curative of AD/HD. Instead, their value lies in their temporary reduction of AD/HD symptom levels and in their reduction of related behavioral or emotional difficulties. When these treatments are removed, AD/HD symptoms often return to pretreatment levels of deviance. Thus, their effectiveness in improving prognosis presumably rests on their being maintained over long periods.

Rationale for Parent Training

On what basis is there justification for including PT in the clinical management of children with AD/HD? Although by no means complete, part of the answer to this question stems from a consideration of the following clinical and theoretical points.

Clinical Considerations

Although stimulant medication therapy is by far the most commonly used treatment in the clinical management of children with AD/HD, 10–20% of those who take such medication do not show clinically significant improvements in their primary AD/HD symptomatology (Greenhill, Halperin, & Abikoff, 1999). Even when a favorable response is obtained, some children experience side effects that are of sufficient frequency and severity to preclude continued use of stimulant medication. Independent of these issues, many parents prefer not to use any form of medication in treating their child. To the extent that there are indeed children with AD/HD for whom stimulant medication therapy, as well as other medications, is not a viable treatment option, alternative treatments must be used. Among these, PT is certainly worthy of further consideration.

PT can also be helpful to children with AD/HD who are stimulant medication responders. For example, in an effort to reduce the risks for insomnia and various other side effects, most physicians limit their stimulant prescriptions to twice- or thrice-daily dosages. For similar reasons, some physicians further limit the child's medication regimen to schooldays only. What this means from a practical standpoint is that there are substantial portions of any given day, usually in the late afternoons and early evening, when children are not deriving any therapeutic benefits from stimulant medication. For parents and other caretakers, this necessitates finding other means for handling their child's behavioral difficulties in the home. Here again, PT can play a useful role.

Additional justification for using PT stems from a consideration of the potential for comorbidity. As noted earlier, children with AD/HD often display oppositional defiant behavior, aggression, conduct difficulties, and other externalizing problems. Because such secondary features cannot be fully addressed through the use of medication, alternative treatment approaches need to be considered. In view of its highly successful track record with noncompliant (Forehand & McMahon, 1981) and conduct-disordered (Patterson, 1982) populations, PT is well suited to this purpose.

Of additional clinical importance is that raising a child with AD/HD can place enormous strains on family functioning. In particular, levels of parenting stress can be quite high, along with a diminished sense of parenting competence (Mash & Johnston, 1990). Such circumstances are not usually due to faulty parenting. On the contrary, many parents of children with AD/HD use parenting strategies that work just fine for normal siblings in the family. Alerting parents to this reality begins the process of alleviating their distress. Teaching them more effective ways of dealing with their difficult child, through the use of PT, can also go a long way toward facilitating their own personal adjustment.

Theoretical Justification

Additional justification for implementing PT comes from a consideration of the following theoretical matters. Many experts view AD/HD as a condition characterized by neurologically based deficits in behavioral inhibition (Barkley, 1998). To the extent that deficits in behavioral inhibition are indeed central to understanding this disorder, it suggests that children with AD/HD will not be adept at thinking through the consequences of their actions. Working from this assumption, it would then seem reasonable to consider increasing the child's awareness of the connection between his or her behavior and the consequences that follow. More than many other forms of treatment, PT lends itself especially well to meeting this therapeutic objective.

Further theoretical justification stems from a consideration of the apparent relationship that exists among AD/HD, ODD, and CD. Specifically, recent findings from the field of developmental psychopathology have implicated the possibility of a developmental pathway, leading from AD/HD to these comorbid conditions (Loeber, Keenan, Lahey, Green, & Thomas, 1993). If having AD/HD greatly increases the risk for developing ODD or CD at a later point in time, it would seem to be of utmost clinical importance to begin treatment as soon as possible to reduce this risk among children not yet affected by these comorbid conditions. Although research of this sort has yet to be conducted, the fact that PT has worked so well with noncompliant (Forehand & McMahon, 1981) and conduct-disordered (Patterson, 1982) populations provides a basis for considering its use in such a preventive role.

Treatment Goals

Based on the preceding discussion, it should come as no surprise that the therapeutic objective of PT is multifaceted in nature. Not only is the child with AD/HD a target for change, so too are his or her parents and other family members. In terms of child objectives, it would be unreasonable to think that neurologically based AD/HD symptoms could be eliminated through the use of an environmentally based treatment such as PT. More realistically, what can be accomplished is greater parental control over such symptoms as they occur in the home. In addition to targeting primary AD/HD symptoms, PT can also prevent, reduce, or eliminate secondary features of oppositional defiant behavior or conduct problems that the child may be displaying. To the extent that such behavior problems come under better control, the child with AD/HD will likely be exposed to less failure, frustration, correction, and criticism. Thus, improvements in the child's self-esteem and mood may also ensue.

Contrary to popular belief, the benefits of PT are not limited to the child. Parents who receive PT learn a great deal about AD/HD. Such knowledge has great potential for altering faulty perceptions of their children and of themselves. Parents also receive supervised instruction and detailed information about behavior management principles, which makes it possible for them to tailor their parenting style to their child's special needs. Together, these changes in parental knowledge of AD/HD and contingency management skills can set the stage for greater control over child behavior, which in turn can lead to changes in the quality of the parent–child bond and in parental psychological adjustment. In two-parent families there may also be less disagreement over parenting issues, thereby reducing marital tensions. Other tensions within the family (e.g., between siblings) may lessen as well.

CHARACTERISTICS OF THE PARENT TRAINING PROGRAM

Although there are many ways to conduct PT programs for children with AD/HD, little is known about their relative efficacy (Newby, Fischer, & Roman, 1991). Thus, it would not be unreasonable to present any one of them to illustrate how PT is applied in clinical practice. For the purposes of this chapter, the program presented here is the one originally developed by Barkley (1987) and later modified (Anastopoulos & Barkley, 1990; Barkley, 1997). Readers interested in learning more about this program can request a detailed session-by-session manual from the first author (Anastopoulos).

Therapist Qualifications

At face value, delivering PT to parents of children with AD/HD might seem to be a relatively easy task. If all that is done is didactic in nature (i.e., simply presenting the program to an attentive and cooperative parent), it can be. More often than not, however, this is not the case. Thus, its delivery typically requires the skills of a qualified therapist.

One's professional degree is perhaps the least important of these qualifications. What is of utmost relevance is the depth of the therapist's understanding of AD/HD, as well as his or her familiarity with and expertise in using behavior management strategies. Having these skills is especially critical to the success of the program because a one-size-fits-all approach just does not work. Finding ways to tailor PT to fit the needs of individual parents requires a great deal of flexibility and creativity, and these attributes typically come from extensive experience and in-depth knowledge.

Although not necessary for many purely behavioral PT applications, possessing cognitive therapy skills can also play an important role in delivering this form of treatment. Such skills can be used to overcome parental difficulties in using recommended PT strategies and in setting realistic expectations for therapeutic change.

Child and Family Characteristics

PT is not necessarily appropriate for all children who receive an AD/HD diagnosis. At the least, there needs to be some indication that the child's AD/HD is contributing to family difficulties. This need not be limited to hard-to-manage child behavior. It may also encompass elevated levels of parenting stress and other types of family disruption that would benefit from PT intervention. Another limitation is that PT is best suited for parents of children with AD/HD between 4 and 12 years of age. Although elements of the program can be adapted for use with adolescents, many teenagers with AD/HD do not respond well to PT, primarily because parental control over the meaningful contingencies in their lives decreases dramatically. For teens with AD/HD, therefore, alternative psychosocial treatments, such as problem-solving communication training (Robin & Foster, 1989), need to be considered.

A parent's capacity for undergoing PT also needs to be taken into account. Parents who are troubled by significant levels of psychological distress or marital discord may not be good candidates for this form of treatment. Depending on the situation, some parents may need to defer starting PT until such clinical matters are resolved. Others may find it more appropriate to address such problems at the same time they are participating in PT.

Specific Training Steps

Although the PT program typically can be completed in 8 to 12 sessions in either a group or individual format, it does not confine clinicians to a specific number of treatment sessions that must be followed inflexibly. Instead, it allows clinicians to guide parents through the 10 phases of treatment in a step-by-step fashion, taking as many sessions as necessary to bring about desired therapeutic change. When delivered to individual families, each session typically lasts 1 hour. When delivered to multiple families in a group format, 90-minute sessions are commonly used. Regardless of whether an individual or group format is employed, the same sequence of treatment steps is followed. Table 11.1 provides a summary of these 10 steps.

To facilitate acquisition of the parenting skills taught throughout the program, parents are given between-session "homework" assignments at the end of every session. To increase the likelihood that they will practice newly learned techniques between sessions, they also receive written handouts summarizing what they are supposed to do. Should unforeseen problems arise in their efforts to practice, they are encouraged to telephone their therapist for assistance. At the beginning of every session, their efforts to complete their homework are reviewed. Parenting knowledge and skills are then fine-tuned as necessary before moving on to whatever new material is presented in that session.

Step 1: Program Orientation and Overview of AD/HD

Following a detailed orientation to the program, an overview of AD/HD is presented. This overview begins with a brief discussion of how AD/HD has evolved from earlier diagnostic conceptualizations and labels with which parents might be more familiar (e.g., ADD, hyperactivity, and minimal brain dysfunction). Against this historical background, the core symptoms of AD/HD and its currently accepted diagnostic criteria are presented next. Also covered are many of the commonly encountered associated features of AD/HD, generally followed by a discussion of what is known about the immediate and extended families of children with AD/HD. Up-to-date information about the developmental course of this disorder is presented as well. Attention is then directed to etiological concerns. In the context of this discussion, emphasis is placed on the view that, for most children, AD/HD is a biologically based inborn temperamental style that predisposes them to be inattentive, impulsive, and physically restless. Special efforts are also made to clarify the confusion surrounding the situational variability of this disorder's primary

TABLE 11.1. Components of Parent Training Program

Step	Therapeutic content
1	Overview of AD/HD
2	Discussion of four-factor model; review of behavior management principles
3	Using positive attending and ignoring skills
4	Promoting appropriate independent play and compliance with simple requests; issuing commands more effectively
5	Setting up a reward-oriented home token or point system
6	Using response cost for noncompliance and minor rule violations
7	Using time-out for serious rule violations
8	Handling child behavior problems in public
9	Handling future problems; fading out home program; discussion of school issues; termination and disposition issues
10	Booster session to review progress and troubleshoot as needed

symptoms. The importance of using a multimethod assessment approach is discussed next. In the ensuing treatment discussion, emphasis is placed on the need for a multimodal intervention approach.

Presentation of this information should be as brief as possible. This brevity allows parents to focus more attentively on the main points that need to be made. It is also helpful for clinicians to limit their references to summary statistics and percentages obtained from the AD/HD population as a whole. As so many parents have so frankly stated, they are not interested in facts and figures that have little to do with their child. The more that the presentation relates to the parents' particular child, the more likely it is that they will grasp the clinical and theoretical points that need to be made. Another precaution for clinicians to bear in mind as they describe the general AD/HD population is that some parents will incorrectly infer that their child is doomed to a life filled with comorbidity, failure, and misery. For this reason, clinicians must be sure to clarify that (1) what applies to the AD/HD population as a whole does not necessarily apply to any one individual, and (2) outcome is determined by a large number and variety of factors, of which AD/HD is just one influence, albeit an important one.

Although it is certainly possible to conduct this first session in a lecture format, most clinicians would agree that its therapeutic impact is much greater when parents have an opportunity to ask questions, to voice their emotional reactions to what they just heard, and to discuss expectations for the program. Should parents feel overwhelmed by the sheer volume of new AD/HD information, they are reminded that processing such information will occur gradually over time. Should they wish to facilitate their acquisition of such knowledge, they are also alerted to the availability of pertinent texts and encouraged to review videotaped presentations on the topic. To the extent that parental feelings of shock, guilt, sadness, or anger arise, therapeutic attention must then be directed to addressing such negative emotions. For this purpose, cognitive restructuring and other cognitive therapy techniques are especially helpful. Similar therapeutic efforts can be used to address unrealistic parental expectations for treatment outcome—unrealistic in the sense that changes in child behavior are expected to occur in a rapid, continuous fashion. As an alternative to this viewpoint, clinicians might instead suggest that therapeutic change will occur in a gradual and variable manner. Moreover, they must remind parents that what they learn needs to become part of their everyday parenting style, not just what they do during the treatment program. To the extent that parents can indeed continue to use these skills after the program ends, their chances for bringing about improvements in their child's behavior increase dramatically.

Step 2: Understanding Parent–Child Relations

After reviewing carryover concerns from the previous session, clinicians provide parents with a conceptual framework for understanding deviant parent–child interactions and their therapeutic management. In this context, parents are alerted to four major factors which, in various combinations, can contribute to the emergence and/or maintenance of children's behavioral difficulties. The first of these involves the child's characteristics. Along with the child's characteristics, a variety of parent characteristics are cited as circumstances that can place children at risk for conflict with their parents. Additional attention is directed to the goodness of fit between various child and parent characteristics. Stresses impinging upon the family are recognized as well. The way that parents respond to child behavior is also discussed. In particular, attention is directed to explaining how certain parenting styles (e.g., excessive or harsh criticism and inconsistency), though not the cause of AD/HD, nevertheless can complicate the management of this disorder and its associated features.

At this point in the session clinicians provide parents with an overview of general behavior management principles as a way of preparing them for later coverage of specific behavioral techniques. This overview may be introduced with a discussion of how antecedent events, as well as consequences, can be altered to modify children's behavior. Included as part of this discussion are different types of positive reinforcement, ignoring, and punishment strategies; the need for using such consequences in combination; and the advantages of dispensing them in a specific, immediate, and consistent fashion. Special attention is also directed to the role played by negative reinforcement via the request–noncompliance cycle—that is, the cycle of multiple parental requests, following multiple instances of child noncompliance, that generally leads to escalating emotions and coercive interactions, not to mention an increased likelihood of further noncompliance from the child.

Step 3: Increasing Positive Attending Skills during Special Time

This step begins with a discussion of the importance of attending positively to individuals of any age. Because children with AD/HD frequently engage in aversive behaviors, many parents prefer not to interact with them. When parent–child interactions do occur, parents often assume that negative child behavior will arise and therefore adopt a parenting style that is overly directive, corrective, coercive, or unpleasant. This in turn contributes to children becoming even less willing to behave in a compliant manner. For reasons such as these, the "special time" assignment is presented. Unlike other types of special time, which simply involve setting aside time with the child, special time in this program requires that parents must remain as nondirective and as noncorrective as possible. Doing so allows them to see their child's behavior in a different light, in particular allowing them the opportunity to "catch them being good." This, of course, leads to opportunities to attend positively to the child, which in turn helps to rebuild positive parent–child relations. Those who have tried special time are well aware of how difficult it is to do. This difficulty, along with various other complications (e.g., busy daily schedules), is called to the attention of parents for the purpose of setting realistic expectations for its implementation. To be sure that parents get sufficient practice, they are encouraged to catch their children being good, not just during special time but throughout the day as well. Such spontaneous opportunities can be used to increase the amount of positive attention that children receive.

Step 4: Extending Positive Attention to Other Situations; Giving Commands More Effectively

Once it is clear that parents have become sufficiently adept at using positive attending strategies in the context of special time, it becomes possible to expand these skills to other situations. In particular, parents are taught how to use positive attending to increase independent play while parents are engaged in home activities, such as talking on the telephone, preparing dinner, or visiting with company. Positive attending skills may also be applied to parental command situations. Although most parents have little trouble pointing out the various ways in which children with AD/HD do not comply with their requests, it is much harder for them to identify request situations that elicit compliance. Some even get to the point of believing that their child "does nothing that I ask him (or her) to do." Although it is certainly true that children with AD/HD are frequently non-compliant, it is equally important for parents to recognize an unintentional tendency on their part to ignore instances of compliance when they occur. In cognitive therapy terms, parents are selectively attending to the negative aspects of their child's responses to their requests. In behavior therapy terms, they are discouraging compliance by ignoring its oc-curence, and encouraging noncompliance through their attention to it. Against this back-ground, clinicians point out the importance of paying positive attention to children whenever they are compliant. In addition, parents are advised to set the stage for practic-ing their use of such positive attending skills by issuing brief sequences of simple house-hold commands that have a high probability of eliciting compliance from their child.

The final topic for this step is the manner in which commands are given. Verbal and nonverbal parameters of how parents communicate commands to children are examined. This includes coverage of the following recommendations: that parents only issue com-mands they intend to follow through on; that commands take the form of direct state-ments rather than questions; that commands be relatively simple; that they be issued in the absence of outside distractions, and only when direct eye contact is being made with the child, to increase the likelihood of the child's attending to such instructions; and that commands be repeated back to the parents, to give them an opportunity to clarify any misunderstanding before the child responds.

Step 5: Establishing a Home Poker Chip/Point System

Setting up a reward-oriented home token system is the major focus of this step. Such a system provides children with AD/HD with the external motivation they need to com-plete parent-requested activities that may be of little intrinsic interest and/or a trigger for their defiance. Another reason for using such a system is because positive attending and ignoring strategies are often insufficient for managing children with AD/HD, who gener-ally require more concrete and meaningful rewards.

Following review and refinement of the therapeutic skills taught in steps 3 and 4, clinicians embark on a somewhat philosophical, yet practical, discussion of children's rights and privileges. Such a discussion often serves to alert parents to how they have in-advertently been treating many of their child's privileges as if they were rights, which in turn makes it easier to set up the home-based poker chip or point system described here.

Parents are initially asked to generate two lists: one of daily, weekly, and long-range privileges that are likely to be interesting and motivating to the child; the other pertain-ing to regular chores and/or household rules that parents would like done better. Such target behaviors should include not only instances of noncompliance and defiance but also those situations in which a child does not follow through because of loss of interest, distractions, and other AD/HD symptoms. Upon returning home, parents may wish to incorporate input from the child as to any other items that should be included in these lists.

Point values are then assigned to items on each list. For children 9 years old and un-der, plastic poker chips are used as tokens. Earned poker chips are collected and stored in a home "bank" that a child has set aside specifically for that purpose. For 9- to 11-year-old children, points are used in place of chips and are monitored in a checkbook register or some other type of notebook of interest to a youngster. Generally speaking, children can earn predetermined numbers of poker chips or points for complying with initial par-ent requests and for completing assigned tasks, which previously may have been left in-complete due to lack of interest or motivation in doing them. In addition, parents can dispense bonus chips or points for especially well-done chores or independent displays of appropriate behavior. At no time, however, should chips or points be taken away for noncompliance in this phase of the training program. Instead, encountered noncompliance should be handled in the same way that parents have dealt with such situations previously.

Parental motivation, which may have been quite high until now, may begin to waver for several reasons. Some parents may once again tell us, "I've done something like this before and it doesn't work." As described earlier, cognitive therapy strategies may be used to correct this type of faulty thinking, which has the potential to interfere with parental efforts to institute a home token system.

Step 6: Adding Response Cost to the Program

This session begins with a careful review of parental efforts to implement the home token system. Because problems inevitably arise, most of this session is set aside for clarifying confusion when necessary and for making suggestions for increasing the effectiveness of this system.

Following this discussion, the response cost technique is introduced, which represents the first time in the treatment program that a penalty or punishment approach has been considered for use. Specifically, parents are instructed to begin deducting poker chips or points for noncompliance with one or two particularly troublesome requests on the list. Similar penalties may be used for one or two "don't behaviors" (i.e., don't hit, don't talk back, etc.) that may be added to the program. At this stage, not only does the child with AD/HD fail to earn chips or points that would have resulted from compliance, but previously earned chips or points are now also removed from the bank for displays of noncompliance. The number of chips or points lost is equal to the number of chips or points that would have been gained had compliance occurred. For many children with AD/HD, who over the past week may have learned how to expend minimal effort to get the privileges that they desire, adding a response cost component to their token system often increases their overall level of compliance with parental requests, because they now have the additional incentive of trying not to lose what they have already earned. Clinicians also routinely caution parents to avoid getting into punishment spirals, whereby so many chips are taken away that a debt is incurred. If needed, backup penalties, such as time out, can be employed instead.

Step 7: Using Time-Out from Reinforcement

After reviewing the home token system and making whatever adjustments are deemed necessary, clinicians begin discussing "time-out from reinforcement," or simply time-out. Although most types of noncompliance will continue to be handled via response cost, parents are encouraged to identify one or two especially resistant or serious types of noncompliance or rule violations (e.g., hitting a sibling) that may become the targets of time-out. Once these are identified, attention is then focused on teaching the mechanics of implementing the time-out procedure. Like the token system, time-out is a rather difficult technique to employ. Its use must be explained carefully before asking parents to practice it at home.

Critical to the success of this technique is that three conditions must be met prior to releasing the youngster from time-out. First, the child must serve a minimum amount of time, generally equal in minutes to the number of years in his or her age. Once this con-

dition is met, parents may approach the time-out area only when the child has been quiet for a brief period. This, of course, avoids the problem of inadvertently dispensing
parental attention for inappropriate behavior. Next, and perhaps most important, parents must reissue the request or command that initially led the youngster to be placed
into time-out. In cases in which the child does not comply with the reissued directive, the
entire three-step time-out cycle is repeated as many times as is necessary, until compliance is achieved. Thus, under no circumstances does the child avoid doing what was
asked.

In addition to covering these facets of time-out, clinicians routinely address other aspects of this procedure, including how to select a location for serving time-out and what
to do if the child defiantly leaves the time-out area. Because time-out is a strategy that
usually has been tried in one form or another, many parents have firm beliefs about its
potential for success, or lack thereof. Such biases therefore will need to be addressed via
cognitive restructuring techniques.

Step 8: Managing Behavior in Public Places

Assuming that the home-based program is running relatively smoothly, attention is then
directed to a discussion of settings outside the home in which problem behaviors arise.
Among the many settings that are often identified by parents as problematic are grocery
stores, department stores, malls, movie theaters, restaurants, churches, and synagogues.
Disciplinary strategies previously employed in such settings are reviewed and analyzed in
terms of their overall ineffectiveness.

Against this background, the importance of anticipating such problems in public is
discussed. In particular, parents are advised to formulate a plan of action before entering
a predictably problematic public situation. This may be accomplished as follows: First,
parents must review their expectations for the child's behavior in this setting. Next, they
must establish some incentive for compliance with these rules. Finally, they must specify
what types of punishment will be applied, should noncompliance with these rules ensue.
Of equal importance to the success of this plan is to have the child state his or her understanding of these rules and consequences prior to entering the public situation. Such a
statement allows parents an opportunity to clarify any misunderstanding on the part of
the child that may result from confusion or from inattentiveness.

Generally speaking, modified versions of the strategies used successfully within the
home are incorporated into this plan. Unfortunately, many parents are less than enthusiastic about experimenting with these techniques in public places. The perceived threat
of public embarrassment is often cited. After all, "What will people think?" The mind-
reading aspects of this particular situation are highlighted as the basis for parents jump-
ing to such a conclusion. Alternative viewpoints of what people might think, and the relative importance of what others think when it pertains to their child's welfare, are
discussed. Addressing parental perceptions of the situation in this manner generally
makes it possible to reduce parents' uneasiness and to increase their motivation for trying
such a new and challenging approach.

Step 9: School Management Issues and Preparing for Termination

This step serves many purposes: to increase parental knowledge of relevant school issues,
to discuss how to handle future problems that might arise, and to begin preparing for
termination, including instructions on how to fade out the home-based program. In addi-

tion to reviewing and fine-tuning parental efforts to deal with problem behavior in public places, clinicians also review and refine all other aspects of the training program. Parental feedback about the training program may be elicited at this time as well. Such comments often serve as a backdrop against which the handling of future behavior problems may be discussed.

Parents also discuss what they believe might be problematic for them in the future and how they might handle such problematic situations. Attention is then directed to the various ways in which many parents slip away from adherence to this program. Although some degree of slippage or departure from the protocol is acceptable, and in fact encouraged, too much may lead to increased behavioral difficulties. For this reason, parents are informed how to run a check on themselves to ascertain where fine-tuning of their specialized child management skills is required. A written handout summarizing this self-check system is distributed at this time.

Another important feature of this session is to discuss the child's current school status, including what modifications, if any, are being employed to deal with the child's AD/HD. This is followed by a description of the legal rights of children with AD/HD within the school system. Emphasis is placed on the child being in the least restrictive educational environment. How and when to consider special education accommodations is covered as well. Independent of placement issues, parents receive numerous suggestions for modifying their child's classroom environment to accommodate the child's AD/HD. Throughout this discussion parents are strongly encouraged to work with school personnel in as collaborative and cooperative a manner as possible. It is in this spirit that particular attention is directed to the mechanics of setting up a daily report card system in which home-based consequences are used in conjunction with written daily feedback from the teacher.

The final portion of this session is used to address termination and/or disposition issues. In addition to agreeing on an appropriate booster session date, efforts are made to determine whether any other types of clinical services are needed. This might include, for example, the need for adding a medication component or for scheduling school consultation visits to address classroom management concerns directly with school personnel.

Step 10: Booster Session

Although any length of time may be deemed acceptable, it is customary to meet with parents for a booster session approximately 1 month after conducting step 9. One objective of this session is to readminister pertinent child behavior and parent self-report rating scales and questionnaires, which serve as indices of any posttreatment changes that may have occurred. Further review and refinement of previously learned intervention strategies are conducted as well. Also established at this time is a mutually agreed-on final clinical disposition. If desired, this may include scheduling of additional booster sessions.

EFFICACY OF TREATMENT

In terms of empirical support, it is somewhat surprising that few studies have actually examined the efficacy of PT with children specifically identified as having AD/HD. What few well-controlled studies exist (Anastopoulos, Shelton, DuPaul, & Guevremont, 1993; Erhardt & Baker, 1990; Pisterman et al., 1992; Pisterman, McGrath, Firestone, & Goodman, 1989; Pollard, Ward, & Barkley, 1983) can be interpreted with cautious optimism as supporting the use of PT with such children (also see Pelham et al., 1998, for a review). Most of these interventions used weekly therapy sessions in either group or individual formats that were short term in nature, spanning 6 to 12 weeks in length. By and large, most of these programs served to train parents in the use of specialized contingency management techniques, such as positive reinforcement, response cost, and/or time-out strategies. Some, however, combined contingency management training with didactic counseling, aimed at increasing parental knowledge and understanding of AD/HD (Anastopoulos et al., 1993). In addition to producing changes in child behavior, PT interventions have also contributed to improvements in various aspects of parental and family functioning, including decreased parenting stress and increased parenting self-esteem.

Information about the efficacy of PT also comes from studies in which this form of treatment was combined with other interventions, such as pharmacotherapy (Abikoff & Hechtman, 1996) and self-control therapy (Horn et al., 1991). In contrast to what is found when used alone, many of these early multimodal intervention studies, especially those involving medication, noted that PT contributes little to outcome, above and beyond that accounted for by the other treatment. Although these initial results were discouraging, findings from the recently completed Multimodal Treatment of AD/HD (MTA) study have shown that the efficacy of psychosocial treatment depends in large part on the type and context of the outcome being assessed (MTA Cooperative Group, 1999; Pelham, 1999; Swanson et al., 2002). When using changes in primary AD/HD symptomatology as a yardstick for therapeutic change, the MTA study found that a rigorously controlled medication regimen was equal to or better than either a psychosocial treatment package that included a PT component or the combination of medication and the PT–psychosocial treatment package. However, in subsequent analyses that used indices of functional impairment (e.g., family functioning) and other ecologically valid measures (e.g., consumer satisfaction) to assess outcome, the combination of medication and the PT–psychosocial treatment package did produce therapeutic benefits above and beyond those from medication alone. Moreover, certain types of children with AD/HD, such as those with comorbid anxiety, also seemed to benefit more from the combination of medication and PT–psychosocial treatment versus medication alone.

Although these MTA findings are most encouraging, many questions about PT remain. Particularly limited is our understanding of how PT works. Most PT programs are multifaceted in nature, typically including some combination of various contingency management techniques and counseling about AD/HD. Which of these components might be responsible for the observed therapeutic benefits of PT is not at all clear. Also limited is our knowledge of the scope of PT benefits. Although research has shown that PT brings about improvements in child behavior, parent–child relations, and parent functioning, little is known about its impact on a child's emotional functioning. Even less information is available regarding the role of fathers.

Although not yet published, our own research has produced some interesting preliminary findings pertaining to these unanswered questions. In particular, a therapeutic component analysis was conducted, comparing the effects of a complete PT program (i.e., contingency management plus AD/HD counseling; Anastopoulos & Barkley, 1990) versus AD/HD counseling alone. It was predicted that both forms of treatment would produce benefits, with the complete PT program clearly being the superior of the two. This study also included child emotional indices as outcome measures, based on the assumption that PT would improve this area of functioning as well. Input from fathers was obtained, with the expectation that their ratings would reflect relatively less therapeutic change than those of mothers.

The sample for this study was drawn from a larger group of 138 clinic-referred children participating in a federally funded project examining comorbidity and AD/HD parent training outcome. All carried a diagnosis of AD/HD, with half also displaying ODD. Sample selection was further determined by parental psychopathology, with relatively equal numbers of mothers displaying either low or high levels. For the current project, a subsample of 59 children (47 boys, 12 girls) and their parents served as participants. The children ranged in age from 6–11 years with a mean of 106 months. All were of at least normal intelligence, with 49% receiving special education services. None was taking medication for behavior management purposes during the active portion of the study. Most were from two-parent (71%), middle class, Caucasian homes.

Participants were randomly assigned to either a group receiving the complete PT program ($N = 35$) or AD/HD counseling ($N = 24$). The PT program followed the 10 steps outlined earlier in this chapter. As summarized in Table 11.2, the therapeutic goal of the AD/HD counseling program was threefold: to provide basic information about AD/HD, to give parents an opportunity to describe how AD/HD affected their child and family, and to encourage parents to generate solutions to their child management problems based on the knowledge they gained. No contingency management training was offered. Both groups received 10 weekly, 1-hour individually delivered treatment sessions over the course of 3 to 4 months. Experienced PhD-level psychologists delivered the treatments in accordance with treatment manuals that had been developed for the project. Treatment integrity was further addressed via expert review of randomly selected audiotapes of the treatment sessions. For both treatment conditions, all the reviewed tapes met the minimum criteria for adherence (i.e., covering at least 85% of the session outline). Assessment data were gathered prior to, immediately following, and 6 months after treatment.

As expected, knowledge of AD/HD increased over time for mothers and fathers in both groups. Also in line with expectations, posttreatment knowledge of behavior management principles was significantly greater for PT mothers and fathers than for parents receiving AD/HD counseling. PT mothers and fathers also reported using more effective parenting strategies at posttreatment, but these differences were not maintained at follow-up.

Contrary to expectations, repeated-measures analyses of the various child, parent, and marital outcome data failed to show significantly better outcomes for PT than for

TABLE 11.2. **Components of AD/HD Counseling Program**

Step	Therapeutic content
1	Overview of AD/HD
2	Four factor model
3	Assessment and treatment issues
4	School history and current functioning
5	Impact of AD/HD on child's home functioning
6	Impact of AD/HD on child's social–emotional functioning
7	School rights of children with AD/HD
8	Overview of pharmacotherapy
9	Overview of social skills training
10	1-month booster session, termination, and final disposition

AD/HD counseling. However, a number of nonsignificant trends did emerge, consistently favoring PT over AD/HD counseling. For example, PT mothers and fathers reported lower rates of ODD symptoms at posttreatment but not at follow-up. Coded observations of PT mothers interacting with their children revealed lower levels of child inattention and anger at posttreatment. PT fathers also reported lower rates of hyperactivity–impulsivity and internalizing symptoms in their children, along with lower levels of parenting stress and greater parenting alliance. Of additional interest is that children in PT reported greater improvement in their self-esteem.

Except for the parental depression and marital satisfaction indices, both groups showed posttreatment improvements on all other parent rating scale measures. The same was true for child self-esteem and for two of the coded behaviors from the mother–child observations (i.e., appropriate parenting and mutual enjoyment). Although not statistically significant, fewer PT parents (6%) dropped out of treatment than those receiving AD/HD counseling (17%).

The obtained findings provided partial support for the study's hypotheses. As expected, PT and AD/HD counseling increased parental knowledge of AD/HD. But PT was clearly superior to AD/HD counseling in terms of increasing parental knowledge of behavior management principles and with respect to parenting effectiveness. Although such changes indicated that the experimental manipulation was in fact successful, statistically significant group differences were not evident on any of the child, parent, or family functional outcome measures. Because both treatment groups produced a number of significant improvements over time, it would appear that giving parents knowledge of AD/HD is far more beneficial therapeutically than previously thought. That said, it would be premature to conclude that AD/HD counseling alone is sufficient. Numerous trends in the data consistently pointed to contingency management training as an important component of PT.

In addition to reducing child behavior problems, there was evidence to suggest that PT produced anticipated changes in the child's emotional functioning. This was seen in terms of parent-reported reductions in internalizing symptomatology and child-reported improvements in self-esteem. Although speculative in nature, such changes may stem from increased parental use of positive attending and positive reinforcement strategies, which are emphasized throughout PT.

Contrary to expectations, input from fathers revealed more treatment-related changes in home functioning than did similar input from mothers. The basis for this discrepancy is unclear. At the very least, this difference of parental opinion highlights the need for including fathers' perspectives in subsequent treatment research.

SUMMARY AND CONCLUSIONS

PT is frequently used in the treatment of children with AD/HD. Although many variations of PT exist, all share a common therapeutic objective—namely, to teach parents specialized child management techniques. Some PT programs, such as the one described in this chapter, incorporate additional therapeutic components that systematically provide parents with factual information about AD/HD and use cognitive therapy techniques to facilitate parental acceptance, understanding, and management of the disorder.

Based on a consideration of the various clinical, theoretical, and empirical issues that were presented in this chapter, there should be little doubt that PT does have a place in the overall clinical management of children with AD/HD. One of the major advantages of using PT is that it can target not only the child's primary AD/HD symptomatology but also many comorbid features, including oppositional defiant behavior and conduct problems. Moreover, because PT interventions use parents as cotherapists, many parents themselves derive indirect therapeutic benefits from their involvement in treatment. Although it remains to be seen what the long-term impact of PT interventions might be, preliminary evidence seems to suggest that treatment-induced improvements in psychosocial functioning can be maintained in the absence of ongoing therapist contact, at least in the short run.

As was noted earlier, much of the research to date has focused on the clinical efficacy of PT interventions when used alone. One benefit of pursuing this type of research is that it has allowed for a better understanding of the unique impact that this form of treatment can have on outcome within an AD/HD population. Examining PT by itself has also provided important insight into its therapeutic limitations, including the fact that not everyone benefits from PT.

Although early multimodal treatment studies suggested that PT did not produce therapeutic benefits above and beyond that accounted for by medication, the recently reported MTA findings have shown that the combination of medication and PT–psychosocial treatment is superior to medication alone for certain types of outcomes (e.g., family functioning) and for certain types of children (e.g., with comorbid anxiety) and their families. Thus, what remains to be clarified is not so much whether PT is an efficacious treatment for AD/HD. Rather, it seems timely for the field to begin conducting research that addresses for which children and for which outcomes the combination of medication and PT is best suited.

NOTE

1. We use a slash mark in the acronym AD/HD to conform with the DSM-IV presentation of this disorder.

REFERENCES

Abikoff, H. B., & Hechtman, L. (1996). Multimodal therapy and stimulants in the treatment of children with attention-deficit hyperactivity disorder. In E. D. Hibbs & P. S. Jensen (Eds.), *Psychosocial treatments for child and adolescent disorders: Empirically based strategies for clinical practice* (pp. 341–369). Washington, DC: American Psychological Association.

American Psychiatric Association. (1994). *Diagnostic and statistical manual of mental disorders* (4th ed.). Washington, DC: Author.

Anastopoulos, A. D., & Barkley, R. A. (1990). Counseling and training parents. In R. A. Barkley, *Attention-deficit hyperactivity disorder: A handbook for diagnosis and treatment* (pp. 397–431). New York: Guilford Press.

Anastopoulos, A. D., & Shelton, T. L. (2001). *Assessing attention-deficit/hyperactivity disorder.* New York: Kluwer Academic/Plenum Press.

Anastopoulos, A. D., Shelton, T. L., DuPaul, G. J., & Guevremont, D. C. (1993). Parent training for attention-deficit hyperactivity disorder: Its impact on parent functioning. *Journal of Abnormal Child Psychology, 21,* 581–596.

Barkley, R. A. (1987). *Defiant children: A clinician's manual for parent training.* New York: Guilford Press.

Barkley, R. A. (1997). *Defiant children: A clinician's manual for parent training* (2nd ed.). New York: Guilford Press.

Barkley, R. A. (1998). *Attention-deficit hyperactivity disorder: A handbook for diagnosis and treatment* (2nd ed.). New York: Guilford Press.

Erhardt, D., & Baker, B. L. (1990). The effects of behavioral parent training on families with young hyperactive children. *Journal of Behavior Therapy and Experimental Psychiatry, 21,* 121–132.

Forehand, R. L., & McMahon, R. J. (1981). *Helping the noncompliant child: A clinician's guide to parent training.* New York: Guilford Press.

Greenhill, L. L., Halperin, J. M., & Abikoff, H. (1999). Stimulant medications. *Journal of the American Academy of Child and Adolescent Psychiatry, 38*(5), 503–512.

Horn, W. F., Ialongo, N., Pacoe, J. M., Greenberg, G., Packard, T., Lopez, M., Wagner, A., & Puttler, L. (1991). Additive effects of psychostimulants, parent training, and self-control therapy with ADHD children: A 9-month follow-up. *Journal of the American Academy of Child and Adolescent Psychiatry, 32,* 182–189.

Jensen, P. S., Martin, D., & Cantwell, D. P. (1997). Comorbidity of ADHD: Implications for research, practice, and DSM-V. *Journal of the American Academy of Child and Adolescent Psychiatry, 36,* 1065–1079.

Loeber, R., Keenan, K., Lahey, B. B., Green, S. M., & Thomas, C. (1993). Evidence for developmentally based diagnoses in oppositional defiant disorder and conduct disorder. *Journal of Abnormal Child Psychology, 21,* 377–410.

Mash, E. J., & Johnston, C. (1990). Determinants of parenting stress: Illustrations from families of hyperactive children and families of physically abused children. *Journal of Clinical Child Psychology, 19,* 313–328.

MTA Cooperative Group. (1999). A 14-month randomized clinical trial of treatment strategies for attention-deficit/hyperactivity disorder. *Archives of General Psychiatry, 56,* 1073–1086.

Newby, R. F., Fischer, M., & Roman, M. A. (1991). Parent training for families of children with ADHD. *School Psychology Review, 20,* 252–265.

Patterson, G. R. (1982). *Coercive family process.* Eugene, OR: Castalia.

Pelham, W. E. (1999). President's message: The NIMH multimodal treatment study for ADHD: Just say yes to drugs? *Clinical Child Psychology Newsletter, 14,* 1–10.

Pelham, W. E., Wheeler, T., & Chronis, A. (1998). Empirically supported psychosocial treatments for attention deficit hyperactivity disorder. *Journal of Clinical Child Psychology, 27,* 190–205.

Pisterman, S., Firestone, P., McGrath, P., Goodman, J., Webster, I., Mallory, R., & Goffin, B. (1992). The effects of parent training on parenting stress and sense of competence. *Canadian Journal of Behavioural Science, 24,* 41–58.

Pisterman, S., McGrath, P., Firestone, P., & Goodman, J. T. (1989). Outcome of parent-mediated treatment of preschoolers with attention deficit disorder with hyperactivity. *Journal of Consulting and Clinical Psychology, 57,* 636–643.

Pollard, S., Ward, E. M., & Barkley, R. A. (1983). The effects of parent training and Ritalin on parent–child interactions of hyperactive boys. *Child and Family Therapy, 5,* 51–69.

Robin, A. L., & Foster, S. (1989). *Negotiating parent–adolescent conflict.* New York: Guilford Press.

Swanson, J. M., Arnold, L. E., Vitiello, B., Abikoff, H. B., Wells, K. C., Pelham, W. E., March, J. S., Hinshaw, S. P., Hoza, B., Epstein, J. N., Elliott, G. R., Greenhill, L. L., Hechtman, L., Jensen, P. S., Kraemer, H. C., Kotkin, R., Molina, B., Newcorn, J. H., Owens, E. B., Severe, J., Hoagwood, K., Simpson, S., Wigal, T., Hanley, T., & the MTA Group (2002). Response to commentary on the Multimodal Treatment Study of ADHD (MTA): Mining the meaning of the MTA. *Journal of Abnormal Child Psychology, 30,* 327–332.

12

Parent–Child Interaction Therapy for Oppositional Children

MARY Y. BRINKMEYER AND SHEILA M. EYBERG

OVERVIEW

Parent–child interaction therapy (PCIT) is an evidence-based treatment for disruptive behavior in preschoolers. Disruptive behaviors range from relatively minor infractions such as talking back to severe acts of aggression. Depending on the severity of their presenting problems, children with disruptive behavior can be diagnosed with either oppositional defiant disorder (ODD) or conduct disorder (CD), often with a comorbid diagnosis of attention-deficit/hyperactivity disorder (ADHD). Disruptive behavior is the most common reason for referral of young children to mental health services.

The development of disruptive behavior in young children has been linked to certain child characteristics, such as difficult infant temperament, neuropsychological abnormalities affecting information processing, and the interaction of the child's genetic makeup with adverse family factors. Family variables associated with disruptive behavior include maternal depression, social isolation, inappropriate anger expression, parental conflict, single-parent status, and poverty.

The presence of disruptive behaviors in young children is often a marker for poor outcomes. Children who show persistently high levels of disruptive behavior early in their lives are at high risk for serious antisocial behavior and criminal activity in adolescence and into adulthood (Hann & Borek, 2002). It appears that children with early disruptive behavior develop along an early onset pathway for conduct problems, failing to learn prosocial behavior and setting the stage for serious problems without treatment.

Conceptual Underpinnings of PCIT

The development of PCIT has been influenced by Baumrind's (1967, 1991) developmental theory associating various parenting styles with different child outcomes. Baumrind described the authoritative parenting style as one in which parents are both highly demanding and highly responsive. Her demonstration of less successful outcomes for children whose parents do not adequately meet their children's needs for both nurturing and limits has been subsequently documented in diverse samples of young children. To change maladaptive parent–child interactions to ones that characterize authoritative parenting, PCIT draws on both attachment and social learning theories.

Attachment theory is based on the premise that children whose parents are able to recognize and respond warmly to their emotional needs are more likely to develop a secure working model of their relationships, leading to more effective emotional regulation. Conversely, parents who are intolerant of their children's emotional expression or unable to respond effectively to their children's distress often have children who are insecurely attached. Maladaptive parent–child attachment has been consistently linked to children's aggressive behavior, low social competence, poor coping skills, low self-esteem, and poor peer relationships. Moreover, an insecure attachment is related to increased maternal stress as well as child abuse and neglect. Thus, in PCIT parents first learn a child-directed interaction (CDI), in which their part is similar to that of a play therapist. The parents use skills that restructure the play interaction in ways designed to create a secure attachment.

Once parents have mastered CDI, they learn parent-directed interaction (PDI), in which they use specific behavior management techniques based on social learning theory. Social learning theory emphasizes the contingencies that shape the dysfunctional interactions of disruptive children and their parents. These interactions are characterized by mutual and escalating aversive behaviors resulting from the attempts of both the parent and child to control the actions (e.g., arguing, criticizing, whining, and aggression) of the other. To interrupt this cycle, parents must change their behavior to incorporate clear limit setting in the context of an authoritative relationship. PDI specifically addresses these processes by implementing firm, consistent consequences in the context of the positive parent–child attachment relationship established through the CDI interactions.

Goals of PCIT

The combination of poor parent–child attachment and poor child behavior management skills predicts more severe disruptive behavior than either factor alone. Thus, the goals of PCIT are to improve both the parent–child attachment relationship and the behavior management skills of the parent.

PCIT assumes that a secure, nurturing relationship is a necessary foundation for establishing effective limit setting and consistency in discipline that will achieve lasting change in the behaviors of the parent and child. Therefore, in the first phase of PCIT, the CDI, the parents learn to follow the child's lead in play. The specific goal of CDI is to increase parental responsiveness and establish a nurturing and secure relationship between parent and child. Once parents have mastered the skills of CDI, treatment moves on to the PDI phase, which resembles clinical behavior therapy. Parents learn to lead the child's behavior when needed. The goal of PDI is to improve parental limit setting and consistency in discipline to reduce the child's noncompliance, aggression, and other negative behavior. Therapists teach parents problem-solving skills to assist them in applying the principles and methods taught in CDI and PDI to new situations and new problems as they arise.

CHARACTERISTICS OF THE TREATMENT PROGRAM

Family Characteristics

Children and their parents are seen together for treatment. PCIT is most often used with families of children between the ages of 3 and 6, although it has also been successfully implemented with older and younger children. PCIT has been used with families from diverse socioeconomic backgrounds. The majority of participating families have been European American, although families from other ethnic groups have also participated in PCIT. Children included in the outcome studies have been clinic-referred by caseworkers, pediatricians, psychiatrists, teachers, other mental health workers, or other families. PCIT has been used most often with children referred for disruptive behavior. It has also been implemented, however, for families that have been reported to state agencies for physical abuse. In these cases, the parent is the identified patient. Treatment may include one or both parents or other significant caregivers in the child's life (e.g., grandparents or parent's companion). If parents are divorced and share custody, the therapist may elect to see them together or at separate sessions, depending on the family dynamics and the parents' wishes.

Therapist Characteristics

PCIT therapists have been psychologists, graduate students in psychology, and social workers. Ideally, new PCIT therapists should be trained using a combination of didactic methods (e.g., attending classes or seminars and reading the PCIT manual) and experiential ones, such as role-playing coaching techniques and observing sessions. To futher assist in training new therapists, the cotherapy training model can be used, in which a less experienced therapist learns from an experienced lead therapist. In this model, the cotherapist helps to prepare the materials for the session and, during the session, tracks the session elements in the treatment manual to prevent omissions. As they become more familiar with PCIT, cotherapists may assume an increasingly active role in teaching, coaching, and dealing with process issues that arise during treatment.

Therapy Format

Each phase of treatment begins with a teaching session in which the therapist explains and models the CDI or PDI skills, followed by coaching sessions, in which parents practice the skills with their child while the therapist prompts them and provides reinforcement to shape the parents' new behaviors. In the coaching sessions, the therapist first briefly reviews the home progress and provides support to parents if indicated. Next, the therapist observes and codes the behaviors of the parent and child during a 5-minute interaction, which helps determine which skills the parents have mastered and which will be important targets for coaching during the session.

Coaching usually takes place in a playroom that is equipped with a one-way mirror and "bug in the ear" system for coaching the parents while they play with the child. If such a system is not available, the therapist coaches the parent in a low voice from inside the playroom. Coaching consists of frequent, brief statements that give parents immediate feedback on their CDI or PDI skills (e.g., "Nice labeled praise" and "Good direct command"), their manner (e.g., "Great enthusiasm" and "Good job staying calm"), or their effect ("He seems to try harder when you praise his effort" and "She quieted right down after you ignored her whining"). The therapist also provides suggestions ("Give her as many praises as you can when she's playing so quietly with the toys") or gentle corrections ("Oops, a question").

At the end of each session, the therapist reviews with parents a summary sheet showing how often they used each skill during the initial 5-minute observation period. This sheet includes data from each session so parents can see their progress. Using this summary sheet, the parents can decide which skill to focus on most during daily home practice sessions the following week.

CONTENT OF THE TREATMENT SESSIONS

Child-Directed Interaction

In the CDI, parents learn specific communication skills, called the PRIDE skills, to give positive attention to their child's positive behaviors as they play together. The basic rule for parents in CDI is to follow the child's lead, much like therapists in client-centered play therapy. The PRIDE skills include *P*raising the child's behavior, *R*eflecting the child's statements, *I*mitating and *D*escribing the child's play, and using *E*nthusiasm. At the same time, parents learn to ignore any negative behaviors that occur. Thus, parents learn to apply the PRIDE skills using the technique called differential social attention. Parents are also taught to avoid behaviors that attempt to lead the play, such as commands, questions, and criticism. After explaining, modeling, and role playing these skills during the CDI teaching session, the therapist provides parents with a handout summarizing the skills. Parents are asked to practice the CDI skills for 5 minutes each day at home and are given a separate handout to record how each home practice session goes (see Table 12.1).

During the first CDI coaching session, therapists focus exclusively on providing positive reinforcement for the PRIDE skills that the parents are using. During subsequent coaching sessions, therapists address specific skills that the parents have not yet mastered. For example, in the second coaching session, therapists typically focus on decreasing the use of questions. The therapist might gently cue the parent when a question occurs ("Oops!") and might suggest a way to restate it as a statement, if needed. The therapist also praises the parent frequently for not asking questions (e.g., "Good catching yourself and restating that question" and "Nice saying that with certainty").

The therapist continues to guide and coach the parents in the use of the PRIDE skills until the parents meet the minimum criteria for mastery during the initial 5-minute observation: (1) 10 behavioral descriptions ("You're putting the red block on top"); (2) 10 reflective statements ("That's right, that *is* a tower"); (3) 10 labeled praises ("I like how you're using your inside voice"), and (4) no more than three total questions, commands, or criticisms. Once the parents have met these criteria, they move to the second phase of treatment, PDI. Because the CDI skills form an important foundation for establishing and maintaining effective discipline, the therapist continues to observe and code 5 minutes of CDI at the beginning of each therapy session. If a parent falls below the criterion on any of the skills, the therapist will coach CDI briefly before beginning PDI. The 5-minute CDI home practice sessions also continue.

Parent-Directed Interaction

Primary goals of PDI include increasing compliance and decreasing inappropriate behaviors that do not respond to ignoring or are too severe to ignore (e.g., destroying toys and hitting). During PDI, parents continue to give positive attention to appropriate behavior and to ignore inappropriate behavior. Rather than exclusively following the child's lead, however, parents learn to give the child specific directions and to follow through consistently. One of the keys to PDI is that it teaches parents to give calm, predictable responses to their child's behavior. Both parents and children know what consequences will fol-

TABLE 12.1. CDI Rules

Rules	Reason	Examples
Praise your child's appropriate behavior	• Causes your child's good behavior to increase • Lets your child know what you like • Increases your child's self-esteem • Makes you and your child feel good	• Good job of putting the toys away! • I like the way you're playing so gently with the toys. • Great idea to make a fence for the horses. • Thank you for sharing with me.
Reflect appropriate talk	• Lets your child lead the conversation • Shows your child that you are listening • Demonstrates that you accept and understand your child • Improves your child's speech • Increases verbal communication between the both of you	• Child: I drew a tree. Parent: Yes, you made a tree. • Child: The doggy has a black nose. Parent: The dog's nose is black. • Child: I like to play with the blocks. Parent: These blocks are fun.
Imitate appropriate play	• Lets your child lead • Shows your child that you approve of the activity • Shows that you're involved • Teaches your child how to play with others and take turns • Increases the child's imitation of the things that you do	• Child: I put a nose on the potato head. Parent: I'm putting a nose on Mr. Potato Head too. • Child (*drawing circles on a piece of paper*). Parent: I'm going to draw circles on my paper just like you.
Describe appropriate behavior	• Lets your child lead • Shows your child that you are interested • Teaches your child concepts • Models speech for your child • Holds your child's attention on the task • Organizes your child's thoughts about the activity	• You're making a tower. • You drew a square. • You are putting together Mr. Potato Head. • You put the girl inside the fire truck.
Be *enthusiastic*	• Lets your child know that you are enjoying the time you are spending together • Increases the warmth of the play	• Child (*carefully placing a blue Lego on a tower*). Parent: (*gently touching the child's back*) You are REALLY being gentle with the toys.
Avoid *commands*	• Takes the lead away from your child • Can cause unpleasantness	*Indirect commands:* • Let's play with the farm next. • Could you tell me what animal this is? *Direct commands:* • Give me the pigs. • Please sit down next to me. • Look at this.

TABLE 12.1. *Continued*

Rules	Reason	Examples
Avoid *questions*	• Leads the conversation • Many questions are commands and require an answer • May seem like you aren't listening to your child or that you disagree	• We're building a tall tower, aren't we? • What sound does the cow make? • What are you building? • Do you want to play with the train? • You're putting the girl in the red car?
Avoid *critical statements*	• Often increases the criticized behavior • May lower your child's self-esteem • Creates an unpleasant interaction	• That wasn't nice. • I don't like it when you make that face. • Do not play like that. • No, sweetie, you shouldn't do that. • That animal doesn't go there.
Ignore negative behavior (unless it is dangerous or destructive) a. Avoid looking at the child, smiling, frowning, etc. b. Be silent c. Ignore every time d. Expect the ignored behavior to increase at first e. Continue ignoring until your child is doing something appropriate f. Praise your child immediately for appropriate behavior • Behaviors to ignore include crying without good reason, whining, and sassing	• Helps your child to notice the difference between your responses to good and bad behavior • Although the ignored behavior may increase at first, consistent ignoring decreases many behaviors	• Child (*sasses parent and picks up toy*). Parent (*ignores sass; praises picking up*).
Stop the playtime for aggressive and destructive behavior • Hitting • Biting • Stomping on toys	• Teaches your child that good behavior is required during special playtime • Shows your child that you are beginning to set limits	• Child (*hits parent*). Parent: (*CDI stops. This can't be ignored.*) Special playtime is stopping because you hit me. Child: Oh, oh, oh Mom. I'm sorry. Please, I'll be good. Parent: Special playtime is over now. Maybe next time you will be able to play nicely during special playtime.

Note. From Querido, Bearss, and Eyberg (2002). Copyright 2002 by John Wiley & Sons, Inc. All rights reserved. Reprinted by permission.

low the child's obedience or disobedience, which reduces parents' anxiety and helps them feel in control of their child's behavior.

Therapists teach parents to give their children clear, direct commands ("Please sit here beside me.") rather than criticisms ("Stop running around the room.") or indirect commands that suggest compliance is optional ("Do you want to put the blocks away now?"). Parents also learn to explain commands either before they are given ("We are leaving for the store soon. Please put on your shoes.") or after they are obeyed ("Thank you for putting on your shoes! Now you are ready to go to the store with me."). Parents learn to avoid arguing with the child by ignoring all delay tactics (e.g., "Why, Mom?") until the command has been obeyed. In addition to practicing commands during the teaching session, parents receive a handout summarizing the rules to review at home (see Table 12.2).

Therapists next teach parents precise steps to follow once they have given a command. Every command is followed by a specific parental response. If the child obeys, the parent gives a labeled praise for compliance (e.g., "Thank you for listening!") and then returns to the CDI until the next command is needed. If the child disobeys, the parent initiates the time-out procedure. Parents are taught never to ignore noncompliance because noncompliant behavior is reinforced if children are not made to do things that they refuse to do.

The time-out procedure provides parents with a standard, concrete set of steps to follow after they have given a command. The procedure has three levels: warning, chair, and room. At each level, the child may choose to obey the parent and end the time-out. The procedure does not end until the child obeys the original command.

The Warning

The warning is given after the child first disobeys a parental command. Before giving the warning, parents may give the child up to 5 seconds to begin obeying the command. This "5-second rule" is used when it is not clear whether the child intends to obey but not when the child is clearly disobeying (e.g., saying "No!"). The warning is the statement: "If you don't [original command] then you will have to sit on the time-out chair." If the child obeys the warning, the parent gives the child a labeled praise and the play continues.

The Chair

After the warning, the parent again has the option of using the 5-second rule. Once it is clear that the child has not obeyed the warning, the parent calmly and quickly takes the child to the time-out chair while saying, "You didn't [original command] so you have to sit on the chair." This statement reminds the child of the reason for the punishment and reiterates the connection between noncompliance and a negative consequence. The parent may lead the child to the chair with just a touch, or may carry the child from behind, if necessary, with arms under the child's arms and crossed over the child's chest. After placing the child on the chair, the parent says only, "Stay here until I tell you that you can get off." This statement has a different meaning than a statement such as "Stay here until you are ready to behave." It is important for the parent to establish control of the time the child spends on the chair. If the child could get off the chair whenever he or she wanted to, time-out would be a much less effective punishment.

Therapists teach parents to ignore all negative behavior as long as the child is on

TABLE 12.2. Eight Rules for Effective Commands in PDI

Rule	Reason	Examples
1. Commands should be *direct* rather than indirect.	• Leaves no question that the child is being told to do something. • Does not imply a choice or suggest that the parent might do the task for the child. • Is not confusing for young children.	• Please hand me the block. • Put the train in the box. • Draw a circle. *Instead of* • Will you hand me the block? • Let's put the train in the box. • Would you like to draw a circle?
2. Commands should be *positively stated.*	• Tells child what *to do* rather than what *not to do*. • Avoids criticism of the child's behavior. • Provides a clear statement of what the child can or should do.	• Come sit beside me. *Instead of* • Don't run around the room! • Put your hands in your pockets. *Instead of* • Stop touching the crystal.
3. Commands should be *given one at a time.*	• Helps child to remember the whole command. • Helps parent to determine if child completed entire command.	• Put your shoes in the closet. *Instead of* • Put your shoes in the closet, take a bath, and brush your teeth. • Put your shirt in the hamper. *Instead of* • Clean your room.
4. Commands should be *specific* rather than vague.	• Permits children to know exactly what they're supposed to do.	• Get down off the chair. *Instead of* • Be careful. • Talk in a quiet voice. *Instead of* • Behave!
5. Commands should be *age appropriate.*	• Makes it possible for children to understand the command and be able to do what they are told to do.	• Put the blue Lego in the box. *Instead of* • Change the location of the azure plastic block from the floor to its container. • Draw a square. *Instead of* • Draw a hexagon.
6. Commands should be given *politely and respectfully.*	• Increases the likelihood that the child will listen better. • Teaches children to obey polite and respectful commands. • Avoids child learning to obey only if yelled at. • Prepares child for school.	• Child (*banging block on table*). • Parent: (*in a normal tone of voice*) Please hand me the block. *Instead of* • Parent: (*loudly*) Hand me that block this instant!

(continues)

TABLE 12.2 *(continued)*

Rule	Reason	Examples
7. Commands should be explained *before* they are given or *after* they are obeyed.	• Avoids encouraging child to ask "why" after a command as a delay tactic. • Avoids giving child attention for not obeying.	Parent: Go wash your hands. Child: Why? Parent (*ignores, or uses time-out warning if child disobeys*). Child (*Obeys.*) Parent: Now your hands look so clean! It is good to be all clean when you go to school!
8. Commands should be used *only when necessary.*	• Decreases the child's frustration (and the amount of time spent in the time-out chair).	(*Child is running around*) • Please sit in this chair. [Good time to use command] *Instead of* • Please hand me my glass from the counter. [Not a good time to use a direct command]

Note. From Querido, Bearss, and Eyberg (2002). Copyright 2002 by John Wiley & Sons, Inc. All rights reserved. Reprinted by permission.

the chair. This skill can be difficult for parents because children often resort to various forms of emotional manipulation (e.g., "I don't love you anymore," "I want my daddy," "My stomach hurts," and "I'm sorry, I'm sorry") or, more rarely, negative physical behavior (e.g., taking off their clothes or wetting their pants). The child is required to sit on the chair for 3 minutes, plus 5 seconds of quiet at the end. These 5 seconds of quiet ensure that the child does not come away with the impression that whatever he or she said or did on the chair immediately before the end of the time-out caused the parent to end it.

Once the child's time on the chair has ended, the parent is instructed to walk over to the child and ask, "Are you ready to [original command]?" If the child says "No," begins to argue, or ignores the parent, the parent says, "All right, then stay on the chair until I tell you that you can get off." The parent then immediately leaves the area of the chair and begins the 3-minute time period again. If the child indicates that he or she is ready, either by saying "yes" or by getting off of the chair in a compliant manner, the parent walks the child back to the task. The parent then indicates that the child should obey the original command (e.g., pointing to the block that the child was originally instructed to put in its box). A child rarely refuses to obey at this point, but if the child does disobey, the parent says again, "You didn't [original command], so you have to sit on the chair," and then follows through as before.

When the child does obey the original command, the parent gives only a brief acknowledgment, such as "fine." The parent does not give the child extensive, labeled praise at this point because the child did not comply until he or she was punished. Instead, the parent immediately gives the child another similar but simple command. The child is also likely to obey this command, and it is at this point that the parent gives the child highly enthusiastic labeled praise for minding and returns to CDI. In this way, the child begins to discriminate between the positive responses that follow immediate compliance and the less reinforcing responses that follow compliance that requires punishment.

The Room

Time-out is the only punishment that therapists teach parents to use for noncompliance. The time-out chair alone is not sufficient, however, if children can get off of the chair before the parent gives them permission. An intended time-out can easily become a positively reinforcing event if the child is chased through the house by an increasingly exasperated parent. For this reason, therapists instruct parents to use a time-out room as a backup tool to teach their child to stay on the chair. Parents rarely need to use the time-out room after the first 2 or 3 weeks of PDI because children quickly learn to stay on the time-out chair once they realize that their parents will take them immediately to the time-out room every time they get off of the chair.

When the child gets off the time-out chair, the parent leads or carries the child to the time-out room. While taking the child to the time-out room, the parent says, "You got off the chair before I told you that you could, so you have to go to the time-out room." Once the child is in the time-out room, the parent closes the door and then keeps close track of the time so that the child stays in the room for 1 minute plus 5 seconds of quiet. The parent then leads the child back to the time-out chair and says, "Stay on the chair until I tell you that you can get off." The child's 3-minute time-out on the chair then starts over. This process may need to be repeated several times during the first time-out, so it is essential that parents and therapists leave enough time to follow through until the child understands that the parent is not going to give in.

The time-out room used in PCIT sessions should be an empty room that is easily accessible from the playroom. The room ideally should have an observation window or camera through which the therapist can monitor the child's behavior, although a room with a window in the door that allows the parent or therapist to check on the child can also be used. The time-out room selected for use in the child's home must be at least 4' by 4' and well lit. Although the time-out room will only be used for a short time, it is important that it is well prepared so it is both safe and effective. The therapist needs to discuss with the parents how to childproof the room so any items that could harm the child or that the child could damage are removed. Common choices for time-out rooms include walk-in closets or pantries because they can be emptied entirely for a few weeks. Use of a utility room or bathroom as a time-out room requires particularly careful review of and advice on safety hazards, such as removing all cleaning solutions and medicines from cabinets and turning down the hot water setting or disconnecting the water supply to a spare bathroom. Some families clear the child's bedroom of all but the bed for use as a time-out room during the first few weeks of PDI.

When children experience the time-out procedure during the first PDI coaching session, the therapist can coach and support the parents through the process the first time they use it. Children often escalate their negative reactions (crying, yelling, kicking) initially when their parents do not give in to them. Coaching the first PDI allows therapists to support parents during the emotionally difficult process of learning consistency so that they do not give up, and it gives therapists many opportunities to teach parents about their own and their child's behavior. Therapists can convey accurate attributions about the reasons for the child's behavior and can provide behavioral interpretations of the change as it is occurring. They can coach parents in relaxation and anger-control techniques *in vivo* and, if the child makes many journeys between the time-out chair and time-out room, they can assure the parents that their child does understand the process, is choosing time-out over obeying, but will complete the procedure and obey the original command within the session.

If the child does not need to go to time-out during the first PDI coaching session, the therapist must make a decision about whether a parent is ready to practice the procedure at home. Parents who demonstrate understanding of the skills and have the ability to remain calm when dealing with their child's misbehavior may go ahead and begin to practice PDI at home if they feel confident in doing so. Many parents wait an additional week so that they will have been coached through the time-out procedure at least once during treatment before beginning to practice PDI at home. Some children never go to time-out during a treatment session because they enjoy playing with their parents so much that they follow every command. In these cases, the therapist may ask parents to practice the time-out procedure and demonstrate it to their child using a large stuffed animal ("Mr. Bear") as a substitute for the child. The therapist will move and speak for "Mr. Bear" while the parent implements PDI, including the complete time-out procedure, with "Mr. Bear." This teaching procedure can also be used before the first PDI coaching session for families in which a parent or child may need extra time or practice to understand the time-out process.

Measuring Therapy Progress

Therapists assess the families' progress through PCIT in several ways. First, the observation and coding of parent–child interactions at the start of each session are used both to select the skills to target during the session and to determine when parents have met the criteria for moving from one phase of treatment to the next and for completing treatment. Before each session, the therapist also asks parents to fill out the Intensity Scale of the Eyberg Child Behavior Inventory (ECBI), which measures the current frequency of disruptive behavior at home. The therapist graphs the score each week to monitor the child's progress outside the session and may, at various points in treatment, share this graph with the parents. One criterion for treatment termination is an ECBI intensity score within ½ standard deviation of the normal mean (114 or lower). Finally, regardless of whether the scores meet criteria, treatment does not end until the parents express confidence in their ability to manage their child's behavior and feel ready for treatment to end. Thus, PCIT is performance based rather than time limited, and the number of treatment sessions can vary widely. Although the average length of treatment is 13 sessions, families attended as few as 8 and as many as 27 sessions before completing treatment in a recent study of 99 families (Werba, Eyberg, Boggs, & Algina, 2002). Werba and colleagues reported a PCIT dropout rate of 33%, which compares favorably to the 40–60% rate commonly cited for child psychotherapy.

EVIDENCE FOR THE EFFECTS OF TREATMENT

Several studies have provided empirical support of the effectiveness of PCIT for treating young children with disruptive behavior. These studies have compared PCIT to wait-list controls (McNeil, Capage, Bahl, & Blanc, 1999; Schuhmann, Foote, Eyberg, Boggs, & Algina, 1998), classroom controls (McNeil, Eyberg, Eisenstadt, Newcomb, & Funderburk, 1991), modified PCIT (Nixon, 2001), and group parent training (Eyberg & Matarazzo, 1980). In addition to changes in children's disruptive behavior, PCIT outcome studies have evidenced changes in parents' behavior toward their children, including increased reflective listening, physical proximity, prosocial verbalization, and decreased criticism and sarcasm (Eisenstadt, Eyberg, McNeil, Newcomb, & Funderburk, 1993). Significant improvements in parent psychopathology, personal distress, and parenting locus of control have been reported after PCIT as well (Schuhmann et al., 1998). The effects of PCIT have been found to generalize to untreated siblings (Brestan, Eyberg, Boggs, & Algina, 1997; Eyberg & Robinson, 1982), to other settings, such as school (McNeil et al., 1991), and across time (Edwards et al., 2002; Eyberg et al., 2001; Funderburk et al., 1998; Hood & Eyberg, in press). Table 12.3 presents a summary of efficacy data.

Treatment Efficacy

In the largest study of treatment efficacy to date, Schuhmann and colleagues (1998) compared families receiving PCIT to wait-list controls. Following an initial assessment, 64 clinic-referred families were randomly assigned to an immediate treatment (IT) or wait-list control (WL) group. After treatment, parents in the IT group interacted more positively with their child and were more successful in gaining their child's compliance than parents in the WL group. These parents also reported less parenting stress and a more internal locus of control than WL parents. They reported clinically as well as statistically significant improvements in their child's behavior at the end of treatment. All families that completed treatment reported high levels of satisfaction with both the content and process of PCIT. Preliminary 4-month follow-up data showed that gains were maintained on all parent-report measures.

Treatment Generalization to School Settings

McNeil et al. (1991) evaluated the generalization of PCIT treatment effects from the clinic to school setting in 10 children with conduct problem behaviors occurring both at home and in the classroom. Families received 14 weeks of PCIT. No advice regarding school problems or direct classroom intervention was provided. Both teacher ratings and school observational measures indicated significantly greater improvements in disruptive behavior for the treated group than for a group of 10 normal controls and a group of 10 behavior problem controls drawn from the classrooms of the treated children. On measures of hyperactivity/distractibility, results were less supportive of generalization. The evidence of school generalization after PCIT was among the first to call into question the behavioral contrast effect—the notion that as children's conduct improves in the home, it worsens in the classroom.

Funderburk et al. (1998) conducted 12- and 18-month follow-up school assessments for 12 children, including those who had completed PCIT in the McNeil et al. (1991) study. At the 12-month follow-up, children in the treatment group maintained posttreatment improvements in teacher ratings and observational measures of disruptive behavior and showed further improvements in social competency. The children were indistinguishable from 72 randomly selected control children from their classrooms on measures of conduct problems and social competence. At the 18-month follow-up, children maintained their improvements in compliance but demonstrated declines on other measures into the range of pretreatment levels.

Treatment Generalization within the Family

Eyberg and Robinson (1982) conducted the first study to examine the effects of PCIT on family functioning. In a sample of seven families that completed PCIT, significant im-

TABLE 12.3. Parent–Child Interaction Therapy Outcome Studies

Study	Participants	Ethnicity and SES	Type of analysis	Findings
Edwards et al. (2002)	46 families (23 dropouts, 23 completers), 78% boys, mean pretreatment age = 4.9, pretreatment diagnosis = ODD	74% Caucasian, 15% African American, 8% other, mean Hollingshead Index = 35	2 (group) × 2 (time) repeated-measures ANOVAs on parent reports of disruptive behavior, diagnostic symptoms, parenting stress, depression, and confidence from pretreatment to follow-up 1–3 years later. Pre- to follow-up effect sizes and Jacobson's index of clinically significant change.	Treatment completers showed statistically and clinically significantly better long-term outcomes than treatment dropouts on most measures. Large effect sizes for treatment completers on all measures.
Hood & Eyberg (in press)	23 families, 70% boys, mean pretreatment age = 5.0, pretreatment diagnosis = ODD	83% Caucasian, 4% African American, 13% other, mean Hollingshead Index = 40	Repeated-measures ANOVAs on parent report of child behavior and parent locus of control comparing pretreatment to follow-up 3–6 years after treatment completion. Pre- to follow-up effect sizes and Jacobson's index of clinically significant change.	Majority of children maintained their treatment gains.
McNeil, Capage, Bahl, & Blanc (1999)	32 families, 75% boys, mean child age = 4.0, children referred for disruptive behavior problems	88% Caucasian	Families assigned to treatment (n = 18) or wait-list condition (n = 14) based on therapist availability. Group × time MANOVA performed on parent report of child and parent functioning.	Families in treatment condition showed clinically and statistically significantly greater improvements over time than families in the wait-list condition.
Nixon, (2001)	37 families, 73% boys, mean child age = 4.0, pretreatment diagnosis = ODD, comparison group of 21 nonproblem preschoolers	Australian families, mean family income between $23,200 and $40,599	Random assignment to standard PCIT, abbreviated PCIT, or wait-list control group. 3 × 2 ANCOVAs of observed behavior, parent report of child and parent functioning, and teacher report from pre- to post-treatment. Repeated-measures ANOVA at 3-month, 6-month, 1-year, and 2-year follow-up.	Both groups made clincally and statistically significant improvements and maintained gains over time. Little statistical difference between outcomes for abbreviated and standard PCIT.
Eyberg et al. (2001)	13 families, 90% boys, mean child age = 4.7, pretreatment diagnosis = disruptive behavior	84% Caucasian, 8% African American, 8% other, median yearly income =	One-way repeated-measures ANOVAs and effect sizes on observed behavior and parent report of child and parent function-ing at pre-, post-, 1-year, and 2-year	Two years after treatment completion, mothers continued to report child behavior problems, child activity level, and parenting stress at posttreatment levels, and the majority

Study	Sample		Methodology	Results
	disorder (85% ADHD)	$15,000, 62% single-parent families	follow-up. Clinically significant change evaluated using published cutoff scores and 30% change for observational measures.	of children remained free of diagnoses of disruptive behavior disorders.
Borrego, Urquiza, Rasmussen, & Zebell (1999)	Single-case study with 35-year-old mother at high risk for physically abusing 3-year-old son (fetal alcohol syndrome, severe internalizing and externalizing problems)	Caucasian, low SES, history of alcoholism and homelessness	Observed behavior and parent ratings of child and parent functioning tracked at pretreatment, posttreatment, 5-month, and 16-month follow-up.	Family moved into normal range of functioning at posttreatment and maintained gains at both follow-up assessments.
Schuhmann, Foote, Eyberg, Boggs, & Algina (1998)	64 families, 81% boys, mean child age = 4.9, pretreatment diagnosis = ODD	77% Caucasian, 14% African American, 9% other, mean Hollingshead Index = 35	Random assignment to treatment versus wait-list, ANCOVAs for observed behavior and parent ratings of child and parent functioning at pre- and posttreatment, t tests on TAI, 4-month follow-up for treatment completers.	Treatment group showed significant improvements in child and parent functioning compared to wait-list group. Treatment gains maintained at 4-month follow-up.
Funderburk et al. (1998)	84 children (12 treatment, 72 controls with high, average, or low teacher ratings of behavior problems), mean child age (treatment group) = 4.7, pretreatment diagnosis = disruptive behavior disorder	Treatment group = 92% Caucasian	Repeated measures ANOVA for treatment group outcome, and pairwise comparisons for treatment versus control groups on teacher ratings and observational measures at pre-, post-, 12-month, and 18-month follow-up.	Treatment group showed clinically significant improvements in school behavior after PCIT. At 12-month follow-up, treatment group maintained improvements. At 18-month follow-up, treatment group maintained improvements in compliance but showed significant declines during second follow-up year.
Brestan, Eyberg, Boggs, & Algina (1997)	30 siblings of children treated for ODD, 63% boys, mean age = 5.8	70% Caucasian, 20% African American, 7% Hispanic, 3% other, mean Hollingshead Index = 33	Random assignment to PCIT versus waitlist, ANCOVA on mother and father ratings for group comparisons of untreated siblings.	Relative to siblings in the wait-list control group, fathers rated behavior problems of siblings in treatment group as occuring less frequently, and mothers rated siblings' behavior as less problematic for them after treatment.
Eisenstadt, Eyberg, McNeil, Newcomb, & Funderburk (1993)	24 families, 92% boys, mean age = 4.5	88% Caucasian, mean family income = $18,274	Families randomly assigned to CDI-first or PDI-first. Between-group ANOVAs performed at mid- and posttreatment. t test comparisons between pre- and posttreatment scores on observed behavior and parent ratings of child and parent functioning.	All families moved into normal range on compliance, disruptive behavior, activity level, and parent stress, child self-esteem, internalizing problems, and parent–child proximity. Gains maintained at 6-week follow-up. Few significant differences between groups at midtreatment or posttreatment.

TABLE 12.3. *Continued*

Study	Participants	Ethnicity and SES	Type of analysis	Findings
McNeil, Eyberg, Eisenstadt, Newcomb & Funderburk (1991)	10 treated children, 10 normal controls, 10 untreated children with school behavior problems, 100% boys, mean age = 4.7, treated group diagnosed with disruptive behavior disorder and presented significant school behavior problems	Treated group = 90% Caucasian, treated group median income = $12,000, control groups = 70% Caucasian	3 × 2 repeated measures ANOVAs for comparison of 3 groups on classroom observation and teacher rating scales.	Treated group displayed significantly greater improvements than control groups on all measures of disruptive behavior in the classroom.
Eyberg & Robinson (1982)	7 treatment families, 86% boys, mean age = 4.9, children referred for disruptive behaviors	Mean parent education = 13 years	t tests comparing pre- and posttreatment scores on observed behavior and parent ratings of child and parent functioning.	Significant pre–post improvements in child and sibling behavior and parent adjustment.
Eyberg & Matarazzo (1980)	29 families enrolled in speech and language program	Not reported	Families assigned to 5-week group parent training, 5-week individual PCIT, or control group. 3 × 2 repeated measures ANOVAs and t tests performed for observational measures and parent ratings at pre- and posttreatment.	Improvements on observational measures and parent ratings for families assigned to individual PCIT. Parent training showed no significant changes. Parents in PCIT reported greater satisfaction with treatment.
Eyberg & Ross (1978)	10 behavior problem children referred for treatment, 90% boys, mean age = 6.2, 42 normal controls, 43 clinic-referred comparison children	Not reported	F test comparing pre- and posttreatment scores on parent ratings of disruptive child behavior; pre- scores compared to comparison children referred for behavior problems, post- scores compared to normal and clinic comparison samples.	Significant pre- and posttreatment improvements on child disruptive behavior. At pretreatment, children at mean of clinic-referred behavior problem sample. At posttreatment children at mean of nonbehavior problem samples, demonstrating clinically significant change.

Note. SES, socioeconomic status; ANOVA, analysis of variance; ODD, oppositional defiant disorder; MANOVA, multivariate analysis of variance; PCIT, parent–child interaction therapy; ANCOVA, analysis of covariance; ADHD, attention-deficit/hyperactivity disorder; TAI, Therapy Attitude Inventory.

provements were seen not only in the behavior of the child but also in several other aspects of family life. Following treatment, mothers in the study showed less anxiety and pessimism, increased involvement and interest in others, and a greater degree of internal control. Marital adjustment ratings also improved, as did observed behavior of the children's untreated siblings.

More recently, Brestan et al. (1997) examined parents' perceptions of untreated siblings. Researchers randomly assigned 30 referred families to an immediate treatment or WL control group. The two groups did not differ initially on their ratings of the target child or the untreated siblings. Following treatment, fathers in the treatment group rated the behavior problems of untreated siblings as occurring less frequently, and mothers in the treatment group rated these behaviors as less problematic.

Treatment Generalization across Time

The effects of PCIT have been shown to last after treatment has ended. For example, in a 6-week follow-up of 14 families, all families maintained treatment gains on observational measures of child compliance, parent-rating scale measures of disruptive behavior, internalizing problems, activity level, maternal stress, and child self-report of self-esteem (Eisenstadt et al., 1993). At a 2-year follow-up with these families, parent ratings of child behavior problems, child activity level, and parenting stress remained similar to posttreatment levels, and most of the children remained free of disruptive behavior diagnoses. Further, these parents continued to report high satisfaction with the process and outcome of PCIT (Eyberg et al., 2001).

Edwards et al. (2002) compared outcomes for families who completed PCIT and those who dropped out of the Schuhmann et al. (1998) study. From each group, 23 families were located that provided data. Telephone and mail assessments included a structured diagnostic interview, several parent-report measures, and, for a subset of families, teacher-report measures. Length of follow-up for both groups ranged from 10 to 30 months after the initial treatment intake, with the average length of follow-up just under 20 months. Results indicated significantly poorer long-term outcomes for those who dropped out of treatment. Children and families that completed treatment maintained treatment gains over this period, whereas the dropouts showed disruptive behavior and parenting stress at pretreatment levels.

Finally, Hood and Eyberg (in press) attempted to locate 50 families that had completed PCIT 4 to 6 years earlier. Of the 29 families that could be located, 23 participated in telephone and mail follow-up assessments of child disruptive behavior and parenting locus of control. Results indicated that the significant changes made during treatment were maintained for the children, now ages 6 to 12, and their mothers. Child behavior at posttreatment assessment and length of time since treatment were strong predictors of child behavior at long-term follow-up. The investigators found that children's disruptive behavior decreased with time since treatment.

DIRECTIONS FOR FUTURE RESEARCH

Treatment Attrition

Continued research is needed to identify the factors that affect successful completion of PCIT. Because treatment is performance based and continues until the treatment goals are met, the only way a family cannot succeed, theoretically, is to drop out. In reality, most families complete PCIT in 16 or fewer sessions (Werba et al., 2002), and those that drop out after 20 sessions are families that would likely not have succeeded with further sessions. Nevertheless, families that meet the criteria for treatment completion are successful treatment completers, and PCIT dropouts are treatment failures. In the first study examining predictors of dropout from PCIT, Werba et al. (2002) found that mothers who were highly critical during parent–child interactions or who were experiencing severe parenting stress were more likely to drop out, which led to increased attention to maternal distress during treatment. Much of the variance in dropout is still unaccounted for, however, and further examination of family factors and therapy process variables that affect treatment attrition is urgently needed.

Treatment Maintenance

More study of the treatment completers is needed as well. For these families, research examining maintenance of the treatment effects has been encouraging. At the group level, important treatment gains have been maintained. Group-level analyses mask individual differences, however, and studies of clinical significance have documented various rates of long-term relapse. Although in the minority, these are the families that must be targeted in future research. It is critical to examine the factors that put certain families at risk for relapse. For these at-risk families, treatment gains may require a period of consolidation to achieve durable effects. Alternatively, disruptive child behavior or a chaotic lifestyle that disrupts effective parenting may be a chronic, recurring condition requiring ongoing monitoring and treatment. Families that have demonstrated the commitment to succeed in treatment once are likely to rally quickly with timely booster treatment.

Moderators of Outcome

The PCIT outcome studies to date have been conducted in psychology clinics at major metropolitan medical centers using culturally heterogeneous samples of referred boys and girls with disruptive behavior and multiple diagnoses. Despite this demographic diversity, with the exception of examining predictors of dropout, these studies have not examined results separately for demographic groups. No study has yet examined moderator effects on treatment length or specific outcomes at treatment completion. Research in this area may reveal ways to refine treatment to improve both retention and long-term outcome; however, the basic conceptual framework of PCIT appears to be consistent with parenting values across a variety of diverse racial and cultural groups. For example, Querido, Warner, and Eyberg (2002) found that the authoritative parenting style predicted optimal child outcomes among African American families, and Calzada and Eyberg (2002) found that Dominican and Puerto Rican parents living in the United States endorsed similar authoritative parenting values. These findings suggest that PCIT may be a successful treatment for children and families from diverse racial/ethnic groups, and research directly addressing this question with homogeneous groups is needed to identify treatment elements that can maximize gains for every child.

Application to New Populations

Although the evidence base of PCIT has been established with children referred for disruptive behavior, principles of parenting that derive from attachment and social learning theories and form the theoretical basis of PCIT have broad application. The treatment has been used clinically to treat behavior problems associated with an array of primary diagnoses including neurological impairments, developmental disorders, chronic medical illness, and separation anxiety disorder. PCIT is also used in treatment with abusive families, where the identified patient is often the parent. The coercive parent–child relationship that characterizes families of disruptive children is central to physically abusive families. Further, because abusive families tend to experience few positive interactions, they seem to benefit greatly from being coached in the positive parenting skills that facilitate warm, enjoyable family experiences (Urquiza & McNeil, 1996). PCIT has been adopted as a standard therapy in several child abuse treatment facilities, and empirical data on its effects with this population are clearly needed.

Treatment Effectiveness

The effectiveness of PCIT also needs to be evaluated in real-world clinics, where clinicians generally provide services without the scrutiny and support that graduate student therapists are accustomed to receive from their supervisors. In disseminating PCIT to nonuniversity settings, it will be important not to lose the critical elements of the treatment (e.g., coding parent–child interactions to guide treatment sessions and requiring skill mastery before parents move from one treatment phase to the next or complete treatment). Without treatment fidelity, treatment effectiveness cannot be assured. It is still unknown, however, how best to ensure adequate fidelity outside the apprenticeship model of the graduate training program. Research examining training models that provide varying levels of instruction (e.g., reading the treatment manual and observing a set number of sessions) to clinicians who have varying levels of prior training is another urgent need.

SUMMARY AND CONCLUSIONS

This chapter has described parent–child interaction therapy for children with disruptive behavior disorders and their families. Key elements of the treatment have been illustrated, such as involving the parents and child together in treatment, using assessment to guide the families' progress, actively coaching the parents in relationship and behavior change skills, and continuing treatment until parents have mastered the skills and their child's behavior is within the normal range. These treatment elements draw on both attachment and social learning principles to produce lasting improvements in the parent–child bond as well as reductions in the child's disruptive behavior.

Studies have been presented that document treatment efficacy and generalization of its effects within the family and across settings and time for the majority of families that complete treatment. These efficacy studies do not address, however, the minority of families that fail to complete treatment. More research on predictors of attrition is needed to identify families that need more specialized interventions to complete treatment. For the families that complete treatment, research on maintenance of treatment gains is needed to identify families at risk for relapse and to determine whether relapse rates can be improved through timely booster treatment.

In view of the high risk of poor lifetime outcomes for young children with disruptive behavior, the need for effectiveness studies in real-world settings is critical. Early intervention has the power to alter the dismal prognosis for these children; however, in disseminating PCIT to a wider range of mental health providers, we cannot overlook the need to ensure proper training and close adherence to essential treatment elements. This challenge—balancing the drive to assist families with the preservation of treatment integrity—demands further study of the training resources necessary for a clinician to become an effective PCIT therapist.

REFERENCES

Baumrind, D. (1967). Child care practices anteceding three patterns of preschool behavior. *Genetic Psychology Monographs, 75,* 43–88.

Baumrind, D. (1991). The influence of parenting style on adolescent competence and substance use. *Journal of Early Adolescence, 11,* 56–95.

Borrego, J., Urquiza, A., Rasmussen, R., & Zebell, N. (1999). Parent–child interaction therapy with a family at high risk for physical abuse. *Child Maltreatment, 4*(4), 331–342.

Brestan, E., Eyberg, S. M., Boggs, S., & Algina, J. (1997). Parent–child interaction therapy: Parent perceptions of untreated siblings. *Child and Family Behavior Therapy, 19,* 13–28.

Calzada, E. J., & Eyberg, S. M. (2002). *Normative parenting in a sample of Dominican and Puerto Rican mothers of young children.* Manuscript submitted for publication.

Edwards, D. L., Eyberg, S. M., Rayfield, A., Jacobs, J., Bagner, D., & Hood, K. K. (2002). *Outcomes of parent–child interaction therapy: A comparison of treatment completers and treatment dropouts one to three years later.* Manuscript submitted for publication.

Eisenstadt, T. H., Eyberg, S. M., McNeil, C. B., Newcomb, K., & Funderburk, B. (1993). Parent–child interaction therapy with behavior problem children: Relative effectiveness of two statges and overall treatment outcomes. *Journal of Clinical Child Psychology, 22,* 42–51.

Eyberg, S. M., Funderburk, B. W., Hembree-Kigen, T., McNeil, C. B., Querido, J., & Hood, K. K. (2001). Parent–child interaction therapy with behavior problem children: One and two year maintenance of treatment effects in the family. *Child and Family Behavior Therapy, 23,* 1–20.

Eyberg, S. M., & Matarazzo, R. G. (1980). Training parents as therapists: A comparison between individual parent–child interactions training and parent group didactic training: *Journal of Clinical Psychology, 36,* 492–499.

Eyberg, S. M., & Robinson, E. A. (1982). Parent–child interaction therapy: Effects on family functioning. *Journal of Clinical Child Psychology, 11,* 123–129.

Eyberg, S. M., & Ross, A. W. (1978). Assessment of child behavior problems: The validation of a new inventory. *Journal of Clinical Child Psychology, 7,* 113–116.

Funderburk, B., Eyberg, S. M., Newcomb, K., McNeil, C., Hembree-Kigin, T., & Capage, L. (1998). Parent–child interaction therapy with behavior problem children: Maintenance of treatment effects in the school setting. *Child and Family Behavior Therapy, 20,* 17–38.

Hann, D. L., & Borek, N. B. (2002). Taking stock of risk factors for child/youth externalizing behavior problems [On-line]. Available from National Institutes of Mental Health: *http://www. nimh.nih.gov/childhp/takingstock.pdf*

Hood, K. K., & Eyberg, S. M. (in press). Outcomes of parent–child interaction therapy: Mothers' report of maintenance three to six years later. *Journal of Clinical Child and Adolescent Psychotherapy.*

McNeil, C. B., Capage, L., Bahl, A., & Blanc, H. (1999). Importance of early intervention for disruptive behavior problems: Comparison of treatment and waitlist control groups. *Early Education and Development, 10,* 445–454.

McNeil, C., Eyberg, S., Eisentadt, T., Newcomb, K., & Funderburk, B. (1991). Parent–child interaction therapy with behavior problem children: Generalization of treatment effects to the school setting. *Journal of Clinical Child Psychology, 20,* 140–151.

Nixon, R. D. V. (2001). *Parent–child interaction therapy: A comparison of standard and abbreviated treatments for oppositional defiant preschoolers.* Paper presented at the Second Annual Parent–Child Interaction Therapy Conference, Sacramento.

Querido, J. G., Bearss, K., & Eyberg, S. M. (2002). Theory, research, and practice of parent–child interaction therapy. In F. W. Kaslow & T. Patterson (Eds.), *Comprehensive handbook of psychotherapy: Vol. 2. Cognitive/behavioral/functional approaches* (pp. 91–113). New York: Wiley.

Querido, J. G., Warner, T. D, & Eyberg, S. M. (2002). The cultural context of parenting: An assessment of parenting styles in African-American families. *Journal of Clinical Child and Adolescent Psychology, 31,* 272–277.

Schuhmann, E. M., Foote, R., Eyberg, S. M., Boggs, S., & Algina, J. (1998). Parent–child interaction therapy: Interim report of a randomized trail with short-term maintenance. *Journal of Clinical Child Psychology, 27,* 34–35.

Urquiza, A. J., & McNeil, C. B. (1996). Parent–child interaction therapy: Potential applications for physically abusive families. *Child Maltreatment, 1,* 134–144.

Werba, B. E., Eyberg, S. M., Boggs, S., & Algina, J. (2002). *Predicting outcome in parent–child interaction therapy: Success and attrition.* Manuscript submitted for publication.

13

The Incredible Years Parents, Teachers, and Children Training Series

A Multifaceted Treatment Approach for Young Children with Conduct Problems

Carolyn Webster-Stratton and M. Jamila Reid

OVERVIEW

The Clinical Problem

The incidence of oppositional defiant disorder (ODD) and conduct disorder (CD) in children is alarmingly high, with reported cases of early-onset conduct problems in young children as high as 35% for low-income families (Webster-Stratton & Hammond, 1998). Between 1988 and 1997, arrests of young offenders (between 7 and 12 years old) for violent crimes increased by 45% and for drug abuse violations by 165% (Snyder, 2001). Research indicates that children with early-onset ODD and CD are at increased risk for abuse by their parents, school dropout, depression, drug abuse, juvenile delinquency, violence, adult crime, antisocial personality, marital disruption, and other diagnosable psychiatric disorders. Conduct problems (hereafter this term is used to refer to young children with ODD and/or CD) are one of the most costly mental disorders to society, because such a large proportion of antisocial children remain involved with mental health agencies or criminal justice systems throughout the course of their lives.

Developmental theorists have suggested that "early starter" delinquents, those who first exhibit ODD symptoms in the preschool years, have a two- to threefold risk of becoming tomorrow's serious violent and chronic juvenile offenders (Loeber et al., 1993; Patterson, Capaldi, & Bank, 1991). These children with early-onset CD also account for a disproportionate share of delinquent acts in adulthood, including interpersonal violence, substance abuse, and property crimes. Indeed, the primary developmental pathway for serious conduct disorders in adolescence and adulthood appears to be established during the preschool period.

Assumptions Underlying Treatment

Theories regarding the causes of child conduct problems include ineffective parenting (e.g., harsh discipline, low parent involvement in school activities, and low monitoring); family factors (e.g., marital conflict, depression, drug abuse, and criminal behavior in parents); child biological and developmental risk factors (e.g., attention deficit disorders, learning disabilities, and language delays); school risk factors (e.g., teachers' use of poor classroom management strategies, classroom level of aggression, large class sizes, and low teacher involvement with parents); and peer and community risk factors (e.g., poverty and gangs).

Because conduct disorder becomes increasingly resistant to change over time, intervention that begins early in the child's life is clearly a strategic way to prevent or reduce later development of CD, violence, substance abuse and delinquency. Our decision to focus our interventions on the preschool and early school years (ages 3–8 years) was based on several considerations. First, there is evidence that children with ODD and CD are clearly identifiable at this age. Our prior studies have revealed that children as young as age 4 have already been expelled from two or more preschools and have experienced considerable peer and teacher rejection. Second, there is evidence that the younger the child at the time of intervention, the more positive the child's behavioral adjustment at home and at school. Third, preschool entry through the first years of elementary school is a major transition and a period of great stress for many children and their parents. Early success or failure in school sets the stage for children's future behavior at school and relationships with teachers and peers, and also for their parents' future attitudes and relationships with the school, teachers, and administrators. Fourth, young children with conduct problems are a chronically underserved population; approximately 70% do not receive any treatment and even fewer receive treatments that are "empirically validated" (Brestan & Eyberg, 1998). It is our belief that early intervention, placed strategically during the high-risk child's first major transition point, can counteract risk factors and strengthen protective factors, thereby helping to prevent a developmental trajectory to increasingly aggressive and violent behaviors, negative reputations, peer rejection, low self-esteem, and spiraling academic failure.

CHARACTERISTICS OF THE TREATMENT PROGRAM

To address the parenting, family, child, and school risk factors, we have developed three complementary training curricula, known as the Incredible Years Training Series, targeted at parents, teachers, and children (ages 2–8 years). This chapter reviews these training programs and their associated research.

Incredible Years Parent Interventions

Goals of the Parent Programs

Goals of the parent programs are to promote parent competencies and strengthen families by doing the following:

- Increasing parents' positive parenting, nurturing relationships with their children, and general self-confidence about parenting.
- Replacing critical and physically violent discipline with positive strategies such as ignoring, natural and logical consequences, redirecting, monitoring, and problem-solving.

- Improving parents' problem-solving skills, anger management, and communication skills.
- Increasing family support networks and school involvement/bonding.
- Helping parents and teachers work collaboratively to ensure consistency across settings.
- Increasing parents' involvement in children's academic-related activities at home.

Content of the BASIC Parent Training Treatment Program

In 1980, we developed an interactive, videotape-based parent intervention program (BASIC) for parents of children ages 2–6 years. Next we developed a school-age version of the BASIC program (with a more culturally diverse population) for use with parents of children ages 6–10 years. The BASIC parent training program takes 26 hours and is completed in 13–14 weekly, 2-hour sessions. The foundation of the program is videotape vignettes of modeled parenting skills (250 vignettes, each lasting approximately 1–2 minutes) shown by a therapist to groups of 8–12 parents. The videotapes demonstrate social learning and child development principles and serve as the stimulus for focused discussions, problem solving, and collaborative learning. The program is also designed to help parents understand normal variations in children's development, emotional reactions, and temperaments.

The BASIC program begins with a focus on enhancing positive relationships between parents and children by teaching parents to use child-directed interactive play, praise, and incentive programs. Next, a specific set of nonviolent discipline techniques is taught, including monitoring, ignoring, commands, natural and logical consequences, and time-out. Finally, parents are taught how they can teach their children problem-solving skills.

Content of the ADVANCE Parent Training Treatment Program

In addition to parenting behavior per se, other aspects of parents' behavior and personal lives constitute risk factors for child conduct problems. Researchers have demonstrated that personal and interpersonal risk factors such as parental depression, marital discord, lack of social support, poor problem-solving ability, and environmental stressors disrupt parenting behavior and contribute to coercive parent–child interactions and relapses subsequent to parent training. This evidence led us to expand our theoretical and causal model concerning conduct problems, and in 1989 we developed the ADVANCE treatment program. We theorized that a broader-based training model (i.e., one involving helping parents with conflict management issues) would help mediate the negative influences of these personal and interpersonal factors on parenting skills and promote increased maintenance and generalizability of treatment effects.

The content of this 14-session videotape program (60 vignettes), which is offered after the completion of the BASIC training program, involves four components:

1. *Personal self-control.* Parents are taught to substitute coping and positive self-talk for their depressive, angry, and blaming self-talk. In addition, parents are taught specific anger management techniques.
2. *Communication skills.* Parents are taught to identify blocks to communication and to learn effective communication skills for dealing with conflict.
3. *Problem-solving skills.* Parents are taught effective strategies for coping with conflict with spouses, employers, extended family members, and children.

4. *Strengthening social support and self-care.* This concept is woven throughout all the group sessions and components by encouraging the group members to ask for support when necessary and to give support to others.

The content of both the BASIC and ADVANCE programs is also provided in the text that parents use for the program, titled *The Incredible Years: A Troubleshooting Guide for Parents* (Webster-Stratton, 1992).

Content of the SCHOOL Parent Training Treatment

In follow-up interviews with parents who completed our parent training programs, 58% requested guidance on issues surrounding homework, communication with teachers, behavior problems at school, and promoting their children's reading, academic, and social skills. These data suggested a need for teaching parents to access schools, collaborate with teachers, and supervise children's peer relationships. In addition, 40% of teachers reported problems with children's compliance and aggression in the classroom and requested advice on how to manage these problems. Clearly, integrating interventions across settings (home and school) and agents (teachers and parents) to target school and family risk factors fosters greater between-environment consistency and offers the best chance for long-term reduction of antisocial behavior.

In 1990 we developed an interactive videotape modeling academic skills training intervention (SCHOOL) as an adjunct to our BASIC and ADVANCE interventions. This intervention consists of four to six additional sessions that are usually offered to parents after the BASIC program. These sessions focus on collaboration with teachers and fostering children's academic readiness and school success through parental involvement in school activities, homework, and peer monitoring.

This program involves six components:

1. *Promoting children's self-confidence.* Parents are taught to lay the foundation for their children's success at school by helping children feel confident about their own ideas and ability to learn. Specifically, we teach parents to facilitate reading using the "dialogic reading" approach, to foster language development and problem solving, and to promote children's reading, writing, and story-telling skills.
2. *Fostering good learning habits.* Parents are taught to establish a predictable homework routine, set limits concerning television and computer games, and follow through with consequences for children who test these limits.
3. *Dealing with children's discouragement.* Parents are taught to set realistic goals for their child, to gradually increase the difficulty of the learning task as the child acquires mastery, and to use praise, tangible rewards, and attention to motivate and reinforce progress.
4. *Participating in homework.* Parents are taught strategies to play a positive and supportive role in their children's homework.
5. *Using teacher–parent conferences to advocate for your child.* This segment helps parents to collaborate with teachers to jointly develop plans that address school difficulties, such as inattentiveness, tardiness, and aggression in school.
6. *Discussing a school problem with your child.* Parents learn to talk with their children about academic problems and set up plans with them to maximize school success.

Incredible Years Teacher Training Intervention

Once children with behavior problems enter school, negative academic and social experiences escalate the development of conduct problems. Aggressive, disruptive children quickly become socially excluded, which leads to fewer opportunities to interact socially and to learn appropriate friendship skills. Over time, peers become mistrustful and respond to aggressive children in ways that increase the likelihood of reactive aggression. Evidence suggests that peer rejection eventually leads to association with deviant peers. Once children have formed deviant peer groups, the risk for drug abuse and antisocial behavior is even higher. Furthermore, teacher behaviors and school characteristics, such as low emphasis on teaching social and emotional competence, low rates of praise, little attention to individualizing goals for particular children, and high student–teacher ratio, are associated with classroom aggression, delinquency, and poor academic performance. Rejecting and nonsupportive responses from teachers further exacerbate the problems of aggressive children. Aggressive children frequently develop poor relationships with teachers and are often expelled from classrooms. In our own studies with conduct problem children, ages 3–7 years, over 50% of the children had been asked to leave three or more classrooms by second grade. Lack of teacher support and exclusion from the classroom exacerbate these children's social problems and academic difficulties, contributing to the likelihood of school dropout.

Goals of the Teacher Training Programs

The goals are to promote teacher competencies and strengthen home–school connections by doing the following:

- Strengthening teachers' effective classroom management skills, including proactive teaching approaches;
- Strengthening positive relationships between teachers and students;
- Increasing teachers' use of effective discipline strategies;
- Increasing teachers' collaborative efforts with parents and promotion of parents' school involvement;
- Increasing teachers' ability to teach social skills, anger management, and problem-solving skills in the classroom; and
- Decreasing levels of classroom aggression.

Content of Teacher Training Intervention

The teacher training program is a 4-day (or 32-hour) group-based program for teachers, school counselors, and psychologists. Training targets teachers' use of effective classroom management strategies for dealing with misbehavior; promoting positive relationships with difficult students; strengthening social skills in the classroom, the playground, bus, and lunchroom; and strengthening teachers' collaborative process and positive communication with parents (e.g., the importance of positive home phone calls, regular meetings with parents, home visits, and successful parent conferences). Teachers, parents, and group facilitators jointly develop "transition plans" that detail successful classroom strategies for the child with conduct problems; goals achieved and goals still to be worked on; characteristics, interests, and motivators for the child; and ways parents would like to be contacted by teachers. This information is passed on to the following year's teachers. In addition, teachers learn to prevent peer rejection by helping the aggressive child learn appropriate problem-solving strategies and helping his or her peers to respond appropriately to aggression. Teachers are encouraged to be sensitive to individual developmental differences (i.e., variation in attention span and activity level) and biological deficits in children (e.g., unresponsiveness to aversive stimuli, heightened interest in novelty) and the relevance of these differences for enhanced teaching efforts that are positive, accepting, and consistent. Physical aggression in unstructured settings (e.g., playground) is targeted for close monitoring, teaching, and incentive programs. A complete description of the content included in this curriculum is described in the book that teachers use for the course, titled *How to Promote Social and Emotional Competence* (Webster-Stratton, 2000).

Incredible Years Child Training Intervention

Research has indicated that some abnormal aspects of the child's internal organization at the physiological, neurological, and/or neuropsychological level are linked to the development of conduct disorders, particularly for children with a chronic history of early behavioral problems. Children with conduct problems are more likely to have certain temperamental characteristics such as inattentiveness, impulsivity, and attention-deficit/hyperactivity disorder (ADHD). Other child factors have also been implicated in early onset conduct disorder. For example, deficits in social-cognitive skills and negative attributions contribute to poor emotional regulation and aggressive peer interactions. In addition, studies indicate that children with conduct problems have significant delays in their peer-play skills—in particular, difficulty with reciprocal play, cooperative skills, taking turns, waiting, and giving suggestions (Webster-Stratton & Lindsay, 1999). Finally, reading, learning, and language delays are also associated with conduct problems, particularly for "early life course persisters" (Moffitt & Lynam, 1994). The relationship between academic performance and ODD/CD is bidirectional. Academic difficulties may cause disengagement, increased frustration, and lower self-esteem, which contribute to the child's behavior problems. At the same time, noncompliance, aggression, elevated activity levels, and poor attention limit a child's ability to be engaged in learning and achieve academically. Thus, a cycle is created in which one problem exacerbates the other. This combination of academic delays and conduct problems appears to contribute to the development of more severe CD and school failure.

These data suggest that children with conduct problems may require added structure and monitoring and overteaching (i.e., repeated learning trials) to learn to inhibit undesirable behaviors and to manage emotion. Parents and teachers need to use consistent, clear, specific limit setting; simple language; concrete cues; and frequent reminders and redirections. In addition, this information suggests the need for direct intervention with children, focusing on their particular social learning needs, such as problem solving, perspective taking, and play skills, as well as literacy and special academic needs.

Goals of the Child Training Programs

The goals are to promote children's competencies and reduce aggressive and noncompliant behaviors by doing the following:

- Strengthening children's social skills and appropriate play skills (turn taking, waiting, asking, sharing, helping, and complimenting).

- Promoting children's use of self-control strategies such as effective problem-solving and anger management strategies.
- Increasing emotional awareness by labeling feelings, recognizing the differing views of oneself and others, and enhancing perspective taking.
- Boosting academic success, reading, and school readiness.
- Reducing defiance, aggressive behavior, and related conduct problems such as noncompliance, peer aggression and rejection, bullying, stealing, and lying.
- Decreasing children's negative cognitive attributions and conflict management approaches.
- Increasing self-esteem and self-confidence.

Content of Child Training Treatment

In 1990 we developed a videotape modeling child treatment program for children with conduct problems (ages 3–8). This 22-week program consists of a series of nine video-tape programs (over 100 vignettes) that teach children problem-solving and social skills. Organized to dovetail with the content of the parent training program, the program consists of seven main components: (1) Introduction and Rules; (2) Empathy Training; (3) Problem-Solving Training; (4) Anger Control; (5) Friendship Skills; (6) Communication Skills; and (7) School Training. The children meet weekly in small groups of six children for 2 hours. To enhance generalization, the videotape scenes selected for each unit involve real-life conflict situations at home and at school (playground and classroom), such as teasing, lying, stealing, and destructive behavior.

Group Process and Methods Used in Parent, Teacher, and Child Training Programs

All three treatment approaches rely on performance training methods including video-tape modeling, role play, practice activities, and live feedback from the therapist and other group members. In accordance with modeling and self-efficacy theories of learning, parents, teachers and children using the program develop their skills by watching (and modeling) videotape examples of key management and interpersonal skills. We theorized that videotape provides a more flexible method of training than didactic instruction or sole reliance on role play; that is, we could portray a wide variety of models and situations. We hypothesized that this flexible modeling approach would result in better generalization of the training content and, therefore, better long-term maintenance. Furthermore, it would be a better method of learning for less verbally oriented learners. Finally, such a method, if proven effective, would have the advantage not only of low individual training cost when used in groups but also of possible mass dissemination.

Heavily guided by the modeling literature, each of the programs aims to promote modeling effects for participants by creating positive feelings about the videotape models. For example, the videotapes show parents, teachers and children of differing ages, cultures, socioeconomic backgrounds, and temperaments, so that participants will perceive at least some of the models as similar to themselves and will therefore accept the tapes as relevant. Whenever possible, videotapes show models (unrehearsed) in natural situations "doing it right" and "doing it wrong" in order to demystify the notion there is "perfect parenting or teaching " and to illustrate how one can learn from one's mistakes. This approach also emphasizes our belief in a coping and interactive model of learning (Webster-Stratton & Herbert, 1994); that is, participants view a videotape vignette of a situation and then discuss and role-play how the individual might have handled the interaction more effectively. Thus participants improve upon the interactions they see on the videotapes. This approach enhances participants' confidence in their own ideas and develops their ability to analyze interpersonal situations and select an appropriate response. In this respect, our training differs from some training programs where the therapist provides the analysis and recommends a particular strategy.

The videotapes demonstrate behavioral principles and serve as the stimulus for focused discussions, problem solving, and collaborative learning. After each vignette, the therapist solicits ideas from group members and involves them in the process of problem solving, sharing, and discussing ideas and reactions. The therapists' role is to support and empower group members by teaching, leading, reframing, predicting, and role playing, always within a collaborative context (Webster-Stratton & Hancock, 1998). The collaborative context is designed to ensure that the intervention is sensitive to individual cultural differences and personal values. The program is "tailored" to each teacher, parent, or child's individual needs and personal goals (identified in the first session) as well as to each child's personality and behavior problems.

This program also implies a commitment to group members' self-management. We believe that this approach empowers participants in that it gives back dignity, respect, and self-control to parents, teachers, and children who are often seeking help at time of low self-confidence and intense feelings of guilt and self-blame (Webster-Stratton, 1996). By using group process, the program not only is more cost-effective but also addresses an important risk factor for children with conduct problems: the family's isolation and stigmatization. The parent groups provide that support and become a model for parent support networks. (For details of therapeutic processes, see Webster-Stratton & Herbert, 1994.) The child groups provide children with conduct problems some of their first positive social experiences with other children. Moreover, it was theorized that the group approach would provide more social support and decrease feelings of isolation for teachers as well as parents and children.

As with the teacher and parent programs, the child treatment program uses videotape modeling examples in every session to foster discussion, problem solving, and modeling of prosocial behaviors. To enhance generalization, the scenes selected for each of the units involve real-life conflict situations at home and at school (playground and classroom), such as teasing, lying, stealing, and destructive behavior. The videotapes show children of differing ages, sexes, and cultures interacting with adults (parents or teachers) or with other children. After viewing the vignettes, children discuss feelings, generate ideas for more effective responses, and role-play alternative scenarios. In addition to the interactive videotapes, the therapists use life-size puppets to model appropriate behavior and thinking processes for the children. The use of puppets appeals to children on the fantasy level so predominant in this preoperational age group. Because young children are more vulnerable to distraction, are less able to organize their thoughts, and have poorer memories, we use a number of strategies for reviewing and organizing the material, such as (1) playing "copy cat" to review skills learned; (2) using many videotape examples of the same concept in different situations and settings; (3) using cartoon pictures and specially designed stickers as "cues" to remind children of key concepts; (4) role playing with puppets and other children to provide practice opportunities and experience with different perspectives; (5) reenacting videotape scenes;

(6) acting out visual story examples of key ideas; (7) rehearsing skills with play, art, and game activities; (8) homework, so children can practice key skills with parents; and (9) letters to parents and teachers that explain the key concepts children are learning and asking them to reinforce these behaviors whenever they see them occurring throughout the week.

EVIDENCE FOR THE EFFECTS OF TREATMENT

Effects of Parent Training Program

The efficacy of the Incredible Years BASIC parent program for treatment for children (ages 3–8 years) diagnosed with ODD/CD has been demonstrated in six published randomized control group trials by the program developer and colleagues at the University of Washington Parenting Clinic (Webster-Stratton, 1981, 1982, 1984, 1990a, 1994, 1998; Webster-Stratton & Hammond, 1997; Webster-Stratton, Hollinsworth, & Kolpacoff, 1989; Webster-Stratton, Kolpacoff, & Hollinsworth, 1988). In all these studies, the BASIC program has been shown to significantly improve parental attitudes and parent–child interactions and significantly reduce parents' reliance on violent and critical discipline and child conduct problems, when compared to waiting-list control groups and other treatment approaches that did not use either the group method or videotape modeling. In the third of these studies, treatment component analyses indicated that the combination of group discussion, a trained therapist, and videotape modeling produced the most lasting results in comparison to treatment that involved only one training component (Webster-Stratton et al., 1988, 1989). In addition, the BASIC program has been replicated in three projects by independent investigators in mental health clinics with families of children diagnosed with conduct problems (Scott, Spender, Doolan, Jacobs, & Aspland, 2001; Spaccarelli, Cotler, & Penman, 1992; Taylor, Schmidt, Pepler, & Hodgins, 1998). Two of these replications were "effectiveness" trials; that is, they were done in applied settings, not a university research clinic, and the therapists were typical therapists at the center (Scott et al., 2001; Taylor et al., 1998).

In our fourth study, we examined the effects of adding the ADVANCE intervention component to the BASIC intervention (Webster-Stratton, 1994) by randomly assigning 78 families to either BASIC parent training or BASIC + ADVANCE training. Both treatment groups showed significant improvements in child adjustment and parent–child interactions and a decrease in parent distress and child behavior problems. These changes were maintained at follow-up. ADVANCE children showed significant increases in the number of prosocial solutions generated during problem solving, in comparison to children whose parents received only the BASIC program. Observations of parents' marital interactions indicated significant improvements in ADVANCE parents' communication, problem solving, and collaboration skills when compared with parents who did not receive ADVANCE. ADVANCE parents reported significantly greater consumer satisfaction than did parents who did not receive ADVANCE, with parents reporting the problem-solving skills to be the most useful and anger management the most difficult.

Next we looked at how clinically significant improvements (30%) in parents' communication and problem-solving skills were related to improvements in their parenting skills. We found that, in the case of fathers, improvement in marital communication skills was related to a significant reduction in number of criticisms in their interactions with their children; fathers' improved marital communication was also related to im-

provements in the child's prosocial skills. These results indicate the importance of fathers' marital satisfaction as a determining factor in their parenting skills.

Overall, these results suggest that focusing on helping families to manage personal distress and interpersonal issues through a videotape modeling group discussion treatment (ADVANCE) is highly promising in terms of (1) improvements in marital communication, problem solving, and coping skills; (2) improvements in parenting skills; (3) improvements in children's prosocial skills; and (4) consumer satisfaction—that is, being highly acceptable and perceived as useful by families (Webster-Stratton, 1994). As a result of these findings we combined BASIC plus ADVANCE plus SCHOOL into an integrated 22–24-week program for parents, which has become our core treatment for parents with children with conduct problems over the past 8 years.

In our sixth study, we compared the effects of combining our child training intervention (Dinosaur School) with the parent training program (BASIC + ADVANCE) to the same parent training program without child training. We replicated our results from the prior ADVANCE study and were able to determine the added advantages of training children and parents. (See description of these study results in the section on child training results.)

Parent Training Treatment: Who Benefits and Who Does Not

We have followed families longitudinally (1, 2, and 3 years posttreatment), and for study three we have completed a 10–15-year follow-up. We have assessed, not only the "statistical significance" of treatment effects but also their "clinical significance." In assessing the clinical significance, three criteria were used: (1 and 2) the extent to which parent and teacher reports indicated that the children were within the normal or the nonclinical range of functioning or showed a 30% improvement if there were no established normative data and (3) whether families requested further therapy for their children's behavior problems at the follow-up assessments. These outcome criteria were chosen to avoid reliance on a single informant or criterion measure, thereby providing greater validity to the findings. In our 3-year follow-up of 83 families treated with the BASIC program, we found that while approximately two-thirds of children showed clinically significant behavior improvements, 25% to 46% of parents and 26% of teachers still reported clinically significant child behavior problems (Webster-Stratton, 1990b). We also found that the families whose children had continuing externalizing problems (according to teacher and parent reports) at our 3-year follow-up assessments were more likely to be characterized by maritally distressed or single-parent status, increased maternal depression, lower social class, high levels of negative life stressors, and family histories of alcoholism, drug abuse, and spouse abuse (Webster-Stratton, 1990b; Webster-Stratton & Hammond, 1990).

Recently Hartman (Hartman, Webster-Stratton, & Stage, 2003) examined whether child ADHD symptoms (i.e., inattention, impulsivity, and hyperactivity) predicted poorer treatment results from the parent training intervention (BASIC). Contrary to Hartman's hypothesis, analyses suggested that the children with ODD/CD who had higher levels of attentional problems showed greater reductions in conduct problems than did children with no attentional problems.

Rinaldi (2001) conducted an 8 to 12 year follow-up of families in the ADVANCE study. She interviewed 83.5% of the original study parents and adolescents (ages 12–19 years). Results indicated that at least 75% of the teenagers were typically adjusted with minimal behavioral and emotional problems. Furthermore, parenting skills taught in the intervention had lasting effects. Important predictors of long-term outcome were mothers' level of critical statements and fathers' use of praise. In addition, the level of coercion between the children and mothers immediately posttreatment was a significant predictor of later teen adjustment.

In the past decade, we have also evaluated the parent programs as a selective prevention program with over 1,000 multiethnic, socioeconomically disadvantaged families in two randomized studies with Head Start families. Results of these studies suggest the program's effectiveness as method of preventing the development of conduct problems and strengthening social competence in preschool children (Webster-Stratton, 1998; Webster-Stratton, Reid, & Hammond, 2001a).

Summary and Significance

In focusing on parenting training over the past two decades, we have hypothesized that because parents are the most powerful, and potentially malleable, influence on young children's social development, intervening with parents would be the strategic first step. Indeed, our studies have shown that parent training is highly promising as an effective therapeutic method for producing significant behavior change in children with high-risk behaviors (i.e., conduct problems) and with high-risk populations (i.e., socioeconomically disadvantaged). These findings provide support for the theory that parenting practices play a key role in children's social and emotional development.

Effects of Teacher Training Program

We recently completed a randomized trial of our teacher training curriculum with teachers targeted because a student in their classroom had been diagnosed with ODD/CD. The trial included 133 clinic-referred families, the majority (85%) of whom were Caucasian. Families were admitted to the study if their children (ages 4–8) met criteria for early-onset ODD or CD according to the fourth edition of the *Diagnostic and Statistical Manual of Mental Disorders* (DSM-IV; American Psychiatric Association, 1994). Families were randomly assigned to one of six groups: (1) parent training only (BASIC + ADVANCE); (2) child training only (Dina Dinosaur Curriculum); (3) parent training, academic skills training, and teacher training (BASIC + ADVANCE + SCHOOL + TEACHER); (4) parent training, academic skills training, teacher training, and child training (BASIC + ADVANCE + SCHOOL + TEACHER + CHILD); (5) child training and teacher training (CHILD + TEACHER); and (6) waiting-list control group.

The parent training (without teacher training) consisted of 22 2-hour weekly sessions covering the BASIC and ADVANCE components. The child training treatment was 18–20 weeks of the Dina Dinosaur curriculum. The parent plus teacher training consisted of BASIC and ADVANCE program, as well as the academic skills (SCHOOL) and teacher training (TEACHER) programs. In this evaluation, the teacher program consisted of four full-day workshops offered monthly, and a minimum of two school consultations, in which the parent and group leader met with the teacher to create an individual behavior plan for the targeted child. Families in the waiting-list control condition were randomly assigned to the parent training condition after nine months.

Results indicated that, as expected, trained teachers were rated as less critical, harsh, and inconsistent, and more nurturing than control teachers. Parents in all three conditions who received parent training were significantly less negative and more positive than parents who did not receive training (although parents who did not receive training but whose children received child training were less negative than controls). Children in all five conditions showed reductions in aggressive behaviors with mothers at home and at school with peers and teachers (Webster-Stratton & Reid, 1999). Treatment effects for children's positive social skills with peers were found in the three conditions with child training compared with controls. The treatments that addressed more than one risk factor resulted in more significant results across multiple outcome domains (e.g., home, school, and peers). Most treatment effects were maintained at 1-year follow-up. In summary, short-term results replicate our previous findings on the effectiveness of the parent and child training programs and indicate that teacher training significantly improves teacher's classroom management skills.

Our second randomized control group study evaluating the teacher training curriculum was conducted with 61 Head Start teachers in 34 classrooms. Following the program, parent–teacher bonding was significantly higher for experimental than for control mothers. Experimental children showed significantly fewer conduct problems at school than control children, and trained teachers showed significantly better classroom management skills than did control teachers (Webster-Stratton et al., 2001a).

Effects of the Child Dinosaur Program

To date, there have been two randomized studies evaluating the effectiveness of the child training program for reducing conduct problems and promoting social competence in children diagnosed with ODD/CD. In the first study, 97 clinic-referred children (72 boys and 25 girls), ages 4–7, and their parents (95 mothers and 71 fathers) were randomly assigned to one of four groups: a parent training treatment group (PT: BASIC + ADVANCE), a child training group (CT), a child and parent training group (CT + PT), or a waiting-list control group (CON). Posttreatment assessments indicated that all three treatment conditions resulted in significant improvements in comparison to controls, as measured by parent reports, mothers' daily observations of targeted behaviors at home, and independent observations of interactions with a best friend. Comparisons of the three treatment conditions indicated that CT and CT + PT children showed significant improvements in problem solving as well as conflict management skills, as measured by observations of their interactions with a best friend; differences among treatment conditions on these measures consistently favored the CT condition over the PT condition. On measures of parent and child behavior at home, PT and CT + PT parents and children had significantly more positive interactions in comparison to CT parents and children.

One-year follow-up assessments indicated that all the significant changes noted immediately posttreatment were maintained over time. Moreover, child conduct problems at home had significantly decreased over time. Analyses of the clinical significance of the results suggested that the combined CT + PT condition produced the most significant improvements in child behavior at 1-year follow-up. However, children from all three treatment conditions showed increases in behavior problems at school 1 year later, as measured by teacher reports (Webster-Stratton & Hammond, 1997). The second randomized control group evaluation of the child Dinosaur School program (described earlier with the addition of teacher training) replicated immediate posttest findings showing the effectiveness of the child program compared to controls but suggests that the addition of teacher training to the child treatment produces greater change. Follow-up analyses on these data are currently being conducted.

Who Benefits from Dinosaur Child Training?

Families of 99 children with ODD/CD, ages 4–8 years who were randomly assigned to either the child training treatment group or a control group, were assessed on multiple risk factors (child hyperactivity, parenting style, and family stress). These risk factors were examined in relation to children's responses to the child treatment. The hyperactivity or family stress risk factors did not have an impact on children's ability to benefit from the treatment program. Negative parenting, on the other hand, did have a negative impact on children's treatment outcome. Fewer children who had parents with one of the negative parenting risk factors (high levels of criticism or physical spanking) showed clinically significant improvements compared to children who did not have a negative parenting risk factor. This finding suggests that for children whose parents exhibit harsh and coercive parenting styles, it may be necessary to offer a parenting intervention in addition to a child intervention (Webster-Stratton, Reid, & Hammond, 2001b). Our latest studies suggest that child training significantly enhances the effectiveness of parent training treatment for children with conduct problems.

DIRECTIONS FOR FUTURE RESEARCH

Although our programs were first designed and evaluated to be used as clinic-based treatments for diagnosed children and their parents and teachers, our recent work has moved away from the clinic-based treatment model to school-based prevention/intervention delivery targeting high-risk populations and children with aggressive symptoms. Both the parent and teacher training programs have been successfully evaluated in this context. We are currently conducting a randomized study evaluating the effects of a school-based intervention beginning in kindergarten. This project involves two levels of intervention: (1) a 2-year universal intervention that includes teacher training and a classroom version of Dinosaur School for all children and (2) an indicated intervention that includes a 2-year parent training (BASIC + SCHOOL + ADVANCE) program for the parents of children who are exhibiting high-risk behaviors. We hypothesize that the most proactive and powerful approach to the problem of escalating aggression in young children will be to offer our programs using a school-based prevention/early intervention model designed to strengthen all children's social and emotional competence. Our reasons for this are threefold: First, offering interventions in schools makes programs more accessible to families and eliminates some of the stigma as well as the barriers (e.g., lack of transportation) associated with services offered in traditional mental health settings. Second, offering interventions in schools integrates programs before children's common behavior problems have escalated to the point that they require extensive clinical treatment. Moreover, when intervention is offered in natural communities, these communities are strengthened as a source of support for teachers and parents. Another advantage of interventions delivered by on-site school staff (nurses, counselors, social workers, or teachers) is the sheer number of high-risk families and children that can be reached at comparatively low cost. Finally, offering a social and emotional curriculum such as our Dinosaur School program to the entire class is less stigmatizing than a "pullout" group and more likely to result in sustained effects across settings and time. Though we have shown that a child can learn new skills in our pullout weekly Dinosaur group sessions, the skills do not necessarily generalize to the classroom. When peers are not involved in the intervention, they may continue to react to the target child in negative ways because of his or her negative reputation. Classroomwide intervention provides opportunities for more prosocial children to model appropriate social and conflict management skills and provides the entire classroom with a common vocabulary and problem-solving steps to use in resolving everyday conflicts. Thus, social competence is strengthened for lower-risk children, children with internalizing problems (e.g., social withdrawal and anxiety), and aggressive children (whose reputation with peers is changed), and the classroom environment fosters students' appropriate social skills on an ongoing basis as well as their understanding and empathy toward others who may have differing temperaments, activity levels, and learning styles, as well as a culture and academic abilities. In addition, with a classroom-based model, the dosage of intervention is magnified as teachers provide reinforcement of the key concepts throughout the day and weeks.

As more is known about the type, timing, and dosage of interventions needed to prevent and treat children's conduct problems, we can further target children and families to offer treatment and support at strategic points. By providing a continuum of services we believe we will be able to prevent the further development of conduct disorders, delinquency, and violence. For example, the prevention versions of the classroom social skills interventions, parent training, and/or teacher training might be offered as universal prevention to all children in a school. Children who continue to exhibit significant behavior problems might be offered the treatment versions of the programs (see Table 13.1 for program recommendations according to child's level of risk). For those children requiring additional treatment, more research is needed to understand what constellation of treatments (parent, teacher, child) would most benefit particular families. For instance, our research indicates that children with conduct problems whose parents are exhibiting consistent and positive parenting will benefit from the child treatment while those with harsh or critical parents will do less well. We might also hypothesize that children with

TABLE 13.1. Program Recommendations Depending on Degree of Risk or Treatment or Prevention Focus

Population and intended use	Minimum "core" program	Recommended supplemental programs for special populations
Prevention programs for selected populations (i.e., "high-risk" populations without overt behavior or conduct problems) Settings: preschool, day care, Head Start, schools (grades K–3), public health centers	BASIC (12–14 2-hour weekly sessions)	• ADVANCE Parent Program for highly stressed families. • SCHOOL Parent Program for children kindergarten to grade 3. • Child Dinosaur Program if child's problems are pervasive at home and school. • TEACHER classroom management program if teachers have high numbers of students with behavior problems or if teachers have not received this training previously.
Treatment programs for indicated populations (i.e., children exhibiting behavior problems or diagnosed conduct disorders) Settings: mental health centers, pediatric clinics, HMOs	BASIC and ADVANCE (22–24 2-hour weekly sessions)	• Child Dinosaur Program if child's problems are pervasive at home and at school. • TEACHER Program if child's problems are pervasive at home and at school. • SCHOOL Program for parents if child has academic problems.

pervasive, comorbid conduct problems and ADHD may need the more comprehensive combination of child, parent, and teacher programs. Alternatively, a young child whose difficult behavior is confined to the home setting may do well with only parent training.

SUMMARY AND CONCLUSIONS

In summary, a review of our own research suggests that comprehensive interactive video-tape family training methods are effective treatments for early-onset ODD/CD. Our most effective parent intervention involved videotape training, not only in parenting skills but also in marital communication, problem solving and conflict resolution, and ways to foster children's academic and social emotional competence. These findings document the need for interventions that strengthen families' protective factors (specifically, parents' interpersonal skills and coping skills) so that they can cope more effectively with the added stress of having a child with conduct problems. Our research has also suggested that child and teacher training is a highly effective strategy for building young conduct-problem children's social skills, problem-solving strategies, and peer relationships. The child training program seems to be particularly helpful for children with conduct problems which are pervasive across settings (school and home) and with peer relationship difficulties.

Our intervention studies, which target different combinations of risk factors, can be seen as an indirect test of the different theoretical models regarding the development of conduct disorders. We started with a simple parenting skills deficit model and have evolved to a more complex interactional model. In our current model, we hypothesize that the child's eventual outcome will be dependent on the interrelationship between child, parent(s), teacher(s), and peer risk factors. Therefore, the most effective interventions should be those that involve schools, teachers, and the child's peer group. Optimally, one would assess these risk factors and determine which programs would be needed for a particular family and child.

Our future plans include continuing research looking at not only what family, child, or parent factors predict a families' success or lack of success with a particular intervention but also how change in a particular variable (e.g., improvements in parent or teacher skills) relates to change in children's behaviors. This analysis promises further insights into the mechanisms contributing to the development of conduct disorders. Given the increasing rates of aggression in younger children and the continuity of the problem from early childhood, through adolescence, and often into adulthood, the chance of breaking the link in the "cycle of aggression and coercion" is a public health matter of the utmost importance.

ACKNOWLEDGMENTS

This research was supported by the NIH National Center for Nursing Research Grant 5 R01 NR01075 and NIMH Research Scientist Development Award MH00988.

REFERENCES

Brestan, E. V., & Eyberg, S. M. (1998). Effective psychosocial treatments of conduct-disordered children and adolescents: 29 years, 82 studies, and 5,272 kids. *Journal of Clinical Child Psychology, 27,* 180–189.

Hartman, R. R., Webster-Stratton, C., & Stage, S. (2003). A growth curve analysis of parent training outcomes: Examining the influence of child inattention, impulsivity, and hyperactivity. *Child Psychology and Psychiatry Journal, 44*(3), 388–398.

Loeber, R., Wung, P., Keenan, K., Giroux, B., Stouthamer-Loeber, M., Van Kammen, W. B., & Maughan, B. (1993). Developmental pathways in disruptive child behavior. *Development Psychopathology, 5*, 103–133.

Moffitt, T. E., & Lynam, D. (1994). The neuropsychology of conduct disorder and delinquency: Implications for understanding antisocial behavior. In D. C. Fowles, P. Sutker, & S. H. Goodman (Eds.), *Progress in experimental personality and psychopathology research* (pp. 233–262). New York: Springer.

Patterson, G. R., Capaldi, D., & Bank, L. (1991). An early starter model for predicting delinquency. In D. J. Pepler & K. H. Rubin (Eds.), *The development and treatment of childhood aggression* (pp. 139–168). Hillsdale, NJ: Erlbaum.

Rinaldi, J. (2001). *A 10-year follow up of children treated for conduct problems.* Unpublished doctoral dissertation, University of Washington, Seattle.

Scott, S., Spender, Q., Doolan, M., Jacobs, B., & Aspland, H. (2001). Multicentre controlled trial of parenting groups for child antisocial behaviour in clinical practice. *British Medical Journal, 323*, 1–5.

Snyder, H. (2001). Epidemiology of official offending. In R. Loeber & D. P. Farrington (Eds.), *Child delinquents: Development, intervention and service needs* (pp. 25–46). Thousand Oaks, CA: Sage.

Spaccarelli, S., Cotler, S., & Penman, D. (1992). Problem-solving skills training as a supplement to behavioral parent training. *Cognitive Therapy and Research, 16*, 1–18.

Taylor, T. K., Schmidt, F., Pepler, D., & Hodgins, H. (1998). A comparison of eclectic treatment with Webster-Stratton's Parents and Children Series in a children's mental health center: A randomized controlled trial. *Behavior Therapy, 29*, 221–240.

Webster Stratton, C. (1981). Modification of mothers' behaviors and attitudes through videotape modeling group discussion program. *Behavior Therapy, 12*, 634–642.

Webster-Stratton, C. (1982). Teaching mothers through videotape modeling to change their children's behaviors. *Journal of Pediatric Psychology, 7*, 279–294.

Webster-Stratton, C. (1984). Randomized trial of two parent-training programs for families with conduct-disordered children. *Journal of Consulting and Clinical Psychology, 52*, 666–678.

Webster-Stratton, C. (1990a). Enhancing the effectiveness of self-administered videotape parent training for families with conduct-problem children. *Journal of Abnormal Child Psychology, 18*, 479–492.

Webster-Stratton, C. (1990b). Long-term follow-up of families with young conduct problem children: From preschool to grade school. *Journal of Clinical Child Psychology, 19*, 144–149.

Webster-Stratton, C. (1992). *The incredible years: A trouble-shooting guide for parents of children aged 3–8.* Toronto: Umbrella Press.

Webster-Stratton, C. (1994). Advancing videotape parent training: A comparison study. *Journal of Consulting and Clinical Psychology, 62*, 583–593.

Webster-Stratton, C. (1996). Parenting a young child with conduct problems: New insights using grounded theory methods. In T. H. Ollendick & R. S. Prinz (Eds.), *Advances in clinical child psychology* (pp. 333–355). Hillsdale, NJ: Erlbaum.

Webster-Stratton, C. (1998). Preventing conduct problems in Head Start children: Strengthening parent competencies. *Journal of Consulting and Clinical Psychology, 66*, 715–730.

Webster-Stratton, C. (2000). *How to promote social and academic competence in young children.* London: Sage.

Webster-Stratton, C., & Hammond, M. (1990). Predictors of treatment outcome in parent training for families with conduct problem children. *Behavior Therapy, 21*, 319–337.

Webster-Stratton, C., & Hammond, M. (1997). Treating children with early-onset conduct problems: A comparison of child and parent training interventions. *Journal of Consulting and Clinical Psychology, 65*, 93–109.

Webster-Stratton, C., & Hammond, M. (1998). Conduct problems and level of social competence in Head Start children: Prevalence, pervasiveness and associated risk factors. *Clinical Child Psychology and Family Psychology Review, 1,* 101–124.

Webster-Stratton, C., & Hancock, L. (1998). Parent training: Content, methods, and processes. In E. Schaefer (Ed.), *Handbook of parent training* (2nd ed., pp. 98–152). New York: Wiley.

Webster-Stratton, C., & Herbert, M. (1994). *Troubled families–problem children: Working with parents: A collaborative process.* Chichester, UK: Wiley.

Webster-Stratton, C., Hollinsworth, T., & Kolpacoff, M. (1989). The long-term effectiveness and clinical significance of three cost-effective training programs for families with conduct-problem children. *Journal of Consulting and Clinical Psychology, 57,* 550–553.

Webster-Stratton, C., Kolpacoff, M., & Hollinsworth, T. (1988). Self-administered videotape therapy for families with conduct-problem children: Comparison with two cost-effective treatments and a control group. *Journal of Consulting and Clinical Psychology, 56,* 558–566.

Webster-Stratton, C., & Lindsay, D. W. (1999). Social competence and early-onset conduct problems: Issues in assessment. *Journal of Child Clinical Psychology, 28,* 25–93.

Webster-Stratton, C., & Reid, M. J. (1999, November). *Treating children with early-onset conduct problems: The importance of teacher training.* Paper presented at the meeting of the Association for Advancement of Behavior Therapy, Toronto, Canada.

Webster-Stratton, C., Reid, M. J., & Hammond, M. (2001a). Preventing conduct problems, promoting social competence: A parent and teacher training partnership in Head Start. *Journal of Clinical Child Psychology, 30,* 283–302.

Webster-Stratton, C., Reid, M. J., & Hammond, M. (2001b). Social skills and problem solving training for children with early-onset conduct problems: Who benefits? *Child Psychology and Psychiatry Journal, 42,* 943–952.

14

Problem-Solving Skills Training and Parent Management Training for Conduct Disorder

Alan E. Kazdin

OVERVIEW

Conduct disorder (CD) refers to a broad pattern of functioning that includes diverse disruptive and rule-breaking behaviors.[1] As a psychiatric disorder, CD requires the presence of at least 3 of the 15 symptoms within the past 12 months (American Psychiatric Association, 1994). The symptoms include bullying others, initiating fights, using a weapon, being physically cruel to people or animals, stealing from others, forcing someone into sexual activity, setting fires, destroying property, lying, truancy, running away, and others. The behaviors come in various combinations and vary markedly in severity, chronicity, and frequency. The significance of the disorder stems from several critical features, including the following:

- A relatively high prevalence rate (conservatively between 2 and 6% or approximately 1.4–4.2 million children in the United States);
- A high rate of clinical referrals (e.g., 33–50% of cases referred for outpatient treatment);
- Untoward long-term outcomes for such children in adulthood (e.g., approximately 80% are likely to meet criteria for a psychiatric disorder in the future);
- Untoward consequences for others including siblings, peers, parents, teachers, as well as strangers who are targets of antisocial and aggressive acts; and
- The monetary costs as youth traverse special education, mental health, juvenile justice, and social services over the course of their lives.

Each of these features could be elaborated to convey more persuasively the scope of the problem. For example, the prevalence rates underestimate the extent of the problem. Youth who do not quite meet diagnostic criteria can still show significant impairment and a poor long-term prognosis. Also, the central features of the disorder fail to convey the scope of the problems of children who come to treatment. Children who meet criteria for CD are likely to meet criteria for other externalizing or disruptive behavior disorders, such as oppositional defiant disorder (ODD) and attention-deficit/hyperactivity disorder (ADHD), and, to a slightly lesser extent, internalizing disorders, such as major depression and anxiety disorders.

Several features associated with CD are relevant to treatment. For example, children with CD are also likely to:

- Show academic deficiencies, as reflected in achievement level, grades, being left behind in school, early termination from school, and deficiencies in specific skill areas such as reading;
- Have poor interpersonal relations, as reflected in diminished social skills in relation to peers and adults and higher levels of peer rejection;
- Show deficits and distortions in cognitive processes related to interpersonal functioning; and
- Live in families in which there is likely to be a history of criminal behavior and psychiatric dysfunction, childrearing practices that contribute to the child's dysfunction (e.g., harsh punishment), unhappy marital relations, interpersonal conflict and aggression between the parents, poor family communications, and pervasive influences such as financial hardship (unemployment, significant debt, bankruptcy of the parent), untoward living conditions (dangerous neighborhood, small living quarters), high levels of parental stress (e.g., in relation to former spouses and living with relatives), and adversarial contact with outside agencies (schools, youth services, courts).

These characteristics of CD convey that the task of treatment is more than addressing the presenting symptoms. The challenge is to address child functioning as well as the parent, family, and contexts that can support prosocial behavior and adaptive functioning.

CHARACTERISTICS OF THE TREATMENT PROGRAM

Setting and Participants

Our treatment is provided at the Yale Child Conduct Clinic, an outpatient service for children and families. The clinic is a freestanding facility integrated with other clinical services and facilities within the community. There is a close affiliation with child psychiatry at the university (Yale Child Study Center) to address multiple issues raised by patient care (e.g., inpatient and outpatient services, emergency services, psychiatric evaluation, and medication evaluation). The needs, presenting, and emerging problems of CD youth and their families often require immediate access to these resources.

Children (range = 2–13 years of age) referred for aggressive and antisocial behavior are seen at the clinic. Children usually meet criteria for a primary diagnosis (using criteria according to the *Diagnostic and Statistical Manual of Mental Disorders* or DSM) of CD or ODD. Approximately 70–75% of the children meet criteria for two or more disorders (range = 0–5 disorders). Most youth fall within the normal range of intelligence, although a broad range is represented (e.g., mean Full Scale IQ = 100–105; range = 60–140 on the Wechsler Intelligence Scale for Children—Revised). The families are European American, African American, or Hispanic American (approximately 60, 30, and 5%, respectively), with mixed or Asian American forming the remainder. Approximately 60% of our cases come from two-parent families. All socioeconomic–occupational levels are represented, although there is a slight skew toward lower socioeconomic classes. Approximately 20–30% of families receive social assistance.[2]

Treatments and Format

The treatments we provide include cognitive problem-solving skills training (PSST) and parent management training (PMT). These are provided individually to children and families rather than in group format. The scope of dysfunction of both the children and families and the concrete implications these often have (failing to meet confirmed appointments, showing up for treatment on the incorrect days or time, quite varied pace in learning and using the treatment material) have led us to abandon a group treatment.

We have explored two treatments based on several considerations. First, in both our inpatient and outpatient treatment work, sometimes no parent is available. The parent cannot or will not participate in treatment (due to mental illness, serving in prison, mental retardation, or simple unwillingness) or engages in practices (e.g., current drug abuse) or occupations (e.g., prostitution) that interfere with participation. For such cases, providing intensive treatment of the child with little or no parent intervention has been important. Thus, we have worked on PSST as a stand-alone treatment. At other times, there may be parents who can participate actively in PMT. Some children referred to us are young and PSST is not feasible. In these cases, too, PMT is a viable treatment. Finally, when the stars are positioned just right, both PSST and PMT can be used with the family, and we do so whenever possible.

Another reason for exploring two treatments is the fact that the conceptual models of the treatments are compatible and complementary. One model focuses on processes internal to the child that can be deployed to address diverse interpersonal situations. The other model focuses on environmental changes to develop new repertoires in diverse situations. We felt that integrating these two treatments would optimize therapeutic change.

Problem-Solving Skills Training

Overview

Cognitive processes refer to a broad class of constructs that pertain to how the individual perceives, codes, and experiences the world. Individuals who engage in conduct-disordered behaviors, particularly aggression, show distortions and deficiencies in various cognitive processes. These distortions and deficiencies are not merely reflections of intellectual functioning. Examples include generating alternative solutions to interpersonal problems (e.g., different ways of handling social situations), identifying the means to obtain particular ends (e.g., making friends) or consequences of one's actions (e.g., what could happen after a particular behavior), making attributions to others of the motivation of their actions, perceiving how others feel, and expectations of the effects of one's own actions (Lochman, Whidby, & FitzGerald, 2000; Shure, 1997; Spivack & Shure, 1982). Deficits and distortion among these processes relate to teacher ratings of disruptive behavior, peer evaluations, and direct assessment of overt behavior.

An example of cognitive processes implicated in CD can be seen in the work on attributions and aggressive behavior. Aggression is not merely triggered by environmental events but, rather, through the way in which these events are perceived and processed. The processing refers to the child's appraisals of the situation, anticipated reactions of others, and self-statements in response to particular events. Attribution of intent to others represents a salient cognitive disposition critically important to understanding aggressive behavior. Aggressive children and adolescents tend to attribute hostile intent to others, especially in social situations in which the cues of actual intent are ambiguous (Crick & Dodge, 1994). Understandably, when situations are initially perceived as hostile, children are more likely to react aggressively. Although many studies have shown that conduct-disordered children experience various cognitive distortions and deficiencies, the specific contribution of these processes to CD, as opposed to risk factors with which they may be associated (e.g., untoward living conditions and low IQ), has not been established. Nevertheless, research on cognitive processes among aggressive children has served as a heuristic base for conceptualizing treatment and for developing specific treatment strategies (Kendall, 2000).

Content of the Treatment Sessions

PSST consists of developing interpersonal cognitive problem-solving skills and includes several characteristics. First, the emphasis is on how children approach situations (i.e., the thought processes in which the child engages to guide responses to interpersonal situations). The children are taught to engage in a step-by-step approach to solve interpersonal problems. They make statements to themselves that direct attention to certain aspects of the problem or tasks that lead to effective solutions. Second, the behaviors (solutions to the interpersonal problems) that are selected are important as well. Prosocial behaviors are fostered through modeling and direct reinforcement as part of the problem-solving process. Third, treatment uses structured tasks involving games, academic activities, and stories. Over the course of treatment, the cognitive problem-solving skills are increasingly applied to real-life situations. Fourth, therapists play an active role in treatment. They model the cognitive processes by making verbal self-statements, apply the sequence of statements to particular problems, provide cues to prompt use of the skills, and deliver feedback and praise to develop correct use of the skills. Finally, treatment combines several different procedures, including modeling and practice, role playing, reinforcement, and mild punishment (loss of points or tokens), to develop increasingly complex response repertoires of the child.

In our program, PSST consists of weekly therapy sessions with the child, with each session usually lasting 30–50 minutes. The core treatment (12–20 sessions) may be supplemented with optional sessions, if the child requires additional assistance in grasping the problem-solving steps (early in treatment) or their application in everyday situations (later in treatment). (In separate projects we have varied the duration of treatment.) Table 14.1 presents the core treatment sessions and their foci. Central to treatment is developing the use of *problem-solving steps* designed to break down interpersonal situations into units that permit identification and use of prosocial responses. Table 14.2 notes the steps and what they intend to accomplish. The steps serve as verbal prompts the children deliver to themselves to engage in thoughts and actions that guide behavior. Each self-prompt or self-statement represents one step in solving a problem.

Early in treatment, the five steps noted in Table 14.2 are trained. We quickly move to combining the steps to emphasize solutions and consequences. In our current treatment, we begin with this combination in which these steps are used: (1) What am I supposed to do? (2) and (3) I need to figure out what to DO and what would HAPPEN,

TABLE 14.1. Problem-Solving Skills Training: Overview of the Core Sessions

1.   *Introduction and learning the steps.* The purpose of this initial session is to establish rapport with the child, to teach the problem-solving steps, and to explain the procedures of the cognitively based treatment program. The child is acquainted with the use of tokens (chips), reward menus for exchange of the chips, and response–cost contingencies. The child is trained to use the problem-solving steps in a game-like fashion in which the therapist and child take turns learning the individual steps and placing them together in a sequence.

2. and 3.   *Applying the steps.* The second session reviews and continues to teach the steps, as needed. The child is taught to employ the problem-solving steps to complete a relatively simple game. The child applies the steps to simple problem situations presented in a board-game fashion in which the therapist and child alternate turns. During the session, the therapist demonstrates how to use the problem-solving steps in decision making, how to provide self-reinforcement for successful performance, and how to cope with mistakes and failure. One of the goals of this session is to illustrate how the self-statements can be used to help "stop and think" rather than respond impulsively when confronted with a problem. The third session includes another game that leads to selection of hypothetical situations to which the child applies the steps. The therapist and child take turns, and further work is provided using prompts, modeling, shaping, and reinforcement to help the child be facile and fluid in applying the steps. The therapist fades prompts and assistance to shape proficient use and application of steps. A series of "supersolvers" (homework assignments) begins at this point, in which the child is asked to identify when the steps could be used, then to use the steps in increasingly more difficult and clinically relevant situations as treatment continues.

4.   *Applying the steps and role playing.* The child applies the steps to real-life situations. The steps are applied to the situation to identify solutions and consequences. Then the preferred solution, based on the likely consequences, is selected and then enacted through repeated role-plays. Practice and role-play are continued to develop the child's application of the steps. Multiple situations are presented and practiced in this way.

5.   *Parent–child contact.* The parent(s), therapist, and child are seen in the session. The child enacts the steps to solve problems. The parents learn more about the steps and are trained to provide attention and contingent praise for the child's use of the steps and for selecting and enacting prosocial solutions. The primary goal is to develop the repertoire in the parent to encourage (prompt) use of the steps and to praise applications in a way that will influence child behavior (i.e., contingent, enthusiastic, continuous, verbal and nonverbal praise). Further contacts with the parents at the end of later sessions continue this aspect of treatment as needed.

6.–11.   *Continued applications to real-life situations.* In these sessions, the child uses the problem-solving steps to generate prosocial solutions to provocative interpersonal problems or situations. Each session concentrates on a different category of social interaction that the child might realistically encounter (peers, parents, siblings, teachers, etc.). Real-life situations, generated by the child or parent or from contacts with teachers and others, are enacted; hypothetical situations are also presented to elaborate themes and problem areas of the child (e.g., responding to provocation, fighting, being excluded socially, and being encouraged by peers to engage in antisocial behavior). The child's supersolvers also become a more integral part of each session; they are reenacted with the therapist beginning in session in order to better evaluate how the child is transferring skills to his daily environment.

12.   *Wrap up and role reversal.* This "wrap up" session is included (1) to help the therapist generally assess what the child has learned in the session, (2) to clear up any remaining confusions the child may have concerning the use of the steps, and (3) to provide a final summary for the child of what has been covered in the meetings. The final session is based on role reversal in which the child plays the role of the therapist and the therapist

(continues)

TABLE 14.1. *Continued*

plays the role of a child learning and applying the steps. The purpose of this session is to have the child teach and benefit from the learning that teaching provides, to allow for any unfinished business of the treatment ("spending" remaining chips, completing final supersolvers), and to provide closure for the therapy.

Optional sessions. During the course of therapy, additional sessions are provided to the child, as needed, if the child has special difficulty in grasping any features of the problem-solving steps or their application. For example, the child may have difficulty in applying the steps, learning to state them covertly, and so on. An additional session may be applied to repeat material of a previous session, so that the child has a solid grasp of the approach. Optional sessions may be implemented at any point that the child's progress lags behind the level appropriate to the session that has been completed. For example, if a facet of treatment has not been learned (e.g., memorization of steps and fading of steps) associated with the particular session that has been completed, an optional session may be implemented. Also, if there is a problem or issue of child or parent participation in supersolvers, a session will be scheduled with parent and child to shape the requisite behaviors in the session and to make assignments to ensure this aspect of treatment is carried out.

(4) I need to make a choice, and (5) I need to find out how I did. Combining steps 2 and 3 requires the child to identify a solution (what to DO) and then the consequence (what would HAPPEN) and to do this with three or more solutions before proceeding to step 4. The steps are taught through modeling; the therapist and child alternate turns in using and applying the steps and each helps the others. Prompting, shaping, practice, and effusive praise develop the child's mastery of the steps usually by the end of the first treatment session. As the child learns the steps, the therapist modeling and prompting are faded and omitted or only used to help (e.g., if needed to craft a third solution or to elaborate the consequences of a poor solution to an interpersonal problem). The steps are not merely a cognitive exercise. The problems and solutions and use of the steps are practiced extensively in the session through role play between the therapist and child and eventually involving the therapists, child, and parent(s). The steps evolve over the course

TABLE 14.2. Problem-Solving Steps and Self-Statements

Self-statement steps to solve a problem	Purpose of the step
1. What am I suppose to do?	This step requires that the child identify and define the problem.
2. I have to look at all my possibilities.	This step asks the child to delineate or specify alternative solutions to the problem.
3. I'd better concentrate and focus in.	This step instructs the child to concentrate and evaluate the solutions he or she has generated.
4. I need to make a choice.	During the fourth step the child chooses the answer which he or she thinks is correct.
5. I did a good job, (or) Oh, I made a mistake.	This final step to verify whether the solution was the best among those available, whether the problem-solving process was correctly followed, or whether a mistake or less than desirable solution was selected and the process should begin anew.

of treatment in multiple ways. Among the most significant changes, the steps move from overt (made aloud) to covert (silent, internal) statements. By the end of treatment, use of the steps cannot be visibly seen; their overt features have been faded completely by this time.

To assist the children in the acquisition and generalization of the problem-solving skills, several tasks are taught sequentially. The early sessions use simple tasks and games to teach the problem-solving steps, to help to deter impulsive responding, and to introduce the reward system and response cost contingencies, noted later. The majority of treatment focuses on the child's use of the problem-solving steps to generate and to enact prosocial solutions to a range of interpersonal problems or situations. The interpersonal problems are presented in a variety of ways using various approaches, materials, and tasks to encourage the child to think about multiple prosocial ways to handle problems with others. Role playing is used extensively to give the child the opportunity to enact what he or she would do in a situation, thus making these interactions similar to real-life exchanges. Sessions concentrate on situations the child actually encounters (i.e., with peers, parents, siblings, teachers, and others) across multiple stimulus characteristics and conditions in an effort to promote generalization and maintenance (Kazdin, 2001).

In a typical session, we address interpersonal problems (e.g., in relation to school). The therapist models application of the steps to one situation, identifies alternative solutions, and selects one of them. The child and therapist enact (role-play) that solution. Throughout, the therapist prompts the child verbally and nonverbally to guide performance, provides a rich schedule of contingent social reinforcement, delivers concrete feedback for performance, and models improved ways of performing. Direct reinforcement of behavior is critical and sessions draw heavily on the contingent and immediate delivery of social reinforcement (smiles, praise, "high five," applause, etc.).

Children begin each session with tokens (small plastic chips) that can be exchanged for small prizes at a "store" after each session. During the session, children can lose chips (response cost) for misusing or failing to use the steps, or gain a few additional chips. In fact, few chips are provided or taken away in most of the sessions. Social reinforcement and extinction are relied on more than token reinforcement to alter child behavior. The chips present opportunities to address special issues or problems with the child such as encouraging a particular type of prosocial solution that the child might find difficult.

Critical to treatment is use of the problem-solving approach outside treatment. *In vivo* practice, referred to as *supersolvers,* consists of systematically programmed assignments designed to extend the child's use and application of problem-solving skills to everyday situations. The parents, as available, are trained to help the child use the problem-solving steps. Parents are brought into sessions over the course of treatment to learn the problem-solving steps and to practice joint supersolver assignments with the child at home. Prompting, shaping, and praise are used by the therapist to develop the parent's behavior. Over time, the child and parent supersolvers increase in complexity and eventually relate to those problem domains that led to the child's referral to treatment.

Parent Management Training

Overview

PMT refers to procedures in which parents are trained to alter their child's behavior in the home. The parents meet with a therapist or trainer who teaches them to use specific procedures to alter interactions with their child, to promote prosocial behavior, and to decrease deviant behavior. Training reflects the general view that conduct problem behavior is inadvertently developed, exacerbated, or sustained in the home by maladaptive parent–child interactions and that altering these interactions can reduce these behaviors.

There are multiple facets of parent–child interaction that promote aggressive and antisocial behavior. These patterns include directly reinforcing deviant behavior, frequently and ineffectively using commands and harsh punishment, and failing to attend to appropriate behavior (Patterson, 1982; Patterson, Reid, & Dishion, 1992). Among the many interaction patterns, those involving coercion have received the greatest attention. Coercion refers to deviant behavior on the part of one person (e.g., the child) that is rewarded by another person (e.g., the parent). Coercive interchanges between parent and child have been shown to operate in such a way as to reinforce aggressive child behavior. Also, parents tend to use punitive practices (e.g., corporal punishment) and many commands in ways that escalate problem behavior and tend to ignore prosocial behavior. Of course, this is not to say that all aggression and antisocial behavior is caused by mismanaged contingencies. Broader conceptual models have been suggested that integrate diverse facets related to parent, family, and peer functioning (e.g., parental stress and marital conflict) and their role in the unfolding of antisocial behavior (e.g., Dumas & Wahler, 1985; Patterson, 1988; Patterson et al., 1992, Reid, Patterson, & Synder, 2002). Parent–child interaction sequences remain pivotal in the models and have served as the basis for treatment of antisocial youth.

The model underlying PMT extends beyond the treatment of antisocial youth or indeed any particular population. PMT draws from the basic and applied operant conditioning research. The main focus of operant conditioning is the *contingencies of reinforcement,* which refer to the relationships between behaviors and the environmental events that influence behavior. Three components are included in a contingency, namely, antecedents (A), behaviors (B), and consequences (C). The notion of a contingency is important not only for understanding behavior but also for developing behavior-change programs. *Antecedents* refer to stimuli, settings, and contexts that occur before and influence behaviors. Examples include instructions, gestures, or looks from others. *Behaviors* refer to the acts themselves, what individuals do or do not do. *Consequences* refer to events that follow behavior and may include influences that increase, decrease, or have no impact on what the individual does.

There has been enormous progress in understanding how to apply contingencies to change behavior, how antecedent events can be used to control behavior, and how to identify factors that account for the maintenance of maladaptive behaviors (see Kazdin, 2001; Luiselli & Cameron, 1998). Contingencies of reinforcement have been used to alter behavior in a wide range of clinic and community samples, in diverse settings (home, school, community, institutions), and among virtually all age groups (infants, geriatric patients) (see Kazdin, 2001). Thus, much of what is used in PMT has a strong basis in adjacent literatures where behavior change has been a goal.

Content of the Treatment Sessions

PMT focuses on altering parent–child interaction and includes several characteristics. First, treatment is conducted primarily with the parent(s) who directly implement several procedures at home. Usually there is no direct intervention of the therapist with the child. Second, parents are trained to identify, define, and observe problem behaviors in new ways. Careful specification of the problem is essential for the delivery of reinforcing or punishing consequences and for evaluating progress. Third, the treatment sessions cover operant conditioning principles and the procedures including positive reinforcement (e.g., the use of social praise and tokens or points for prosocial behavior), prompting and shaping, mild punishment (e.g., use of time out from reinforcement and loss of privileges), negotiation, and contingency contracting. Fourth, the sessions provide opportunities for parents to see how the techniques are implemented, to practice using the techniques, and to review the behavior-change programs in the home.

In our program, the core treatment consists of 12–16 weekly sessions, with each session usually between 45 and 60 minutes. Table 14.3 presents the core treatment sessions and their foci. As with the child, optional sessions are interspersed as needed to convey the approach, to develop or to ensure the procedures are being implemented at home and at school, and to alter specific behavior-change programs. Meetings with the parent develop behavior-change skills and programs that can be implemented at home and at school. The program begins with relatively simple tasks for the parent. These build over the course of treatment to develop increasingly complex proficiencies in the parent's childrearing repertoire and practices in everyday life.

The general format of the individual sessions is to convey content, to teach specific skills, and to develop use of the skill in the home in relation to child behavior. Thus, the session usually begins by discussing the general concept (e.g., positive reinforcement) and how it is to be implemented. Typically, a specific program is designed for implementation at home. Programs take into account special features of the family situation (others in the home, schedules), target behaviors of the child (e.g., noncompliance and fighting), available incentives, and parameters that are required for effective implementation (e.g., rich reinforcement schedule, shaping, and immediate and contingent consequences). The bulk of the treatment session is devoted to modeling by the therapist and role playing and rehearsal of the parent for such tasks as presenting the program to the child, providing prompts, and delivering consequences. As part of this rehearsal, therapist and parent may alternate roles of parent and child to develop proficiency of the parent. For example, delivery of reinforcement (e.g., praise) by the parent is likely to be infrequent, flat, delayed, and connected to parental nagging. Shaping begins with the initial parent repertoire and moves progressively to obtain more consistent, enthusiastic, and immediate praise, reduced nagging, clearer prompts, and so on.

A token reinforcement system is implemented in the home to provide the parent with a structured way of implementing the reinforcement contingencies. The tokens vary from stars, marks, points, coins, and other materials based on age of the child, ease of delivery for the parent, and other practical issues. The tokens, paired with praise, are contingent upon specific child behaviors. Among the many advantages of token reinforcement is the prompting function they serve for the parent to reinforce consistently. Also, tokens facilitate tracking of reinforcement exchanges between parent and child (earning and spending the tokens). The token reinforcement programs reflect an effort to shape both child (e.g., prosocial behaviors) and parent behavior (e.g., childrearing practices). At the beginning of each treatment session, the therapist reviews precisely what occurred in the previous week or since the previous phone contact and in many cases reenacts what the parent actually did in relation to the child.

PMT also focuses on child performance at school. Teachers are contacted to discuss individual problem areas, including deportment, grades, and homework completion. A home-based reinforcement system is devised in which child performance at school is monitored with consequences provided at home by the parents. The teachers may also implement programs in the classroom. Monitoring of the school program is maintained

TABLE 14.3. Parent Management Training Sessions: Overview of the Core Sessions

1.	*Introduction and overview.* This session provides the parents with an overview of the program and outlines the demands placed on them and the focus of the intervention.
2.	*Defining and observing.* This session trains parents to pinpoint, define, and observe behavior. The parents and trainer define specific problems that can be observed and develop a specific plan to begin observations.
3.	*Positive reinforcement (point chart and praise).* This session focuses on learning the concept of positive reinforcement, factors that contribute to the effective application, and rehearsal of applications in relation to the target child. Specific programs are outlined where praise and points are to be provided for the behaviors observed during the week. An incentive (token/point) chart is devised and the delivery praise of the parent is developed through modeling, prompting, feedback, and praise by the therapist.
4.	*Time-out from reinforcement.* Parents learn about time-out and the factors related to its effective application. Delivery of time-out is extensively role-played and practiced. The use of time-out is planned for the next week for specific behaviors.
5.	*Attending and ignoring.* In this session, parents learn about attending and ignoring and choose undesirable behavior that they will ignore and a positive opposite behavior to which they will attend. These procedures are practiced within the session. Attention and praise for positive behavior are key components of this session and are practiced
6.	*Shaping/school intervention.* Parents are trained to develop behaviors by reinforcement of successive approximations and to use prompts and fading of prompts to develop terminal behaviors. Also, in this session, plans are made to implement a home-based reinforcement program to develop school-related behaviors. These behaviors include individually target academic domains, classroom deportment, and other tasks (e.g., homework completion). Prior to the session, the therapist identifies domains of functioning, specific goals, and concrete opportunities to implement procedures at school. The specific behaviors are incorporated into the home-based reinforcement program. After this session, the school-based program continues to be developed and monitored over the course of treatment, with changes in foci as needed in discussion with the teachers and parents
7.	*Review of the program.* Observations of the previous week as well as application of the reinforcement program are reviewed. Details about the administration of praise, points, and backup reinforcers are discussed and enacted so the therapist can identify how to improve parent performance. Changes are made in the program as needed. The parent practices designing programs for a set of hypothetical problems. The purpose is to develop skills that extend beyond implementing programs devised with the therapist.
8.	*Family meeting.* At this meeting, the child and parent(s) are bought into the session. The programs are discussed along with any problems. Revisions are made as needed to correct misunderstandings or to alter facets that may not be implemented in a way that is likely to be effective. The programs are practiced (role-played) to see how they are implemented and to make refinements.
9. and 10.	*Negotiating, contracting, and compromising.* The child and parent meet together to negotiate new behavioral programs and to place these in contractual form. In the first of these sessions, negotiating and contracting are introduced and parent and child practice negotiation. In the second of these sessions, the child and parent practice

(continues)

TABLE 14.3. *Continued*

___

	with each other on a problem/issue in the home and develop a contract that will be used as part of the program. Over the course of the sessions, the therapist shapes negotiating skills in the parent and child, reinforces compromise, and provides less and less guidance (e.g., prompts) as more difficult situations are presented.
11.	*Reprimands and consequences for low-rate behaviors.* Parents are trained in effective use of reprimands and how to deal with low-rate behaviors such as setting fires, stealing, or truancy. Specific punishment programs (usually chores) are planned and presented to the child, as needed for low-rate behaviors.
12. and 13.	*Review, problem solving, and practice.* Material from other sessions is reviewed in theory and practice. Special emphasis is given to role-playing application of individual principles as they are enacted with the trainer. Parents practice designing new programs, revising ailing programs, and responding to a complex array of situations in which principles and practices discussed in prior sessions are reviewed.

___

through phone contact with the school as well as in discussions in the treatment sessions with the parent.

Over the course of treatment, the child is brought into the PMT sessions to ensure that the child understands the program and that the program is implemented as reported by the parent, and to negotiate behavioral contracts between parent and child. The review of the program focuses on concrete examples of what was done, by and to whom, and with what consequences. An effort is made to identify how parent and child behavior can be improved (shaping), to practice and to provide feedback to the parent, and to refine or alter programs as needed. Modeling, rehearsal, and role-play are used here as well.

Treatment Implementation

Common Treatment Characteristics

Both PSST and PMT emphasize changing how individuals perform (i.e., what they do in everyday life). In the case of PSST, treatment is directed specifically at changing how the child responds in interpersonal situations at home, at school, and the community and in interactions with teachers, parents, peers, siblings, and others. In the case of PMT, treatment focuses on altering a number of specific child–parent interaction practices in relation to developing behavior and responding to inappropriate behavior. Both treatments emphasize the development of behavior and generality of that behavior across situations. Much of treatment is conducted in everyday life (i.e., outside the treatment sessions). Tasks for the children (e.g., PSST) and behavior-change programs implemented by parents and teachers in everyday life are central. These are monitored carefully between sessions and repaired or revised as needed regularly as a function of developing repertoires in the child and parents.

PSST and PMT draw heavily on learning theories and research findings. For example, within each treatment session, whether for child or parent, there is extensive use of modeling, prompting and fading, shaping, positive reinforcement, practice and repeated rehearsal, extinction, and mild punishment (e.g., time out from reinforcement and response cost). The demands for effective implementation of each of these are more complex than they appear and research here too has provided useful guidelines. For example, delivering social reinforcement is not merely a matter of praising good behavior. Reinforcement is optimized by delivering the consequences that are contingent, immediate, continuous (rich reinforcement schedule), and of high quality and that are associated with antecedents (prompts, establishing operations) as needed to develop the behavior (see Kazdin, 2001).

Another feature of treatment pertains to monitoring of patient progress. As child and parent are trained, one can readily assess how well the person is doing in everyday life. The child and parent use of the skills and their efforts are monitored in the session to see if a program is being implemented, is having the desired effects, has obstacles, and so on. If there is little or no progress, the obstacles usually can be attended to immediately within the treatment sessions. Programs are revised, requirements placed on parent or child are reduced or altered, and changes are made to improve implementation and to move toward the goals. Feedback from external sources (e.g., teachers and principal) is also obtained during treatment. Monitoring of progress also comes from telephone contact with parents during the week.

Finally, both PSST and PMT are manualized and individualized. There is a core set of themes and skill domains for each treatment and treatment session. Within the core sessions, child, parent, and family circumstances, including problem areas, domains of dysfunction, and special conditions of the family (e.g., living conditions, job schedules, custody issues, and presence of extended family members), are accommodated. Also, flexibility is achieved by providing optional sessions for the child or family to address specific problems or to work on a theme that was not sufficiently well conveyed in the core session. Scores of manuals are available for these treatments.[3] The availability of other manuals for research and practice has allowed us to use our own manuals as working documents that we can revise based on data and clinical experience. Thus, we have routinely tinkered with better ways of presenting, sequencing, and individualizing materials, even though the core themes and ways in which they are developed in the parents have not materially changed.

Therapist Training and Supervision

Full-time therapists provide treatment. Typically, therapists have a master's degree in one of the mental health professions and training in psychotherapy. Therapists undergo an additional period of training of approximately 6–12 months. We know that training can be readily achieved in this period but have not tested different or abbreviated training methods. Repeated practice, viewing of sessions of others, and simulated treatment is completed before a therapist is assigned a patient. The treatment manuals focus on the content of the session and provide the flow of the presentation, dialogue, and procedures to be used. Supervision of the initial treatment case consists of viewing live sessions (through video system) and discussing concretely all facets of the session. Modeling, role playing, practice, shaping, and reinforcement are used individually and in group format to train therapists. For PMT, we include a brief academic component or individualized seminar in applied behavior analysis to cover diverse concepts and techniques (e.g., establishing operations, different types of prompts, and response priming).

Therapist supervision, training, and feedback are ongoing. All sessions are videotaped, and routine as well as difficult sessions are reviewed. In addition, all treatment can be observed live from video monitor stations in the clinic. Review of tapes and live observation of treatment improve the quality of treatment because the entire treatment team can assist in addressing a difficult clinical issue.

EVIDENCE FOR THE EFFECTS OF TREATMENT

Assessment and Treatment Evaluation

The goals of treatment are to reduce antisocial behavior and to improve the children's functioning at home, at school, and in the community; to reduce parental stress and dysfunction; and to improve family functioning. Several measures are administered immediately before and after treatment and at follow-up 1 year later. Table 14.4 notes the primary measures related to our outcome studies.

Children who participate in our clinic are assigned randomly to alternative treatment conditions. Children up to age 6 receive PMT only; children 7 years and older receive PSST and PMT, alone or in combination. The different treatments have been based on reading level of the children given the format of our PSST, evidence that PSST may be

TABLE 14.4. **Primary Measures Related to Treatment Evaluation**

Measures	Domains assessed
Intake measures	
General Information Sheet	Subject and demographic characteristics
Research Diagnostic Interview	Child DSM diagnosis, number of conduct disorder symptoms, total number of symptoms
Risk Factor Interview	Child, parent, family, and contextual factors related to conduct disorder
Child functioning	
Wechsler Intelligence Scale for Children	Verbal and performance scores, overall IQ
Wide Range Achievement Test	Reading ability
Interview for Antisocial Behavior	Child aggressive and antisocial behavior
Self-Report Delinquency Checklist	Child delinquent acts
Children's Action Tendency Scale	Child aggressiveness, assertiveness, submissiveness
Parent Daily Report	Parent evaluation of problems at home
Child Behavior Checklist (Parent)	Diverse behavior problems and social competence
Child Behavior Checklist—TRF (Teacher)	Diverse behavior problems and adaptive functioning
Peer Involvement Inventory	How well child gets along with peers in school
Parent and family functioning	
Dyadic Adjustment Scale	Perceived quality of marital relation
Family Environment Scale	Domains of family functioning
Parenting Stress Index	Perceived parental stress and life events
Beck Depression Inventory	Parent depression
Hopkins Symptom Checklist	Overall parent impairment
Quality of Life Inventory	Parent evaluation of quality of life
Treatment-related measures	
Parent Expectancies for Child Therapy	Parents' expectancies about treatment, their role, and child improvement
Barriers to Participation in Treatment	Barriers, obstacles, stressors that parents experience specifically in relation to treatment
Child, Parent, and Therapist Evaluation Inventories	Acceptability of and progress in treatment

Note. Details of, and references for, individual measures can be found in the citations in Table 14.5.

more effective with older children (see Durlak, Fuhrman, & Lampman, 1991), and the availability of the parent to participate in treatment. When both PSST and PMT are provided to a family, two therapists are involved with each case. Child and parent are seen during the same visit.

Treatment Effects

Table 14.5 highlights studies on the effects of treatment and the factors that contribute to outcome. Overall, the main findings are as follows:

1. PSST alone and PSST in combination with PMT produce reliable and significant reductions in antisocial behavior and increases in prosocial behavior among children;

TABLE 14.5. Main Studies to Evaluate Treatment Outcome and Therapeutic Change

Investigation	Sample	Objective
Kazdin, Esveldt-Dawson, French, & Unis (1987a)	Inpatient children (ages 7–13, $n = 56$)	Evaluated PSST, Relationship therapy, and treatment-contact control
Kazdin, Esveldt-Dawson, French, & Unis (1987b)	Inpatient children (ages 7–12, $n = 40$)	Evaluated PSST and PMT combined and treatment-contact control
Kazdin, Bass, Siegel, & Thomas (1989)	Inpatient and outpatient children (ages 5–13, $n = 112$)	Compared PSST, PSST with *in vivo* practice, and Relationship therapy
Kazdin, Siegel, & Bass (1992)	Outpatient children (ages 7–13, $n = 97$)	Evaluated effects of PSST, PMT, and both combined on child and parent functioning
Kazdin, Mazurick, & Siegel (1994)	Outpatient children (ages 4–13, $n = 75$)	Evaluated therapeutic change of completers and dropouts and factors that account for their different outcomes
Kazdin (1995a)	Outpatient children (ages 7–13, $n = 105$)	Replication of effects of combined treatment and child, parent, and family moderator of outcome
Kazdin & Crowley (1997)	Outpatient children (ages 7–13, $n = 120$)	Examined relation of intellectual functioning and severity of symptoms on responsiveness to treatment
Kazdin & Wassell (2000a)	Outpatient children (ages 2–14, $n = 169$)	Examined relation of parent psychopathology and quality of life as moderators of therapeutic changes in children
Kazdin & Wassell (2000b)	Outpatient children (ages 2–14, $n = 250$)	Examined therapeutic changes in children, parents, and families and the predictors of these change
Kazdin & Whitley (in press)	Outpatient children (ages 6–14, $n = 127$)	Examined the effects of addressing parental stress in treatment and the impact on perceived barriers to treatment and therapeutic change

2. The combined treatment (PSST + PMT) tends to be more effective than either treatment alone;

3. Improvements are not plausibly explained by the passage of time, repeated contact with a therapist, or nonspecific (common) treatment factors associated with participation in treatment, given comparisons of treatment with other intervention and control conditions;

4. Youth referred for antisocial behavior and who do not receive PSST or PMT or who receive relationship-based treatment usually do not change or deteriorate over time in relation to their conduct problem symptoms;

5. The effects of treatment are evident in performance at home, at school, and the community both immediately after treatment and up to a 1-year follow-up assessment;

6. The effects of treatment have been obtained with both inpatient and outpatient cases;

7. Treatment outcome is influenced by multiple moderators; greater severity of child deviance, parent psychopathology and stress, and family dysfunction at pretreatment are associated with less therapeutic change;

8. Adding a treatment component to address parent sources of stress in everyday life improves treatment outcome of the child; and

9. Treatment effects are not only evident in child behavior but also in reductions in stress and maternal depression and improved family relations.

Overall Evaluation

Many fundamental questions are yet to be resolved. Two especially salient questions are whether the impact of treatment alters the lives of the children and families in palpable ways and whether these effects are long term. Our studies have shown that statistically significant improvements are made with treatment and that the magnitude of these changes (pre–post) is rather large (e.g., mean effect size of change > 1.2; Kazdin & Wassell, 2000b). Yet, do the gains make a difference to the youth or to others in everyday life? Clinical significance refers to the practical value or importance of the effect of an intervention—that is, whether it makes any "real" difference to the clients or to others with whom they interact. There are many measures of clinical significance, and they have become more sophisticated (Kendall, 1999). The most commonly used index of clinical significance in child therapy is whether treatment returns to normative levels of functioning, based on data from same-age and -sex youths who are functioning well in the community. Our treatment has demonstrated such changes.

However, a major obstacle that qualifies enthusiasm stems from the fact that standard measures of clinical significance have unclear meaning. For example, demonstrating that children return to normative levels of symptoms on a standardized measure (e.g., Child Behavior Checklist) does not necessarily mean that a genuine difference is evident in everyday life or that functioning is palpably improved. It might; there is just little evidence to support the view that it does. The entire matter of symptom change raises issues regarding clinical significance of an outcome. It is easy to show that little, no, or a lot of change could mean clinically significant or no significant change depending on the clinical problem, goals of treatment, and contextual influences in the life of the client (Kazdin, 1999). Much more work is needed to permit interpretation of measures of clinical significance currently in use.

No less significant is whether treatment effects are maintained. Obviously, follow-up assessment is critically important because developmental change is a strong competitor with treatment for many problems and because treatments that appear effective or more effective at one point in time (e.g., posttreatment assessment) may not be at another point in time (e.g., follow-up assessment) (Kazdin, 2000). Follow-up assessment in our program has focused primarily on evaluation of child functioning at home and at school 1 year (and occasionally 2 years) after completing the program. Therapeutic changes usually are maintained, as reflected in symptoms as well as prosocial functioning. Clearly, a limitation is not knowing the long-term impact (e.g., 5–10 years after the intervention).

Special Issues Regarding Implementation

There are many obstacles in moving from research findings to implementation in clinical practice. First and perhaps most salient, few training opportunities exist for mental health professionals to learn these techniques. The training issue is dramatically illustrated by PMT, probably the most well studied and supported treatment of all therapies for children and adolescents (see Brestan & Eyberg, 1998; Kazdin, 1997). In training mental health professionals in psychology, child psychiatry, social work, and nursing, it is unlikely that PMT is mentioned or covered. Many treatment manuals are available and an occasional convention workshop here or there. Reading the manuals and attending a workshop are only a beginning and not sufficient if one wants to learn how to fly an airplane, play a musical instrument, or provide PMT or PSST.

Second, the success of extending treatment techniques from research to practice has focused on the interventions themselves. I believe that several procedures used routinely in research and considered to be unique to research may be as critical for use in clinical practice. I have in mind some of the features of controlled clinical trials that are designed to augment treatment implementation and therapeutic effects. To begin, therapist training in the techniques is extensive. There is no doubt a great deal of art in the delivery of treatment. In clinical work outside the confines of research, "clinical experience" is a concept frequently flaunted. Experience is important for all sorts of reasons. However, experience is not to be confused with competence and skill. We would like to believe that experience (e.g., years on the job) and competence and skill are positively correlated, but I know of no data in the context of psychotherapy that suggest the correlation is high. Indeed, in clinical work the lack of initial training to mastery (however defined for a treatment), lack of ongoing feedback to therapists about performance, and the tendency to combine multiple treatments or to introduce new treatments based on quite abbreviated "training" (e.g., attending a workshop, reading a book) are quite likely to reduce fidelity of and dilute treatments with known efficacy.

In our own program, and other programs as well, therapists can be trained to a level of mastery and supervised to sustain and improve that level. All treatment is videotaped and also can be viewed live to provide immediate feedback to a therapist and to problem-solve with the therapist regarding how to redress a problem. This kind of supervision not only maintains the integrity of treatment but also enhances quality of the treatment for the individual case. The precise procedures we use to train and to supervise therapists, to monitor treatment integrity, and to manage patient care may not be essential. However, some features to help establish and sustain the quality and integrity of treatment in clinical work are likely to have salutary effects in clinical practice.

Third, extension of effective treatments to clinical practice probably requires better assessment. Indeed, some practices could improve both clinical research and practice.

Systematic assessment of patient progress during treatment, rather than merely at the end of treatment, would be helpful in establishing the effects of treatment in research and clinical work. The absence of systematic evaluation in most clinical practice is a great deficiency. Even if evidence-based treatments were used, the treatments are not likely to be effective, or optimally effective, for all cases. Some monitoring procedures are needed to provide an evaluation of progress during treatment and to provide the basis for decision making about continuing, changing, augmenting, or ending treatment. A number of resources are available to suggest procedures that can be used in clinical work to evaluate treatment progress (see Kazdin, 2003). Ultimately, the quality of clinical work will depend not only on using techniques with evidence in their behalf but also on systematically examining their impact on individual patients.

DIRECTIONS FOR FUTURE RESEARCH

There are several areas of research we consider important in light of findings to date and their limitations. Let me mention four that are especially high priorities. First, we are exploring *novel models for delivering treatment*. The current dominant model in use in therapy consists of brief and time-limited treatment. It is likely that clinical dysfunction (e.g., CD, depression, and ADHD) will require more enduring interventions. We are currently exploring alternative models of delivering treatment that are designed to improve impact. Central to this work is evaluation of treatment of the usual duration, designed to address crises and to alter functioning at home, at school, and in the community. After initial treatment and demonstrated improvement in functioning in everyday life, treatment is suspended. At this point, the child's functioning begins to be monitored systematically and regularly (e.g., every month). Treatment is then provided as-needed based on the assessment data or emergent issues raised by the family, teachers, or others. The approach might be likened to the more familiar model of dental care in the United States in which regular "checkups" are recommended; an intervention is provided if and as needed based on these periodic checks.

Second, we are trying to *elaborate and understand treatment outcome* and the interrelations among domains. For example, we know now that treatment of the child has an impact on parent and family functioning (e.g., decreases in stress, depression, and other symptoms of psychopathology and improved family relationships). There are likely to be intricate and reciprocal relations among the domains. For example, parent quality of life at pretreatment probably influences child deviance and also is influenced by child deviance (Crowley, & Kazdin, 1998). A given domain might well serve as a moderator and important treatment outcome.

Third, and related, we are *focusing in treatment more on parent sources of stress*. Parent and family sources of stress can play a role in child dysfunction as well as treatment. Socioeconomic disadvantage, marital conflict, parent psychopathology, stress, and social isolation are among the many characteristics of the families of children with CD. Families that show adversity in one or more of these domains are more likely to drop out of treatment prematurely, more likely to show fewer gains in treatment (among those who remain), and less likely to maintain therapeutic gains (see Kazdin, 1995b for a review). Also, stress can disrupt discipline practices of the parent in ways that promote deviant child behavior (Dumas & Wahler, 1985; Patterson, 1988; Patterson et al., 1992). We are evaluating a component of our treatment designed to aid parents by increasing the time they have for themselves, developing friendships, reestablishing a relationship that has gone awry, or pursuing something they consider personally fulfilling.

Finally, we have been evaluating patient *attrition*. Dropping out of treatment prematurely is an enormous problem and occurs among 40–60% of children, adolescents, and adults who begin therapy (Wierzbicki & Pekarik, 1993). We completed a few studies to predict who drops out of treatment (Kazdin, 1990; Kazdin, Mazurick, & Bass, 1993), to examine the outcomes of families that drop out (Kazdin, Mazurick, & Siegel, 1994), to distinguish different types of families and circumstances among dropouts (Kazdin & Mazurick, 1994; Kazdin, Stolar, & Marciano, 1995), and to develop and test a conceptual model about why families drop out (Kazdin, 1996; Kazdin, Holland, & Crowley, 1997; Kazdin, Holland, Crowley, & Breton, 1997; Kazdin & Wassell, 1999, 2000a). Of special interest, perhaps, is the fact that many families that drop out of treatment often are functioning well. For example, approximately 34% of dropouts have made important changes in their seemingly all-too-brief treatment period, as compared with 79% of those who complete treatment, based on parent evaluations (Kazdin & Wassell, 1998). There are several facets of interest here, including who changes and why, what are or ought to be the criteria for terminating therapy, when is dropping out of treatment not premature, and, of course, when is completion of treatment (finishing the fixed regimen) premature.

There are other areas of research that are at a preliminary stage of development in our program. Among them are (1) the role of the therapeutic alliance in treatment and therapeutic change, (2) factors that influence patient adherence to treatment prescriptions, and (3) the role of parent expectancies about the effects of treatment on participation in treatment and therapeutic change. Each of these has emerged as a theme in the application of treatment with children and families or has been stimulated by specific findings in other work cited here and the work of other investigators conducting similar work.

Treatment outcome studies in the context of clinical work with patient samples require long-term investigations. Even so, in many ways the outcome studies are the easy part of the challenge. The task is to integrate the range of pertinent variables and influences on the treatment process and outcome in ways that at once improve understanding and clinical care. In the treatment of CD, we have been compelled to study all sorts of influences because of their clear relevance to implementing treatment and achieving therapeutic change.

SUMMARY AND CONCLUSIONS

Our program is devoted to the treatment of CD children and their families. We have focused on combined cognitive-behavioral procedures to address interpersonal cognitive processes of the child (PSST) and parent–child interactions (PMT). The treatments focus on facets within the individual (e.g., cognitive and behavioral repertoires and predisposition to respond to potentially problematic situations), as well as external and interactional events (e.g., antecedents and consequences from others) to promote prosocial behavior. With both treatments, emphasis is placed on altering performance at home, at school, and in the community. Although formal treatment sessions form the basis of the intervention, most treatment is conducted outside the sessions. The child, parent, and teacher have separate but interrelated activities outside the sessions that consist of practicing activities and strategies learned in the treatment sessions.

Treatment outcome studies, our own and those of others, indicate that clinically referred patients improve with PSST and PMT and that effects are maintained at least to 1-year follow-up assessment. Several moderators of treatment have been identified and include characteristics of the children, parents, and families. Many of these are as would be expected, including severity of child and parent dysfunction, stress in the home, and harsh punishing practices, as assessed at pretreatment. Our research also shows that the effects of treatment extend beyond multiple outcomes of the child. Parent dysfunction and stress decline and family relations improve.

CD represents a special challenge, given the multiple domains of functioning that are affected. Indeed, we consider CD a pervasive developmental disorder precisely because of the scope of dysfunction children present. Even this characterization is inadequate in the context of clinical work, because broader influences (parental, familial, and contextual) often must be considered in treatment. These influences have a demonstrated relation to child antisocial behavior, to participation and completion of treatment, and to therapeutic change. In the process of developing treatment, we have been drawn into many other areas that are related to dysfunction and change.

ACKNOWLEDGMENTS

Research in this chapter was facilitated by generous research support of a Research Scientist Award (MH00353) and a MERIT Award (MH35408) from the National Institute of Mental Health. Projects currently underway are facilitated by support from the Leon Lowenstein Foundation, the William T. Grant Foundation (98–1872–98), the National Institute of Mental Health (MH59029), and Yale University. I am very grateful for the support. No less essential to the work has been the remarkable staff that has served at the Yale Child Conduct Clinic. I am pleased to acknowledge several staff members and interns whose contributions in providing and evaluating treatment and running the clinic have been enormous: Wayne Ayers, Susan Breton, Elizabeth Brown, Susan Bullerdick, Mary Cavaleri, Michael Crowley, Lisa Holland, Bernadette Lezca, Erin Levix, Paul Marciano, Molly McDonald, Jennifer Mazurick, Francheska Perepletchikova, Elif Tongul, Gloria Wassell, and Moira Whitley. The clinic has thrived through the support of others, especially the late Donald J. Cohen, MD, and Paula Armbruster, MSW, at the Yale Child Study Center.

NOTES

1. In this chapter, conduct disorder refers generally to clinically severe antisocial behavior, including aggression, lying, stealing, truancy, running away, and other behaviors. The term (when in lower case or abbreviated as CD) is used generically to refer to the constellation of symptoms rather than specifically to the diagnostic category (as when capitalized and spelled out).
2. The Child Conduct Clinic and the research reported in this chapter initially began at the Western Psychiatric Institute and Clinic, University of Pittsburgh School of Medicine (1981–1989) and continued at Yale University (1989–present). Although screening criteria for the clinic have not changed appreciably over time, the demographic characteristics have changed to match the change in geographical locale. Further descriptions of samples of individual studies can be obtained from the primary references themselves (Table 14.5).
3. Several manuals with variants of cognitive skills training (e.g., Feindler & Ecton, 1986; Finch, Nelson, & Ott, 1993; Santostefano, 1985; Shure, 1992) and parent management training (e.g., Cavell, 2000; Forehand & McMahon, 1981; Forgatch, 1994; Sanders & Dadds, 1993) are available, only a small sample of which can be noted here. We are currently preparing our manuals for dissemination. In advance of their completion, a description of our treatments is available from the author.

REFERENCES

American Psychiatric Association. (1994). *Diagnostic and statistical manual of mental disorders* (4th ed.). Washington, DC: Author.

Brestan, E. V., & Eyberg, S. M. (1998). Effective psychosocial treatments of conduct-disordered children and adolescents: 29 years, 82 studies, and 5,272 kids. *Journal of Clinical Child Psychology, 27,* 180–189.

Cavell, T. A. (2000). *Working with aggressive children: A practitioner's guide.* Washington, DC: American Psychological Association.

Crick, N. R., & Dodge, K. A. (1994). A review and reformulation of social information processing mechanisms in children's social adjustment. *Psychological Bulletin, 115,* 74–101.

Crowley, M. J., & Kazdin, A. E. (1998). Child psychosocial functioning and parent quality of life among clinically referred children. *Journal of Child and Family Studies, 7,* 233–251.

Dumas, J. E., & Wahler, R. G. (1985). Indiscriminate mothering as a contextual factor in aggressive oppositional child behavior: "Damned if you do and damned if you don't." *Journal of Applied Behavior Analysis, 13,* 1–17.

Durlak, J. A., Fuhrman, T., & Lampman, C. (1991). Effectiveness of cognitive-behavioral therapy for maladapting children: A meta-analysis. *Psychological Bulletin, 110,* 204–214.

Feindler, E. L., & Ecton, R. B. (1986). *Adolescent anger control: Cognitive-behavioral techniques.* Elmsford, NY: Pergamon Press.

Finch, A. J., Jr., Nelson, W. M., & Ott, E. S. (1993). *Cognitive-behavioral procedures with children and adolescents: A practical guide.* Needham Heights, MA: Allyn & Bacon.

Forehand, R., & McMahon, R. J. (1981). *Helping the noncompliant child: A clinician's guide to parent training.* New York: Guilford Press.

Forgatch, M. S. (1994). *Parenting through change: A training manual.* Eugene: Oregon Social Learning Center.

Kazdin, A. E. (1990). Premature termination from treatment among children referred for antisocial behavior. *Journal of Child Psychology and Psychiatry, 3,* 415–425.

Kazdin, A. E. (1995a). Child, parent, and family dysfunction as predictors of outcome in cognitive-behavioral treatment of antisocial children. *Behaviour Research and Therapy, 33,* 271–281.

Kazdin, A. E. (1995b). *Conduct disorder in childhood and adolescence* (2nd ed.). Thousand Oaks, CA: Sage.

Kazdin, A. E. (1996). Dropping out of child psychotherapy: Issues for research and implications for practice. *Clinical Child Psychology and Psychiatry, 1,* 133–156.

Kazdin, A. E. (1997). Parent management training: Evidence, outcomes, and issues. *Journal of the American Academy of Child and Adolescent Psychiatry, 36,* 1349–1356.

Kazdin, A. E. (1999). The meanings and measurement of clinical significance. *Journal of Consulting and Clinical Psychology, 67,* 332–339.

Kazdin, A. E. (2000). *Psychotherapy for children and adolescents: Directions for research and practice.* New York: Oxford University Press.

Kazdin, A. E. (2001). *Behavior modification in applied settings* (6th ed.). Pacific Grove, CA: Wadsworth.

Kazdin, A. E. (2003). *Research design in clinical psychology* (4th ed.). Needham Heights, MA: Allyn & Bacon.

Kazdin, A. E., Bass, D., Siegel, T., & Thomas, C. (1989). Cognitive-behavioral treatment and relationship therapy in the treatment of children referred for antisocial behavior. *Journal of Consulting and Clinical Psychology, 57,* 522–535.

Kazdin, A. E., & Crowley, M. (1997). Moderators of treatment outcome in cognitively based treatment of antisocial behavior. *Cognitive Therapy and Research, 21,* 185–207.

Kazdin, A. E., Esveldt-Dawson, K., French, N. H., & Unis, A. S. (1987a). The effects of parent management training and problem-solving skills training combined in the treatment of antisocial child behavior. *Journal of the American Academy of Child and Adolescent Psychiatry, 26,* 416–424.

Kazdin, A. E., Esveldt-Dawson, K., French, N. H., & Unis, A. S. (1987b). Problem-solving skills training and relationship therapy in the treatment of antisocial child behavior. *Journal of Consulting and Clinical Psychology, 55,* 76–85.

Kazdin, A. E., Holland, L., & Crowley, M. (1997). Family experience of barriers to treatment and premature termination from child therapy. *Journal of Consulting and Clinical Psychology, 65,* 453–463.

Kazdin, A. E., Holland, L., Crowley, M., & Breton, S. (1997). Barriers to Participation in Treatment Scale: Evaluation and validation in the context of child outpatient treatment. *Journal of Child Psychology and Psychiatry, 38,* 1051–1062.

Kazdin, A. E., & Mazurick, J. L. (1994). Dropping out of child psychotherapy: Distinguishing early and late dropouts over the course of treatment. *Journal of Consulting and Clinical Psychology, 62,* 1069–1074

Kazdin, A. E., Mazurick, J. L., & Bass, D. (1993). Risk for attrition in treatment of antisocial children and families. *Journal of Clinical Child Psychology, 22,* 2–16.

Kazdin, A. E., Mazurick, J. L., & Siegel, T. C. (1994). Treatment outcome among children with externalizing disorder who terminate prematurely versus those who complete psychotherapy. *Journal of the American Academy of Child and Adolescent Psychiatry, 33,* 549–557.

Kazdin, A. E., Siegel, T., & Bass, D. (1992). Cognitive problem-solving skills training and parent management training in the treatment of antisocial behavior in children. *Journal of Consulting and Clinical Psychology, 60,* 733–747.

Kazdin, A. E., Stolar, M. J., & Marciano, P. L. (1995). Risk factors for dropping out of treatment among white and black families. *Journal of Family Psychology, 9,* 402–417.

Kazdin, A. E., & Wassell, G. (1998). Treatment completion and therapeutic change among children referred for outpatient therapy. *Professional Psychology: Research and Practice, 29,* 332–340.

Kazdin, A. E., & Wassell, G. (1999). Barriers to treatment participation and therapeutic change among children referred for conduct disorder. *Journal of Clinical Child Psychology, 28,* 160–172.

Kazdin, A. E., & Wassell, G. (2000a). Predictors of barriers to treatment and therapeutic change in outpatient therapy for antisocial children and their families. *Mental Health Services Research, 2,* 27–40.

Kazdin, A. E., & Wassell, G. (2000b). Therapeutic changes in children, parents, and families resulting from treatment of children with conduct problems. *Journal of the American Academy of Child and Adolescent Psychiatry, 39,* 414–420.

Kazdin, A. E., & Whitley, M. K. (in press). Treatment of parental stress to enhance therapeutic change among children referred for aggressive and antisocial behavior. *Journal of Consulting and Clinical Psychology.*

Kendall, P. C. (Ed.) (1999). Special section: Clinical significance. *Journal of Consulting and Clinical Psychology, 67,* 283–339.

Kendall, P. C. (Ed.). (2000). *Child and adolescent therapy: Cognitive-behavioral procedures* (2nd ed.). New York: Guilford Press.

Lochman, J. E., Whidby, J. M., & FitzGerald, D. P. (2000). Cognitive-behavioral assessment and treatment with aggressive children. In P. C. Kendall (Ed.), *Child and adolescent therapy: Cognitive-behavioral procedures* (2nd ed., pp. 31–87). New York: Guilford Press.

Luiselli, J. K., & Cameron, M. J. (Eds.). (1998). *Antecedent control: Innovative approaches to behavioral support.* Baltimore: Brookes.

Patterson, G. R. (1982). *Coercive family process.* Eugene, OR: Castalia.

Patterson, G. R. (1988). Stress: A change agent for family process. In N. Garmezy & M. Rutter (Eds.), *Stress, coping, and development in children* (pp. 235–264). Baltimore: Johns Hopkins University Press.

Patterson, G. R., Reid, J. B., & Dishion, T. J. (1992). *Antisocial boys.* Eugene, OR: Castalia.

Reid, J. B., Patterson, G. R., & Snyder, J. (Eds.). (2002). *Antisocial behavior in children and adolescents: A developmental analysis and model for intervention.* Washington, DC: American Psychological Association.

Sanders, M. R., & Dadds, M. R. (1993). *Behavioral family intervention.* Needham Heights, MA: Allyn & Bacon.

Santostefano, S. (1985). *Cognitive control therapy with children and adolescents.* Elmsford, NY: Pergamon Press.

Shure, M. B. (1992). *I can problem solve (ICPS): An interpersonal cognitive problem solving program.* Champaign, IL: Research Press.

Shure, M. B. (1997). Interpersonal cognitive problem solving: Primary prevention of early high-risk behaviors in the preschool and primary years. In G. W. Albee & T. P. Gulotta (Eds.), *Primary prevention works* (pp. 167–188). Thousand Oaks, CA: Sage.

Spivack, G., & Shure, M. B. (1982). The cognition of social adjustment: Interpersonal cognitive problem solving thinking. In B. B. Lahey & A. E. Kazdin (Eds.), *Advances in clinical child psychology* (Vol. 5, pp. 323–372). New York: Plenum Press.

Wierzbicki, M., & Pekarik, G. (1993). A meta-analysis of psychotherapy dropout. *Professional Psychology: Research and Practice, 24,* 190–195.

15

Anger Control Training for Aggressive Youth

John E. Lochman, Tammy D. Barry,
and Dustin A. Pardini

OVERVIEW

Childhood aggression has become a central focus of many prevention and treatment efforts due to its relative stability over time and consistent linkage with a variety of negative outcomes including delinquency, substance use, conduct problems, academic difficulties, and poor adjustment (Loeber, 1990). Early hostile behavior has also received considerable attention because youth who engage in the most persistent, severe, and violent antisocial behavior are most likely to initiate their deviant behavior in childhood rather than adolescence. As a result, childhood aggression is often viewed as an indication of a broader-based syndrome that is characterized by various norm-violating behaviors in adolescence. Although there is no commonly accepted definition of aggressive behavior, various conceptualizations have included behaviors such as starting rumors, excluding others, arguing, bullying, the use of strong-arm tactics, threatening, striking back in anger, and engaging in physical fights. The diversity of these aggressive activities, as well as the tendency for some children to exhibit only certain types of combative behavior, has prompted many researchers to devise classification systems aimed at identifying clinically meaningful subgroups of aggressive children (e.g., Dodge, Lochman, Harnish, Bates, & Pettit, 1997; Lochman & Dodge, 1994). These complexities aside, aggressive behavior has an aversive effect on others, leading children who exhibit this behavior to develop poor relations with their peers, parents, and teachers.

Contextual Social-Cognitive Model

The development of adolescent antisocial behavior is often conceptualized as the result of a set of familial and personal factors (Patterson, Reid, & Dishion, 1992), with children's aggressive behavior representing a substantial part of that developmental course

(Lochman & Wells, 2002b). Because this developmental course is set within the child's social environment, an ecological framework is needed to guide preventive efforts (Conduct Problems Prevention Research Group, 1992). Loeber (1990) theorized that poor parenting practices contribute to children's aggressive behavior, and as these aggressive behavior patterns become entrenched, they lead to the development of substance abuse and conduct disorder. In early to middle childhood, increasingly oppositional children can experience highly negative reactions from teachers and peers and develop impaired social-cognitive processes. As their academic progress and social bond to school weakens, they become more susceptible to deviant peer group influences. By adolescence, this trajectory results in a heightened risk of substance use, delinquent acts, and school failure (Loeber, 1990). Thus, the contextual social-cognitive model of prevention presented here focuses on two relevant sets of potential mediators of adolescent antisocial behavior: (1) child-level factors including their lack of social competence and poor social-cognitive skills and (2) parent-level contextual factors including poor caregiver involvement and discipline of the child.

Children's Social-Cognitive Processes

The anger arousal model that served as the conceptual framework for the child component of the Anger Coping Program was initially derived from Novaco's work with aggressive adults (Lochman, Nelson, & Sims, 1981; Lochman, Whidby, & FitzGerald, 2000). This model stresses the cognitive processes that occur as the child responds to interpersonal conflicts or frustrations with environmental obstacles. This first stage of cognitive processing consists of the child's perceptions and attributions of the problem event, which in turn influences the child's subsequent anger. The second stage of processing consists of the child's cognitive plan for his or her response to the perceived threat or provocation. The anger arousal model proposed that children's cognitive and emotional processing of the problem and their planned response led to their behavioral response (ranging from aggression to assertion, passive acceptance, or withdrawal).

The more recent development of the Coping Power Program, which is an extension of the Anger Coping Program, was influenced by research supporting Crick and Dodge's (1994) six-stage model of social information processing. In the first three stages (Lochman, FitzGerald, & Whidby, 1999), children encode relevant details in the immediate environment, generate interpretations about the nature of the situation, and then formulate a social goal that will influence their response to the situation (e.g., gaining revenge and avoiding conflict). During the encoding stage, aggressive children are more likely to attend to hostile cues, remember fewer cues, and attend only to the most recent cues in comparison to their nonaggressive peers. Higher levels of aggression are associated with an increased tendency to view others' actions as hostile (Lochman & Dodge, 1994), suggesting that aggressive children have problems interpreting the information they have encoded. When generating interpersonal goals, aggressive children also tend to endorse those goals associated with dominance, disruption, and troublemaking more often than their peers, even in fairly benign conflict situations.

The final three stages of Crick and Dodge's (1994) model involve generating a mental list of possible behavioral responses, systematically evaluating the quality of each response, and then enacting the chosen response. Aggressive children have been shown to have problems at each of these social information-processing stages (Lochman et al., 1999). When asked to generate solutions to interpersonal conflicts, aggressive children demonstrate deficiencies in the overall number and quality of solutions generated, and they produce fewer verbal solutions and more direct-action solutions involving physical aggression. Youth exhibiting deviant behavior are also more confident that aggressive solutions will produce positive outcomes and less likely to believe that negative consequences will result from hostile actions. Even when aggressive children choose to enact positive responses, evidence suggests that they are less adept at carrying them out. The entire process is said to be circular in nature because the outcome of the enacted response often influences the child's future response choices.

These social-cognitive processes are affected by children's acquired schemas for social interactions. Aspects of aggressive children's schemas, such as their expectations for others and their social goals, have been found to have an impact on their social information processing (Lochman et al., 2000). Aggressive children's attributions and social problem solving have been found to become more hostile and less adaptive as they become more physiologically aroused and as they engage in more automatic, rather than deliberate, information processing.

Contextual Parenting Behaviors

Patterson et al. (1992) proposed that childhood aggressive behavior arises out of early contextual experiences with parents who provide harsh or irritable discipline, poor problem solving, vague commands, and poor monitoring of children's behavior. Parental risk factors such as a lack of maternal involvement and inconsistent discipline have been linked to childhood aggression and the development of adolescent antisocial behavior. There is also evidence suggesting that parents who use irritable and ineffective discipline are more likely to have children who exhibit overt (oppositional behavior, physical aggression) and covert (stealing, lying, and truancy) antisocial behavior. These results suggest that parent factors exert a direct effect on adolescent antisocial behavior and an indirect effect via their association with factors such as childhood aggression, poor social competence, and academic failure. The relation between poor parenting and children's aggressive behavior is also viewed as bidirectional, with poor parenting stimulating children's negative behavior and deteriorating in response to increasingly negative child behaviors.

Goals of Anger Coping and Coping Power Programs

Using the contextual social-cognition model as a guide, the Anger Coping and Coping Power programs are designed to prevent the development of antisocial behavior in adolescence by modifying the maladaptive parenting practices and child social information-processing problems that have been associated with childhood aggressive behavior. Anger Coping and the Coping Power Program's child component include group sessions addressing issues such as anger management, perspective taking, social problem solving, emotional awareness, relaxation training, social skills enhancement, positive social and personal goals, and dealing with peer pressure. The Coping Power Program also has a parent component with group sessions designed to address such issues as social reinforcement and positive attention, the importance of clear house rules, behavioral expectations and monitoring procedures, the use of appropriate and effective discipline strategies, family communication, positive connection to school, and stress management. During parent group meetings, parents are also informed of the skills their children are working on during their sessions, and parents are encouraged to facilitate and reinforce children for using these new skills at home and school.

CHARACTERISTICS OF THE TREATMENT PROGRAM

Anger Coping Program: Format and Clients

The Anger Coping Program was developed to address the model of anger arousal and social-cognitive processes associated with aggression in children. In earlier empirical research, the program was implemented with boys only. However, the practical application of the Anger Coping Program has included both boys and girls. Likewise, both boys and girls have been included in research investigating the effectiveness of the Coping Power Program (an extension of Anger Coping). The Anger Coping Program is designed for five to seven children in a group format; however, the content can be delivered in individual sessions as well. A group format has several advantages over individual sessions, providing opportunities to address children's difficulties with social competence through modeling, role playing, group problem solving, and feedback/reinforcement of children's social behavior with peers and adult group leaders (Lochman et al., 1999). The program has been successfully implemented in both a school and clinical setting.

Ideally, each anger coping group has two coleaders, who alternate between leading specific group activities and monitoring children's behaviors. This minimizes the behavioral management difficulties that can arise with an aggressive population and allows for frequent feedback, redirection, and reinforcement. The modal coleader has at least a master's degree in social work, counseling, school psychology, or clinical psychology. The program consists of 18 sessions and generally meets weekly for 60 to 90 minutes in a large room with chairs and a table. Posterboards (with group rules, point charts, etc.) are hung around the room, and a chalkboard or dry erase board is often used for session-specific reminders and activities.

Although children demonstrating high levels of anger and aggressive behaviors are targeted for the groups, research findings suggest that specific client characteristics are associated with greater improvement following involvement in the Anger Coping Program. Specifically, aggressive children who are extremely poor social problem-solvers, have lower perceived levels of hostility, and who are more rejected by their peers tend to exhibit better treatment-related outcomes (Lochman et al., 1999). Likewise, children with a more internalized attributional style and higher levels of anxiety symptoms and somatic complaints tend to benefit more from the intervention. The most successful groups include children who have some level of understanding that their aggressive behavior is problematic and have some desire to change this behavior (Lochman et al., 1999).

Given the differential outcomes associated with client characteristics, it is recommended that various assessment techniques be used prior to treatment. Examples include structured diagnostic interviews and behavioral rating forms, such as the Achenbach Child Behavior Checklist (Lochman et al., 2000). Finally, an assessment of characteristics and skills related to the model of anger arousal and social information processing (e.g., problem-solving skills, attributional biases, and emotional regulation) can be conducted. Data from these assessment instruments can also be used to individualize the treatment targets for the specific difficulties of the children in the group (Lochman et al., 1999).

Sequence and Content of Therapy Sessions

The following overview of the Anger Coping Program is adapted from Lochman et al. (1999) and includes the objectives outlined for each session (see Table 15.1 for a list of

TABLE 15.1. Sessions for the Anger Coping Program

Session No.	Title
1	Introduction and Group Rules
2	Understanding and Writing Goals
3	Anger Management: Puppet Self-Control Task
4	Using Self-Instruction
5	Perspective Taking
6	Looking at Anger
7	What Does Anger Feel Like?
8	Choices and Consequences
9	Steps for Problem Solving
10	Problem Solving in Action
11–18	Video Productions I–VIII and Review

program sessions). The program uses cognitive-behavioral procedures; however, rigid adherence is not necessary. Rather, leaders are encouraged to implement the structured program in a flexible manner, so that the agenda can be shifted to address specific problems and issues that arise for group members. Nevertheless, the overall objectives of the program and the specific objectives of each session should be considered to ensure that the social-cognitive difficulties of aggressive children are affected.

• *Review main points from previous session.* Beginning with session 2, the first portion of the session is used to review information from the previous session in a group discussion format. Each group member is asked to recall one point from the previous session, and group leaders use reminders and encouragement to shape the discussion.

• *Review goals.* Beginning with session 3, each child's goal sheet (see discussion in Session 2) from the previous week is reviewed and a point is rewarded if the goal has been met. Leaders should help members discuss what led to their success or problem-solve ways to help the child reach his or her goal if he or she was not successful.

• *Session 1, Objective 1.* Explain the group purpose and set the group structure: (1) The group discusses general difficulties with anger management, as well as specific problems among group members. The Anger Coping Program is presented as a way to learn anger control. (2) The time, frequency, number of meetings, and general agenda items are presented. (3) Group rules are generated (e.g., confidentiality and paying attention), with input from group members and guidance by leaders. Rules should be displayed at all subsequent sessions. (4) The group contingency management system is discussed (e.g., earn points for goal sheets, following rules, and positive participation; lose points if break rules and receive too many "strikes").

• *Session 1, Objective 2.* Group members and leaders get better acquainted (e.g., play the "pass the ball" game with each person naming the person to his or her right when that person has the ball).

• *Session 1, Objective 3.* Focus on individual perceptual processes: (1) Continue to play the "pass the ball" game with each person stating something alike and something different between him- or herself and the person who threw the ball. (2) Children are shown a stimulus picture displaying a somewhat ambiguous social problem, and each member describes (in a tape recorder) what he or she sees. Members listen to the tape and discuss what they saw that was alike and different.

• *Session 2, Objective.* Introduce the concept of setting and realizing goals: (1) A "goal" is defined. (2) The overall goal of the program is reviewed (i.e., to learn problem-solving and anger coping skills). (3) Goal sheets are introduced; each member works on one goal related to anger coping or self-control per week in the classroom. (4) Group members generate a goal for the coming week; goals should be described as an observable behavior and should be relevant and challenging but within reachable limits. Group members vote to approve all goals. (5) A level of performance needed to reach the goal (e.g., 3 of 5 days) is determined and written on the sheet. (6) Members are told they are solely responsible for their goal sheet. (7) Leaders explain that each member can earn a point for meeting his or her goal. Individual rewards can also be combined with group rewards (e.g., 10 minutes in a fun activity if all members meet their goal for the week).

- *Session 3, Objective 1.* Assess group problem-solving skills: (1) Members are asked to get a puppet from a central location, whereas leaders have provided enough puppets for all but one group member. Members' problem-solving skills for this situation are observed. (2) Each member states how he or she tried to solve the problem, and alternative solutions are discussed.

- *Session 3, Objective 2.* Introduce the concepts of self-talk, distraction techniques, and relaxation methods as affecting feelings and reactions: (1) One of the leaders uses a puppet to model self-talk and distraction techniques when being teased. (2) Each member selects a puppet for the "practicing self-control game" and uses self-talk and other techniques to control anger while the puppet is being teased by other group members. The self-control techniques used are discussed. (3) The activity is repeated with an emphasis on what the puppet says to himself to stay calm.

- *Session 4, Objective 1.* Review concepts of anger coping or self-control (i.e., have members relate the puppet "practicing self-control" game to real-life experiences).

- *Session 4, Objective 2.* Practice using anger coping or self-control: (1) Members try to remember 10 playing cards in 5 seconds while being teased by other group members; the member with the most correct numbers wins. (2) Group members discuss how difficult or easy it was to keep attention focused on the cards while being teased. (3) Members build a domino tower using one hand while being teased by other group members; the member with the highest tower in 30 seconds wins. (4) Group members discuss how one could be successful at this activity, with an emphasis on self-talk. (5) Leaders model using self-control while being teased and then members play the "practicing self-control" game with teasing directed at group members rather than puppets. (6) Feelings and coping techniques for this activity should be discussed, with an emphasis on self-talk that helps members "stay cool."

- *Session 5, Objective 1.* Establish the concept of perspective taking: (1) A stimulus picture is presented and different perceptions of the problem are elicited, with each member thinking of at least one new problem that could be happening. (2) Differences in interpretations are discussed.

- *Session 5, Objective 2.* Problem recognition is discussed: (1) Members role-play a problem from a stimulus picture, starting with what led up to the problem. Prior to the solution, group members "freeze," and a leader assumes the role of a roving reporter asking each member's perspective on the situation. (2) Differences in perspectives are discussed with an emphasis on the fact that it is often difficult to tell what others' intentions are. (3) Group members summarize what they have learned on perspective taking and are encouraged to look for real-life situations in the next week.

- *Session 6, Objective.* Elaborate the possibility for differing interpretations of a situation, focusing on how anger gets involved: (1) Members role-play a problem and repeat the roving reporting exercise. (2) Group members exchange roles and repeat the role-play.

(3) Group members discuss different perspectives in the role-play. (4) The role-play is repeated again, and leaders ask for "Academy Award-winning" portrayals of anger (both verbal and nonverbal indicators). (5) The concept of anger and how it may range from mild irritation to intense rage is discussed. (6) Group members generate real-life examples of anger and how it affects social situations.

• *Session 7, Objective 1*. Identify physiological reactions to anger: (1) Discuss how we can recognize anger within ourselves and within others. (2) View a videotape that portrays the physiological aspects of anger arousal. (3) Group members discuss bodily changes that occur when one gets angry and how they can serve as signals that one is angry.

• *Session 7, Objective 2*. Explore the role of self-statements in coping with anger and redirecting behavior in a problem-solving manner: (1) Discuss the thought processes that usually accompany anger. (2) View a videotape that portrays two different types of self-statements, pausing after each set to discuss if members use these types of statements and whether they help solve the problem. (3) Discuss real-life experiences when members have become angry, including how body signals helped them know they were angry and what kinds of things they said to themselves.

• *Session 8, Objective 1*. Encourage the process of alternative generation, including all possible alternatives: (1) Brainstorm all possible solutions to a problem occurring for a group member in the past week (both positive and negative). (2) Determine if each solution involved anger coping or self-control.

• *Session 8, Objective 2*. Establish the idea of consequences as what happens after a choice is made and as something to be considered in deciding on a choice: (1) Leaders generally discuss what a consequence is and that a consequence can be positive or negative. (2) Group members determine a possible consequence for each solution choice for one of the previous problems. (3) Members then rate each consequence as either good or bad and discuss.

• *Session 9, Objective*. Review the steps of social problem solving beginning with identifying that there is a problem through consideration of consequences: (1) Write down the steps of the problem-solving process (e.g., using a flow chart format). (2) Apply the problem-solving process to problems group members had during the week.

• *Session 10, Objective*. Present the problem-solving model in action: (1) Tell members that they will make a videotape to show how anger coping works. (2) View a videotape of a conflict between a boy and his teacher. Stop the tape and discuss after each alternative. (3) Encourage group members to generate ideas for their own videotape.

• *Session 11, Objective 1*. Identify a school problem for videotaping: (1) Ask group members for ideas for problem situations in school involving anger arousal. (2) Determine three or four choices for solving the problem and what consequences would follow (have choices involving anger coping and at least one that does not). (3) Decide which problem to videotape.

• *Session 11, Objective 2*. Desensitize the group to being on camera (i.e., give each group member an opportunity to be on camera informally so that he or she will be less likely to "act silly" when the actual taping of the problem stem occurs).

• *Session 12, Objective*. Tape the problem situation, leading into an initial inappropriate, aggressive action with a negative consequence for the aggressive child: (1) Write a script for the problem stem, assign roles, and arrange scenery. (2) Provide several dress rehearsals of role-plays of the problem stem. (3) Allow the group to watch and critique their videotaped rehearsals. (4) A roving reporter or narrator can comment on the action while the actors are frozen in place.

- *Session 13, Objective 1.* Prepare for taping of alternatives and consequences: (1) Watch the final taped version of the problem stem. (2) Prepare needed additional props.
- *Session 13, Objective 2.* Videotape a clear representation of each alternative solution (i.e., those that involve self-control and anger coping) and its subsequent consequence.
- *Sessions 14–18.* During the closing sessions, concepts presented during the previous sessions are reviewed and techniques are applied to the group members' real-life situations. Goal sheets and the point system continue throughout the remainder of the program.
- *Sessions 14–18, Objective 1.* View the finished videotape with comments.
- *Sessions 14–18, Objective 2.* Produce videotapes of other problems, alternatives, and consequences (e.g., a focus on conflicts with adults rather than with peers). Alternatively, members can create a cartoon scenario/comic book for a problem-solving situation.
- *Sessions 14–18, Objective 3.* Social problem solving is reviewed, and other members (rather than leaders) should be encouraged to aid with recall.
- *Sessions 14–18, Objective 4.* Leaders review the progress that group member have made in anger coping, using specific examples such as their progress on their goal sheets.
- *Sessions 14–18, Objective 5.* Preview how anger coping skills can be used in the future.
- *Positive feedback and optional free time.* Although each session has certain objectives, all 18 sessions end with positive feedback and free time. During positive feedback, group members are asked to identify one positive thing about themselves and/or one positive thing about another group member. Leaders should shape comments to focus on positive behaviors and good use of problem-solving skills rather than vague compliments or concrete statements about physical characteristics. At this time, points earned during group are tallied and added to the total, and children have the option of purchasing a prize from the prize box.

Free play is optional (if time allows). Leaders should monitor the children's activities and encourage "problem solving in action" if conflict arises (i.e., identify the problem, discuss choices and consequences, select a solution, and plan ways to avoid the problem in the future). Free play also provides an opportunity for leaders to reinforce prosocial behavior (e.g., sharing and following group rules).

Skills and Accomplishments Emphasized in Treatment

With a focus on anger arousal and social-cognitive processes, the Anger Coping Program targets development of several skills found to be poorly developed in angry and aggressive children. Such skills include awareness of negative feelings, use of self-talk and distraction techniques to decrease anger arousal and perspective-taking, goal-setting, and problem-solving skills. The concepts presented in session 8 are the most critical components of the anger coping model in terms of leading to behavior change (Lochman et al., 1999). Given their predisposition to believe that angry behaviors lead to desired outcomes, it is important for members to come to view anger as a problem with which they need to cope and to begin to look at alternative solutions, which will lead to better consequences when they are angry. Use of weekly goal sheets promotes generalization of skills learned in group sessions to other environments such as the classroom.

Duration and How to Determine When Treatment Is "Finished"

The Anger Coping Program is a manualized treatment lasting 18 sessions with approximately one session per week. Ideally, following treatment, group members will show improvements in the targeted skills as outlined previously. An individual child's improvements can be tracked across his or her weekly goal sheets and can be observed through the child's behavior in group, including his or her ability to generate nonaggressive solutions to problems. In addition, assessment techniques used to collect data prior to group can be readministered to determine individual change following the intervention. A child may require some follow-up, including possible individual "booster sessions" to continue improvements and/or to maintain gains. If a child exhibits significant behavioral difficulties after participation in the group, a decision regarding a referral for therapy services should be made. Approximately one-third of children receiving the Anger Coping Program in clinical settings have needed some type of continued involvement in treatment following the conclusion of the program.

Related Program: The Coping Power Program—Child and Parent Components

The Coping Power Program is an extension of the Anger Coping Program and includes 33 child sessions to be delivered over a 15-month period, as well as a 16-session parent component delivered during the same period. The additional child group sessions allows for coverage of other problem areas associated with aggression in children, such as advanced emotional awareness skills, relaxation training, and positive social and personal goals (Lochman & Wells, 1996; Lochman, Wells, & Murray, in press). Likewise, the additional child sessions focus on enhancing social skills, involving methods of entering new peer groups, and using positive peer networks (focus on negotiations and cooperation during structured and unstructured interactions with peers) and coping with peer pressure. In addition, the group sessions are augmented with regular individual meetings (at least monthly) to aid in generalization of skills.

Parent group sessions address use of social learning techniques, such as identifying prosocial and disruptive behavioral targets for children using specific operational terms, rewarding and attending to appropriate child behaviors, giving effective instructions and establishing age-appropriate rules and expectations for children in the home, and applying effective consequences to negative child behaviors (Lochman & Wells, 1996; Lochman et al., in press). Parents also learn ways to manage child behavior outside the home and to establish ongoing family communication structures (such as weekly family meetings). In addition to these "standard" parenting skills, parents learn additional techniques that support the social-cognitive and problem-solving skills that their children learn in the child component. For example, parents learn techniques for managing sibling conflict in the home and to apply the problem-solving model to family problem solving, as well as how to set up homework support structures and to reinforce organizational skills around homework completion. Finally, the parent component includes sessions on stress management for parents. Part of the rationale for this component is to help parents learn to remain calm and in control during stressful or irritating disciplinary interactions with their children (Lochman & Wells, 1996). Periodic home visits to parents are also used to generalize skills.

In an enhanced version of the Coping Power Program, a third component involving teacher intervention has been added. This component involves five 2-hour teacher inservice meetings and ongoing teacher consultation. The teachers learn about the Coping

Power Program and how they can reinforce the skills being presented in the program to the children. Each meeting includes a combination of didactic presentation of information on the topic of that day, as well as time for teacher problem solving around the topic. The didactic content is designed to promote children's bonding to school and to peers, to prevent early antisocial behavior, and to enhance the home–school connections.

The manual for the Anger Coping Program can be found in Lochman et al. (1999) and in Larson and Lochman (2002). The manuals for the Coping Power Program are being prepared for dissemination.

EVIDENCE FOR THE EFFECTS OF TREATMENT

The Anger Coping Program has been evaluated in two studies that included random assignment of children to an anger coping condition and to an untreated control condition (Lochman, Burch, Curry, & Lampron, 1984; Lochman, Lampron, Gemmer, Harris, & Wyckoff, 1989). In addition, one study has compared two versions of the program, using random assignment (Lochman & Curry, 1986), and one study has used a quasi-experimental design to compare different treatment lengths (Lochman, 1985). Two studies have examined follow-up effects of the program (Lochman, 1992; Lochman & Lampron, 1988), and one study has examined moderator variables (Lochman, Lampron, Burch, & Curry, 1985). More recent variants of the Anger Coping Program which have been studied with randomized designs include the Social Relations Program (Lochman, Coie, Underwood, & Terry, 1993) and the Coping Power Program (e.g., Lochman & Wells, 2002b). Treatment effects have been evaluated, in different studies, with behavioral checklists completed by teachers and by parents, by behavioral observations of children's behaviors in classrooms, by peer sociometric ratings, and by measures of the child and parent processes which were the targets of the intervention. The following sections provide an overview of the results of these studies.

Anger Coping Outcome Effects

A preliminary uncontrolled study of a school-based Anger Control Program for 12 aggressive children (11 boys and 1 girl) in the second and third grades (age range = 7–10 years) showed significant posttreatment reductions in teacher-reported aggressive behavior and trends for reductions in teacher checklist ratings of acting-out behavior (Lochman et al., 1981). These improvements in children's aggressive behavior were accompanied by increases in teachers' daily ratings of children's on-task behavior in the classroom. All the children were African American and lived in single-family homes in a low-income urban neighborhood. The children met with a graduate student therapist twice a week for 12 sessions. These findings spurred a programmatic series of subsequent studies comparing the further-refined Anger Coping Program to alternative interventions and untreated control conditions.

In a subsequent study, 76 aggressive boys were randomly assigned to anger coping (AC), goal setting (GS), anger coping plus goal setting (AC + GS), or untreated control (UC) cells (Lochman et al., 1984). The boys were identified as aggressive based on teacher checklist ratings. The boys were in fourth through sixth grades (age range = 9–12 years), and 53% were African American, 47% Caucasian. They participated in a 12-week AC group program, based on the earlier Anger Control Program. Boys met in weekly group sessions, lasting 45–60 minutes, in their elementary schools. Groups were co-led by university-based project staff (psychologists, social workers, psychology interns) and by school counselors based at each school. Goal setting was conceptualized as a minimal treatment condition and included eight group sessions in which boys set weekly goals for classroom behaviors and received contingent reinforcements for goal attainment. In comparison to the UC and GS conditions, aggressive boys in the AC cells (AC, AC + GS) displayed less parent-reported aggressive behavior, had lower rates of independent observers' time-sampled ratings of boys' disruptive classroom behavior, and tended to have higher levels of self-esteem at posttreatment. The addition of a GS component, in the AC + GS cell tended to enhance the treatment effects of the program (Lochman et al., 1984), indicating that behavioral goal setting can increase the generalization of cognitive-behavioral intervention effects.

The Anger Coping Program effects have been found to be augmented by the use of an 18-session version of the program, in comparison to the earlier 12-session version (Lochman, 1985). In this quasi-experimental study, 22 teacher-identified aggressive boys (55% African American; 45% Caucasian; mean age = 10 years, 4 months) received an 18-session version of the Anger Coping Program (with more emphasis on perspective taking, role playing, and more problem solving about anger-provoking situations) and were compared to the boys who had received the 12-session program in the Lochman et al. (1984) study. With the longer 18-session program, aggressive boys displayed significantly greater improvement in on-task behavior and greater reduction in passive off-task behavior, illustrating the need for longer intervention periods for children with chronic acting-out behavior problems.

However, in two other studies of the effects of variations in delivery of the Anger Coping Program, the addition of a five-session teacher consultation component (Lochman et al., 1989) and a self-instruction training component focusing on academic tasks (Lochman & Curry, 1986) did not enhance intervention effects. Lochman et al. (1989) had randomly assigned 32 boys (31% African American; 69% Caucasian; mean age = 11 years, 0 months) to AC, to AC plus Teacher Consultation, or to a UC condition. Lochman and Curry (1986) assigned 20 teacher-identified aggressive boys (50% African American; 50% Caucasian; mean age − 10 years, 3 months) either to AC or to AC plus Self-Instruction Training. In both studies, the school-based groups lasted for 18 weekly sessions, and the boys in the AC conditions did display reductions in parent-rated aggression (Lochman & Curry, 1986), reductions in teacher-rated aggression (Lochman et al., 1989), improvements in perceived social competence and self-esteem (Lochman & Curry, 1986; Lochman et al., 1989), and reductions in off-task classroom behavior (Lochman & Curry, 1986; Lochman et al., 1989). The Lochman et al. (1989) findings, in comparison to an untreated control condition, replicated the earlier positive effects for the Anger Coping Program evident in the Lochman et al. (1984) study.

Two other studies have examined the follow-up effects of the Anger Coping Program. Lochman and Lampron (1988) conducted a partial follow-up of the Lochman et al. (1984) sample in four of the eight schools. In the follow-up sample, 21 boys had received the Anger Coping Program, and 10 had been in the UC condition (39% African American; 61% Caucasian; mean age = 11 years, 7 months). When children's classroom behavior was examined at a 7-month follow-up, the AC boys had significantly improved levels of independently observed on-task classroom behavior and significant reductions in passive off-task behavior.

At a 3-year follow-up when boys were 15 years old on average, boys who received the Anger Coping Program training (n = 31) exhibited lower levels of marijuana and drug involvement and lower rates of alcohol use and maintained their increases in self-esteem and problem-solving skills (Lochman, 1992) in comparison to a UC condition ($n = 52$). Boys who were followed up were highly similar on peer aggression nominations and social status ratings to boys who were not available for follow-up. These results indicate that the Anger Coping Program produced long-term maintenance of social-cognitive gains and important prevention effects of adolescent substance use. The AC boys functioning in these domains were within the range of a nonaggressive comparison group ($n = 62$), indicating the clinical significance of these positive effects. However, the AC boys did not have significant reductions in delinquent behavior at follow-up, and their reductions in independently observed off-task behavior and parent-rated aggression were maintained only for a subset of AC boys who had received a brief six-session booster intervention for themselves and their parents in the school year following their initial AC group. Thus, across multiple controlled intervention studies, this child-centered cognitive-behavioral intervention reduced children's disruptive behaviors immediately after treatment and provided important preventive effects on adolescent substance use. Booster interventions in subsequent years may lead to less dissipation of treatment effects on children's overtly aggressive–disruptive behavior.

Moderation of Anger Coping Program Effects

AC boys who had the greatest reductions in parent-rated aggression in the Lochman et al. (1984) study were boys who initially had higher levels of peer rejection, more comorbid internalizing symptoms, and the poorest problem-solving skills (Lochman et al., 1985). The latter variable was a particularly important predictor of treatment effectiveness because boys with the poorest social problem-solving skills in the UC condition were likely to have increasingly higher levels of aggressive behavior by the end of the school year.

Social Relations Program Outcome Effects

In another study of child characteristics which predict intervention outcomes, Lochman et al. (1993) found that a social relations program which included the AC components addressing anger management and social problem-solving skills along with additional social skill training components had significant impact at postintervention and at a 1-year follow-up with aggressive-rejected fourth-grade children but not with rejected-only children. Relative to control conditions, the intervention aggressive-rejected children had reductions in peer-rated and teacher-rated aggressive behavior. This study involved an African American sample of fourth-grade children from an inner-city area. The intervention appeared to influence the mediator variables associated with children's aggressive behavior but did not influence mediator variables associated with nonaggressive peer rejection.

Coping Power Program Outcome Effects

The Coping Power Program (Lochman & Wells, 1996) is a lengthier, multicomponent version of the Anger Coping Program designed to enhance outcome effects by providing an accompanying parent intervention component and by providing for stronger maintenance of gains over time by lengthening the intervention period to 15–18 months. Four grant-funded studies are currently in process to examine the efficacy of the Coping Power Program, and initial results have been obtained in two of these studies.

In the first of these studies (Lochman & Wells, 2002c), 183 boys (61% African American; 39% Caucasian) who had high rates of teacher-rated aggression in fourth or

fifth grade were randomly assigned to either a school-based Coping Power child component, to a combination Coping Power Program including both child and parent components, or to a UC condition. Intervention took place over two academic years (fourth and
fifth grades for some children; fifth and sixth grades for others). Outcome analyses have
indicated that the Coping Power intervention in this study produced lower rates of delinquent behavior and of parent-rated substance use at a 1-year follow-up than did the control cell, and these intervention effects were most apparent for the full Coping Power
Program with child and parent components (Lochman & Wells, 2002c). Boys also displayed teacher-rated behavioral improvements in school during the follow-up year, and
these effects were evident in both intervention conditions and appeared to be primarily
influenced by the Coping Power child component. The intervention effect on substance
use was stronger with boys from moderate-income families than boys from low-income
families, and the intervention-produced improvements in school behavior functioning
were more apparent for Caucasian boys than for African American boys. Normative
comparison analyses, with a nonrisk sample of 63 boys from the same schools, indicate
that the intervention has moved at-risk boys into normative ranges for substance use,
delinquency, and school behavior, in contrast to at-risk control boys who significantly
differ from the normative group on the latter two outcomes. The Coping Power intervention also had significant or trend effects at postintervention on variables assessing constructs that were central to the contextual social-cognitive model, including boys' social-
cognitive processes and schemas and caregivers' parenting behaviors. The intervention
effects at the Time 2 period immediately after the intervention indicated, in general, that
both intervention conditions had immediate impact on the potential mediator variables.

Path analyses with these outcome data indicate that the intervention effects were at
least partly mediated by changes in boys' social-cognitive processes, schemas, and parenting processes (Lochman & Wells, 2002a). Changes in social-cognitive appraisal
processes, involving boys' hostile attributions and resulting anger, and decision-making
processes, involving reductions in the boys' expectations that aggressive behavior would
lead to good outcomes for them, contributed to the boys' reduced risk for antisocial behavior. Similarly, changes in boys' schemas involving their beliefs about their degree of
internal control over successful outcomes and the complexity of their internal representa-
tions of others and changes in their perceptions of the consistency of the parents' discipline efforts led to lower levels of delinquency, substance use, and school behavioral
problems. Consistent with the assumptions of the contextual social-cognitive model used
here, boys' engagement in serious problem behavior in the year following their involvement in the Coping Power intervention was affected in part by the improvements in the
ways that they perceived and processed their social world and in their expectations of
more consistent and predictable responses from their parents.

In the second ongoing study of the Coping Power Program we are examining
whether the effects of the Coping Power Program, offered as an indicated prevention intervention for targeted high-risk aggressive children, can be enhanced by combining the
indicated intervention with a universal prevention intervention (Lochman & Wells,
2002b). The universal intervention was randomly offered to half of the fifth-grade teachers and consisted of in-service training for teachers and large-scale parent meetings for all
parents of children in universal intervention classrooms. The sample consisted of 245
male (66%) and female (34%) aggressive fourth-grade students (78% African American;
20% Caucasian) who were randomly assigned to one of four conditions: Indicated Intervention + Universal Intervention (II + UI), Indicated Intervention + Universal Control (II
+ UC), Indicated Control + Universal Intervention (IC + UI), and Indicated Control +

Universal Control (IC + UC). Intervention began in the fall of the fifth-grade year and continued midway through the sixth-grade year. Analyses of postintervention effects (Lochman & Wells, 2002b), comparing intervention to control conditions, indicate that the combined Coping Power Program plus the UI produced lower rates of self-reported substance use, lower teacher-rated aggression, higher perceived social competence, and greater teacher-rated behavioral improvement, indicating the value of nesting the Coping Power Program within a universal prevention program. The Coping Power intervention by itself produced reduced ratings of parent-rated proactive aggression, lower activity level by children, better teacher-rated peer acceptance of target children, and increased parental supportiveness. At a 1-year follow-up, all the intervention cells produced reductions in substance use and delinquency in comparison to the control condition, and the reduction in delinquency was most apparent for children who had received both interventions (Lochman & Wells, 2001).

Overall Evaluation of Anger Coping and Coping Power Programs

This series of research studies has indicated that a cognitive-behavioral intervention, using the Anger Coping framework, can have immediate effects at postintervention on children's aggressive behavior at home and at school, according to parent, teacher, and independent observer ratings. The effect sizes are typically in the moderate range, and moderators such as initial levels of problem-solving skills and family income level can affect the intervention effects on certain outcomes, indicating that not all children respond to this form of intervention. The Anger Coping Program can have lasting preventive effects on children's later substance use, up to 3 years later, but it appears to be necessary to include an adjunctive parent intervention component to have longer-term effects on children's delinquency. The most robust effects have been evident when teacher inservice training has also been offered as an adjunctive component. The results emphasize that this form of cognitive-behavioral intervention can be useful not only for short-term treatment purposes but also for longer-term prevention purposes, and that the program can be effectively delivered in school settings as an outreach program.

Implementation Issues

The next stage of evaluation with the Anger Coping Program has assessed the program's impact with an uncontrolled pre–post design, when the program is conducted in the field by trained school personnel rather than by the program developer's trained staff. In this dissemination phase, training consisting of three full-day workshop training sessions in the spring and summer prior to the implementation of the program, monthly 2-hour large-group consultation sessions during the implementation of the program, and two telephone "hot-line" hours per week during the implementation of the program was offered to all the psychologists and counselors in a school system (Lochman et al., 1998). The 161 students in 41 Anger Coping groups with at least partial pre–post data were an average of 9.8 years, ranging in age from 8 to 12 years. One hundred fifty of these children were male, and 11 were female. Eighty-one were of minority racial status (primarily African American). Forty-six percent of these children received free or reduced lunch, and 41% received special education services. Pre–post analyses indicated that changes in teacher ratings of children's social competence and in children's social problem-solving skills, with increases in their verbal assertion and compromise solutions and reductions in irrelevant solutions, were accompanied by positive improvements in the children's behavior. Parents reported that children's externalizing problem behaviors had declined by postintervention, and teachers' ratings indicated that children's social and attention problems had decreased. Teachers reported that 85% of the children had displayed at least some reduction in aggressive and disruptive behaviors. Because parents had also rated the children as having significant reductions in attention problems, the Anger Coping Program appears to assist children in better focusing their attention in appropriate ways at home and at school. These changes in attentional control may have partially mediated the reductions in externalizing behavior problems, as indicated by the significant correlation between these change scores.

Children's academic achievement was assessed by a state-created achievement measure. AC children had a 12% improvement at the 1-year follow-up in their rates of grade-level achievement in mathematics and reading, and this improvement was significantly higher than the systemwide improvement rate over the same period. The AC children also were found to have a significantly lower rate of increase in school suspensions than was evident for other children their age in this school system.

This dissemination evaluation has all the weaknesses of a design without a randomized control group, but it provides initial evidence that the Anger Coping Program can be effectively disseminated. Successful dissemination of the program will likely be affected by the ability of the practitioners to gain adequate parent and teacher involvement in the program, by practitioners' desire to implement the program, and by their degree of understanding of the underlying conceptual model, which will allow them to individualize the intervention appropriately as it is delivered.

DIRECTIONS FOR FUTURE RESEARCH

The clearest needs for the next steps in research on the Anger Coping and Coping Power programs will be ongoing studies of moderation and mediation effects and of longer-term follow-up. Although initial research has been conducted on each of these topics, it will be important to understand the longer term adjustment of individuals who have received these programs as they move through the adolescent years and into early adulthood to determine whether the intervention effects on children's social-cognitive processes and on their parents' behaviors, at the time of the middle school transition, can have meaningful impact on serious antisocial outcomes years later. Similarly, although suggestive information has been gathered about mediating and moderating processes, it is apparent that current efforts have accounted for only a small fraction of the variance in mediation and moderation processes. It will be necessary to consider, for example, how larger contextual factors such as the degree of violence and crime in the child's neighborhood can limit intervention effects. In addition, a clear strength of cognitive-behavioral interventions for conduct problem children has been that the intervention model for the Anger Coping and Coping Power Programs is based on a clear conceptual model of what the mutable mediating processes should be. However, despite interesting recent findings (Lochman & Wells, 2002a), limited research has attempted to confirm the mediational effects of changes in social-cognitive and parenting processes on change in behavior, as a result of the Anger Coping or Coping Power intervention. Thus, further research needs to examine whether the interventions have had an immediate proximal effect on an array of social-cognitive and parenting practices, and then whether these proximal effects lead to distal reductions in conduct disorder, delinquency, and substance abuse.

SUMMARY AND CONCLUSIONS

The next steps for intervention development and intervention research for these anger-management interventions include a focus on methods for maintaining and generalizing the effects over time, of maximizing effects by recognizing the multiple causal factors at multiple contextual levels contributing to children's aggressive behavior and then by addressing the children's contexts more broadly, of examining and controlling negative group processes, and of exploring and understanding the processes that lead to successful dissemination and implementation of the Anger Coping and Coping Power programs.

Our existing research (Lochman, 1992) has suggested in a preliminary, uncontrolled way that booster interventions can play a critical role in maintaining intervention effects with children's externalizing behaviors. Further intervention development needs to examine the optimal timing, intensity, and focus of booster interventions, as an effort to promote relapse prevention. Booster interventions can reinforce children's and parents' use of skills that they have learned during the intervention period and help them to problem-solve with their current social difficulties. These efforts will likely involve methods for assessing an individual child's level of current risk, because children who have completed intervention will represent a broad band of functioning ranging from clearly normal behavior to unimproved and quite seriously disturbed behavior, and then, as a result, for individualizing the planned booster intervention in a systematic way. When children begin discussing a current or recent social problem they have encountered, practitioners can respond by shifting to a problem-solving set and modeling and reinforcing problem-solving skills directly rather than rigidly sticking to planned activities for that day. It is critical that practitioners keep the overall objectives of the programs in mind, so that the practitioners' flexible responses can still have direct, strategic impact on the targeted social-cognitive difficulties of aggressive children and on the parenting behaviors of their parents.

Intervention research with aggressive children, including our own research on the Coping Power Program, indicates that cognitive-behavioral interventions with components that address both children's social-cognitive processes and parents' parenting practices produce broader positive effects and better maintenance of behavioral improvements over time than do interventions that focus on children or parents alone. In addition, our findings that the inclusion of a teacher-focused universal intervention can augment the effects of the Coping Power Program indicates the need for development and research on an integrated teacher-training component. Interventions that have child, parent, and teacher components can address a wider set of risk and protective factors, in a broader set of the children's interpersonal contexts, than can an intervention with single components (Conduct Problems Prevention Research Group, 1992). It will be critical to have teacher training that is tightly linked to the other components of the intervention and which will encourage teachers to facilitate parents' active, positive involvement in their children's academic development, as well as to reinforce the early, often fragile efforts by children to try out new methods for emotional regulation and negotiation of conflicts with peers and adults.

When cognitive-behavioral interventions, such as the Anger Coping and Coping Power programs, are delivered within the context of group therapy, the therapists have to be attentive to the development of negative group process among children and of possible iatrogenic effects which can occur when group members reinforce each others' deviant beliefs (Dishion & Andrews, 1995). Clearly, group processes and children's bonding to their therapists and to other children in the group need to be further researched, and methods for controlling deviancy training and for managing negative group process need to be refined. Structurally, to proactively minimize deviancy training, we have two group leaders with a small group of children (four to six), clear expectations and consequences for negative behavior during group (including deviant talk), and the potential to break into subgroups or into individual sessions if deviancy promotion by group members is chronic. During the course of group sessions, we attempt to enhance a positive group process by including positive feedback time from all group members at the end of group sessions; we include groupwide contingencies for earning group reinforcements which thus promote positive cooperative behavior among group members; and we encourage the group to plan prosocial group activities which can positively impact others outside the group (e.g., creating drug prevention posters which focus on handling peer pressure that can be mounted in their school). When disagreements and conflicts develop between group members during sessions, they can provide opportunities to directly model and reinforce the social-cognitive skills which are the focus of these cognitive-behavioral interventions, including finding ways to cool down, listening to the other person's point of view, getting a better understanding of the perspective of their peers, and using verbal assertion and negotiation skills under controlled conditions, while the group leaders provide coaching.

The next generation of intervention research should begin to examine factors in the training process and in the host systems (clinics, community agencies, schools) that affect the implementation and dissemination of the Anger Coping and Coping Power programs. Organizational climate (including openness of communication, leadership, and decision-making style) and readiness to change within agencies can have a direct impact on the enthusiasm and care with which new programs are implemented. Agency acceptance may be affected by the level of support for the program by key administrative personnel and by the staff's ability to review the program critically and to participate in its acceptance. Elements of the training process also may have a direct impact on the effectiveness of the intervention as it is delivered within the agency. One-shot workshops may not be optimal. Without ongoing training and consultation, practitioners may not be able to cope adaptively with the expected and unexpected problems which arise during the delivery of the Anger Coping and Coping Power programs. Research needs to examine these implementation and dissemination processes with a similar degree of scientific rigor as is apparent in clinical trial research.

ACKNOWLEDGMENTS

The intervention research on the Anger Coping and Coping Power programs has been supported by grants from the National Institute for Drug Abuse, the Center for Substance Abuse Prevention, the Centers for Disease Control and Prevention, the Department of Justice, and the National Institute of Mental Health.

REFERENCES

Conduct Problems Prevention Research Group. (1992). A developmental and clinical model for the prevention of conduct disorder: The Fast Track Program. *Development and Psychopathology, 4,* 509–527.

Crick, N. R., & Dodge, K. A. (1994). A review and reformulation of social information-processing mechanisms in children's social adjustment. *Psychological Bulletin, 115,* 74–101.

Dishion, T. J. & Andrews, D. W. (1995). Preventing escalation in problem behaviors with high-risk young adolescents: Immediate and 1-year outcomes. *Journal of Consulting and Clinical Psychology, 63,* 538–548.

Dodge, K. A., Lochman, J. E., Harnish, J. D., Bates, J. E., & Pettit, G. S. (1997). Reactive and proactive aggression in school children and psychiatrically-impaired chronically-assaultive youth. *Journal of Abnormal Psychology, 106,* 37–51.

Larson, J., & Lochman, J. E. (2002). *Helping school children cope with anger: A cognitive-behavioral intervention.* New York: Guilford Press.

Lochman, J. E. (1985). Effects of different treatment lengths in cognitive-behavioral interventions with aggressive boys. *Child Psychiatry and Human Development, 16,* 45–56.

Lochman, J. E. (1992). Cognitive-behavioral interventions with aggressive boys: Three-year follow-up and preventive effects. *Journal of Consulting and Clinical Psychology, 60,* 426–432.

Lochman, J. E., Burch, P. P., Curry, J. F., & Lampron, L. B. (1984). Treatment and generalization effects of cognitive-behavioral and goal setting interventions with aggressive boys. *Journal of Consulting and Clinical Psychology, 52,* 915–916.

Lochman, J. E., Coie, J. D., Underwood, M., & Terry, R. (1993). Effectiveness of a social relations intervention program for aggressive and nonaggressive rejected children. *Journal of Consulting and Clinical Psychology, 61,* 1053–1058.

Lochman, J. E., & Curry, J. F. (1986). Effects of social problem-solving training and self-instruction training with aggressive boys. *Journal of Clinical Child Psychology, 63,* 549–559.

Lochman, J. E., & Dodge, K. A. (1994). Social-cognitive processes of severely violent, moderately aggressive, and nonaggressive boys. *Journal of Consulting and Clinical Psychology, 62,* 366–374.

Lochman, J. E., FitzGerald, D. P., & Whidby, J. M. (1999). Anger management with aggressive children. In C. Schaefer (Ed.), *Short-term psychotherapy groups for children* (pp. 301–349). Northvale, NJ: Jason Aronson.

Lochman, J. E., & Lampron, L. B. (1988). Cognitive behavioral intervention for aggressive boys: Seven month follow-up effects. *Journal of Child and Adolescent Psychotherapy, 5,* 15–23.

Lochman, J. E., Lampron, L. B., Burch, P. R., & Curry, J. E. (1985). Client characteristics associated with behavior change for treated and untreated boys. *Journal of Abnormal Child Psychology, 13,* 527–538.

Lochman, J. E., Lampron, L .B., Gemmer, T. C., Harris, S. R., & Wyckoff, G. M. (1989). Teacher consultation and cognitive-behavioral interventions with aggressive boys. *Psychology in the Schools, 26,* 179–188.

Lochman, J. E., Nelson, W. M., & Sims, J. P. (1981). A cognitive behavioral program for use with aggressive children. *Journal of Clinical Child Psychology, 13,* 146–148.

Lochman, J. E., Rahmani, C. H., Flagler, S. L., Nyko-Silva, I., Ross, J. J., & Johnson, J. L. (1998). *Dissemination of the Anger Coping Program.* Unpublished manuscript, University of Alabama, Tuscaloosa, AL.

Lochman, J. E., & Wells, K. C. (1996). A social-cognitive intervention with aggressive children: Prevention effects and contextual implementation issues. In R. Peters & R. J. McMahon (Eds.), *Prevention and early intervention: Childhood disorders, substance use and delinquency* (pp. 111–143). Thousand Oaks, CA: Sage.

Lochman, J. E., & Wells, K. C. (2001, August). *Coping Power prevention program for preadolescent children: Intervention effects at a one-year follow-up.* Paper presented at the annual convention of the American Psychological Association, San Francisco.

Lochman, J. E., & Wells, K. C. (2002a). Contextual social cognitive mediators and child outcome: A test of the theoretical model in the Coping Power Program. *Development and Psychopathology.*

Lochman, J. E., & Wells, K. C. (2002b). The Coping Power Program at the middle school transition: Universal and indicated prevention effects. *Psychology of Addictive Behaviors, 16,* 540–554.

Lochman, J. E., & Wells, K. C. (2002c). *The Coping Power Program for preadolescent aggressive boys and their parents: Outcome effects at the one-year follow-up.* Manuscript submitted for publication.

Lochman, J. E., Wells, K. C., & Murray, M. (in press). The Coping Power Program: Preventive intervention at the middle school transition. In J. Szapocznik, P. Tolan, & S. Sambrano (Eds.), *Preventing substance abuse: 3 to 14.* Washington, DC: American Psychological Association.

Lochman, J. E., Whidby, J. M., & FitzGerald, D. P. (2000). In P. C. Kendall (Ed.), *Child and adolescent therapy* (2nd ed., pp. 31–87). New York: Guilford Press.

Loeber, R. (1990). Development and risk factors of juvenile antisocial behavior and delinquency. *Clinical Psychology Review, 10,* 1–42.

Patterson, G. R., Reid, J. B., & Dishion, T. J. (1992). *Antisocial boys.* Eugene, OR: Castalia.

16

Antisocial Behavior in Children and Adolescents

The Oregon Multidimensional Treatment Foster Care Model

PATRICIA CHAMBERLAIN AND DANA K. SMITH

OVERVIEW

Disruptive behavior is the most frequent reason children are brought into mental health clinics and accounts for more than half of the referrals to such clinics in the United States. It has been estimated that between 1 and 4 million children and adolescents in the United States today exhibit conduct problems, and that delinquent individuals between the ages of 12 and 19 represent the most violent age group in the nation when arrests for assault, rape, and theft are calculated (U.S. Department of Justice, 1994). Severely delinquent acts by adolescents and young adults are quite prevalent in the United States, where the homicide rate for 15- to 24-year-olds is four times the rate of other industrialized countries (Fingerhut & Kleinman, 1990; World Health Organization, 1992). These statistics are alarming and make evident that such behaviors are disruptive to individuals, families, and communities. The good news is that researchers have made substantial progress in understanding the development and treatment of antisocial behavior, and scholars have identified a predictable developmental course (e.g., Patterson, Reid, & Dishion, 1992).

The Oregon Multidimensional Treatment Foster Care (MTFC) Program is a community-based treatment program that is based on over 30 years of longitudinal research on the development and treatment of antisocial behavior. The Oregon MTFC model was first developed in the early 1980s as an alternative to institutional-, residential-, and group-care placements for youth with severe and chronic delinquent behavior and has since been extended to work with children and adolescents (and their families) referred from both mental health and child welfare service systems. Four randomized trials have been completed on MTFC, and three additional randomized trials are currently under way. In this chapter, we focus on describing the studies with youth referred from the juvenile justice system. Applications of MTFC to child welfare and mental health populations are discussed only briefly here (additional details can be found in Chamberlain, Moreland, & Reid, 1992; Chamberlain & Price, 2002; Chamberlain & Reid, 1991; Fisher, Gunnar, Chamberlain, & Reid, 2000; Smith, Stormshak, Chamberlain, & Bridges-Whaley, 2001). This chapter briefly reviews the theory underlying the MTFC model, the goals of the intervention, and the characteristics of the youth from juvenile justice who have participated. We examine staff roles and present data on the evidence for effectiveness of the model. Finally, we provide findings from a cost–benefit analysis, and briefly discuss issues relating to dissemination and replication of MTFC.

Conceptual Model and Underlying Assumptions

The MTFC model is based on social learning theory. Within that theory, the individual's behavior, attitudes, and emotions are thought to be highly responsive to influences provided by the contexts in which they live. New behaviors are thought to be most effectively taught and learned through *in vivo* experiences. In this light, MTFC was designed as a "naturalistic" method of providing treatment to severely troubled youths through intensive daily support and carefully guided interventions that take place in a relatively nonrestrictive, family-style, community-based setting.

Over the past 20 years, empirically supported, community-based models such as MTFC have gained in popularity as cost-efficient, effective alternatives for treating youth needing out-of-home care (e.g., Mendel, 2000; Rivera & Kutash, 1994), yet group homes, residential treatment facilities, and state training schools continue to be the most common placements for such youth, especially for those with chronic and severe antisocial behavior (Elliott, 1998). Although residential programs typically provide on-site treatment in preparation for a youth's inevitable return to the community, residential treatment approaches tend to focus on group therapies and operate with minimal family involvement (see Chamberlain, 1999, for review). In addition, the majority of the time that youth spend in such settings is in the company of other youth with similar problems. This provides a lot of time for youth with problem behaviors to associate with other troubled youth. Unfortunately, such contexts create and extend opportunities for further bonding, socialization, and delinquency skill training by an antisocial peer group. Association with delinquent peers has been shown in several studies to result in increased risk for the maintenance and enhancement of delinquent behavior (e.g., Dishion, McCord, & Poulin, 1999; Elliott, Huizinga, & Ageton, 1985).

In addition to evidence demonstrating the negative effects of deviant peer association, there is also ample evidence that effective parenting can have a powerful socializing role and positive influence on troubled youth (see Smith, Sprengelmeyer, & Moore, in press, for review). Researchers at Oregon Social Learning Center and elsewhere (Prinz & Miller, 1994; Webster-Stratton & Hammond, 1997) have conducted extensive research detailing the processes by which social-interactional learning takes place in the family context. Parent–child interactions have been shown to shape the development of both prosocial and antisocial behaviors. In families with children who have high levels of antisocial behavior, parents have been shown to be more likely to reinforce their child inadvertently for negative behaviors. For example, if a parent fails to follow through on a consequence (e.g., if you grab at the candy, you cannot have it) in the face of a child pushing limits (e.g., child screams and grabs at the candy, parent gives her the candy), both the behavior of the child (screaming and grabbing) and the behavior of the parent (giving in) are reinforced. The parent is reinforced because the child quits screaming when the parent gives in and the child is reinforced for pushing limits by getting his or her way. This mutually reinforcing dynamic results in a coercive family process that facilitates the escalation of negative and coercive behaviors that, over time, become entrenched and amplified in the family setting.

As a youth reaches school age, the antisocial behaviors and coercive processes in which they engaged in their families begin to spread out to their school and peer relations. By the time such youth reach adolescence, they are associating with other youth who engage in antisocial behavior and are becoming more and more immune to the typical socializing processes that teach teens the skills they need to be successful young adults. Without effective intervention, such youth are at high risk for delinquency, school failure and dropout, chronic family problems, and drug use (Reid & Eddy, 1997).

The MTFC model was designed to take advantage of the potential positive socializing influence of the family and as an alternative to treating delinquent youth in aggregate-care settings. Although the MTFC model focuses initially on treating youth while they are in out-of-home care, the model clearly provides components that address the difficulties of reintegrating seriously troubled youth back into their homes and communities. Youth are placed one per foster home and are provided with intensive support and treatment within a setting that closely mirrors the "real world" (i.e., community-based, foster family setting). In addition, intensive parent management training is provided weekly to biological parents (or other after-care resource) beginning at the outset of their child's MTFC placement. By providing treatment in a family setting and focusing treatment on the youth and his or her family, MTFC not only reduces difficulties associated with generalizing treatment gains to a new setting (i.e., foster care is a smaller "jump" to the home setting than an inpatient facility) but also capitalizes on the power of the family environment to increase prosocial behavior by providing moment-by-moment teaching and reinforcement in the foster and biological home, all of which increase the likelihood that treatment gains will be maintained long term.

Goals of MTFC for Youth Referred from Juvenile Justice

There are two major aims of MTFC: (1) To create opportunities for youth to live successfully in their communities while providing them with intensive supervision, support, and skill development, and (2) to simultaneously prepare their parents (or other after-care resource) to provide effective parenting that will increase the chance for positive reintegration into the family following placement.

Placements in MTFC typically last from 6 to 9 months. The aim is to implement an intensive, well-coordinated set of interventions (e.g., family and individual therapy, skill training, academic support, case management, and psychiatric consultation for medication management) across multiple settings (e.g., home, school, peer group, and community). Involvement of each youth's family or after-care resource is emphasized from the beginning of the youth's placement in MTFC in an effort to maximize training and prepare for posttreatment. Four key elements of treatment are targeted during placement and aftercare: (1) providing youth with a consistent reinforcing environment where they are mentored and encouraged to perform specific behaviors or tasks designed to increase their skill base, (2) providing daily structure with clear expectations and limits, as well as well-specified consequences delivered in a teaching-oriented manner, (3) providing close supervision of youth's whereabouts, and (4) avoiding deviant peer associations while providing support and assistance in establishing prosocial peer contacts.

Populations Where MTFC Has Been Tested

Four randomized trials have been conducted on the MTFC model, including a study with boys referred from juvenile justice (Chamberlain & Reid, 1998; Eddy & Chamberlain, 2000), a study with girls referred from juvenile justice (Chamberlain & Leve, 2002; Chamberlain & Moore, 2002), a study with children and adolescents leaving a state mental hospital (Chamberlain & Reid, 1991), and a study with children from three Oregon counties in state-supported foster care (Chamberlain et al., 1992). In addition, three randomized trials are currently under way (see section "Dissemination and Replication of the MTFC Approach"). Referrals to MTFC are made by community agencies (i.e., departments of juvenile justice, child welfare, and mental health) and typically involve cases with complex comorbid conditions and histories of multiple placement failures.

Youth referred to MTFC from juvenile justice departments are between the ages of 12 and 17 and have been involved in serious criminal offending behavior in the community (mean offenses for boys = 14, girls = 11). All youth are court-mandated to out-of-home placement prior to referral to MTFC. Most of these youth have been involved in numerous treatment efforts prior to their referral to MTFC, and most have experienced at least one failed out-of-home placement prior to referral (means = 1.3 previous placements for boys and 3.1 for girls). Table 16.1 presents other youth characteristics and risk factors.

The Treatment Program

A team consisting of the MTFC parent(s), program supervisor, family therapist (for the biological, adoptive, or other after-care family), individual therapist (for the youth), be-

TABLE 16.1. Sample Description and Risk Factors for Boys and Girls at Baseline

	Boys (n = 79)	Girls (n = 61)
Age in years	14.4	15.1
Single parent family at present (%)	57.0	71.2
Adopted (%)	9.1	8.2
Family income less than $10,000 (%)	37.3	35.7
Number of crimes committed (by self)	13.5	13.1
Biological mother was convicted of crime (%)	21.6	46.7
Biological father was convicted of crime (%)	31.3	63.2
At least one parent convicted of crime (%)	41.1	70.0
At least one sibling was institutionalized (%)	20.0	37.3
Experienced (documented) physical abuse (%)	5.7	65.6
Experienced (documented) sexual abuse (%)	6.8	72.1
Attempted suicide (%)	2.6	58.3
Characterized as heavy drug or alcohol user (%)	9.3	82.0
Pregnant at least once (%)	N/A	29.3
Number of prior treatment placements	1.33	3.03
Ran away at least once (%)	73.7	91.7

Note. Unless otherwise noted, data are from referral agent and/or parent. Significance tests compare boys to girls.

havioral support specialist, and consulting psychiatrist conducts the treatment intervention. The foster parent recruiter/trainer provides support to the team as well as to the foster parents through daily telephone calls with the foster parents that measure youth daily behaviors and levels of foster parent stress. Implementation of the program will be discussed in the context of each team member's role.

MTFC Treatment Team Roles

Interventions are implemented across multiple settings (i.e., in the MTFC home, school, family home, and community). The goal is to coordinate and time interventions to gradually increase youth skill levels (i.e., positive functioning in the foster home, academic achievement, and prosocial peer and adult relationships) and decrease problem behaviors across each setting in which a youth is involved. Youth are provided with close supervision, consistent limit setting and contingencies, and positive adult mentoring. Simultaneously, the aim is to prepare the youth's family for reunification. Due to the potentially complex nature of implementing interventions in multiple settings using a number of different modes (e.g., individual therapy, family therapy, contingency management in the MTFC home, and psychiatric consultation), the roles of treatment team and staff members are clearly defined and involve little overlap.

Role of the MTFC Parents

MTFC parents are recruited, screened, trained, and supervised by the foster parent recruiter/trainer and program supervisors. They participate in a 20-hour preservice training conducted by experienced MTFC foster parents. Program supervisors provide MTFC parents with ongoing support and supervision in the form of weekly foster parent meetings and daily telephone contact. Training follows a social learning and behavioral model, where foster parents are taught to provide youth with frequent reinforcement and clear and consistent limits. Treatment foster parents have extensive contact with youth, making their role an extremely important and integral part of the overall treatment process. Treatment foster parents are taught methods for turning problem situations into teaching opportunities, for giving feedback to youth on a daily basis through the use of the point-and-level system, and for responding to youth aggression in nonreactive ways.

MTFC parents implement a daily behavior management system that has been tailored to meet the needs of each youth. MTFC parents are trained and supervised to use this system to provide feedback to youths on their behavior for a variety of daily expectations (e.g., getting up on time, attending school, positive behavior in class and at home, following directions, maturity, and positive attitude). Youth earn points for positive behaviors and lose points for negative, undesirable, or maladaptive behaviors. MTFC parents exchange points for privileges that increase as a youth progresses through the program. Consequences for rule violations and minor behavior problems consist of privilege removal (e.g., loss of phone or TV for short periods) or work chores (e.g., raking leaves). Each day, point levels are reported to the program supervisor via a telephone interview using the Parent Daily Report Checklist (PDR; Chamberlain & Reid, 1987). Privilege removal and work chores are typically prescribed for short durations in an effort to teach and encourage youth to "recover" from negative instances and quickly resume positive and adaptive behaviors. Short stays in detention can be used as a response to extreme problem behaviors, such as violent behavior or other serious probation or parole violations.

No educational requirements have been specified for MTFC foster parents; however, we have found that successful MTFC foster parents have many things in common—in particular, the willingness to work as part of a team and implement a structured daily program, the ability to take another's perspective and avoid emotionally reactive responses, basic knowledge of child development (i.e., age-appropriate expectations for behavior), and the flexibility and humor to maintain a positive outlook in the midst of managing complex situations and behaviors.

Program Supervisor

Program supervisors are trained in social learning theory, developmental psychology, and behavioral treatment methods. They are responsible for coordinating all aspects of the treatment program. Program supervisors carry small caseloads (i.e., approximately 10 youth and families) so that high levels of contact, support, and intervention can be maintained. They serve as consultants to the foster parents and provide support and supervision in the form of weekly foster parent meetings and daily telephone contact (through PDR). They are available to the foster parents for support and backup 24 hours a day. Program supervisors work with the foster parents to establish a treatment plan for each youth and to incorporate a point-and-level system into the family's daily routine. Supervision and review of each youth's progress are provided in the context of weekly foster parent meetings, where the program supervisor provides feedback to the foster parents on areas of strength for each youth, as well as areas to target for intervention. In addition, the program supervisor gathers information on levels of support needed by foster parents and coordinates each youth's involvement in school, community activities, and psychiatric consultation during weekly foster parent meetings.

Program supervisors review PDR daily, and data are used to guide treatment interventions across settings and adjust treatment plans as needed. The program supervisor also uses PDR data to inform caseworkers, parole and probation officers, and psychiatrists of a youth's progress. Weekly clinical meetings are conducted by the program supervisor and clinical director and are attended by all treatment staff (i.e., individual and family therapists and behavioral skill specialists). During clinical meetings, each youth's progress is reviewed using PDR data, and interventions are planned and coordinated.

Program supervisors are also responsible for providing regular consultation with school personnel and parole/probation officers. Each youth carries a school card that is completed and signed daily by each teacher, where information is obtained regarding the status of homework assignments, tardiness, and behavior in class. The format of the school card is simple (homework assignments complete/not complete; behavior in class good/poor) so that necessary information is gathered relatively quickly. The purpose of the school card is twofold. First, the school card is used to track the youth's whereabouts so that unsupervised time is kept to a minimum. Second, tracking daily progress at school allows for early identification of potential problems (e.g., skipping class and poor behavior) so that interventions can occur in a preventative fashion (e.g., implementing academic interventions when one or two assignments are overdue rather than waiting until a youth is failing a course). In addition, weekly consultation occurs between the program supervisor and the parole/probation officer, where progress in all aspects of treatment (i.e., foster home, school, community, family involvement, and after-care planning) is discussed. In the event of a major rule or parole/probation violation, program supervisors coordinate and orchestrate interventions using parole/probation officers (i.e., meeting with parole/probation officer; short stays in detention) so that interventions are seamless and occur in the least disruptive manner possible.

The program supervisor is central to the MTFC program's running in a smooth, planful, and well-coordinated manner. The role of the program supervisor is complex because he or she is required to balance the agendas of the youth and family participants and members of the treatment team and community in order to provide youths and their families with integrated treatment plans. In this light, key characteristics of effective program supervisors are that they are flexible thinkers with good social and managerial skills and are adept at problem solving complex treatment issues. Program supervisors are typically master's-level clinicians who receive weekly individual supervision from the program director.

Family Therapist

Youth are returned to their family or relatives' homes following MTFC in 85% of the cases. For the remaining 15%, long-term foster care is the most common placement. Other options include placement in a more restrictive setting, such as a locked residential facility. Family therapy begins immediately after referral and follows a parent management training (PMT) model. The effectiveness of PMT has been empirically supported, especially for the management of antisocial behavior in children and adolescents (Patterson, Chamberlain, & Reid, 1982; Prinz & Miller, 1994; Webster-Stratton & Hammond, 1997). In line with PMT approaches, a primary goal of family therapy in MTFC is to develop a positive relationship or "alliance" with the family. Because many families of chronically delinquent youth have been involved with the juvenile justice system, courts, and various treatment agencies prior to the youth's placement in MTFC, a family's experience with "helping professionals" or "the system" can vary widely. Many families report negative or frustrating experiences during the course of their parenting as they struggle to find support in managing the difficult behaviors exhibited by their youth. With this in mind, family therapists are taught to get the parents' perspective on the youth's developmental course, including the parents' "theory" of the youth's problem behavior, successful and unsuccessful attempts at intervention, and the parents' views on supportive versus unsupportive interventions from community agencies and previous treatment professionals. These elements of "joining" and understanding the family are viewed as important groundwork on which successful parenting practices are taught and reinforced by the therapist.

As the youth is placed in the foster home and progresses with treatment, the parents are kept informed of the youth's progress and problems and are simultaneously taught to use the same parenting strategies used in the foster home. In addition to focusing on managing chaos and general family struggles (e.g., managing behavior of siblings in the home, employment, and financial demands), parents are taught strategies to provide thorough supervision and consistent and fair discipline and to encourage and ensure that the youth associates with prosocial peers and adults in the community.

The parents' attempts to use specific parenting skills are practiced during home visits, and strategies to improve these skills are reviewed and reinforced in weekly family therapy sessions. Visits with the youth begin slowly (e.g., supervised visit at the center) and progress to lengthier visits (e.g., day visit in the community) as parents improve their ability to apply appropriate supervision and discipline strategies. This tempered approach is used in an effort to provide parents with extensive support and to monitor the youth's progress in the family so that neither the family nor the youth revert to "old" behaviors. As parents begin to improve their skills, home visits extend to overnight and weekend visits and continue on this course until reunification. The family therapist maintains weekly sessions with the family into aftercare to increase the chances of successfully transferring treatment gains to the home setting. Family therapists are typically master's-level clinicians. They receive individual supervision by senior clinicians and attend weekly clinical meetings to assist in designing and implementing intervention strategies.

Research on MTFC shows that outcomes (i.e., decreases in offending behavior) are significantly related to parents' successful implementation of the family management strategies used in MTFC (i.e., thorough supervision, reinforcement for appropriate/prosocial behaviors, fair and consistent discipline for misbehavior and rule violations, and decreased association with delinquent peers). Although it may be tempting to think that successful intervention with youth alone will change their antisocial patterns of behavior, our data do not support this point of view and, in contrast, highlight the central role that parents must play in maintaining treatment gains by actively practicing effective parent management strategies (e.g., Eddy & Chamberlain, 2000).

Individual Therapist

Individual therapy is provided for youth at least weekly and is focused on providing support and advocacy for each youth, as well as on implementing interventions for target behaviors specific to each youth. In general, individual therapy is focused on the development and practice of problem-solving skills, modulation of anger expression, social skill development, and development of an educational and/or occupational plan incorporating each youth's unique individual strengths. For example, many youth in MTFC have poor social skills at the time of placement and when faced with a demand requiring compliance (e.g., request to do homework, limit setting, and hearing "no") are inclined to argue or become oppositional and refuse to comply. In such a situation, the individual therapist works under the guidance of the program supervisor to assist the youth in using effective problem-solving and coping skills to manage his or her frustration. With the help of the therapist, a youth is able to practice using new skills to respond to common situations while receiving reinforcement in multiple formats (e.g., encouragement and praise from the individual therapist and foster parents and bonus points on the daily point-and-level system). Such a well-coordinated intervention system not only improves the power of the intervention (i.e., reinforcement comes from multiple individuals and in multiple forms) but also encourages desired behaviors to generalize across settings.

Several months before reunification, family therapy with the youth and his or her biological parents, adoptive parents, or other after-care individuals begins to take place weekly. During these sessions, the individual therapist and family therapist work under the guidance of the program supervisor to design appropriate topics and interventions to be addressed in weekly sessions. The individual therapist functions as an advocate and "coach" to the youth during role-plays designed to practice appropriate responses to parent management strategies.

Although most of the youth in MTFC have histories of significant abuse and/or trauma, individual or family therapists do not push them to explore these issues. Based on information indicating that youth placed in MTFC have highly unstable lives (e.g., highly chaotic families with multiple adult and placement transitions), it is our primary goal to provide a stable and predictable environment for each youth such that he or she may learn adaptive and effective coping and problem-solving skills. It is our experience that once youth become stable in their placements, they may then have the emotional support necessary to effectively process past trauma experiences. In these instances, careful attempts are made to tailor this therapy to match the cognitive processing stage of each youth (i.e., taking into account coping skills, emotional support systems, and careful monitoring of emotional and behavioral responses) so that interventions are aimed at improving functioning and specifically avoid the possibility of retraumatizing or exacerbating the troubles the youth has experienced. Above all, the processing of past abuse and/or trauma is conducted only at the initiation of the youth.

Individual therapists are typically master's-level clinicians. They receive weekly individual supervision by senior clinicians and attend weekly clinical meetings to review each youth's progress and to coordinate treatment interventions.

Behavioral Support Specialist

Behavioral support specialists (BSS) are "bridging" individuals who teach youth effective ways of interacting in the community. The work of the BSS usually occurs during one or two sessions a week (approximately 2–6 hours per week) and is focused on teaching, practicing, and reinforcing prosocial behaviors through intensive one-on-one interaction, role playing, and modeling. Interventions typically occur in general community settings (e.g., restaurants and libraries), at school, or during community activities (e.g., sports teams and art classes) where youth may benefit from assistance and "coaching" to interact with other individuals in a positive manner. BSSs are trained to use applied behavior analysis to examine potential antecedents and reinforcers of problem behavior during *in vivo* experiences with youth. In addition, they are taught shaping techniques (i.e., reinforcement strategies) to teach and encourage new behaviors. BSSs attend weekly group supervision meetings led by a senior clinician and weekly clinical meetings conducted by the program director and program supervisor to review each youth's progress and design targets for intervention.

Foster Parent Recruiter, Trainer, and PDR Caller

The foster parent recruiter, trainer, and PDR caller is typically a paraprofessional who is well versed in the MTFC treatment approach and who, ideally, has experience as a successful MTFC foster parent. This person provides daily contact to foster parents through a telephone interview (i.e., the Parent Daily Report Checklist; PDR; Chamberlain & Reid, 1987) where data are collected on each youth's daily behaviors, as well as on levels of foster parent stress. This telephone call serves to monitor the daily progress of each youth in an effort to identify possible problems before they arise, as well as to provide daily support to foster parents. This person also participates in the recruiting and preservice training of new foster parents, attends the weekly foster parent meetings, and provides backup coverage to the program supervisor.

Consulting Psychiatrist

Youth referred from both juvenile justice and child welfare have typically received multiple diagnoses prior to their placement in MTFC, and many of these youth are on multiple medications at the time of placement. Due to the complex nature of dual diagnoses (especially combinations of internalizing and externalizing disorders and developmental delays), consultation with the youth's psychiatrist is necessary to effectively coordinate medication management and psychosocial interventions. Although it is possible to consult with primary care physicians or individual psychiatrists on an individual basis, such an approach can be inefficient and ineffective. We have found it most effective to work with a psychiatrist who is experienced in treating severely emotional and behaviorally disordered youth and who is knowledgeable concerning the complex coordination of information and intervention associated with MTFC. In an effort to facilitate communication and collaboration regarding treatment planning, we have arranged for our psychiatrist to come to our office each week to see youth. Program supervisors set up appointment times for youth, MTFC parents, and occasionally a youth's parents, and regular medication is managed in this way. After a youth is stabilized in an MTFC placement, medications can often be significantly decreased and, in some cases, discontinued altogether.

Role Separation

There are clearly defined roles for each treatment team member and the distinction of these roles is carefully maintained. There are several reasons for clearly defining roles and allowing minimal overlap between team members. First, youth who have severe emotional and behavioral problems and/or chronic offending behaviors typically demonstrate complex responses to individuals and the environment (e.g., difficulty coping with emotional and behavioral expectations and limit setting). The intensity and duration of the emotions or behaviors displayed by youth with severe emotional and behavioral problems can make it challenging to intervene in an immediate yet therapeutic manner. To increase predictability, the treatment team outlines a clear order of responding for youth. For example, the program supervisor is frequently called on to set limits for youth in care, and individual therapists and BSSs are carefully protected from taking on a limit-setting role. Because limits are typically difficult for delinquent and emotionally/behaviorally troubled youth to accept, an extra degree of freedom is provided that allows the foster parents (as well as individual therapists and behavioral support specialists) to play a supportive role when a youth is upset by a limit set by the program supervisor. Such role separation can assist in diffusing the emotionality of a particular circumstance and can allow youth to access support and take feedback (e.g., applying new coping skills or problem-solving strategies) from others in a less defensive manner.

EVIDENCE FOR THE EFFECTS OF TREATMENT

A series of studies have examined the effectiveness of the MTFC approach with a range of children, adolescents, and their families, including children and adolescents leaving a state mental hospital (Chamberlain & Reid, 1991), children in "regular" state-supported foster care (Chamberlain et al., 1992; Chamberlain & Price, 2002; Smith et al., 2001), preschool children with challenging behaviors (Fisher et al., 2000), and preschoolers who are part of a prevention study (Fisher, Ellis, & Chamberlain, 1999). In addition, two major studies have been completed on the treatment of chronically delinquent youth (Chamberlain & Leve, 2002; Chamberlain & Reid, 1998; Eddy & Chamberlain, 2000), and a third study is under way. Although a number of studies have been completed on MTFC, data on the effectiveness of MTFC with juvenile offenders are the focus here.

Outcomes for Juvenile Justice Youth

In the first of these clinical trials (Chamberlain & Reid, 1998), males ($n = 79$) between the ages of 12 and 17 were randomly assigned to MTFC or to group care (GC) placements. GC is the typical "treatment as usual" community placement condition used in the United States for chronically delinquent youth. Youth in the GC condition were placed in one of 11 GC facilities located throughout the state. Their parole/probation officers determined which GC program they attended. GC programs varied slightly in terms of theoretical orientation, but all had the commonality of relying on variations of the positive peer culture approach (Vorrath & Brendtro, 1985). Individual and group therapy were provided as part of GC treatments, and family therapy was provided in 55% of the cases. Most youth in GC (i.e., 83% of cases) attended on-site schools.

Prior to referral, participating boys had an average of 14 previous criminal referrals ($SD = 8.7$) and 4 previous felonies ($SD = 3.8$). Each of the 79 youth had been placed in a locked detention facility prior to placement in MTFC or GC settings (average number of days in detention = 76), and boys had experienced an average of at least one prior out-of-home placement in addition to detention (mean number of previous placements = 1.3). The average age of participating boys was 14.4 years ($SD = 1.3$) and the mean age at their first arrest was 12.6 years ($SD = 1.8$). Of the participants, 85% were white, 6% African American, 6% Hispanic, and 3% American Indian.

The study addressed two primary questions. First, could chronically delinquent boys be safely maintained in a community setting? Second, would the MTFC intervention be effective in reducing posttreatment crime and delinquent activity compared to group care? In addition, we were interested in examining theoretical questions about the role of key factors that were thought to mediate the effects of the MTFC treatment model (i.e., Eddy & Chamberlain, 2000).

Boys assigned to MTFC were shown to have more positive outcomes on program completion and incarceration rates than boys in GC. Significantly fewer boys in MTFC than in GC ran away from their placements (30.5% vs. 57.8%, respectively), and a significantly greater portion of MTFC boys completed their placements than did GC boys (73% vs. 36%). During the year after referral, boys in MTFC spent significantly fewer days in locked settings, including local detention and state training schools, than did GC boys (means = 53 and 139 days). In terms of the effectiveness of the model for reducing criminal behavior, official arrest rates and self-reports of delinquency were examined. All referrals for criminal activity were examined for two time periods; the year prior to enrollment in the study and from placement through 1-year postdischarge. MTFC boys showed significantly larger drops in official criminal referral rates. Figure 16.1 shows the means for criminal referral rates.

In addition to examining program effectiveness, analyses were also conducted to examine three youth variables that have been noted in the literature to predict juvenile offending; these were age at first offense, age at baseline, and number of prior referrals. The only significant univariate predictors of posttreatment offending were group assignment and prereferral rate, with MTFC youngsters showing significantly fewer postplacement criminal referrals. These results were replicated with boys' self-reported data on participation in delinquent activities. In addition, youth who were treated with MTFC were found to be significantly less likely to self-report committing violent offenses compared to youth who were treated with group care, even when preplacement control factors were considered (i.e., age at first arrest, age at placement, official and self-reported prior offenses, and time) (Eddy, Bridges-Whaley, & Chamberlain, 2002).

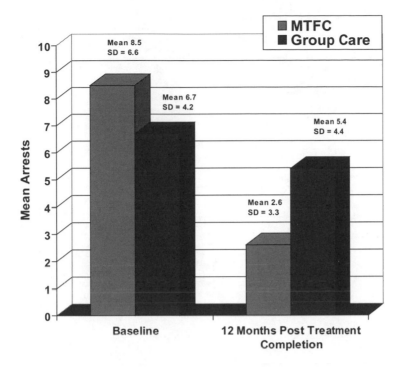

FIGURE 16.1. Total number of criminal referrals at baseline and from placement in either multidimensional treatment foster care or group care to exit plus 1 year.

Evidence showing that the MTFC approach was effective in reducing later offending behavior (i.e., Chamberlain & Reid, 1998) led to the second-level evaluation of the components of the intervention that were hypothesized to be related to differences in intervention effects for the two groups (i.e., Eddy & Chamberlain, 2000). Two sets of factors that guided the theory underlying the design of the MTFC intervention were examined (i.e., family management and deviant peer associations). Measures of family management and deviant peer associations were obtained after boys had been in their placement settings for 3 months. Multiagent, multimode measures of four factors were used to define key constructs of the three family management variables of interest (i.e. supervision, discipline, and positive reinforcement) and association with deviant peers.

These key factors are directly targeted as part of the MTFC intervention and were left free to vary in the GC condition. It was hypothesized that, regardless of study condition (i.e., MTFC or GC), the extent to which family management skills were increased and association with deviant peers was decreased, outcomes for youth would be more positive (e.g., lower levels of arrests and self-reports of delinquency) in follow-up. As hypothesized, results showed that family management (supervision, discipline, positive reinforcement) and deviant peer association mediated the impact of treatment condition on youth antisocial behavior at 1 year posttreatment for youth in both groups. However, as can be seen in Figure 16.2, treatment condition (GC) was significantly related to scores on the mediators such that boys in MTFC were shown to have received higher levels of parent management and lower levels of association with delinquent peers compared to GC boys at the midtreatment assessment. Boys' scores on the mediators at midtreatment

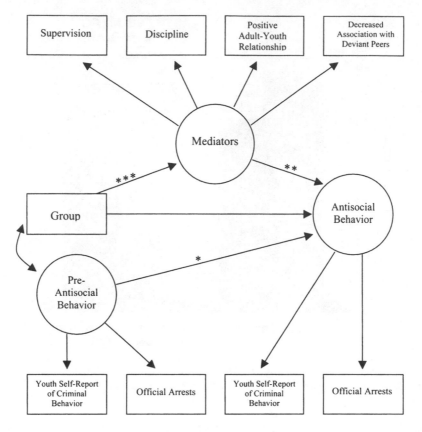

FIGURE 16.2. Mediational model. * $p < .05$; ** $p < .01$; *** $p < .001$.

were significantly related to their levels of antisocial behavior in follow-up (i.e., 15 months later). The effect of group on antisocial behavior was not significant in the presence of the mediators (Eddy & Chamberlain, 2000). These findings suggest that MTFC was not only more effective in treating youth with severe antisocial behavior and criminality but that a significant part of the influence on youth behavior was due to the level and type of family management (i.e., the use of fair, consistent, nonphysical forms of discipline, effective supervision, and a positive relationship with a mentoring adult) and decreased association with delinquent peers provided in the foster home (Eddy & Chamberlain, 2000).

Females Referred from Juvenile Justice

In an effort to examine possible gender differences in the treatment of chronically delinquent youth with MTFC, Chamberlain and Reid (1994) first examined pretreatment family and child risk factors, patterns of previous delinquency, and response to MTFC for 88 consecutive referrals of male and female juvenile offenders. Findings from this pilot study revealed several significant gender differences for pretreatment risk factors; females had been placed outside their families more often, had experienced sexual abuse at a rate four times that of males, were more likely to have attempted suicide, and were more likely to have run away at least twice prior to treatment. Results indicated no significant differences for males and females on successful program completion or for overall arrest rates during the year following treatment. Although there were no significant outcome differences for males and females, their responses to treatment were unique. In particular, the mean number of problem behaviors exhibited by females showed a significant increase during the first 6 months of treatment while males showed a slight decrease. Results of this study led to a 5-year randomized trial of females that was completed in 2002.

In that study (Chamberlain & Leve, 2002), participating female adolescents ranged from 12 to 17 years old (mean = 15.1; SD = 1.1) and had an average of more than 11 police offenses prior to referral. Of the participants, 75% were Caucasian, 1% African American, 7% Hispanic, 7% American Indian, 3% Asian, and 7% of mixed ethnic heritage. Girls were screened and recommended for out-of-home care by their local juvenile justice department parole or probation workers. Following referral and consent from each girl's parent or guardian, girls were randomly assigned to MTFC or treatment-as-usual settings (e.g., residential treatment, group home, hospital, or inpatient drug and alcohol program).

Many of the goals for treating girls are similar to those identified in the previous work with delinquent boys—namely, decreasing delinquent, aggressive, and antisocial behaviors by providing placement and structured treatment in a well-supervised family setting in which contact with delinquent peers is minimized and preparing their aftercare families for their return home. As with their male counterparts, short-term outcomes of interest included decreased contact with delinquent peers, increased academic success, and increased placement stability (i.e., reduced disruptions in placement). Longer-term outcomes of interest were decreased delinquency and drug/alcohol use, increased school success and completion, increased occupational opportunities, and improved relationships with family, adults, and prosocial peers. In addition to these targets that apply to both genders, girls appear to have some unique needs that have implications for specialized treatment approaches.

Examination of differences between boys and girls on preplacement risk factors led to identification of some of these needs (see Table 16.1). For example, females referred from juvenile justice appear to come from families with even greater levels of chaos and distress than those of delinquent males. In particular, a significantly greater number of female youth in this study have mothers who have been convicted of a crime (46.7% of females compared to 21.6% of males) and fathers who have been convicted of a crime (63.2% of females compared to 31.3% of males). Overall, 70% of female adolescents in this study have at least one parent who has been convicted of a crime (compared to 41.1% of males). The girls in this study also have a significantly higher rate of documented physical abuse (65.6% of females compared to 5.7% of males) and sexual abuse (72.1% of females compared to 6.8% of males). In addition, females have been placed out of the home significantly more (3.03 placements compared to 1.33 placements for males), have significantly more documented suicide attempts (58.3% of females compared to 2.6% of males), have run away significantly more (91.7% of females compared to 73.7% of males), and have been characterized as heavy drug or alcohol users (82% of females compared to 9.3% of males). Females also reported higher rates of symptoms for mental health disorders (i.e., depression, anxiety, paranoid/psychotic, somatization, hostility, and general psychopathology) measured at the onset of treatment using the Behavior Symptom Inventory (BSI; Derogatis, 1975).

These findings concur with others showing that antisocial girls tend to come from adverse and dysfunctional backgrounds (e.g., Henry, Moffitt, Robins, & Silva, 1993) and often have parents with criminal histories (Rosenbaum, 1989). The rates of sexual and physical abuse are extremely high, as are girls' endorsements of mental health symptoms. In addition, many of these girls have not attended school for a number of years and have no experience participating in sports, organized prosocial activities, or hobbies. These factors contribute to the challenging nature of designing and implementing a gender-responsive, community-based treatment program and to planning for after-care services. In this light, we have emphasized several factors of treatment to respond to girls' unique needs during their placement in MTFC. We have found that initially it is important to promote a high level of stability for girls and to characterize their early days in MTFC with participation in successful, prosocial activities. We specifically train MTFC parents in strategies for responding to relational/indirect aggression, which has been shown to be more common in girls than the overt forms of aggression typically used by boys (Björkqvist, Lagerspetz, & Kaukiainen, 1992; Underwood, 1998). Although rates of previous abuse are extremely high for study girls, we have found that dealing with past abuse issues in therapy requires both sensitivity and timing. Most girls have had multiple abuse experiences. Opening this area as a topic for therapy can lead to a significant increase in girls' levels of anxiety, which can increase their symptoms of trauma and/or the potential for running away. We allow girls to initiate and control the intensity of therapy around abuse issues rather than taking a more aggressive approach.

Preliminary follow-up data for the first 61 girls (60% of the sample) show that girls in MTFC have spent more days in treatment and fewer days in lockup between placement and 12 months following the end of their placement in MTFC or GC. In addition, 12-month follow-up data suggest a greater decrease in arrests for females treated with MTFC than for those in GC. MTFC girls also are spending significantly fewer days in the hospital for mental health-related problems than are GC girls. Despite these promising initial findings, girls continue to have problems in follow-up that are likely to undermine their adjustment in young adulthood. For example, girls continue to report that they participate in health-risking sexual activities, select partners who are antisocial, and use alcohol and other drugs at high rates following treatment completion. Identification of these continuing problems has led us to revise the MTFC model in an attempt to broaden the focus from reduction of antisocial behaviors alone to the inclusion of interventions designed to prevent health-risking behaviors and foster healthy adult lifestyles. A recently funded study is currently in place to examine the effectiveness of adding components to prevent participation in health-risking sexual behavior and drug use to MTFC for treating chronically delinquent female youth.

Relative Costs of MTFC

Cost comparisons for treating youth from juvenile justice indicate that MTFC costs approximately one-third less than placement and treatment in group care. This is because there are far fewer facility costs in MTFC (offices for staff only, no facility to house youth). The Washington State Institute for Public Policy (Aos, Phipps, Barnoski, & Lieb, 1999) recently conducted an evaluation of the cost-effectiveness of MTFC. They compared MTFC to 31 violence prevention programs and other approaches and identified MTFC as one of the programs that resulted in the greatest savings to taxpayers. Specifically, the MTFC model was estimated to save taxpayers $43,661 per participant in criminal justice and avoided victim costs. For every dollar spent on MTFC, $22.58 of taxpayer benefits were estimated when compared to more commonly used programs such as Boot Camps and Juvenile Intensive Supervision (i.e., parole/probation).

DISSEMINATION AND REPLICATION OF THE MTFC APPROACH

Since 2000, we have been conducting a randomized clinical trial to test the transferability of specific components of MTFC in six regions of health and human services in San Diego County. This project was developed following positive results from a pilot study that provided elements of MTFC to foster parents working with emotionally and behaviorally troubled youths referred from the child welfare system in three counties in Oregon (Chamberlain et al., 1992). In that study we found that training and ongoing supervision with foster parents resulted in decreased child problem behaviors, decreased foster parent stress, decreased rates of placement disruption, and fewer foster parents dropping out of providing care for the child welfare system. The focus of the San Diego study is to examine the effectiveness of moving this intervention into a large, diverse urban child welfare system.

Foster parents who are randomly assigned to the MTFC enhanced support and training intervention receive 16 weeks of foster family support and parent management training provided by a paraprofessional facilitator and a cofacilitator who is trained and supervised in the MTFC model. In addition, foster parents in the intervention group receive weekly telephone contacts from the group's facilitator. Telephone contacts are used to debrief and collect data on daily child behavior problems, provide support to foster parents, and encourage the application of parent management strategies presented and practiced in the weekly foster parent meetings.

Outcomes are being evaluated at multiple levels, including child symptoms, functional behavior, environments, consumer perspectives, and system, using a multimethod/multiagent strategy. Implementation fidelity and contextual factors (e.g., organizational climate and social isolation/insularity of foster parents) are also being assessed. It is hypothesized that foster parents in the MTFC enhanced training and support group will demonstrate improvements in effective parenting skills, will feel more supported, and experience less stress, which, in turn, will result in more positive child outcomes (i.e., decreased behavior problems, improved adjustment, and lower rate of placement disruption). Paraprofessional staff members who receive ongoing supervision from MTFC program supervisors in Oregon are delivering the intervention. In the second phase of this project, San Diego intervention staff will provide training and supervision to a second cohort of paraprofessionals who will deliver the intervention in another three regions of San Diego County.

A similar set of goals (i.e., increased support and training of foster parents, decreased rates of foster parent dropout and child placement disruption, and improved child functioning) is being targeted in a current study of preschoolers in "regular" foster care in Oregon (Fisher et al., 1999). In that randomized trial, child stress and level of emotional regulation (measured in salivary cortisol) are added to the typical behavioral, functioning, and psychological measures obtained in MTFC studies.

In addition, MTFC is currently being implemented with juvenile justice populations by private nonprofit organizations in six sites around the United States and in Sweden. The first agency to implement MTFC on a large scale was Youth Villages in Tennessee. Currently, Youth Villages serves over 400 children and adolescents per day in MTFC (Mendel, 2000), making it the largest site that we know of to implement the MTFC model. Although, to our knowledge, Youth Villages has not conducted a formal outcome study, Youth Villages reports it is able to serve more youth in less restrictive placements and that youths are more successful at remaining at home postplacement than they had been prior to implementing the MTFC model. In addition to reporting more positive outcomes with MTFC placements (compared to their previous attempts at using residential care beds), Youth Villages reports that the costs for MTFC are substantially less.

Another more recent implementation of the MTFC model has been with the Laurel Youth Services Program in Williamsport, Pennsylvania. The program director and three staff members from Laurel were trained at the Oregon site in January 2001. They began implementation at their site soon afterward. By 6 months after the initial training, they had served nine youth and an additional two had completed the program and were successfully returned home. The Laurel program serves youth referred from juvenile justice who are in need of out-of-home placement. The program director reports that MTFC is working well at the Laurel site, particularly in dealing with difficult youth who would have been placed in more restrictive residential programs prior to their implementing MTFC. We continue to conduct weekly telephone consultations with Laurel staff, view videotapes of their family therapy sessions, and review daily PDR data they collect on program youth.

An international application of MTFC is also being conducted in Lund, Sweden. There, a private agency serves youth referred from child welfare who have severe emotional and behavioral problems. Training for that site has involved two weeklong intensive workshops in Sweden and two visits from their staff to the Oregon site. Preliminary data on outcomes for children served in that program appear to be promising (Hansen, personal communication, August 2001). Although anecdotal reports of implementations at these sites are positive, there is an obvious need for well-designed studies to test key theoretical constructs and practical aspects of dissemination of the MTFC model.

SUMMARY AND CONCLUSIONS

The Oregon MTFC Program is a community-based treatment program that was first developed in the early 1980s as an alternative to institutional, residential, and group care placements for youth with severe and chronic delinquent behavior and has since been extended to work with children and adolescents (and their families) referred from both mental health and child welfare service systems. The MTFC approach has been empirically validated in a number of studies with a variety of populations of youth and families. The initial feasibility of the model has been established; however, it is not yet understood what factors could facilitate or inhibit the deployment of this approach on a wider basis within child welfare or juvenile justice systems. The ongoing study in San Diego County is a first step. In that study, the implementation is conducted by paraprofessionals who have not been part of the research team that developed MTFC. Within the context of a large urban child welfare system, the "Cascading Dissemination" design being used there allows for examination of effect sizes when the intervention is implemented under two conditions—first, when the original developers of the intervention train and provide ongoing supervision to the paraprofessional interventionists, and second when the initial cohort of paraprofessional implementers train and supervise the second, generation of interventionists. Although this dissemination study clearly does not address many of the potential barriers that are likely to occur when implementing a program focused on trying to impact practice in a large social service system such as child welfare, it is a first attempt to use the MTFC model as a starting place to bridge the gap between research and practice that has been well documented by researchers and policymakers over the last decade.

ACKNOWLEDGMENTS

Support for this research was provided by grants from NIMH (MH 54257, MH 60195, MH 59127) and from NIMH and the Office of Research on Minority Health (MH 46690).

REFERENCES

Aos, S., Phipps, P., Barnoski, R., & Leib, R. (1999). *The comparative costs and benefits of programs to reduce crime: A review of national research findings with implications for Washington state.* Olympia: Washington State Institute for Public Policy.

Björkqvist, K., Lagerspetz, K. M. J., & Kaukiainen, A. (1992). Do girls manipulate and boys fight? *Aggressive Behavior, 18,* 117–127.

Chamberlain, P. (1999). Residential care for children and adolescents with conduct disorders. In H. C. Quay & A. E. Hogan (Eds.), *Handbook of disruptive behavior disorders* (pp. 495–505). New York: Kluwer Academic/Plenum Press.

Chamberlain, P., & Leve, L. D. (2002). *Preventing health-risking behaviors in delinquent girls.* Grant No. R01 DA15208, National Institute on Drug Abuse, National Institutes of Health, U.S. Public Health Service.

Chamberlain, P., & Moore, K. J. (2002). Chaos and trauma in the lives of adolescent females with antisocial behavior and delinquency. In R. Geffner (Series Ed.) & R. Greenwald (Vol. Ed.), *Trauma and juvenile delinquency: Theory, research, and interventions* (pp. 79–108). Binghamton, NY: Haworth Press.

Chamberlain, P., Moreland, S., & Reid, K. (1992). Enhanced services and stipends for foster parents: Effects on retention rates and outcomes for children. *Child Welfare League of America, 71,* 387–401.

Chamberlain, P., & Price, J. M. (2002). *Cascading dissemination of a foster parent intervention.* Manuscript in preparation.

Chamberlain, P., & Reid, J. B. (1987). Parent observation and report of child symptoms. *Behavioral Assessment, 9,* 97–109.

Chamberlain, P., & Reid, J. B. (1991). Using a specialized foster care community treatment model for children and adolescents leaving the state mental hospital. *Journal of Community Psychology, 19,* 266–276.

Chamberlain, P., & Reid, J. B. (1994). Differences in risk factors and adjustment for male and female delinquents in treatment foster care. *Journal of Child and Family Studies, 3,* 23–39.

Chamberlain, P., & Reid, J. B. (1998). Comparison of two community alternatives to incarceration for chronic juvenile offenders. *Journal of Consulting and Clinical Psychology, 66,* 624–633.

Derogatis, L. R. (1975). *Brief Symptom Inventory.* Foothill Ranch, CA: NCS Pearson.

Dishion, T. J., McCord, J., & Poulin, F. (1999). When interventions harm: Peer groups and problem behavior. *American Psychologist, 54,* 755–764.

Eddy, J. M., Bridges-Whaley, R., & Chamberlain, P. (2002). *The prevention of violent behavior by chronic and serious male juvenile offenders: A randomized clinical trial.* Manuscript submitted for publication.

Eddy, J. M., & Chamberlain, P. (2000). Family management and deviant peer association as mediators of the impact of treatment condition on youth antisocial behavior. *Journal of Consulting and Clinical Psychology, 68,* 857–863.

Elliott, D. S. (Series Ed.). (1998). *Blueprints for violence prevention.* Boulder: Institute of Behavioral Science, University of Colorado at Boulder.

Elliott, D. S., Huizinga, D., & Ageton, S. S. (1985). *Explaining delinquency and drug use.* Beverly Hills, CA: Sage.

Fingerhut, L. A., & Kleinman, J. C. (1990). International and interstate comparisons of homicides among young males. *Journal of the American Medical Association, 263,* 3292–3295.

Fisher, P. A, Ellis, H., & Chamberlain, P. (1999). Early intervention foster care: A model for preventing risk in young children who have been maltreated. *Children's Services: Social Policy, Research, and Practice, 2,* 159–182.

Fisher, P. A., Gunnar, M. R., Chamberlain, P., & Reid, J. B. (2000). Preventive intervention for maltreated preschool children: Impact on children's behavior, neuroendocrine activity, and foster parent functioning. *Journal of the American Academy of Child and Adolescent Psychiatry, 39,* 1356–1364.

Henry, B., Moffitt, T., Robins, L., & Silva, P. (1993). Early family predictors of child and adolescent antisocial behaviour: Who are the mothers of delinquents? *Criminal Behaviour and Mental Health, 3,* 97–118.

Mendel, R. A. (2000). *Less hype, more help: Reducing juvenile crime, what works - and what doesn't.* Washington, DC: American Youth Policy Forum.

Patterson, G. R., Chamberlain, P., & Reid, J. B. (1982). A comparative evaluation of parent training procedures. *Behavior Therapy, 13,* 638–650.

Patterson, G. R., Reid, J. B., & Dishion, T. J. (1992). *A social learning approach: IV. Antisocial boys.* Eugene, OR: Castalia.

Prinz, R. J., & Miller, G. E. (1994). Family-based treatment for childhood antisocial behavior: Experimental influences on dropout and engagement. *Journal of Consulting and Clinical Psychology, 62,* 645–650.

Reid, J. B., & Eddy, J. M. (1997). The prevention of antisocial behavior: Some considerations in the search for effective interventions. In D. M. Stoff, J. Breiling, & J. D. Maser (Eds.), *Handbook of antisocial behavior* (pp. 205–21). New York: Wiley.

Rivera, V. R., & Kutash, K. (1994). *Components of a system of care: What does the research say?* Tampa: Research and Training Center for Children's Mental Health, University of South Florida, Florida Mental Health Institute.

Rosenbaum, J. L. (1989). Family dysfunction and female delinquency. *Crime and Delinquency, 35,* 31–44.

Smith, D. K., Sprengelmeyer, P. G., & Moore, K. J. (in press). Parenting and antisocial behavior. In M. Hoghughi & N. Long (Eds.), *Sage handbook of parenting: Theory, research and practice.* London: Sage.

Smith, D. K., Stormshak, E., Chamberlain, P., & Bridges-Whaley, R. (2001). Placement disruption in treatment foster care. *Journal of Emotional and Behavioral Disorders, 9,* 200–205.

Underwood, M. K. (1998). Competence in sexual decision-making by African-American, female adolescents: The role of peer relations and future plans. In A. Colby, J. James, & D. Hart (Eds.), *Competence and character through life* (pp. 57–87). Chicago: University of Chicago.

U.S. Department of Justice. (1994). *Federal Bureau of Investigation: Crime in the United States, 1993: Uniform Crime Reports.* Washington, DC: U.S. Department of Justice.

Vorrath, H., & Brendtro, L. K. (1985). *Positive peer culture.* Chicago: Aldine.

Webster-Stratton, C., & Hammond, M. (1997). Treating children with early-onset conduct problems: A comparison of child and parent training interventions. *Journal of Consulting and Clinical Psychology, 65,* 93–109.

World Health Organization. (1992). *Annual report on homicide.* Geneva, Switzerland: Author.

17

Multisystemic Treatment of Serious Clinical Problems

Scott W. Henggeler and Terry Lee

OVERVIEW

Clinical Problem and Population Addressed

Multisystemic therapy (MST) is an intensive family- and community-based treatment for adolescent youth who engage in severe willful misconduct that places them at risk for out-of-home placement and their families. "Willful misconduct" is a term with broad meaning, and in a corresponding fashion, MST has been applied to a wide range of youth presenting serious clinical problems including chronic and violent juvenile offenders, substance-abusing juvenile offenders, adolescent sexual offenders, youth in psychiatric crisis (i.e., homicidal, suicidal, and psychotic), and maltreating families. Such youth present significant personal and societal (e.g., crime victimization) costs, and due to their high rates of expensive out-of-home placements, they consume a grossly disproportionate share of the nation's mental health treatment resources. Across these clinical populations, the overarching goals of MST programs are to decrease rates of antisocial behavior, improve functioning (e.g., family relations and school performance), and reduce use of out-of-home placements (e.g., incarceration and residential treatment).

Theoretical Framework

With roots in social ecological (Bronfenbrenner, 1979) and family systems (Haley, 1976; Minuchen, 1974) theories, MST views youths as embedded within multiple interconnected systems, including the nuclear family, extended family, neighborhood, school, peer culture, and community. The juvenile justice, child welfare, and mental health systems may also be involved. In assessing the major determinants of identified problems, the clinician considers the reciprocal and bidirectional nature of the influences between a youth and his or her family and social network as well as the indirect effects of more distal influences (e.g., parental workplace). For a treatment to be effective, the risk factors across these systems must be identified and addressed. Hence, the "ecological validity" of assessing and treating youth in the natural environment is emphasized under the assumption that favorable outcomes are more likely to be generalized and sustained when skills are practiced and learned where the youth and family actually live.

Conceptual Assumptions

Several assumptions are critical to the design and implementation of MST interventions.

Multidetermined Nature of Serious Clinical Problems

As suggested from the social ecological theoretical model and supported by decades of correlational and longitudinal research in the area of youth antisocial behavior, such behavior is multidetermined from the reciprocal interplay of individual, family, peer, school, and community factors. As such, MST interventions assess and address these potential risk factors in a comprehensive, yet individualized, fashion.

Caregivers Are Key to Long-Term Outcomes

The caregiver is viewed as the key to long-term positive outcomes for the youth. Ideally the caregiver is a parent, but another adult (e.g., grandparent, aunt, uncle, or sibling) with an enduring emotional tie to the youth can serve in this role. Often, other caring adults from the youth's ecology are also identified to provide social support as well (Werner & Smith, 2001). Professional supports are introduced only after exhausting resources in the family's natural ecology. Paid professionals may genuinely care but invariably leave the youth's life for reasons such as professional advancement or termination of treatment. Thus, by focusing clinical attention on developing the caregiver's ability to parent effectively and strengthening the family's indigenous support system, treatment gains are more likely to be maintained.

Integration of Evidence-Based Practices

MST incorporates empirically based treatments insofar as they exist. Thus, MST programs include cognitive-behavioral approaches, the behavior therapies, behavioral parent training, pragmatic family therapies, and certain pharmacological interventions that have a reasonable evidence base (U.S. Department of Health and Human Services [DHHS], 1999). As suggested by other assumptions noted in this section, however, these treatments are delivered in a considerably different context than usual. For example, consistent with the view that the caregiver is key to long-term outcomes, a MST cognitive-behavioral intervention would ideally be delivered by the caregiver under the consultation of the therapist. Similarly, as noted next, the therapist would also be accountable for removing barriers to service access.

Intensive Services That Overcome Barriers to Service Access

In light of the serious clinical problems presented by youth and their families in MST programs (i.e., referral criteria include high risk of out-of-home placement) and the high dropout rates of such youth and families in traditional mental health programs, clinicians provide intensive services with a commitment to overcome barriers to service access. Thus, MST clinicians have a relatively low caseload to facilitate the implementation of quality multifaceted interventions and to meet with family members and multiple agency representatives at consumer-friendly times and in consumer-friendly settings. To contain costs and for reasons of clinical efficiency, the average duration of treatment is about 3 to 5 months.

Rigorous Quality Assurance System

Rigorous quality assurance is required to promote the level of treatment fidelity needed to achieve desired clinical outcomes. Hence, intensive quality assurance protocols are built into all MST programs, which differentiates MST from most mental health practices. MST therapist education starts with a 5-day overview of the MST treatment model. Therapists participate in weekly group supervision with their on-site MST-trained supervisor, and weekly consultation is provided with an off-site expert MST consultant. Quarterly on-site consultant booster training is provided to address targeted training needs of the entire MST team. In addition, caregiver ratings of therapist adherence to MST principles are monitored monthly through an Internet-based system. Together, these quality assurance components aim to enhance clinical outcomes through promoting treatment fidelity. Empirical validation of several key aspects of the MST quality assurance system is described in more detail subsequently.

CHARACTERISTICS OF THE TREATMENT PROGRAM

Treatment Principles

The complexity of willful misconduct and related problems requires considerable flexibility in the design and delivery of interventions. As such, MST is operationalized through adherence to nine core treatment principles that guide treatment planning (see Table 17.1) and implementation.

Treatment Format

MST works with youth, family members, and all pertinent systems in which the youth is involved including peers, school, extended family, family supports, the neighborhood, community groups, and other involved agencies such as child welfare or juvenile justice. In the early phase of treatment, specific measurable overarching goals and functionally meaningful outcomes are set in collaboration with the family and, as appropriate, other stakeholders. MST overarching goals are broken down into measurable weekly goals. Any person or agency that may influence attainment of these goals is engaged by the therapist and caregiver with specific interventions designed to encourage actions that will facilitate goal achievement.

Strong engagement with the family is essential for successful outcomes, and the MST treatment model incorporates strategies to encourage cooperative partnering. Families are treated with respect and are assumed to be doing the best they can. Other youth-associated systems are also viewed as vital partners in the treatment process. The MST team focuses on system strengths (Principle 2) and is responsive to families' needs. Barriers to engagement are continuously evaluated and addressed (Principles 1 and 8).

TABLE 17.1. MST Treatment Principles

1. *Finding the fit:* The primary purpose of assessment is to understand the "fit" between identified problems and their broader systemic context and how identified problems "make sense" in the context of the youth's social ecology.

2. *Positive and strength focused:* Therapeutic contacts emphasize the positive and use systemic strengths as levers for positive change. Focusing on family strengths has numerous advantages, such as decreasing negative affect, building feelings of hope, identifying protective factors, decreasing frustration by emphasizing problem solving, and enhancing caregivers' confidence.

3. *Increasing responsibility:* Interventions are designed to promote responsible behavior and decrease irresponsible behavior among family members. The emphasis on enhancing responsible behavior is contrasted with the usual pathology focus of mental health providers and kindles hope for change.

4. *Present focused, action oriented and well defined:* Interventions are present focused and action oriented, targeting specific and well-defined problems. Such interventions enable treatment participants to track the progress of treatment and provide clear criteria to measure success. Family members are expected to work actively toward goals by focusing on present-oriented solutions (vs. gaining insight from or focusing on the past). Clear goals also delineate criteria for treatment termination.

5. *Targeting sequences:* Interventions target sequences of behavior within and between multiple systems that maintain the identified problems. Treatment is aimed at changing family interactions in ways that promote responsible behavior and broaden family links with indigenous prosocial support systems.

6. *Developmentally appropriate:* Interventions are developmentally appropriate and fit the developmental needs of the youth. A developmental emphasis stresses building youth competencies in peer relations and acquiring academic and vocational skills that will promote a successful transition to adulthood.

7. *Continuous effort:* Interventions are designed to require daily or weekly effort by family members, presenting youth and family frequent opportunities to demonstrate their commitment. Advantages of intensive and multifaceted efforts to change include more rapid problem resolution, earlier identification of treatment nonadherence, continuous evaluation of outcomes, more frequent corrective interventions, more opportunities for family members to experience success, and family empowerment as members orchestrate their own changes.

8. *Evaluation and accountability:* Intervention effectiveness is evaluated continuously from multiple perspectives, with MST team members assuming accountability for overcoming barriers to successful outcomes. MST does not label families as resistant, not ready for change, or unmotivated. This approach avoids blaming the family and places the responsibility for positive treatment outcomes on the MST team.

9. *Generalization:* Interventions are designed to promote treatment generalization and long-term maintenance of therapeutic change by empowering caregivers to address family members' needs across multiple systemic contexts. The caregiver is viewed as the key to long-term success. Family members make most of the changes, with MST therapists acting as consultants, advisers, and advocates.

Model of Service Delivery

MST is provided via a home-based model of service delivery, and the use of such a model has been crucial to the high engagement and low dropout rates obtained in recent outcome studies (e.g., Henggeler, Pickrel, Brondino, & Crouch, 1996). While the particular treatment used in home-based programs can vary, critical service delivery characteristics are shared (Nelson & Landsman, 1992) and include the following:

1. *Low caseloads* to allow intensive services: A MST team consists of three to five full-time therapists, a halftime supervisor per team, and appropriate organizational support. Each therapist works with four to five families at a time. The therapist is the team's main point of contact for the youth, family, and all involved agencies and systems.
2. *Delivery of services in community settings* (e.g., home, school, and neighborhood center) to overcome barriers to service access, facilitate family engagement in the clinical process, and provide more valid assessment and outcome data.
3. *Time-limited duration of treatment* (3–5 months) to promote efficiency, self-sufficiency, and cost-effectiveness.
4. *24-hour/day and 7-day/week availability of therapists* to provide services when needed and to respond to crises. MST is proactive, and plans are developed to prevent or mitigate crises. Crisis response can be taxing, but most families are appreciative, and a supportive response can enhance engagement. Moreover, the capacity to respond to crises is critical to achieving a primary goal of MST programs—preventing out-of-home placements.

Skills and Achievements Emphasized in Treatment

Interventions are designed to be consistent with the nine core principles of MST, to be empirically based whenever possible, and to emphasize behavior change in the youth's natural environment that empowers caregivers and youth. A more extensive description of the range of problems addressed and clinical procedures used in MST can be found in the MST treatment manual (Henggeler, Schoenwald, Borduin, Rowland, & Cunningham, 1998).

Family Interventions

Engagement and assessment usually begin with meeting the family and youth to explain MST philosophies and principles. In the MST model, the therapist is more closely aligned with the caregivers, relative to the youth. Allying and engaging with caregivers is a critical component of the initial phase of treatment. Youth are also involved in the intake process, but as might be expected, some are reluctant to engage in a process that usually aims to place them under increased parental control. Each household member's perspective of the presenting problem and goals for treatment is solicited. A genogram is created, and information is obtained about the family, other people living in the home, extended family members, family supports, and the quality of important relationships. Each system is assessed for strengths and weaknesses, and values of the family are incorporated into the treatment plan with measurable goals. Guided by information obtained from the initial family meeting and other referring agencies, the MST therapist meets with individuals representing the interests of other organizations to gain their perspectives. Based on these initial data, hypotheses are generated concerning the factors that might facilitate goal achievement, serve as barriers to progress, and maintain negative behaviors. Hypotheses are testable, and hypothesis testing establishes the basis for interventions.

The MST therapist and treatment team must be well informed about research pertaining to family patterns and effective interventions relevant to youth antisocial behavior and other clinical problems. Family risk factors for antisocial behavior, for example, include low caregiver monitoring, low warmth, ineffective discipline, high conflict, caregiver psychopathology, and family criminal behavior, whereas protective factors include secure attachment to caregivers, supportive family environment, and marital harmony. Thus, the therapist must be capable of assessing the affective bond between caregiver and youth, parental control strategies on a permissive to restrictive continuum, and instrumental aspects of parenting such as structure and consistency. These family processes are assessed with direct questioning, observation, and response to homework assignments. Subsequent interventions aim to optimize strengths that already exist and develop competencies in critical areas that are lacking.

The MST therapist chooses specific parenting interventions with the assistance of the MST supervisor and expert consultant. The assessment of the fit of the particular problem to be addressed and the process of the implementation is pivotal to the selection. In a supportive and nonblaming manner, MST therapists praise positive aspects of parenting (Principle 2), while diplomatically identifying current parenting practices that might be changed for the benefit of all. For example, in a situation in which increased disciplinary structure is needed, interventions would likely occur in three stages. First, the caregivers learn to develop clearly defined rules for observable youth behavior. Second, the caregivers establish rewards and consequences that are closely, consistently, and naturally connected to youth behavior. Third, caregivers learn to monitor their child's compliance with the rules, including when the youth is not directly observable by the caregiver. In so doing, guidelines specified by Munger (1993, 1998) are often followed. Rules are developed to clearly delineate desired and undesired behaviors and are related to the goals of treatment. Expected behaviors are clearly defined and specified so others involved with the youth can determine whether the behavior has occurred. The rules should be posted in a public place and reinforced 100% of the time, in an emotionally neutral manner. Praise should accompany the dispensation of rewards. When two caregivers are involved, rules should be mutually agreed upon and enforced by both caregivers. Consequences need to be meaningful and appropriate to the specific youth. That is, rewards need to be items or activities that the particular youth is motivated to earn, while negative consequences should be disliked. Basic privileges, such as food, clothing, shelter, and love, are to be provided unconditionally and are not withheld or varied in their availability to the youth. Activities that promote prosocial development (e.g., sports teams) are considered growth activities and typically should not be withheld. Because of changes in the system or understanding of the fit, components of the behavior plan, such as the target behaviors, rewards, and consequences need to be continuously assessed and modified when appropriate.

Importantly, frequent barriers to the success of these family interventions pertain to caregiver difficulties, such as substance abuse or untreated mental illness. In such cases, the therapist's primary task is to remove these barriers to caregiver effectiveness by treating them directly. For example, a substance-abusing parent might be treated with a variation of the community reinforcement approach (Budney & Higgins, 1998), which has a strong empirical base in the area of adult substance abuse. Similarly, when caregiver effectiveness is compromised due to high levels of stress, the therapist works closely with the caregiver to identify sources of stress that might be modified and to develop strategies for such change. For example, a single working parent might have significant daily demands from employment responsibilities, caring for younger children, and providing support for an elderly relative. This parent might not have the time and energy needed to provide the high level of monitoring and supervision a problem adolescent often requires. Hence, the therapist would collaborate with the parent in developing and implementing strategies to achieve the desired goals (e.g., engaging the adolescent in structured after school activities and enlisting other supports to help with the elderly relative).

When barriers to effectiveness are removed, the caregiver is then in a position to function as the key change agent.

Peer Interventions

Peer relations affect youth functioning in many ways. Socialization with antisocial or substance-using peers is associated with these respective behaviors, while involvement with prosocial peers is a protective factor. Assessment of peer relations involves interviewing caregivers, school personnel, siblings, and the youth. The MST therapist attends to the number and quality of the peer relations, reputations of peers, social and academic functioning of peers, homogeneity versus heterogeneity of peer group, monitoring of peers by their respective caregivers, and the caregivers' familiarity with youths' peers and their parents.

Limited or poor social skills will contribute to rejection and isolation from peers. The MST therapist should assess the caregiver's social skills and address any caregiver factors that may be contributing to youth socialization difficulties. Some awkwardness may be due to a basic lack of skills or cognitive distortions. Depending on the problem, youth may respond to direct instruction, coaching techniques, and role playing as described by Forman (1993), for example, and the MST therapist will help the caregiver to assist the youth as indicated.

Conversely, youth who are actively rejected are at risk for externalizing behaviors. Peer groups can directly contribute to the youth's disruptive behavior by diverting the youth from more socially acceptable activities, endorsing antisocial behavior as the group norm, providing access to drugs, and encouraging resistance to caregiver monitoring. If the youth is socializing with negative peers, the MST therapist will help the caregiver to have calm discussions about potential negative consequences and avoid criticizing the peers valued by the youth. Interventions to back up these conversations may include systemic monitoring of the youth, caregiver and supportive adults searching places where the deviant peer group tends to socialize if the youth is unaccounted for, asking law enforcement to assist with checking and monitoring, and disallowing telephone contact with antisocial peers. Thus, a relatively stringent plan is put into place to provide significant sanctions for continuing association with problem peers. Concomitantly, MST therapists support caregivers to encourage and reinforce youth contact with prosocial peers and participation in socially accepted and monitored activities. Critical to the success of these interventions is the proactive development of plans to ensure implementation of positive and negative consequences contingent upon the youth's peer interactions. Such plans often include the therapist and several adults in the family's social network.

School Interventions

School is critical for both academic and social development. Risk factors for disruptive behavior in school include limited intellectual functioning, low achievement, learning disabilities, chaotic family functioning, negative family–school linkage, low commitment to education, and chaotic school environment. Protective factors include high intellectual functioning, commitment to schooling, and good caregiver–school communication. During all school interventions, MST therapists must respect the school's policies and procedures.

A frequent goal of treatment is to develop a collaborative relationship between the youth's caregivers and school personnel, in a context that has typically grown conflict-ual. The therapist supports the caregiver in interacting with the school but becomes di-rectly involved if necessary. For instance, when there is a family–school conflict impasse, the MST therapist might intervene in a diplomatic manner, emphasizing the best interests of the youth. The MST therapist performs a careful assessment of the nature of the con-flict and understands the views of all involved parties to help establish trust with both the family and the school. Unseen efforts of the school can be conveyed to the caregivers, and vice versa, while some misperceptions can be gently challenged. Common ground is highlighted, with a goal of setting up collaborative interactions between the school and caregivers. Ideally, these collaborations emphasize positive constructive changes that can help the youth and avoid revisiting prior decisions that cannot be changed or assigning blame for any real or perceived negative events. Importantly, arrangements are often made in which the parent is responsible for implementing contingencies at home based on youth behavior in school.

Individually Oriented Interventions

Whether for youth or caregivers, MST individually oriented interventions always occur in the context of a larger systemic treatment plan. Individually oriented interventions can be categorized as those addressing continued problematic behaviors after the implemen-tation of systemic interventions, continued problematic behaviors that occur in the face of psychiatric disorders that are being optimally treated from medication and systems perspectives, sequelae of victimization that relate to the presenting problems, and situa-tions in which extensive efforts to engage caregivers in changing their behavior are un-successful and the youth will continue to live in the home.

Cognitive-behavioral therapy (CBT) is an individual treatment approach that is fre-quently used in MST individual interventions. Considering the range of all individual treatments provided to youth, the empirical support for CBT for anxiety, depression, and externalizing conditions is relatively strong (Weisz & Jensen, 1999). CBT is consistent with MST in that it is present focused and action oriented (Principle 4), individualized to the developmental level of the youth (Principle 6), evaluated from multiple perspectives (Principle 8), and provides a skill that is potentially generalizable (Principle 9). Briefly, CBT involves first evaluating the youth's cognitions in areas related to the identified problem. This may include examining the youth's planning in achieving an objective, at-tributions regarding the motivation of others, social problem solving, perspective taking, or assessment of consequences of actions. The relationships between these cognitions and the youth's feelings and behaviors are also evaluated. Cognitive deficiencies and distor-tions are assessed as they apply to the presenting problem. Cognitive deficiencies are ad-dressed with the acquisition of additional skills. When cognitive distortions are identi-fied, they are tested; underlying maladaptive assumptions are delineated, and the validity of the maladaptive assumptions is tested. More adaptive cognitions and behaviors are then learned. Fortunately, several excellent resources for CBT interventions for various conditions are available (e.g., Forman, 1993; Kendall et al., 1992), and MST therapists are referred to and supervised in the implementation of these works as appropriate.

Psychiatric Interventions

MST therapists must be familiar with and able to recognize youth and adult conditions that may respond to psychiatric medication. For example, attention-deficit/hyperactivity disorder (ADHD) is often comorbid with disruptive behaviors, and the prognosis of comorbid ADHD and conduct disorder is associated with a more negative outcomes than conduct disorder or ADHD alone. Stimulant medications are well studied, and positive effects have been demonstrated for on-task behavior and various externalizing behaviors, while side effects are also well characterized and generally manageable.

If the MST treatment team feels that symptoms consistent with ADHD are interfering with goal achievement, a stimulant trial may be indicated. If the family is reluctant to follow through on the referral, their feelings should be respected while determining the fit and appropriate interventions. MST teams should seek child and adolescent psychiatrists who are systems oriented and well versed in empirically based treatments. The MST therapist can promote a positive working relationship by supporting youth and family follow-through with appointments and medication compliance while helping empower youth and caregivers to actively and assertively collaborate with the psychiatrist. After establishing a diagnosis of ADHD, a double-blind placebo trial may address some family concerns regarding efficacy and short-term side effects. Research suggests that for optimal pharmacological treatment of ADHD, ongoing medication management is needed (Vitiello et al., 2001).

Interventions for Increasing Family Social Supports

A major goal of MST is to develop and maintain social supports for the youth and family in order to promote sustainability of treatment gains. Youth disruptive behavior is associated with increased need for family supports and resources, yet many of the families referred to MST have few resources. Low socioeconomic status, social disorganization, and lack of supportive structures in and of themselves are risk factors for disruptive behavior (Loeber & Farrrington, 1998). Conversely, resources can help families manage the challenges of raising children as well as mitigate the negative effects of many hardships (Wolkow & Ferguson, 2001).

Assessment of family social supports occurs during the assessment of other youth-involved systems. Social supports can be characterized by type of support—instrumental, emotional, appraisal, and informational (Unger & Wandersman, 1985)—and also on a continuum ranging from informal, proximal relationships, to more distal, professional, and formal systems. The preference is to develop more proximal informal supports, as these are likely to be more responsive, accessible, and maintained over time. To maintain long-term informal social supports, families that receive support must reciprocate. For example, a neighbor might be enlisted to help monitor the after-school time of a problem adolescent with working parents; in return, the adolescent might cut the neighbor's lawn each week. Even with strong indigenous support, however, family needs can sometimes overwhelm the informal support system, necessitating the use of more formal supports. Hence, the MST treatment team should have a good understanding of the available formal supports in the community and the inner workings of each agency.

Treatment Termination

The average duration of MST treatment is 3 to 5 months. MST typically ends in one of two ways. Either the goals are met, by mutual agreement of the therapist, family, and, as appropriate, stakeholders; or the goals are unmet, but it is felt that treatment has reached a point of diminishing returns for time invested. It is important for the MST team to recognize situations in which progress is not being made, despite varied attempts to address barriers to effective change. In such cases, the decision to terminate MST services will contribute to the cost-effectiveness of MST and provide the family an opportunity to try another type of treatment that might be helpful.

Approximately two-thirds of MST cases in community settings end with successful achievement of the goals specified by the family and influential stakeholders. The latter stage of MST is spent preparing the youth, family, and stakeholders for the withdrawal of MST services, and termination is openly discussed. Caregiver competence is highlighted, and mechanisms for maintaining progress are identified. If there is a need for further services, appropriate referrals are made. However, it should not be assumed that families need ongoing services.

Quality Assurance System

In light of the importance of treatment fidelity to MST outcomes (Henggeler, Melton, Brondino, Scherer, & Hanley, 1997; Henggeler, Pickrel, & Borduin, 1999; Huey, Henggeler, Brondino, & Pickrel, 2000; Schoenwald, Henggeler, Brondino, & Rowland, 2000), considerable attention has been devoted to the development of quality assurance mechanisms aimed at enhancing treatment fidelity (Henggeler & Schoenwald, 1999).

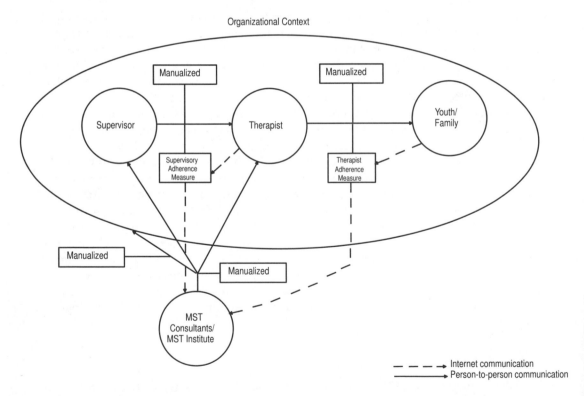

FIGURE 17.1. MST Continuous Quality Assurance System. From Henggeler, Schoenwald, Rowland, and Cunningham (2002). Copyright 2002 by The Guilford Press. Reprinted by permission.

Figure 17.1 provides a representation of the MST quality assurance system. As described extensively in by Henggeler, Schoenwald, Rowland, and Cunningham (2002), the therapist's interactions with the family are viewed as primary because of their critical role in achieving outcomes. Several structures and processes are used to support therapist adherence to MST when interacting with families. These processes include manualization of key components of the MST program, training of clinical and supervisory staff, ongoing feedback to the therapist from the supervisor and MST expert consultant, objective feedback from caregivers on a standardized adherence questionnaire, and organizational consultation. By providing multiple layers of clinical and programmatic support and ongoing feedback from several sources, the system aims to optimize favorable clinical outcomes through therapist support and adherence.

Manualization of Program Components

All components of the quality assurance system are manualized. The treatment manuals for antisocial behavior (Henggeler et al., 1998) and serious emotional disturbance (Henggeler, Schoenwald, Rowland, & Cunningham, 2002) are available from the publisher, The Guilford Press. The other manuals are available only to MST sites. Sites are licensed through MST Services, Inc. (*www.mstservices.com*), which has the exclusive license for the transport of MST technology and intellectual property through the Medical University of South Carolina.

Treatment (Henggeler et al., 1998): specifying MST clinical protocols based on the nine core treatment principles.

Supervision (Henggeler & Schoenwald, 1998): specifying the structure and processes of the weekly onsite supervisory sessions and ongoing development of therapist competences.

Expert consultation (Schoenwald, 1998): specifying the role of the MST consultant in helping teams achieve youth outcomes and in building the competencies of team therapists and supervisors.

Organizational support (Strother, Swenson, & Schoenwald, 1998): addressing administrative issues in developing and sustaining a MST program.

Training

Training in MST, which is provided to MST sites by MST Services, Inc., is ongoing and consists of several components.

Site assessment: The development of a new MST program is a process that requires significant community collaboration and often takes up to 12 months to complete.

Initial orientation: A 5-day training aimed at orienting clinical staff to program philosophy and intervention methods is provided prior to startup.

Expert consultation: Weekly telephone clinical consultations aimed at promoting treatment fidelity and youth outcomes and building team competencies are ongoing.

Quarterly booster training: Quarterly boosters are provided by expert consultants to address challenging clinical (e.g., caregiver cocaine abuse) or system (e.g., low referral rate) problems that are impeding the success of the program.

Outcome Monitoring Components

As discussed subsequently, considerable research efforts are underway to develop and validate a MST quality improvement system. Components that are currently validated include the following:

Therapist Adherence Measure (TAM; Henggeler & Borduin, 1992): This 26-item measure uses caregiver reports to track therapist adherence to MST treatment principles.
Supervisory Adherence Measure (SAM; Schoenwald, Henggeler, & Edwards, 1998): Based on therapist reports, this 43-item measure assesses supervisor adherence to the MST supervisory protocol (Henggeler & Schoenwald, 1998).
Youth Outcome Measure: A brief measure of ongoing youth outcomes is in development.

RESEARCH EMPHASES: OUTCOMES, QUALITY ASSURANCE, AND CURRENT TRIALS

Outcomes and findings from published clinical trials, findings from research on the components of the quality assurance system, and emerging research areas are described.

Evidence for the Effects of Treatment

Federal entities such as the Surgeon General (U.S. Department of Health and Human Services, 1999; U.S. Public Health Service, 2001), National Institute on Drug Abuse (1999), Center for Substance Abuse Prevention (2000), and leading reviewers (e.g., Burns, Hoagwood, & Mrazek, 1999; Elliott, 1998; Farrington & Welsh, 1999; Kazdin & Weisz, 1998; Stanton & Shadish, 1997) have identified MST as demonstrating considerable promise in the treatment of youth criminal behavior, substance abuse, and emotional disturbance. These conclusions are based on the findings from eight published outcome studies (seven randomized, one quasi-experimental) with youth presenting serious clinical problems and their families. As presented in Table 17.2, these studies included approximately 800 families, and, as discussed subsequently, approximately 4,000 additional families will have participated in MST research by 2004.

The following summary of juvenile justice, substance abuse, and mental health outcomes is based on the three randomized trials with chronic and violent juvenile offenders (Borduin et al., 1995; Henggeler et al., 1997; Henggeler, Melton, & Smith, 1992), one with substance-abusing juvenile offenders (Henggeler, Pickrel, & Brondino, 1999), one with youth presenting psychiatric crises (i.e., suicidal, homicidal, or psychotic) (Henggeler, Rowland, et al., 1999), one with maltreating families (Brunk, Henggeler, & Whelan, 1987), one with juvenile sexual offenders (Borduin, Henggeler, Blaske, & Stein, 1990), and one with inner-city delinquents (Henggeler et al., 1986). These projects were conducted in Memphis, several sites in South Carolina, and Columbia, Missouri.

Juvenile Justice Outcomes

Three randomized trials of MST with violent and chronic juvenile offenders were conducted in the 1990s. In the Simpsonville, South Carolina, Project, Henggeler et al. (1992) studied 84 juvenile offenders who were at imminent risk for out-of-home placement because of serious criminal activity. Youth and their families were randomly assigned to receive either MST or the usual services provided by the Department of Juvenile Justice

TABLE 17.2. Published MST Outcome Studies

Study	Population	Comparison	Follow-up	MST outcomes
Henggeler et al. (1986) $n = 57^a$	Delinquents	Diversion services	None	Improved family relations; decreased behavior problems; decreased association with deviant peers
Brunk, Henggeler, & Whelan (1987) $n = 33$	Maltreating families	Behavioral parent training	None	Improved parent–child interactions
Borduin, Henggeler, Blaske, & Stein (1990) $n = 16$	Adolescent sexual offenders	Individual counseling	3 years	Reduced sexual offending; reduced other criminal offending
Henggeler et al. (1991)^b	Serious juvenile offenders	Individual counseling Usual community Services	3 years	Reduced alcohol and marijuana use; decreased drug-related arrests
Henggeler, Melton, & Smith (1992) $n = 84$	Violent and chronic juvenile offenders	Usual community services— high rates of incarceration	59 weeks	Improved family relations; improved peer relations; decreased recidivism (43%); decreased out-of-home placement (64%)
Henggeler et al. (1993)	Same sample		2.4 years	Decreased recidivism (doubled survival rate)
Borduin et al. (1995) $n - 176$	Violent and chronic juvenile offenders	Individual counseling	4 years (10-year outcomes forthcoming)	Improved family relations; decreased psychiatric symptomatology; decreased recidivism (69%)
Henggeler, et al. (1997) $n = 155$	Violent and chronic juvenile offenders	Juvenile probation services— high rates of incarceration	1.7 years	Decreased psychiatric symptomatology; decreased days in out-of-home placement (50%); decreased recidivism (26%, nonsignificant); treatment adherence linked with long-term outcomes
Henggeler, Rowland, et al. (1999) $n = 116$ (final sample = 156)	Youths presenting psychiatric emergencies	Psychiatric hospitalization	None (2-year outcomes forthcoming)	Decreased externalizing problems (CBCL); improved family relations; increased school attendance; higher consumer satisfaction
Schoenwald et al. (2000)	Same sample			75% reduction in days hospitalized; 50% reduction in days in other out-of-home placements

(continues)

TABLE 17.2 (*Continued*)

Study	Population	Comparison	Follow-up	MST outcomes
Henggeler, Pickrel, & Brondino (1999) *n* = 118	Substance-abusing and dependent delinquents	Usual community services	1 year	Decreased drug use at posttreatment; decreased days in out-of-home placement (50%); decreased recidivism (26%, nonsignificant); treatment adherence linked with decreased drug use
Schoenwald et. al. (1996)	Same sample		1 year	Incremental cost of MST nearly offset by between-groups differences in out-of-home placement
Brown et al. (1999)	Same sample		6 months	Increased attendance in regular school settings
Henggeler et al. (2002)	Same sample		4 years	Decreased violent crime; increased marijuana abstinence

Note. From Henggeler, Schoenwald, Rowland, and Cunningham (2002). Copyright 2002 by The Guilford Press. Reprinted by permission.
[a]Quasi-experimental design (groups matched on demographic characteristics); all other studies are randomized.
[b]Based on participants in Henggeler et al. (1992) and Borduin et al. (1995).

(DJJ). At posttreatment, youth who participated in MST reported less criminal activity than their counterparts in the usual services group, and at a 59-week follow-up, MST had reduced rearrests by 43%. In addition, usual-services youth had an average of almost three times more weeks incarcerated (average = 16.2 weeks) than MST youth (average = 5.8 weeks). Moreover, treatment gains were maintained at long-term follow-up (Henggeler, Melton, Smith, Schoenwald, & Hanley, 1993). At 2.4 years post-referral, twice as many MST youth had not been rearrested (39%) as usual-services youth (20%).

In the Columbia, Missouri, Project (Borduin et al., 1995), participants were 200 chronic juvenile offenders and their families who were referred by the local DJJ. Families were randomly assigned to receive either MST or individual therapy (IT). Four-year follow-up arrest data showed that youth who received MST were arrested less often and for less serious crimes than counterparts who received IT. Moreover, while youth who completed a full course of MST had the lowest rearrest rate (22.1%), those who received MST but prematurely dropped out of treatment had better rates of rearrest (46.6%) than IT completers (71.4%), IT dropouts (71.4%) or treatment refusers (87.5%).

In the Multisite South Carolina Study, Henggeler et al. (1997) examined the role of treatment fidelity in the successful dissemination of MST. In contrast with previous clinical trials in which the developers of MST provided ongoing clinical supervision and consultation (i.e., quality assurance was high), MST experts were not significantly involved in treatment implementation and quality assurance was low. Participants were 155 chronic or violent juvenile offenders who were at risk of out-of-home placement because of serious criminal involvement and their families. Youth and their families were randomly assigned to receive MST or the usual services offered by DJJ. Not surprisingly,

MST treatment effect sizes were smaller than in previous studies that had greater quality assurance. Over a 1.7-year follow-up, MST reduced rearrests by 25%, which was lower than the 43% and 70% reductions in rearrest in the previous MST studies with serious juvenile offenders. Days incarcerated, however, were reduced by 47%. Importantly, high therapist adherence to the MST treatment protocols, as assessed by caregiver reports on the TAM, predicted fewer rearrests and incarcerations. Thus, the modest treatment effects for rearrest in this study might be attributed to considerable variance in therapists' adherence to MST principles.

In summary, across the three trials with violent and chronic juvenile offenders, MST produced 25% to 70% decreases in long-term rates of rearrest, and 47% to 64% decreases in long-term rates of days in out-of-home placements. These outcomes have resulted in considerable cost savings. The Washington State Institute on Public Policy (Aos, Phipps, Barnoski, & Lieb, 1999) concluded that MST produced more than $60,000 per youth in savings in placement, criminal justice, and crime victim costs.

Substance Use Outcomes

Two trials have demonstrated short-term reductions in adolescent substance use (Henggeler et al., 1992; Henggeler, Pickrel, & Brondino, 1999); Borduin et al. (1995) have demonstrated long-term reductions in substance-related arrests; and Henggeler, Clingempeel, Brondino, and Pickrel (2002) have demonstrated treatment effects on rates of marijuana abstinence in a 4-year follow-up. In addition, MST has made an important contribution to the substance abuse literature regarding family engagement and retention in treatment. In a study with diagnosed substance-abusing or dependent juvenile offenders (Henggeler et al., 1999), fully 100% (58 of 58) of families in the MST condition were retained in treatment for at least 2 months and 98% were retained until treatment termination at approximately 4 months postreferral. Moreover, Schoenwald, Ward, Henggeler, Pickrel, and Patel (1996) showed that the incremental costs of MST in this trial were nearly offset by the savings incurred as a result of reductions in days of out-of-home placement during the year.

Mental Health Outcomes

MST has demonstrated favorable decreases in psychiatric symptoms in three studies with juvenile offenders (Borduin et al., 1995; Henggeler et al., 1997; Henggeler et al., 1986). A recent study, however, examined the clinical effectiveness of MST with an extremely challenging mental health population—youth in psychiatric crisis approved for emergency hospitalization (Henggeler, Rowland, et al., 1999). Here, MST was more effective than hospitalization at decreasing externalizing symptoms and as effective at decreasing internalizing symptoms. With regard to out-of-home placements, over the first 4 months postreferral, MST produced a 72% reduction in days hospitalized and a 49% reduction in other out-of-home placements (Schoenwald, Ward, Henggeler, & Rowland, 2000).

Mediating and Moderating Variables

MST treatment theory posits that improved caregiver and family functioning are key factors in achieving desired short- and long-term outcomes. This assumption was directly tested and supported by Huey et al. (2000), who showed that improved family functioning predicted decreased association with deviant peers, which, in turn, predicted decreased adolescent antisocial behavior. Indirect support for this treatment theory is provided in the multiple MST studies demonstrating improved family functioning, two recent studies demonstrating increased attendance in regular school classrooms (Brown, Henggeler, Schoenwald, Brondino, & Pickrel, 1999; Henggeler, Rowland et al., 1999), and a recent study showing significantly higher levels of consumer satisfaction for caregivers and youth in the MST condition (Henggeler, Rowland, et al., 1999).

Regarding moderating variables, with few exceptions, favorable MST outcomes have not been moderated by case seriousness or demographic (e.g., race, social class, and gender) characteristics. Hence, outcomes have not varied as a function of such variables. This general absence of moderating influences most likely reflects the intended individualization of MST services to the particular needs, circumstances, and contexts of the youth and families.

Testing the MST Quality Assurance System

One of the long-term goals of this system is to develop strategies that enable continuous tracking of therapist adherence and youth outcomes. Such a system, however, requires the demonstration of empirical linkages between key components of quality assurance. This section describes the empirical status of the linkages shown in Figure 17.1.

Four published studies have demonstrated significant associations between therapist fidelity and youth outcomes. Analyses of data collected in two randomized trials showed that caregiver reports of high adherence on the aforementioned TAM during treatment were associated with low rates of rearrest and incarceration of chronic juvenile offenders at a 1.7-year follow-up (Henggeler et al., 1997) and with decreased criminal activity and out-of-home placement in substance-abusing juvenile offenders approximately 12 months postreferral (Henggeler, Pickrel, & Brondino, 1999). Using data from these two randomized trials, findings from Huey et al. (2000) and Schoenwald et al. (2000) supported the view that therapist adherence to MST principles influences those processes (e.g., family relations and association with deviant peers) that sustain adolescent antisocial behavior.

In addition, A recent nine-site study has demonstrated significant associations between therapist reports of supervisor adherence to the MST supervisory protocol and caregiver reports of therapist adherence to MST treatment principles. (Henggeler, Schoenwald, Liao, Letourneau, & Edwards, 2002). Hence, as assumed in the quality assurance model, supervisor behavior predicts therapist behavior.

Although, two of the key associations in the MST quality assurance system (i.e., the therapist–family linkage and the supervisor–therapist linkage) have been supported empirically, the influence of other aspects of the system remains to be determined. A 41-site study is currently under way that will provide important data regarding the remaining linkages. This study (Schoenwald, PI) is examining the relationship of therapist adherence to child outcomes in 41 community-based MST programs as well as the impact of therapist, supervisory, organizational, and interagency factors on therapist fidelity to MST. Data regarding consultation provided to these programs is being collected, such that potential links between consultation, supervision, and therapist adherence can be examined for the first time.

Ongoing Research

Investigators in numerous states and several countries are conducting studies that will expand the MST knowledge base in several important directions.

Multisite Effectiveness Trials

As Weisz (2000) has emphasized, the distinctions between efficacy and effectiveness research are considerable—demonstrating efficacy is quite a different thing than the effective implementation of an evidence-based practice in real-world settings. Multisite effectiveness studies are being conducted with juvenile offenders in Canada (Alan W. Leshied, PI), Norway (Terje Ogden, PI), Washington state (Robert Barnoski, PI), and New York (Reese Satin, PI). Findings from these studies will provide important information regarding the transport of MST to real world settings.

Adaptations to New Populations and Replications

Several randomized trials are examining the effectiveness of MST adaptations with populations that have not been the traditional focus of the model. Deborah Ellis and her colleagues (Detroit) are adapting MST to treat children and adolescents with insulin-dependent diabetes mellitus who are under poor metabolic control. Charles Borduin (Columbia, Missouri) has recently completed a replication of MST with juvenile sexual offenders. Bahr Weiss, Tom Catron, and Vicki Harris (Nashville) are conducting a randomized trial of MST with middle school and high school students enrolled in classrooms designed for students with serious behavior problems. In addition, faculty at the Family Services Research Center in Charleston, South Carolina, are directing several randomized trials to extend the model, including a study integrating MST into juvenile drug court for treating substance-abusing juvenile offenders (Henggeler, PI), a randomized trial of MST with physically abused youth and their families (Cindy Swenson, PI), and a trial in Philadelphia evaluating the clinical and cost-effectiveness of an MST-based continuum of care as an alternative to out-of-state residential placement (Sonja Schoenwald, PI).

DIRECTIONS FOR FUTURE RESEARCH

Although MST is relatively well validated in the treatment of serious criminal behavior in adolescents, such validation represents a necessary but far from sufficient step in improving the nation's health. Currently, licensed MST programs are operating in 30 states and several countries. In the United States, these programs serve approximately 1% of juvenile offenders at imminent risk of incarceration. In light of the fact that MST is probably the most widely disseminated evidence-based treatment for juvenile offenders in the United States, the vast majority of such youth are not receiving services that have a reasonable probability of improving outcomes. Numerous challenges and research opportunities are posed by these circumstances, and they can be subsumed in one question: "At the levels of consumers, practitioners, agency administrators, policy makers, and funders, what are the barriers to the adoption, implementation, and sustainability of evidence-based practices and what are effective strategies for overcoming these barriers?" This question is consistent with emphases of the Surgeon General's Action Agenda for Children's Mental Health (U.S. Public Health Service, 2000) and reflects a major thrust of several state and National Institutes of Health initiatives.

MST is less well validated in the treatment of several other serious clinical problems, including serious emotional disturbance, child maltreatment, and substance abuse. As indicated previously, several randomized trials are currently in progress addressing these clinical populations. If favorable outcomes are achieved, population specific adaptations of the model might be ready for dissemination (currently, MST has been transported solely for youth presenting serious antisocial behavior and their families). For example, MST for youth with serious emotional disturbance has required adaptation to provide considerably more psychiatric support and increased clinical resources (and cost) than standard MST programs. Similarly, the integration of another evidence-based treatment (i.e., contingency management) with MST in the treatment of adolescent substance abuse seems to be improving substance-related outcomes. These adaptations require specification and integration into all components of the MST quality assurance protocols before transport to field settings can be attempted.

Interestingly, another line of research is examining the potential application of MST for medically related problems. The work of Ellis, Naar-King, Frey, Greger, and Arfken, noted previously, best exemplifies this work. This research group is funded by the National Institute on Diabetes and Kidney Disease to conduct a randomized trial on an adaptation of MST to treat children and adolescents with insulin-dependent diabetes mellitus. Funding was based, in part, on favorable pilot data. Similarly, a proposal is in preparation to adapt the model for youth at high risk of transplant rejection due to low medication compliance. Such work is made possible because MST is not a "treatment" per se. It is a set of strategies aimed at using existing knowledge bases as the foundation for critical analysis of specific costly behavioral problems, within the context of organizational commitments to accountability, service access, and consumer empowerment.

A final area of research is more traditional in focus: aiming to identify the mechanisms of change in MST services. This work is best exemplified by Stan Huey's (Huey et al., 2000) study of the mediators of MST outcomes. Similar analyses are planned for current MST trials and additional studies are being planned to examine associations between in session behavior, based on audiorecordings, and client outcomes. Hence, MST research is ranging from the micro (e.g., therapist–family interaction during sessions) to the macro (e.g., Schoenwald study examining the effects of funding structures on MST programs).

SUMMARY AND CONCLUSIONS

MST is a family-based treatment for youth presenting serious clinical problems, including criminal behavior and violence, substance abuse, and serious emotional disturbance. The evidence base for MST, especially in treating serious antisocial behavior in adolescents, is relatively strong, with several published randomized trials with violent and chronic juvenile offenders showing reductions in recidivism and out-of-home placement. On the strength of this record, MST programs focusing on adolescent antisocial behavior have been adopted by provider organizations in 30 states and 7 nations. Indeed, multisite research is currently examining the capacity of MST programs in community-based settings to achieve outcomes comparable to those attained in clinical trials, and several large multisite effectiveness trials are under way as well. In addition, the fundamental MST model is being adapted to treat other challenging clinical problems that present significant costs to the juvenile justice, mental health, social welfare, and health care service systems. These adaptations are being examined within the context of randomized trials with maltreating families, youth presenting serious emotional disturbance, adolescents with serious medical problems, and substance-abusing youths. If these projects are successful and replicated, plans will be developed to transport such MST adaptations to the field.

Importantly, the success of MST has been based largely on research literatures developed across several disciplines during the past 20–30 years. For example, decades of correlational and longitudinal research have delineated key risk factors in the development and maintenance of antisocial behavior in adolescents. MST interventions focus on these risk factors. Similarly, a cadre of outstanding efficacy researchers have developed and validated models of intervention for particular well-defined clinical problems. MST intervention protocols make extensive use of this evidence base. On the other hand, the MST model has gone against the traditions of much of the mental health treatment community by, for example, emphasizing the importance of provider accountability for outcomes and quality assurance systems to facilitate program fidelity, viewing caregivers as the key to long-term outcomes, and making programmatic commitments to overcome barriers to service access. Nevertheless, careful review of major federal reports (e.g., Surgeon General's reports on mental health and youth violence) and the conclusions of leading theorists and researchers, such as the editors of this volume, suggest that such programmatic emphases represent a direction in which the field is heading.

ACKNOWLEDGMENTS

Work on this chapter was supported by Grants DA10079 and DA99008 from the National Institute on Drug Abuse; MH59138, MH51852, and MH60663 from the National Institute of Mental Health; AA122202 from the National Institute on Alcohol Abuse and Alcoholism, and the Annie E. Casey Foundation.

REFERENCES

Aos, S., Phipps, P., Barnoski, R., & Lieb, R. (1999). *The comparative costs and benefits of programs to reduce crime: A review of national research findings with implications for Washington state, Version 3.0.* Olympia: Washington State Institute for Public Policy.

Borduin, C. M., Henggeler, S. W., Blaske, D. M., & Stein, R. (1990). Multisystemic treatment of adolescent sexual offenders. *International Journal of Offender Therapy and Comparative Criminology, 35,* 105–114.

Borduin, C. M., Mann, B. J., Cone, L. T., Henggeler, S. W., Fucci, B. R., Blaske, D. M., & Williams, R. A. (1995). Multisystemic treatment of serious juvenile offenders: Long-term prevention of criminality and violence. *Journal of Consulting and Clinical Psychology, 63,* 569–578.

Bronfenbrenner, U. (1979). *The ecology of human development: Experiments by design and nature.* Cambridge, MA: Harvard University Press.

Brown, T. L., Henggeler, S. W., Schoenwald, S. K., Brondino, M. J., & Pickrel, S. G. (1999). Multisystemic treatment of substance abusing and dependent juvenile delinquents: Effects on school attendance at posttreatment and 6-month follow-up. *Children's Services: Social Policy, Research, and Practice, 2,* 81–93.

Brunk, M., Henggeler, S. W., & Whelan, J. P. (1987). A comparison of multisystemic therapy and parent training in the brief treatment of child abuse and neglect. *Journal of Consulting and Clinical Psychology, 55,* 311–318.

Budney, A. J., & Higgins, S. T. (1998). *A community reinforcement plus vouchers approach: Treating cocaine addiction.* (Pub. No. NIH 98-4309). Washington, DC: U.S. Department of Health and Human Services, National Institutes of Health.

Burns, B. J., Hoagwood, K., & Mrazek, P. J. (1999). Effective treatment for mental disorders in children and adolescents. *Clinical Child and Family Psychology Review, 2,* 199–254.

Center for Substance Abuse Prevention. (2000). *Strengthening America's families: Model family programs for substance abuse and delinquency prevention.* Salt Lake City: Department of Health Promotion and Education, University of Utah.

Elliott, D. S. (Series Ed.). (1998). *Blueprints for violence prevention* Boulder, CO: University of Colorado, Center for the Study and Prevention of Violence, Blueprints Publications.

Farrington, D. P., & Welsh, B. C. (1999). Delinquency prevention using family-based interventions. *Children and Society, 13,* 287–303.

Forman, S. G. (1993). *Coping skills interventions for children and adolescents.* San Francisco: Jossey-Bass.

Haley, J. (1976). *Problem solving therapy.* San Francisco: Jossey-Bass.

Henggeler, S. W., & Borduin, C. M. (1992). *Multisystemic Therapy Adherence Scales.* Unpublished instrument, Department of Psychiatry and Behavioral Sciences, Medical University of South Carolina.

Henggeler, S. W., Borduin, C. M., Melton, G. B., Mann, B. J., Smith, L., Hall, J. A., Cone, L., & Fucci, B. R. (1991). Effects of multisystemic therapy on drug use and abuse in serious juvenile offenders: A progress report from two outcome studies. *Family Dynamics of Addiction Quarterly, 1,* 40–51.

Henggeler, S. W., Clingempeel, W. G., Brondino, M. J., & Pickrel, S. G. (2002). Four-year follow-up of multisystemic therapy with substance abusing and dependent juvenile offenders. *Journal of the American Academy of Child and Adolescent Psychiatry, 41,* 868–874.

Henggeler, S. W., Melton, G. B., Brondino, M. J., Scherer, D. G., & Hanley, J. H. (1997). Multisystemic therapy with violent and chronic juvenile offenders and their families: The role of treatment fidelity in successful dissemination. *Journal of Consulting and Clinical Psychology, 65,* 821–833.

Henggeler, S. W., Melton, G. B., & Smith, L. A. (1992). Family preservation using multisystemic therapy: An effective alternative to incarcerating serious juvenile offenders. *Journal of Consulting and Clinical Psychology, 60,* 953–961.

Henggeler, S. W., Melton, G. B., Smith, L. A., Schoenwald, S. K., & Hanley, J. H. (1993). Family preservation using multisystemic treatment: Long-term follow-up to a clinical trial with serious juvenile offenders. *Journal of Child and Family Studies, 2,* 283–293.

Henggeler, S. W., Pickrel, S. G., & Brondino, M. J. (1999). Multisystemic treatment of substance abusing and dependent delinquents: Outcomes, treatment fidelity, and transportability. *Mental Health Services Research, 1,* 171–184.

Henggeler, S. W., Pickrel, S. G., Brondino, M. J., & Crouch, J. L. (1996). Eliminating (almost) treatment dropout of substance abusing or dependent delinquents through home-based multisystemic therapy. *American Journal of Psychiatry, 153,* 427–428.

Henggeler, S. W., Rodick, J. D., Borduin, C. M., Hanson, C. L., Watson, S. M., & Urey, J. R. (1986). Multisystemic treatment of juvenile offenders: Effects on adolescent behavior and family interactions. *Developmental Psychology, 22,* 132–141.

Henggeler, S. W., Rowland, M. R., Randall, J., Ward, D., Pickrel, S. G., Cunningham, P. B., Miller, S. L., Edwards, J. E., Zealberg, J., Hand, L., & Santos, A. B. (1999). Home-based multisystemic therapy as an alternative to the hospitalization of youth in psychiatric crisis: Clinical outcomes. *Journal of the American Academy of Child and Adolescent Psychiatry, 38,* 1331–1339.

Henggeler, S. W., & Schoenwald, S. K. (1998). *The MST supervisory manual: Promoting quality assurance at the clinical level.* Charleston, SC: MST Services.

Henggeler, S. W., & Schoenwald, S. K. (1999). The role of quality assurance in achieving outcomes in MST programs. *Journal of Juvenile Justice and Detention Services, 14,* 1–17.

Henggeler, S. W., Schoenwald, S. K., Borduin, C. M., Rowland, M. D., & Cunningham, P. B. (1998). *Multisystemic treatment of antisocial behavior in children and adolescents.* New York: Guilford Press.

Henggeler, S. W., Schoenwald, S. K., Liao, J. G., Letourneau, E. J., & Edwards, D. L. (2002). Transporting efficacious treatments to field settings: The link between supervisory practices and therapist fidelity in MST programs. *Journal of Clinical Child Psychology, 31,* 155–167.

Henggeler, S. W., Schoenwald, S. K., Rowland, M. D., & Cunningham, P. B. (2002). *Serious emotional disturbance in children and adolescents: Multisystemic therapy.* New York: Guilford Press.

Huey, S. J., Henggeler, S. W., Brondino, M. J., & Pickrel, S. G. (2000). Mechanisms of change in multisystemic therapy: Reducing delinquent behavior through therapist adherence and improved family and peer functioning. *Journal of Consulting and Clinical Psychology, 68,* 451–467.

Kazdin, A. E., & Weisz, J. R. (1998). Identifying and developing empirically supported child and adolescent treatments. *Journal of Consulting and Clinical Psychology, 66,* 19–36.

Kendall, P. C., Chansky, T. E., Kane, M. T., Kim, R., Kortlander, E., Ronan, K. R., Sessa, F. M., & Siqueland, L. (1992). *Anxiety disorders in youth: Cognitive-behavioral interventions.* Needham Height, MA: Allyn & Bacon.

Loeber, R., & Farrington, D. P. (1998). *Serious and violent juvenile offenders: Risk factors and successful interventions.* Thousand Oaks, CA: Sage Publications.

Minuchin, S. (1974). *Families and family therapy.* Cambridge, MA: Harvard University Press.

Munger, R. L. (1993). *Changing children's behavior quickly.* Lanham, MD: Madison Books.

Munger, R. L. (1998). *The ecology of troubled children: Changing children's behavior by changing the places, activities and people in their lives.* Cambridge, MA: Brookline Books.

National Institute on Drug Abuse. (1999). *Principles of drug addiction treatment: A research-based guide* (NIH Publication No. 99-4180). Rockville, MD: Author.

Schoenwald, S. K. (1998). *Multisystemic therapy consultation guidelines.* Charleston, SC: MST Institute.

Schoenwald, S. K., Henggeler, S. W., Brondino, M. J., & Rowland, M. D. (2000). Multisystemic therapy: Monitoring treatment fidelity. *Family Process, 39,* 83–103.

Schoenwald, S. K., Henggeler, S. W., & Edwards, D. (1998). *MST Supervisor Adherence Measure.* Charleston, SC: MST Institute.

Schoenwald, S. K., Ward, D. M., Henggeler, S. W., Pickrel, S. G., & Patel, H. (1996). MST treatment of substance abusing or dependent adolescent offenders: Costs of reducing incarceration, inpatient, and residential placement. *Journal of Child and Family Studies, 5,* 431–444.

Schoenwald, S. K., Ward, D. M., Henggeler, S. W., & Rowland, M. D. (2000). MST vs. hospitalization for crisis stabilization of youth: Placement outcomes 4 months post-referral. *Mental Health Services Research, 2,* 3–12.

Stanton, M. D., & Shadish, W. R. (1997). Outcome, attrition, and family–couples treatment for drug abuse: A meta-analysis and review of the controlled, comparative studies. *Psychological Bulletin, 122,* 170–191.

Strother, K. B., Swenson, M. E., & Schoenwald, S. K. (1998). *Multisystemic therapy organizational manual.* Charleston, SC: MST Institute.

Unger, D.G., & Wandersman, A. (1985). The importance of neighbors: The social, cognitive, and affective components of neighboring. *American Journal of Community Psychology, 13,* 139–169.

U.S. Department of Health and Human Services. (1999). *Mental health: A report of the Surgeon General.* Rockville, MD: National Institutes of Health, National Institute of Mental Health.

U.S. Public Health Service. (2000). *Report of the Surgeon General's Conference on Children's Mental Health: A national action agenda.* Washington, DC: Author.

U.S. Public Health Service. (2001). *Youth violence: A report of the Surgeon General.* Washington, DC: Author.

Vitiello, B., Sever, J. B., Greenhill, L. L., Arnold, L. E., Abikoff, H. B., Bukstein, O. G., Elliott, G. R., Hechtman, L., Jensen, P. S., Hinshaw, S. P., March, J. S., Newcorn, J. H., Swanson, J. M., & Cantwell, D. P. (2001). Methylphenidate dosage for children with ADHD over time under controlled conditions: Lessons from the MTA. *Journal of the American Academy of Child and Adolescent Psychiatry, 40*(2), 188–196.

Weisz, J. R. (2000). Agenda for child and adolescent psychotherapy research: On the need to put science into practice. *Archives of General Psychiatry, 57,* 837–838.

Weisz, J. R., & Jensen, P. S. (1999). Efficacy and effectiveness of child and adolescent psychotherapy and pharmacotherapy. *Mental Health Services Research, 1,* 125–157.

Werner, E. E., & Smith, R. S. (2001). *Journey from childhood to midlife: Risk, resiliency, and recovery.* Ithaca, NY: Cornell University Press.

Wolkow, K. E., & Ferguson, H. B. (2001). Community factors in the development of resiliency: Considerations and future directions. *Community Mental Health Journal, 37*(6), 489–498.

C

Other Disorders and Special Applications

18

Early and Intensive Behavioral Intervention in Autism

O. Ivar Lovaas and Tristram Smith

OVERVIEW

Autism begins in the first 3 years after birth and is almost always lifelong without treatment. According to recent estimates, it occurs in about 1 in 750 children (Chakrabarti & Fombonne, 2001). It is three or four times more common in boys than girls. Children receive a diagnosis of autism based on difficulties in communication, social interaction, and repetitive or ritualistic behaviors.

Many children with autism are nonverbal; others simply repeat what others say instead of using language to communicate. A few use language to state their wishes or describe favorite topics but not to engage in a reciprocal conversation. The children tend to have one-sided relationships with caregivers. They may make frequent demands and protest when caregivers leave them yet refuse physical affection, avoid eye contact, wander away from caregivers in public, and make little effort to share enjoyment (e.g., showing caregivers something they have done). They often ignore or actively distance themselves from peers. Rather than playing creatively with toys, they may engage in repetitive activities or routines such as feeling textures on objects, watching objects move back and forth, or insisting on a particular arrangement of household furniture. Interrupting these behaviors or making requests may trigger tantrums or aggression. At times, such children may be so inattentive to their surroundings that caregivers worry that they have sensory impairments, yet, at other times, the same children may be acutely sensitive. For example, despite ignoring a loud banging noise right next to them, they may jump up when a candy bar is unwrapped out of sight in another room. Most score in the range of mental retardation on standardized intelligence tests and have delays in self-care skills such as toileting and dressing.

Two Conceptualizations of Autism

Some investigators view autism as a distinct disorder with an etiology, symptom presentation, and course that clearly set it apart from other disorders and from typical development. However, other investigators view autism as simply a term describing children who lie at one extreme of a continuous dimension of behavior (Lovaas & Smith, 1989). In the dimensional view, while some children diagnosed with autism are markedly different from typically developing children, others "shade into the eccentric end of the wide range of normal behavior" (Wing, 1992, p. 138). Stated differently, everyone has difficulty with communication, reciprocal interaction, and repetitive behavior at one time or another, and it remains unclear whether the high level of difficulty displayed by children diagnosed with autism reflects a distinct disorder or one end of a spectrum of behavior (Beglinger & Smith, 2001).

These two different approaches to conceptualizing autism have important ramifications for treatment research. If the hypothesis that autism is a distinct disorder is correct, an appropriate research strategy is to specify the characteristics and course of the disorder, search for the etiology, and develop interventions based on the etiology. However, if the "distinct disorder" view is incorrect, this strategy may fail. For instance, if autism is not a distinct disorder, it may not have a specific etiology. Also, it may be possible to identify effective treatments without knowing the etiology. In other developmental disabilities such as phenylketonuria, investigators developed effective interventions long before isolating the etiology. Thus, the view of autism as a distinct disorder is a hypothesis that has the potential to guide research but also to be misleading. Indeed, many interventions based on this hypothesis have been unsuccessful. As an example, investigators have proposed that autism results from problems in processing sensory information or from inability to bond with caregivers, but research on treatments derived from these proposals consistently yields discouraging results (Smith, 1996).

BEHAVIORAL APPROACHES TO AUTISM

Because no one yet knows whether autism is a distinct disorder and whether conceptualizing it as such will help identify effective treatments, many investigators, particularly behaviorists, use a more inductive data-driven research strategy in contrast to theory-driven research. Instead of proposing an etiology and treatment for autism and then testing this proposal, behaviorists (sometimes also called applied behavior analysts) aim to build up interventions piece by piece, with each study adding to previous ones in a cumulative manner.

Behavioral investigators have developed methodologies to facilitate this process (Lovaas & Smith, 1989). First, they shift the focus of study from etiology to events in children's current environments. Such events are much easier to observe and alter than are etiological variables such as genetic factors or early history. As a result, investigators can systematically present or remove these events and examine the effects of these changes in experimentally controlled studies.

Second, to assess effects precisely, behaviorists break down the construct of autism into its separate behavioral delays and excesses. Each of these deviant behaviors allows for the investigator to obtain objective, sensitive measures of each behavior. For example, they can count the frequency of communicative speech and classify this speech into categories (e.g., making requests vs. labeling objects). Therefore, when they alter features of the environment, they can detect even small changes in a child's behavior.

Third, instead of hypothesizing that autistic behaviors arise from a process unique to children with autism (e.g., a certain underlying cognitive disturbance), behaviorists emphasize well-studied principles of learning and behavior that apply to a wide range of individuals. Principles of operant conditioning have proved especially useful, as discussed later.

Finally, because large individual differences exist among children diagnosed with autism (e.g., some are nonverbal while others have extensive language), behaviorists emphasize intensive studies of individual children using single-case experimental designs such as ABAB reversal or multiple baseline design. The goal is to discover interventions that have reliable, clinically meaningful benefits for each child. Children may then be classified into groups based on a common response to intervention rather than a common set of behaviors; thus, the classification is functional rather than topographical. For example, one group of children may have tantrums that serve to escape or avoid requests made by others and that may be treated by teaching appropriate responses to requests and preventing escape. In contrast, another group may have tantrums that serve to obtain access to preferred objects or activities and that may be treated by teaching appropriate ways to communicate wishes.

Development of Behavioral Treatment

Behavioral studies of children with autism began in the early 1960s when investigators successfully applied operant conditioning to teach simple behaviors such as pulling levers. Although this teaching had no therapeutic benefit, it was important because it showed that children with autism could learn in a manner like that of other individuals. Soon, investigators discovered that they could also use operant conditioning to teach important skills such as communication and management of aggression. In the late 1960s and 1970s, they extended these findings to other behavioral problems but, at the same time, detected shortcomings in the interventions they designed. Teaching one skill did not by itself lead to improvements in others skills. For example, teaching language skills did not usually improve peer interaction unless peer interaction skills were also taught. Also, gains tended to be situation specific; despite improving with therapists in clinical settings, children's behavior often remained unchanged with caregivers in everyday settings such as home or school (Lovaas, Koegel, Simmons, & Long, 1973).

To overcome these shortcomings, investigators sought to make intervention comprehensive, addressing every behavioral problem that a child exhibited (communication, social interaction, toy play, etc.) as opposed to any one area of difficulty. In addition, to generalize gains across environments, they moved treatment into children's homes and communities, with the active participation of people in those settings such as parents, peers, and teachers (Lovaas & Smith, 1989). More recently, investigators have refined procedures for teaching skills during children's daily activities instead of separate therapy sessions and for tailoring interventions to meet the needs of individual children with autism (Matson, Benavidez, Comptom, Paclawskyj, & Baglio, 1996).

Overview of Behavioral Treatment

The overall goal is to maximize children's functioning so that they can develop meaningful relationships with others and take better advantage of learning opportunities in their homes, schools, and communities. Specific goals consist of reducing excesses (behaviors done too often or too intensely) and alleviating deficits or delays (behaviors done too seldom). From the description of these children at the outset of this chapter, two main types of excesses are evident: repetitive or ritualistic behaviors and tantrums or aggression. The main areas of delay are communication, cognitive skills, interaction with caregivers, peer play, toy play, attention, and self-care. Some children with autism display additional excesses or delays such as eating or sleeping disturbances. Investigators have developed numerous approaches for assessing and treating these excesses and delays, and behavioral treatment has become the main empirically supported intervention for children with autism (Newsom, 1998).

Behavioral intervention is useful for children (and adults) with autism at all ages but probably has most impact during the toddler and preschool years. Studies indicate that, when implemented early (beginning prior to 5 years of age) and intensively (more than 20 hours a week for 2 or more years), the treatment enables some children with autism to make major gains such as large IQ increases, although other children derive much less benefit (Lovaas, 1987). From a learning theory perspective, it makes sense that early, intensive behavioral intervention (EIBI) would be especially beneficial. Because young children with autism have not fallen as far behind their typically developing peers or become as set in their ways as older children with autism, they may require less time to learn skills needed to catch up.

Even in young children, however, the intervention may need to be intensive to match the learning opportunities available to typically developing children. Typically developing children learn from their everyday environment all of their waking hours, 7 days a week, 365 days a year, by exploring, playing with peers, modeling, conversing, and so on. Unfortunately, however, children with autism have little skill or inclination to learn in this manner. Thus, a mismatch arises between these children and environments designed for typically developing children, with the result that children with autism fail to learn except when their environment is redesigned. Different EIBI programs use somewhat different models for redesigning children's environments (Smith, 1999), but the most extensively studied program is the one developed by the UCLA Young Autism Project (YAP).

CHARACTERISTICS OF THE UCLA YOUNG AUTISM PROJECT

Intervention in UCLA YAP is intended to optimize children's functioning in all areas of development. UCLA YAP accepts children who are under 4 years old at intake and have completed a comprehensive diagnostic and assessment protocol. They must also be free of major medical problems such as severe hearing or vision loss, as program personnel are not trained in appropriate interventions for such problems. Children in UCLA YAP average 2 years, 10 months at intake. Consistent with the general population of children with autism, UCLA YAP enrolls about four times as many boys as girls, and the mean income and education level of families is close to the national average. About half the children are White, with the next largest group being Hispanic, followed by Asian Americans and blacks (Smith, Groen, & Wynn, 2000).

Most children in UCLA YAP receive 40 hours per week of one-to-one intervention. However, fewer hours may be appropriate for (1) children under 3 years old, who may start with only 20 hours per week; (2) children near the end of intervention, for whom the number of intervention hours is gradually reduced; and (3) children for whom 40 hours per week is counterindicated for other reasons such as a history of slow progress with this level of intensity. Intervention usually lasts approximately 3 years, though the precise length is determined on a case-by-case basis.

UCLA YAP makes every effort to construct teaching situations that maximize success and prevent failure. Because of their mismatch with the environment, children with autism have already encountered continual frustration in learning situations by the time they enroll in our early intervention program. Understandably, they react to such frustration with tantrums and other attempts to escape or avoid future failures. During the first year of intervention, discrete trial training is the main method we use to overcome this problem. This format is characterized by (1) one-to-one interaction with a therapist, (2) short and clear instructions from the therapist, (3) carefully planned procedures for prompting children to succeed in following instructions and for fading such prompts, and (4) immediate reinforcement for each correct response made by children. As children progress, therapists gradually decrease the use of this format and increase their emphasis on naturalistic instruction, much of which takes place in group settings such as classrooms. An intervention manual (Lovaas, 2002) outlines particular instructional programs as well as ways to individualize programs for particular children. We discuss key programs in the section "Stages of Intervention."

Staffing

UCLA YAP employs four levels of service providers: student therapists, senior therapists, case supervisors, and program directors. Student therapists do most of the one-to-one behavioral intervention. A prerequisite for becoming a student therapist is to obtain a high grade in a college-level course on learning theory or applied behavior analysis. Novice student therapists work alongside experienced therapists for about 25 hours, or until observations by senior personnel indicate that they are qualified to conduct sessions themselves. Intervention teams of approximately five student therapists are assigned to each child, with every student therapist working a minimum of 5 hours per week. In addition, each student therapist must attend a weekly 1-hour clinic meeting with the child, parents, senior therapist, and case supervisor.

After a minimum of 6 months as a student therapist, those who excel are eligible to become senior therapists. Senior therapists work full time and provide additional one-to-one intervention of up to 10 hours per week. Each oversees one to two treatment teams and works closely with the case supervisor. Case supervisors are selected from the group of senior therapists. Criteria for selection include (1) accumulating a minimum of 1,500 supervised hours of intervention experience, (2) being highly rated by families and student therapists, and (3) passing objective tests of their skill at implementing instructional programs, identifying which skills to teach next and critiquing others' therapy (Davis, Smith, & Donahoe, in press).

UCLA program directors are typically doctoral-level personnel who are licensed in a mental health profession (usually psychology), have many years of experience implementing the UCLA YAP, and must complete 9 months of full-time postgraduate training in behavioral intervention and its application to children with autism. Program directors have daily contact with case supervisors, as well as weekly contact with all other intervention personnel, clients, and families.

Program directors and supervisors meet weekly with each child, as well as the child's parents, student therapists, and senior therapist to review the child's progress. They ask student therapists to demonstrate programs during the meeting to make sure that all team members are clear on intervention procedures and receive feedback regarding their performance. They also answer questions from parents and staff. Based on information obtained during this meeting, they modify children's intervention (introducing new instructional programs when children have mastered existing ones, altering and assessing the format of instructional programs when children's progress is slow, etc.).

Family Participation

Parents are an integral part of their children's intervention teams. Prior to enrolling their children into UCLA YAP, they have a 1- to 2-hour intake interview with the project director. In this interview, the project director becomes acquainted with families, confirms information from outside agencies on children's medical and developmental history, and encourages questions from parents. Parents also view a videotape on the UCLA intervention (Anderson & Aller, 1988), receive publications on outcomes achieved by children in the program (e.g., McEachin, Smith, & Lovaas, 1993), and, if they wish, schedule a time to accompany a case supervisor to observe another child's intervention program, with written permission from that child's parents. The parents then review an informed consent form, which outlines the UCLA intervention, the parents' role, and the range of outcomes that children achieve following intervention (some making substantial progress, but others deriving little or no benefit). In addition to exchanging information, the intake interview affords an opportunity to address the anxiety and stress that parents invariably express about their child's condition. The program director attempts to identify the specific concerns that the parents raise, express empathy and support, and describe how the intervention may help. The director also emphasizes that parents' active participation in intervention is likely to contribute to the child's progress and ease their own stress.

Throughout the intervention, parents attend all intervention related meetings and approve in advance all intervention procedures. Also, for the first 3–4 months of intervention, parents are asked to work alongside an experienced therapist for 5 hours per week. During this time, the therapist and parent take turns implementing the child's one-to-one, discrete trial training programs, and they give each other feedback on their work. Thus, parents learn to become effective therapists for their child and make informed decisions about their child's intervention.

Subsequently, many parents reduce their involvement in discrete trial training but continue to generalize and expand skills that children acquire in intervention. For example, they implement incidental teaching procedures to encourage their children to use communication skills in everyday settings, incorporate self-help skills into children's daily routines, and arrange activities that promote further skill development, such as outings where children can learn new labels for objects or events. Parents also recruit peers to participate in play dates with their child and often oversee the play dates with assistance from the case supervisor. In addition, they contact school districts about placements for their child, visit the placements that are offered (often accompanied by the case supervisor), and communicate with teachers about the child's progress.

Stages of Intervention

Large individual differences exist in children's rate of progress. Nevertheless, the intervention, summarized in Table 18.1, generally follows a predictable sequence:

Stage 1—Establishing a Teaching Relationship

We aim to schedule the first hour of intervention within 2 weeks of the intake interview. This hour tends to be the most upsetting for the child, parents, and team. As noted, the child has already learned to escape or avoid teaching situations. This avoidance usually takes the form of intense tantrums that include screaming, crying, and attempting to run away; the child may also hit him- or herself, try to bite therapists, and display other aggression. To address this problem and optimize the child's success, therapists select one

TABLE 18.1. Treatment Stages in the UCLA Young Autism Project

Stage	Length	Teaching method(s)	Goals
1. Establishing a teaching relationship	~2–4 weeks	Primarily discrete trial training (DTT)	Following one-step directions such as "sit" or "come here," reducing interfering behaviors such as tantrums
2. Teaching foundational skills	~1–4 months	Primarily DTT	Discriminating between one-step directions, imitating gross motor actions, matching, receptively identifying objects, dressing, beginning play with toys
3. Beginning communication	~6+ months	DTT, incidental teaching	Imitating speech sounds, expressively labeling objects, receptively identifying actions and pictures, expanding self-help and play skills, starting visual communication for children who are slow to acquire speech (picture communication systems or reading and writing)
4. Expanding communication, beginning peer interaction	~12 months	DTT, incidental teaching, dyads with typical peers	Labeling colors and shapes, beginning language concepts such as big/little and yes/no, recognizing emotions, beginning sentences such as "I want _____" and "I see _____," beginning pretend play and peer interaction, toilet training
5. Advanced communication, adjusting to school	~12 months	DTT, incidental teaching, small group, regular education preschool	Using language concepts (e.g., prepositions, pronouns, past tense), conversing with others, describing objects and events, comprehending stories, understanding perspective of others, learning from models, working independently, helping with chores

action that the child is likely to perform successfully (e.g., putting a block in a bucket or sitting down in a chair) and request this action. By prompting and reinforcing successful completion while withholding reinforcement for escape or avoidance behavior, therapists increase the child's attentiveness and motivation in the teaching situation while reducing tantrums. Each team member and parent takes a turn requesting the action selected by the team.

Every new student therapist and parent must learn correct procedures for teaching in the early stages of intervention because the child's intervention will soon become much more complex and difficult to implement. Program directors and case supervisors, who have considerable experience starting intervention, are present during the first hour to demonstrate how to implement procedures accurately, point out signs of improvement, and reassure the team and family that the child is being successful. By the end of the hour, almost all children have made some progress that is apparent to everyone present. Therapists help transfer this progress by requesting the same action at home later in the day. Over the next 2 to 4 weeks, they slowly add other requests that the child can also carry out successfully. At this stage, choosing requests that increase the child's skill level is not as important as choosing ones that help the child develop trust in the therapists and bolster the parents' confidence that their child can learn.

Stage 2—Teaching Foundational Skills

Once the child has become more responsive to the teaching situation, the intervention moves to new and more challenging programs that provide a foundation for learning complex behaviors. This stage usually lasts 1 to 4 months. One focus is on basic receptive language skills such as coming to an adult upon request. Another is on imitation of actions such as clapping or waving, standing up, and sitting down. Mastery of a dozen or so gross motor actions is followed by imitation of fine motor actions such as facial expressions. Imitation is a powerful tool in treatment because it enables the child to pick up a variety of new skills such as how to play with toys simply by observing others perform them. An additional focus is matching and sorting. Although many children with autism already have some matching skills, such as completing inset puzzles when they enter treatment, extending these skills (e.g., teaching the child to match increasingly complex pictures and three-dimensional objects) helps the child attend to a variety of instructional materials and may facilitate language instruction. Teaching self-care tasks such as dressing also begins at this stage.

Instruction proceeds in small steps. For example, in teaching early receptive language such as "come here," the child initially receives a prompt such as a gentle nudge on the back to carry out the instruction and travels only a couple of feet to the adult. As the child progresses, the prompt is gradually removed so that the child is responding to the verbal request by itself, and the distance to travel increases. To facilitate generalization, the child practices this skill with each therapist and parent in multiple settings (at home, in our clinic, etc.). Once the child masters an instruction, therapists introduce new instructions one at a time and teach the child to discriminate between them (e.g., coming when the therapist says, "Come here" but not when the therapist says, "Wave," or selecting the toy named by the therapist from a group of toys that are on a table). To provide this teaching, therapists must be familiar with empirically validated approaches to discrimination training such as procedures for giving instructions, prompting the child to follow instructions, randomizing presentation of instructions, fading, and reinforcing correct behaviors. Learning to discriminate is vital for children because it indicates that they are truly attending to and differentiating among instructions.

Stage 3—Beginning Communication

In this stage, which lasts six months or longer, children continue to receive instruction in receptive language, imitation, and matching. They also learn new self-care skills such as toileting. Further, they begin working on expressive language. Therapists begin by first teaching the child to imitate speech sounds, then separate words, and finally strings of words (Lovaas, Berberich, Perloff, & Schaeffer, 1966). They then use verbal imitation to prompt expressive labeling of objects and events (e.g., the therapist holds up an object such as ball and says "Ball"). Verbal imitation is often the most difficult skill for therapists to teach and children to master. Only about half the children in UCLA YAP master imitation of speech sounds within the first few months of treatment. This mastery is an important predictor of eventual outcome (Smith, Groen, & Wynn, 2000). Although some children who quickly master verbal imitation encounter difficulties in later stages of the program, most continue to make rapid progress and achieve favorable outcomes such as IQ in the average range and successful functioning in regular education classes (Lovaas, 1987). Those who do not acquire verbal imitation are unlikely to have such favorable outcomes, though they still learn other skills such as using alternative communication systems. Interestingly, reading and writing may be an especially effective form of communication for some of these children (Lovaas & Lovaas, in press).

Stage 4—Expanding Communication and Beginning Peer Interaction

When the child receptively and expressively identifies everyday objects and behaviors, instruction proceeds to abstract concepts and grammatically correct sentences (see Table 18.2). Also, children enter a preschool for typically developing children. Although we recognize that many will eventually go into special education classes (as discussed in Stage 6), we emphasize regular classes at this stage because research indicates that these classes provide more appropriate peer models and higher academic expectations (Smith, Lovaas, & Lovaas, 2002). Therapists help prepare children at home by teaching pretend play skills, age-appropriate games such as "ring around the rosie," songs such as "Wheels on the Bus," and other group activities such as "show and tell." An aide accompanies the child to school to facilitate transfer of skills from home to school. At first, classroom time may be as little as 5–10 minutes per day so that the child is successful and not perceived by teachers and peers as having disabilities. The time is then gradually lengthened to half an hour and more until the child stays for the full preschool session. The relationship between the child's parents and teacher almost always becomes close and positive, and parents may ask the teacher's help in contacting other parents to arrange play dates at home.

Stage 5—Promoting Inclusion in Peer Groups

Therapists teach advanced language concepts and preacademic skills, as shown in Table 18.1. Moreover, they conduct extensive training in social skills such as engaging in sociodramatic play with peers, conversing, making appropriate requests for asssitance, and following school rules (e.g., raising hands). Even at this stage, most children in the UCLA YAP still learn new skills best by receiving one-to-one instruction and then transferring

TABLE 18.2. IQ and Classification for the Intensive Treatment Group ($n = 19$), Minimal Treatment Group ($n = 19$), and Special Education Group ($n = 21$) (Lovaas, 1987; McEachin et al., 1993)

| | IQ[a] | | | | | | Best outcome[b] | |
| | Pretreatment | | Age 7 | | Age 12 | | | |
Group	M	SD	M	SD	M	SD	Age 7	Age 12
Intensive treatment	63	13.7	83	28.6	85	32.4	9	8
Minimal treatment	57	14.5	52	22.4	55	29.1	0	0
Special education	60	15.0	59	20.6	n.a.		1	n.a.

[a]Ratio IQ at intake, deviation IQ at ages 7 and 12 (see Lovaas, 1987, for testing procedures)
[b]Number of children who obtained (1) deviation IQ above 85 and (2) unassisted placement in regular education classrooms

the skills to everyday settings. Therefore, a key goal is to increase their ability to learn while in such settings. Accordingly, therapists help children respond more to the class-room teacher and peers, and less to the aide. They teach observational learning so that children acquire information from peer models in group settings. They also teach inde-pendent work skills so that children start and finish tasks with little direct supervision.

In addition, parents work with the teacher to identify specific tasks he or she will ask children to perform without assistance from the aide (e.g., making transitions be-tween activities). As children become less reliant on the aide, the aide gradually fades out. For example, the aide may be assigned partly to the child with autism and partly to classmates, or may attend only part time.

Stage 6—Termination of Intervention

Intervention ends as children enter elementary school. At age 5, children proceed from preschool to a kindergarten class for typically developing children if they display most of the skills that their classmates do and are ready to begin fading the aide. Otherwise, they repeat preschool in order to be with peers closer to their developmental level, have addi-tional time to adjust to the school setting, and continue receiving one-to-one instruction at home. This extra year enables many children to catch up to typically developing chil-dren who are entering kindergarten, as evidenced by skills such as engaging in sociodra-matic play, cooperating in small groups, having a vocabulary of over 5,000 words, and speaking in complex sentences. For such children, the process of fading the aide and en-hancing socialization is complex. Kindergarten may be repeated if the child continues to experience problems in interacting with peers. However, our research indicates that most children function without an aide by the end of kindergarten and remain in regular class-es for many years without special assistance (McEachin et al., 1993). Therefore, we grad-ually reduce services for these children and terminate these services during first grade.

If, after repeating preschool and kindergarten, children continue to be delayed rela-tive to their classmates, our research indicates that they are likely to need ongoing special services throughout their lives (Lovaas, 1987). Therefore, we evaluate alternative place-ment options, seeking ones in which (1) teachers are willing to collaborate with us (most are quite willing, but a few are not); (2) peers model appropriate, adaptive skills for the child with autism (Smith et al., 2002); and (3) the class has a clear structure and rules. Potential placements include classes with typically developing children where the child with autism receives assistance from an aide, behavioral classrooms for children with autism, or other special education classes. In any of these placements, it is often impor-tant to supplement classroom instruction with one-to-one discrete trial instruction (10 hours per week or more if parents are involved in treatment), as children may still learn most efficiently in this format. Therapists from the home program assist in making the transition to these placements.

Because of all the complex issues associated with identifying appropriate placements for children who continue to have special needs, such children may be at greater risk for losing skills, developing new maladaptive behaviors, or having other difficulties than are children who are fully integrated into regular classes. Therefore, program directors dis-cuss this risk with parents and service providers, and they are available for periodic fol-low-up consultations, as needed. Apart from these consultations, services from the UCLA YAP for special-needs children usually stop during first grade but sometimes con-tinue for another year (until the child is about 8 years old) to enhance skill retention and adjustment to school.

EVIDENCE FOR THE EFFECTS OF TREATMENT

Investigators have published hundreds of peer-reviewed studies on the use of behavioral interventions to reduce specific excesses and delays in children and adults with autism (Matson et al., 1996; Newsom, 1998). Much fewer studies have centered on the long-term, overall outcome of behavioral intervention programs. These outcome studies need to be interpreted cautiously because of methodological limitations but indicate that EIBI programs such as the UCLA YAP may be effective for some children with autism. In most studies, personnel provide clinic-directed intervention as the UCLA YAP, but some findings on applications of the intervention in the community are also available and are reviewed next.

Clinic-Directed Intervention

Lovaas (1987) studied three groups of children with autism: (1) an intensive treatment group of 19 children with autism who received 40 hours per week of intervention for 2 or more years, (2) a minimal treatment group of 19 children who received 10 hours per week or less of behavioral treatment, and (3) a special education group of 21 children enrolled in a university-based classroom. Assignment to intensive or minimal treatment was based on a quasi-experimental procedure: If sufficient student therapists were available, children were assigned to the intensively treated group; if not, children were assigned to minimal treatment. The special education group consisted of children who obtained pretreatment scores similar to those in the intensively treated group but who were not referred to UCLA YAP. As shown in Table 18.2, although the three groups did not significantly differ prior to treatment, the intensively treated group obtained substantially higher IQ scores and less restrictive school placements at age 7 years than did the minimal treatment and special education children. The intensively treated group maintained these gains in a follow-up conducted at an average age of 12 years (McEachin et al., 1993; see Table 18.2).

Nine of the 19 intensively treated children (47%) were described as "best outcome" because they obtained average IQs (above 85) and performed satisfactorily in school placements for typically developing children at 7 years old. Only 1 of the 40 minimally treated children (3%) achieved such a favorable outcome. The best-outcome children accounted for most of the gains in IQ and other measures in the intensive group. Therefore, although some children made remarkable progress, others did not, highlighting the need for continued efforts to improve the intervention.

Replications

Smith, Groen, and Wynn (2000) tested the UCLA YAP using the same kind of intervention, an improved research methodology (a fully randomized clinical trial) and enrollment of lower-functioning children. Children who received an average of 25 hours per week of treatment in the UCLA YAP were compared to 13 children who received only parent training. Results confirmed that children who received the UCLA intervention benefited, but gains averaged only about half what Lovaas (1987) found. For example, at follow-up, the mean IQ in the UCLA YAP group was 16 points higher than in the control group, compared to 31 points in Lovaas (1987); 27% (4 of 15) met criteria for normal functioning, compared to 47% in Lovaas (1987). Possible reasons for the smaller gains were the decreased intervention hours (25 instead of 40) and enrollment of lower-functioning children (e.g., mean IQ of 51 at intake vs. 63 in Lovaas, 1987). Smith (1999) reviewed other replications of the UCLA YAP with reduced treatment hours; these studies yielded results comparable to those of Smith, Groen, and Wynn (2000).

Given the complexity and intensity of the UCLA YAP, we are currently completing a large-scale, multisite study that we anticipate will provide a more definitive test of whether the UCLA YAP can be replicated (Multi-site Young Autism Project). The study is intended to improve the research methodology over previous studies by incorporating randomized assignment to intensive treatment or parent training, comparison groups of children treated at outside agencies, standardized diagnostic procedures, comprehensive assessments conducted yearly, and objective measures of treatment fidelity. Preliminary results are consistent with those of recent outcome studies such as Smith, Groen, and Wynn (2000) but are necessarily tentative given that they are incomplete and have not yet undergone peer review.

Replications with Other Populations

Lovaas (1987) excluded children with autism if they performed in the range of severe or profound mental retardation at preintervention. However, Smith, Eikeseth, Klevstrand, and Lovaas (1997) compared 11 such children who received 30 hours per week of intervention to 10 similar children who received minimal intervention. As in Lovaas (1987), assignment was based on therapist availability. Smith et al. (1997) found that intensively treated children made clinically important gains, but these gains were smaller than those reported for higher-functioning children. Children who had received 30 hours per week achieved a higher mean IQ at age 7 than minimally treated children (36 vs. 24) and were more likely to have communicative speech (10 of 11 vs. 2 of 10), though the groups did not significantly differ in the number of behavioral problems that children displayed.

Lovaas (1987) also excluded children who were older than 4 years at intake. Eikeseth, Smith, Jahr, and Eldevik (2002) implemented the UCLA intervention with 13 such children who had intake IQ above 50 and compared these children to 12 similar children who received eclectic intervention. Assignment to groups was based on therapist availability. Children in both groups received an average of 28 hours per week of intervention. At a 1-year follow-up, the behaviorally treated groups made larger gains than those in the eclectic group (e.g., IQ increase of 16 points vs. 3 points). This result suggests that some older children, particularly those who are higher functioning at pretreatment, may derive significant benefit from the UCLA YAP.

Community Treatment

Parental advocacy has led to a dramatic rise in requests from families for EIBI. This demand poses at least two major practical problems for service providers and families. First, the demand far exceeds the supply of professionals who have the training and experience necessary to provide high-quality, intensively supervised clinic-directed intervention as in the Lovaas (1987) study. Second, because of the intensity of services, it is prohibitively expensive to employ professionals to deliver all of the intervention. The most common solution to these problems is for professionals to assist parents in setting up their own intervention programs. In such programs, parents recruit paraprofessional therapists (often college students) to be trained and provide intervention for their children. The professional then trains the parents and therapists in EIBI techniques and develops an intervention plan for the child. Subsequently, the professional conducts monthly or bimonthly follow-up consultations to provide further training and update the intervention plan (Smith, Buch, & Gamby, 2000).

By delegating much of the responsibility for intervention to parents, professionals can increase the number of families they serve. By relying on paraprofessionals to implement the intervention, they can keep costs down. Given that parents and paraprofessionals can be highly effective in implementing behavioral techniques (e.g., Anderson, DiPietro, Edwards, & Christian, 1987), parent-directed programs with paraprofessional therapists may substantially enhance children's functioning. Despite these potential advantages, however, such programs must be evaluated carefully. Factors such as extensive demands on parents, infrequent training and supervision from consultants, reliance on therapists who may have little background in learning theory and EIBI, and high staff turnover may reduce intervention effectiveness, relative to professionally administered treatment.

In a study of 66 children with autism in parent-initiated intervention, Bibby, Eikeseth, Martin, Mudford, and Reeves (2001) found that outcomes were much less favorable than those reported for clinic-directed programs. Scores on a standardized test of adaptive behavior increased significantly ($M = 9$ points), but scores on tests of intelligence and language did not. No child met Lovaas's (1987) definition of best outcome (IQ > 85 and unassisted placement in regular elementary school classrooms), though 10 did meet the IQ criterion. Consultants had diverse backgrounds ranging from doctorates and extensive EIBI experience to no formal credentials, but this background did not predict children's outcome. Bibby et al. (2001) suggested that the poor results may stem from factors such as the amount of intervention (an average of 30 hours per week instead of the 40 recommended by Lovaas), sporadic supervision from consultants (once every 3 months instead of once weekly as in the UCLA YAP), low quality of therapy, and widespread use of unvalidated supplemental interventions such as megavitamins and elimination diets (81% of the sample). Though further study is needed to clarify these issues, Bibby et al.'s (2001) findings show that, as typically applied in community settings, EIBI is probably less effective than in clinic-directed programs.

DIRECTIONS FOR FUTURE RESEARCH

In many parts of the United States and Europe, EIBI is becoming standard, because of parental advocacy, recent legislation, or professional endorsement (Jacobson, 2002). As a result, the need for studies to fill in gaps left by previous studies has grown. In addition to completing ongoing studies such as the Multi-site Young Autism Project, investigators should analyze treatment components. For example, as discussed in the introduction, early studies on behavioral interventions showed little generalization (e.g., changes in one behavior did not lead to changes in other behaviors). However, for unclear reasons, more recent studies revealed more extensive response generalization (McEachin et al., 1993). For example, children improved on measures such as IQ tests for which they received no direct training, and they continued to progress after treatment ended. Studies of instructional programs for helping children enter classroom settings, form peer friendships and gain confidence, and use observational learning may help explain this improved generalization.

More comprehensive evaluations of EIBI are essential. To illustrate, although much information exists on intellectual and academic gains resulting from EIBI, little information exists regarding emotional and social functioning. Almost no research has been conducted on family variables that may affect, or be affected by, treatment response. Although there are large individual differences in response to EIBI, no reliable preintervention predictors of outcome have been identified. Also, more effective interventions for children who derive little benefit from current EIBI programs need to be developed. For this purpose, investigations of brain–behavior relationships may hold the most promise. For example, neurological investigations may reveal problems that hinder some children from acquiring vocal imitation, which is critical for success in EIBI. As shown by Bibby et al. (2001), studies on how to implement EIBI effectively in the community are required. In this regard, we are validating objective procedures for identifying qualified supervisors (Davis et al., in press).

One area of research may test whether interventions devised for autistic children are applicable to other diagnostic groups. Perhaps what is now called autism represents a random collection of behaviors, each behavior occurring with relatively low frequency in the typical population. The same may hold true for other diagnostic categories such as pervasive developmental disorder not otherwise specified (PDD-NOS) and Asperger syndrome. If so, this intervention would address the various diagnostic entities on a behavior-by-behavior basis but would not be unique to each diagnosis except in extent (Lovaas & Smith, 1989). Preliminary evidence indicate that EIBI may be more effective for PDD-NOS than autism (Smith, Groen, & Wynn, 2000), but research on this issue is at a very early stage.

Traditional research has centered on discovering the causes and treatment of autism. Despite extensive efforts, answers to such questions have not been forthcoming. The construct of autism does not constitute a syndrome based on scientific research but more likely is an illustration of what Kuhn (1970) means by a "social construct." Perhaps this is why traditional research has failed to provide answers.

An emphasis has been placed on the scientific merit and efficiency of behavioral intervention while neglecting to mention the humanistic and ethical respects of this approach. Two such aspects are worth mentioning. First, behavioral treatment gave evidence of increasing variability both within the client and between clients. Such an outcome contrasts the concerns expressed in the public media such as Huxley's *Brave New World* and Carl Rogers (1956). Second, all living organisms possess variability, which is essential for survival. We came to view atypical persons as belonging to this continuum of variability, as different in degree rather than kind, and not as instances of pathology.

SUMMARY AND CONCLUSIONS

Behavioral investigators devised a distinctive methodology that fostered steady progress in identifying effective interventions for children with autism. With EIBI, many children with autism now improve substantially. In the UCLA Young Autism Project, children with autism begin treatment prior to age 4 years and receive 40 hours per week of intervention for about 3 years. The treatment is designed to maximize children's successes and minimize their failures by proceeding in carefully planned steps that children can master. By the end of this intervention, many children achieve average levels of intellectual and academic functioning, although others make much smaller gains. Future research should focus on analyzing treatment components, evaluating effects of treatment on families, identifying predictors of treatment response, studying brain–behavior relationships that may enhance understanding of how best to help children who derive little benefit from current treatments, and implementing treatment effectively in community settings. Behavioral investigators should be in a favorable position to contribute to this research.

ACKNOWLEDGMENTS

This study was supported by Grant MH–51156 from the National Institute of Mental Health.

REFERENCES

Anderson, E. L. (Producer), & Aller, R. (Director). (1988). *Behavioral treatment of young autistic children* [Videotape] (Available from Cambridge Center for Behavioral Studies, http:store.ccb-sstore.com).

Anderson, S. R., DiPietro, E. K., Edwards, G. L., & Christian, W. P. (1987). Intensive home-based early intervention with autistic children. *Education and Treatment of Children, 10,* 352–366.

Beglinger, L., & Smith, T. (2001). Subtypes in autism: Review and proposed dimensional model. *Journal of Autism and Developmental Disorders, 31,* 411–422.

Bibby, P., Eikeseth, S., Martin, N. T., Mudford, O. C., & Reeves. D. (2001). Progress and children with autism receiving parent-managed intensive interventions. *Research in Developmental Disabilities, 22,* 425–447.

Chakrabarti, S., & Fombonne, E. (2001). Pervasive developmental disorders in preschool children. *Journal of the American Medical Association, 285,* 3093–3099.

Davis, B. J., Smith, T., & Donahoe, P. (in press). Evaluating supervisors in the UCLA treatment model for children with autism: Validation of an assessment procedure. *Behavior Therapy.*

Eikeseth, S., Smith, T., Jahr, E., & Eldevik, S. (2002). Intensive behavioral treatment at school for 4- to 7-year-old children with autism: A 1-year comparison controlled study. *Behavior Modification, 26,* 49–68.

Jacobson, J. W. (2002). Early intensive behavioral intervention: Emergence of a consumer-driven service model. *Behavior Analyst, 23*(2), 149–171.

Kuhn, T. S. (1970). *The structure of scientific revolutions.* Chicago: University of Chicago Press.

Lovaas, O. I. (1987). Behavioral treatment and normal educational and intellectual functioning in young autistic children. *Journal of Consulting and Clinical Psychology, 55,* 3–9.

Lovaas, O. I., Berberich, J. P., Perloff, B. F., & Schaeffer, B. (1966). Acquisition of imitative speech by schizophrenic children. *Science, 151,* 705–707.

Lovaas, O. I., Koegel, R. L., Simmons, J. Q., & Long, J. S. (1973). Some generalization and follow-up measures on autistic children in behavior therapy. *Journal of Applied Behavior Analysis, 6,* 131–166.

Lovaas, O. I., & Smith, T. (1989). A comprehensive behavioral theory of autistic children: Paradigm for research and treatment. *Journal of Behavior Therapy and Experimental Psychiatry, 20*(1), 17–29.

Lovaas, N. W., & Lovaas, E. E. (in press). *The reading & writing program: An alternative form of communication for students with developmental delays.* Austin, TX: Pro-Ed.

Matson, J. L., Benavidez, D. A., Compton, L. S., Paclawskyj, T., & Baglio, C. (1996). Behavioral treatment of autistic persons: A review of research from 1980 to the present. *Research in Developmental Disabilities, 17,* 433–465.

McEachin, J. J., Smith, T., & Lovaas, O. I. (1993). Long-term outcome for children with autism who received early intensive behavioral treatment. *American Journal on Mental Retardation, 97,* 359–372.

Newsom, C. B. (1998). Autistic disorder. In E. J. Mash & R. A. Barkley (Eds.), *Treatment of childhood disorders* (2nd ed., pp. 416–467). New York: Guilford Press.

Rogers, C.R. (1956). Some issues concerning the control of human behavior. *Science, 124,* 1057–1066.

Smith, T. (1996). Are other treatments effective? In C. Maurice (Ed.), *Behavioral treatment of autistic children* (pp. 45–67). Austin, TX: PRO-ED.

Smith, T. (1999). Outcome of early intervention for children with autism. *Clinical Psychology: Science and Practice, 6,* 33–49.

Smith, T., Buch, G. A., & Gamby, T. (2000). Parent-directed, intensive early intervention for children with pervasive developmental disorder. *Research in Developmental Disabilities, 21,* 297–309.

Smith, T., Eikeseth, S., Klevstrand, M., & Lovaas, O. I. (1997). Outcome of early intervention for autistic-like children with severe mental retardation. *American Journal on Mental Retardation, 102,* 228–237.

Smith, T., Groen, A., & Wynn, J. W. (2000). Randomized trial of intensive early intervention for children with pervasive developmental disorder. *American Journal on Mental Retardation, 4,* 269–285.

Smith, T., Lovaas, N. W., & Lovaas, O. I. (2002). Behaviors of children with high-functioning autism when paired with typically developing versus delayed peers: A preliminary study. *Behavioral Interventions, 17*(3), 129–143.

Wing, L. (1992). Manifestations of social problems in high-functioning autistic people. In E. Schopler & G. B. Mesibov (Eds.), *High-functioning individuals with autism* (pp. 129–142). New York: Plenum Press.

19

Empirically Supported Pivotal Response Interventions for Children with Autism

Robert L. Koegel, Lynn Kern Koegel,
and Lauren I. Brookman

OVERVIEW

In 1943, Kanner coined the term "autism" to describe a group of children who displayed similar behavioral characteristics related to difficulties with social communication and social interaction (Kanner, 1943). To date, there is not yet a known cause of autism, and individuals are diagnosed based on three general behavioral categories: impairments in social interaction; impairments in verbal and nonverbal communication; and restricted, repetitive, and stereotyped patterns of behaviors, interests, and activities (American Psychiatric Association, 2000). These symptoms often result in numerous disruptive behaviors, such as tantrums, aggression, and self-injury. Further, almost all parents of children with autism, regardless of severity level, experience clinical levels of stress relating to the challenges of having a child with a severe disability (Koegel, 2000; Koegel & Koegel, 1995; Koegel, Schreibman, Loos, & Dirlich-Wilhelm, 1992). Prevalence rates of autism vary considerably with current rates most typically estimated to be approximately 1 case per 500 individuals, and have been reported as high as 1 in every 160 children (Chakrabarti & Fombonne, 2001) for all pervasive developmental disorders. Males are four to five times more likely to receive a diagnosis of autism than females (American Psychiatric Association, 2000). A significant increase in prevalence rates may reflect actual increases in occurrence or increased awareness and detections of signs of autism. Regardless of the reason for the increased incidence, professionals in many settings are likely to encounter children with autism and should remain informed of current, empirically supported interventions for this population.

Conceptual Model Underlying Treatment

Intervention procedures for children diagnosed with autism have changed considerably over time. Early theory-driven (rather than data-based) psychoanalytic treatments for these children were developed based on a parental causation theory. Children were often removed from their parents and treatment was designed to repair a hypothesized faulty mother–child bond. Parents who sought professional help for their children were usually devastated when they were told that they were the cause of their child's serious problems. Not only were they told that they could not help their child, but they often were told that their children would be better off, at least initially, without any parental involvement in their child's life. However, data failed to support this etiological perspective. In fact, systematic studies from our clinics and others have demonstrated that parents of children with autism do not differ from those who have children without psychiatric disorders (Koegel, Schreibman, O'Neill, & Burke, 1983). In addition, research directly contradicts psychoanalytic theory, suggesting that active involvement of parents in assisting with delivery of the intervention is valuable, and generally critical, for successful outcomes for children with autism.

Because of the little success in improving the condition of autism with non–data-based, theory-driven interventions, beginning in the early 1960s researchers began to focus on behavioral intervention techniques that were empirically supported. With these techniques the children made systematic and measurable improvements in many targeted behaviors; however, the intervention was extremely time-consuming and costly (Lovaas, Koegel, Simmons, & Long, 1973). In an attempt to refine and improve the efficiency of this effective intervention approach, we began to focus on the identification and teaching of pivotal responses. The theoretical underpinning of a pivotal response treatment was related to defining pivotal areas of functioning or areas that, once developed, would result in widespread collateral changes in numerous other behaviors. This concept has also been described in the literature as response covariation (Kazdin, 1982). That is, because pivotal responses appear to be central to wide areas of functioning, positive changes in such behaviors result in widespread positive effects on many other behaviors that are not targeted during intervention (Burke & Cerniglia, 1990; Koegel & Koegel, 1995; Koegel, Koegel, Harrower, & Carter, 1999; Koegel et al., 1989). This chapter focuses on two pivotal areas, motivation and child initiations, that appear to be especially important in producing widespread improvements for children with autism.

Motivation

Motivation to respond to social and environmental stimuli appears to be an essential pivotal area and is generally lacking in children with autism. Pivotal response interventions that focus on enhancing the relationship between social communication responses and the consequent reinforcers of such responses appear to increase behaviors characteristic of motivation, such as rate and latency of responding, correct responses, response attempts, and positive affect. Such improvements in environmental and social interactions appear to be important for language and cognitive and social development (Koegel, Koegel, & McNerney, 2001). That is, once children are motivated to respond, they are more likely to be provided with the complex stimulus input and learning opportunities throughout the day that are necessary for developing cognitive, communicative, and social competence.

The current procedures used to increase motivation are extensions of earlier techniques described in the applied behavior analysis (ABA) literature that have repeatedly been reported to be effective in improving behaviors of children with autism. The earlier traditional ABA interventions developed for children with autism focused on providing repetitive drill practice in a stimulus–response–consequence discrete trial format, teaching one target behavior at a time. Generally, instructions or commands were provided for specific child responses, which were then followed by food reinforcers for correct responses and punishment or extinction for incorrect responses. Like the traditional, individual target behavior ABA format, teaching pivotal behaviors can be described within the context of a discrete trial format. That is, antecedent stimuli (e.g., teaching instructions) are provided, and consequences are delivered contingent upon the child's response. The differences between a discrete trial analogue teaching paradigm that focuses on teaching individual target behaviors one at a time and a pivotal response format is that a pivotal area, such as motivation, is the focus of the intervention.

Several specific variables have been identified that increase the motivation of children with autism to respond to multiple types of stimuli. Specifically, these variables include child choice, task variation, interspersal of maintenance tasks, reinforcement of response attempts, and the use of natural and direct reinforcers (described later). The goal of pivotal response teaching is to incorporate all these variables, simultaneously, into teaching opportunities in the natural environment. These techniques have been shown to produce significant improvements in the core symptoms of autism.

Self-Initiations

In addition to increasing the children's motivation to respond, another area that appears to be pivotal in producing widespread improvements in autism is teaching self-initiated social interactions. This area closely relates to the motivational area described previously because similar variables are incorporated into the teaching procedures used to motivate the child to engage in self-initiations. Self-initiations have been defined in the literature as the individual beginning a new verbal or nonverbal social interaction (e.g., bringing a toy to a parent or pointing to a toy), self-initiating a task that results in social interactions (e.g., Saying "Play" or taking a toy to a parent), or changing the direction of an interaction (e.g., a parent is playing with the child and the child brings a new toy to the parent) (Koegel, Koegel, Harrower, & Carter, 1999). A variety of such social initiations occurs frequently in typically developing children; however, they occur infrequently or do not occur at all in children with autism. Even when children with autism are verbal and exhibit some initiations, their language is often limited to protests (e.g., "no") and requests (e.g., "I want water") rather than reflecting the variety of language functions (child-initiated questions, comments, etc.) needed for communicative competence. Recent research from our center indicates that the presence of frequent self-initiations appears to be an important prognostic indicator, associated with extremely favorable long-term language, social, and educational outcomes (Koegel, Koegel, Shoshan, & McNerney, 1999). That is, our preliminary research suggests that preschool children with autism who demonstrate high levels of self-initiations tend to have more favorable long-term outcomes than those who exhibit few or no initiations. In addition, our research suggests that self-initiations can be taught to children who do not exhibit initiations. Furthermore, focusing on teaching a variety of child initiations appears to result in considerably more favorable intervention outcomes.

This promising research suggests that when children with autism make improvements in self-initiated social interactions, concomitant changes are likely to occur in numerous areas of functioning. These changes may include not only improvements in appropriate academic, social, and communicative behaviors but also reductions in aggression, self-stimulation, self-injury, and tantrums. Targeting this pivotal area also appears to result in self-learning that increases autonomy as a child is less reliant on structured, adult-directed learning opportunities. Teaching initiations not only targets the language needs of the children but also increases the appearance of normalcy during social interactions (Koegel, Koegel, Shoshan, & McNerney, 1999). Besides the obvious importance of improving child language and social targets, teaching initiations may also be important in producing positive affect changes in the family environment. Teaching initiations transfers responsibility to the child, thus having the potential to reduce parental stress associated with continuous teaching responsibility throughout the child's waking hours.

Goals of Treatment

The goal of our program is to provide comprehensive intervention in key pivotal areas that will lead to independence and self-education throughout the day, without the need for constant vigilance from an intervention provider. The underlying assumption is that teaching pivotal areas is an effective and efficient mode of intervention in overcoming the number of difficulties that exist for children with autism (Koegel, Koegel, Harrower, & Carter, 1999). In our approach, the teaching of pivotal behaviors is coordinated throughout the child's day with parents serving as key coordinators and interventionists. It is recommended that the children participate in inclusive settings (i.e., participate in the same settings and activities as they would if they did not have a disability) as much as possible so that their curriculum and activities parallel those that a child without a developmental disorder would experience. Comprehensive programs are developed by individuals with extensive experience (e.g., persons with published expertise and/or in consultation with other professionals) in areas of autism, inclusion, and behavior management.

Parent education programs and parent empowerment are an important focus of the program, as parents spend a considerable amount of time with their children and are a stable influence over time. Specifically, within a parent education model, a "practice with feedback" format is used wherein parents work with their children and are provided with feedback regarding procedures for improving pivotal response areas such as motivation and child initiations in the context of teaching communication, academics, and so on. This type of coordinated model, with the families' active involvement, and the child's self-initiating interactions, increases the total amount of intervention available for the child (cf. McClannahan, Krantz, & McGee, 1982). Parent education programs have been effective in increasing communication skills, decreasing disruptive behaviors, and increasing generalization of treatment gains (Koegel, Koegel, Kellegrew, & Mullen, 1996; Koegel, Stiebel, & Koegel, 1998; Laski, Charlop, & Schreibman, 1988; Moes, 1995). In addition to expanding the skills acquired by children through parent education, these programs have numerous other positive effects on the family (Koegel, Bimbela, & Schreibman, 1996). For example, incorporating interventions that are blended into daily routines and match family values have been shown to reduce family stress (Moes, 1995).

CHARACTERISTICS OF THE TREATMENT PROGRAM: INTERVENTION FORMAT

Who Is Seen in Treatment

Most of the families that participate in our intervention program through the UCSB Autism Research and Training Clinic are referred by local regional centers which provide services for children with developmental delays. These families typically live within 90 miles of our center. In addition, we receive referrals from a variety of treatment agencies both nationally and internationally. Families that visit from geographically distant areas typically attend an intensive, 1-week parent education program, whereas our local families receive less intensive services over an extended period. The ages of the children range from 1½ to adulthood and reflect a complete range of severity and SES backgrounds. The ethnic composition of our families traditionally represents the proportions of ethnic groups in the population as a whole.

Individual child and family characteristics determine the intervention setting and target behaviors for each child. Specifically, the target behaviors are determined based on the individual child's needs, and intervention programs are developed to be consistent with a family's goals, values, and cultural identity (Santarelli, Koegel, Casas, & Koegel, 2001). Much of the focus of intervention is on communication skills and appropriate social communication interactions. These targets are generally taught using natural stimulus items found in the child's everyday settings (e.g., toys and games) and usually do not include analogue drill-type activities (e.g., rote repetition of flash cards). The setting in which the parent education program occurs is individualized for each family. For example, sessions may take place in our clinic playrooms, the nearby playground, McDonald's, the zoo, the child's home, and so on.

Parent Education and Motivation

The first steps in the parent education program are to introduce parents to the basics of behavioral interventions (i.e., the antecedent, behavior, and consequence pattern of behavior), the characteristics of the pivotal area of motivation, and how to identify learning opportunities in the natural environment. Parents are then given the manual, *Pivotal Response Teaching: A Training Manual* (Koegel et al., 1989), in which each of the motivational procedures (described later) is outlined and teaching examples are provided.

Throughout the intervention sessions, the clinician provides the parents with immediate and specific feedback on the parent's implementation of each procedure, while the parent works with his or her child. Initially, the focus of the sessions is for the parent to learn to implement the motivational strategies to improve the child's responsivity to instructions. For most children, communication is targeted. After the child is responding at a high rate, self-initiations are targeted using the motivational procedures the parent has learned. (The procedures for teaching self-initiations are described in the next section.) Each of the techniques involves strategies for increasing the child's motivation to engage in verbal communication, appropriate social interactions, and/or engagement in learning interactions from the natural environment. Specifically, the parents are taught each of the following points.

1. *Presentation of clear instructions and questions, the use of child-selected stimulus materials, and the use of direct natural reinforcers.* While each of these points has been researched extensively and individually in its own right (cf. Koegel & Koegel, 1995), the points are highly interrelated. For example, procedures that involve child-preferred activities typically increase a child's attention to the task and the use of natural reinforcers that are integrally related to the target behavior can direct the child's attention to the relevant cues in the activity (cf. Kazdin, 1977). Therefore, while parents are taught to provide instructional stimuli only when the child is attending, they are also taught to increase the child's motivation to respond, by using child-selected materials, topics, and

toys, and following the child's lead during interactions. Giving the child input into determining the stimuli to be used during instruction maximizes the child's interest in the
learning situation and improves the rate and generalization of learning (e.g., Carter,
2001; Koegel, Dyer, & Bell, 1987). Choice may include allowing the child to choose the
topic of conversation or the order of an activity (i.e., who goes first while playing a
board game or the order of academic tasks during homework). Some degree of choice is
incorporated into all activities or topics. Parents are also encouraged to follow their
child's interest in activities—that is, allowing the child to move on to another task when
he or she loses interest in the current one. Direct and natural reinforcers are employed
whenever possible. A direct, natural reinforcer is one that is directly and functionally related to the task. In contrast, an arbitrary, or indirect, reinforcer is one that is not within
the chain of behaviors required to produce the positive consequence. As a simple example, a direct and natural reinforcer for saying "ball" would be throwing the child a ball,
as opposed to giving the child a food item or token reinforcer. Research suggests that the
response–reinforcer relationship can be enhanced by providing direct and natural reinforcers, thus improving overall motivation to respond to the interaction (Kazdin, 1977;
Koegel & Williams, 1980; Saunders & Sailor, 1979; Williams, Koegel, & Egel, 1981).

    For typically developing children, these types of teaching situations may occur fre-
quently throughout the day. However, for children with severe disabilities such as
autism, such activities may not occur frequently and may need to be specifically
arranged. Thus, parents and other intervention providers are taught to implement such
teaching opportunities throughout the day, while employing stimulus materials that are
readily available in the natural environment.

    2. *Interspersing maintenance trials.* This strategy involves interspersing previously
learned tasks with new acquisition tasks. The goal here is to increase the success that a
child experiences, thereby increasing the likelihood that the child will attempt the task
again. Previous literature has described this phenomenon as behavioral momentum (e.g.,
Singer, Singer, & Horner, 1987), referring to the fact that the child is provided with a
target acquisition task trial within the context of a string of rapid correct responses on
previously mastered task trials. Others have described the procedures as employing task
interspersal (e.g., Dunlap, 1984), referring to the fact that the procedures involve a mix-
ture of presenting previously acquired tasks and new acquisition tasks. In both conceptualizations, the procedures differ from other techniques that focus exclusively on presenting successive trials on acquisition tasks; the results suggest that providing a number of
easy tasks results in a high probability of appropriate child responses on more difficult
tasks, with very rapid learning.

    3. *Reinforcing attempts.* "Reinforcing attempts" refers to rewarding the child's
clear, appropriate attempts to respond to instructional materials or natural learning opportunities. Such response attempts are reinforced, even if the response is not a correct
approximation of the targeted behavior. Interestingly, when response attempts are reinforced, the children increase their subsequent correct productions of the target behaviors,
and they do so with a considerable amount of positive affect (e.g., Koegel, O'Dell, &
Dunlap, 1988). This component of teaching may be particularly important for children
with autism who experience repeated difficulties when they attempt a difficult task and
therefore may have been extinguished for trying.

    Table 19.1 shows a comparison of applied behavior analysis procedures. Specifically,
a teaching intervention that incorporates the foregoing motivational variables is compared
with a discrete trial teaching intervention that does not incorporate those variables.

TABLE 19.1. Differences between the Individual Target Behavior and Pivotal Response Treatment Paradigms

	Analogue individual target behavior paradigm	Motivational pivotal response treatment paradigm (NLP/PRT)
Stimulus items	1. Chosen by clinician 2. Repeated until criterion is met 3. Phonologically easy to produce, irrespective of whether they were functional in the natural environment	1. Chosen by child 2. Varied every few trials 3. Age-appropriate items that can be found in the child's natural environment
Prompts	1. Manual (e.g., touch tip of tongue or hold lips together)	1. Clinician repeats item
Interaction	1. Clinician hold up the stimulus item; stimulus item not functional within interaction	1. Clinician and child play with stimulus item (i.e., stimulus item is functional within interaction)
Response	1. Correct responses or successive approximations reinforced	1. Looser shaping contingency so that attempts to respond verbally (except self-stimulation) are also reinforced
Consequences	1. Edible reinforcers paired with social reinforcers	1. Natural reinforcer (e.g., opportunity to play with the item) paired with social reinforcers

Note. Adapted from Koegel, O'Dell, and Koegel (1987).

Amount of Treatment

At this point, there appears to be little doubt that children with autism require intensive intervention throughout the day. However, in the field as a whole there has been considerable ambiguity about how to feasibly accomplish such intensive intervention. Our approach to intervention can result in large amounts of intervention interspersed throughout the children's everyday lives. However, the actual amount of effort required on the part of any given individual can be quite small because the efforts are magnified through ongoing consultation, training, and coordination with other agencies (schools, parents, regional centers, in-home therapists, etc.).

For example, our research suggests that most parents can reach our required 80% criterion for correct use of the motivational procedures within their everyday environments within approximately 25 hours, although the exact number of hours varies across children and families. Several research studies have demonstrated the widespread positive effects of incorporating such motivational procedures into a child's intervention plan through parent training in that learning is accelerated (Koegel, O'Dell, & Dunlap, 1988; Koegel, O'Dell, & Koegel, 1987), disruptive behavior is greatly reduced or eliminated (Koegel, Koegel, & Surratt, 1992), and general family affect is improved (Koegel, Bimbela, & Schreibman, 1996). However, only some of the children in our research programs were reaching a high level of communicative, social, and academic competence. This led us to conduct retrospective studies assessing possible prognostic indicators that may affect the long-term outcome of children with autism. Although this was preliminary research, the data suggested that one aspect of the children's behavior might be an especially important prognostic indicator. That is, the retrospective data analysis suggested that children who engaged in social self-initiations appeared to have more favorable long-term outcomes. Perhaps this is because child initiations have the potential to increase natural teaching opportunities for the child throughout the day, thereby greatly magnifying the quantity of intervention. Therefore, we have developed a number of strategies for teaching a variety of child initiations that may serve as an especially important pivotal skill.

Self-Initiations and Increased Amount of Naturally Occurring Intervention

Typically developing children use a variety of self-initiated queries that result in access to further learning throughout the day. These types of verbal responses appear within a typically developing child's first lexicon and continue throughout life. In contrast, most children with autism and other language disabilities use a limited number of such initiations or none at all. Therefore, we specifically target a variety of child-initiated interrogatives, such as "What's that?" "Where is it?" and "Whose is it?" Typically, "what" and "where" questions emerge in about the second year of life, whereas "whose" appears within the third year of life. These queries (and other types of spontaneous initiations such as "look," "help," etc.) can serve as a means for the child to obtain additional linguistic information from others throughout the day, without our having to program instruction specifically. The strategies we use in our intervention program incorporate the motivational components previously described into teaching child-initiated queries. The procedures that follow are described in more detail in Koegel, Koegel, & Brookman (in press).

Examples of Treatment Interactions for Self-Initiations

"What's That?"

This component of teaching children to initiate learning activities includes the interrogative "What's that?" to provide the child with a self-initiation to access and acquire vocabulary words. The initial goal of this procedure is to teach the children the target of information seeking in order to evoke information from a variety of communicative partners encountered in everyday environments throughout the child's waking hours. To teach children this important strategy, we first identify highly desired items, such as favorite snacks, action figures, and so on. The purpose of starting with highly desired items is to provide a motivational context so that when the child is taught the initial queries, positive consequences will occur. The items are then hidden in an opaque bag in order to facilitate curiosity. Parents typically obtain their child's attention by shaking the bag. Once the children are interested and attending to the learning situation, they are prompted to ask "What's that?" and then are given a (highly desired) item contained in the bag. Parents respond by labeling the item, "It's a _____ [item name]." The prompt is gradually faded until the children are frequently asking the question during the session.

Once the children are both asking the question and repeating the label regularly, neutral (less desired) items are gradually faded into the bag. It is interesting to note that while these neutral items (e.g., a Kleenex tissue) may initially have little interest for the children, it is common for children to begin to develop imaginative play activities with many of the stimulus items. We speculate that this intervention (child-initiated question asking) may produce a situation in which the children are being reinforced on a partial reinforcement schedule for exhibiting curiosity about and socially interacting with items, and that their new strategy of asking questions as an information-seeking tool is being reinforced with partial reinforcement. The bag is also slowly faded so that a variety of unknown items are merely located naturally around the room. This transition from the use of only highly desired items to including a large number of both desired and neutral items may be particularly important in increasing the children's general curiosity about their environment.

"Where Is It?"

Teaching "What's that?" aims to teach children to self-initiate the acquisition of nouns, but this next procedure focuses on teaching children a later developing interrogative ("where" questions) to access preposition use. To teach this interrogative, the child's favorite items are hidden in a variety of different locations. The child is prompted to ask "Where is it?" and the parent responds by telling the child the location of the item. The parent also labels the location with a preposition (e.g., "in the box," "on the dresser," and "beside the refrigerator"). Being allowed to take the favored item from the location then reinforces the child. Throughout this process, the child is being naturally reinforced both for exhibiting curiosity and for learning new prepositions.

"Whose Is It?"

Teaching children to self-initiate this later developing interrogative provides a technique for increasing the child's opportunities to learn pronouns and possessives. Initially, to accomplish this learning, parents bring to the clinic a variety of items that their children clearly associate with a particular member of the family. The child is prompted to ask "Whose is it?" The parent then responds and gives the item to the child. Eventually, the child is prompted to repeat the possessive form. The same general teaching format is used to teach "yours" and "mine." Because this reversal of pronouns is typically difficult for children with autism, we typically employ highly desired stimulus items. For example, we may use a toy or candy item that the child desires, and when the parent responds to the child's initiation of "Whose is it?" by saying "It's yours," the child is prompted to say "mine," and then receives the desired item. Again, with this procedure the child is being reinforced both for exhibiting curiosity and for learning pronouns. Because this reinforcement results in a large number of spontaneous learning interactions throughout the child's day, the procedure is not only an effective teaching technique in its own right but has the effect of greatly increasing the amount of intervention.

EVIDENCE FOR THE EFFECTS OF TREATMENT

Treatment Evaluations

We, along with other researchers in the field, have used a number of different strategies to evaluate the effectiveness of the aforementioned types of pivotal response interventions. The dependent measures in many of the outcome studies usually fall into one of two categories: (1) child variables and (2) parent and family variables. Although the primary focus is on improving child skills, parent and family variables are also important to assess because our research suggests that parents are not likely to use the techniques if the interventions are too burdensome, require one-on-one time to be set aside for teaching, increase stress, or do not fit with a particular family's values. Specific child outcome measures may include, for example, number of child responses, amount of disruptive behavior, amount of spontaneous speech, quality of friendships, academic improvement, and generalization of treatment gains. Parent outcome measures that are typically measured include parents' use of the procedures, parental stress, quality of parent–child interactions in everyday settings, positive affect, and depression. Recently, we also have begun developing measures of parent empowerment as an important additional parent outcome.

Empirical Evidence for Pivotal Response Training

Empirical evidence related to the pivotal areas of *motivation* and *child initiations* is presented next. These studies have used a variety of interrelated terminologies to describe the pivotal response interventions. A number of studies have documented the efficacy of using the natural language paradigm (NLP, or pivotal response training as it was applied to speech and language intervention specifically) and pivotal response training (PRT) as a broadly applied intervention for deficits characteristic of children with autism. Because the procedures more closely resembled the types of interactions adults had with typically developing children (as contrasted to a more analogue approach that has been used for children with autism), the pivotal response language intervention procedure was described as the "natural language paradigm." The NLP package of motivational procedures was initially researched at a time when about 50% of children diagnosed with autism were not developing expressive words and language, even with intensive intervention (Prizant, 1983). The NLP procedures produced rapid results in establishing a first lexicon in nonverbal children, and approximately 90% of nonverbal children were able to learn to use expressive verbalizations as a primary mode of communication (Koegel, 2000). Table 19.1 outlines the differences in the procedures for the two models as applied to language intervention. Subsequent research demonstrating the applicability of these NLP procedures to broader areas of nonlanguage behaviors led us to describe the technique as a "pivotal response treatment."

Components of PRT

Empirical support for the use of each PRT component has been widely documented in numerous research studies both within our laboratories and in independent laboratories (e.g., Matson, Benavidez, Compton, Paclawskyj, & Baglio, 1996; Romaniuk & Miltenberger, 2001). For example, allowing children to make choices in activities or order of activities was shown to reduce social avoidance behaviors (Carter, 2001; Koegel, Dyer, & Bell, 1987), increase accuracy and productivity, and decrease disruptive behaviors when embedded within teaching activities (Moes, 1998). Similarly, interventions in which the child responds to a combination of maintenance and acquisition tasks have resulted in improved correct responding (Dunlap & Koegel, 1980), increased rate of target behavior acquisition, and positive child affect (Dunlap, 1984). In addition, a number of studies have also investigated the response–reinforcer relationship in the intervention interactions. For example, when a child makes target response *attempts,* which are reinforced, as opposed to only successive motor approximations, improved speech production and increased interest, enthusiasm, and happiness occur (Koegel et al., 1988). Similarly, child responses that are directly or naturally related to the reinforcer have been shown to produce immediate increases in target behavior acquisition, rather than when the child responds for an arbitrary reinforcer. That is, when a child makes a response that is direct part of the chain leading to the reinforcer, rapid acquisition immediately follows (Koegel & Williams, 1980; Saunders & Sailor, 1979; Williams et al., 1981). Finally, studies show that the presence of child initiations is related to highly favorable outcomes, and that these initiations can be taught to children who do not initially demonstrate them (Koegel, Koegel, Shoshan, & McNerney, 1999; Koegel, Camarata, Valdez-Menchaca, & Koegel, 1998). In sum, these studies provide strong empirical support for the use of each of the individual motivational components of PRT, as well as empirical support for the importance of motivating the child to exhibit child-initiated social interactions.

PRT as a Package Intervention

In addition to the foregoing research providing empirical support for individual components of pivotal response interventions, other studies have compared the use of a package combining all the motivational components described previously versus a similar package of teaching procedures that does not incorporate the motivational variables. Table 19.2 provides a summary of the empirically based evidence supporting the PRT model. This body of literature reflects the increased efficacy of the motivational PRT procedures over a traditional, analogue individual target behavior approach. Further, improved treatment gains also are seen when parents, rather than clinicians, implement the treatment. In addition to the positive child outcomes of PRT, the collateral effects (i.e., reduction of family stress) of the PRT interventions on the families are documented in multiple studies. Finally, the most recent empirical research in this area has investigated both the importance of self-initiations as a prognostic indicator and the efficacy of teaching such self-initiations to children who lack them.

Summary of Empirical Studies

The characteristics of the studies summarized in Table 19.2 on pivotal response interventions reflect the necessary criteria for an empirically supported treatment for children with autism (Kazdin & Weisz, 1998). The experimental literature on PRT included group design studies that used random assignment to intervention conditions, single-subject studies that employed multiple baseline designs and/or ABA experimental designs, and replication designs both within and outside our laboratories. The procedures in these studies have been manualized and adherence measures (fidelity of implementation) were employed in all studies. The participants in each of the studies were diagnosed by outside agencies with autism based on nationally accepted standards for the diagnosis of autism (e.g., Ritvo & Freeman, 1978; American Psychological Association, 1994). This body of literature also represents studies from three different investigatory laboratories, using the same treatment manual. The preponderance of evidence shows that PRT leads to greater treatment gains in targeted behaviors and nontreated, collateral behaviors than the control treatments commonly used with children diagnosed as having autism.

SUMMARY AND CONCLUSIONS

To achieve widespread, long-term, generalized improvements across a child's environments and behavioral repertoire, a number of researchers have focused on investigating whether children with autism could learn certain pivotal responses that might have a broad impact on their disability and overall development. By treating pivotal areas that have widespread collateral effects, the intervention also can be less time-consuming, burdensome, and costly than those focused exclusively on individual target behaviors. For

TABLE 19.2. Studies Documenting Empirical Evidence for Pivotal Response Interventions

Study	Treatment sample	Design	Treatment/independent variable	Dependent variables	Treatment outcomes
Koegel, O'Dell, & Koegel (1987)	n = 2 Ages 4.5 and 5.8	Multiple baseline across participants	Analogue treatment (baseline) vs. NLP (pivotal response intervention)	Number of utterances (spontaneous and imitative) inside and outside (generalization) of clinic room	Children produced more imitative and spontaneous utterances in NLP condition. Generalization of treatment gains occurred outside treatment room only in NLP condition.
Laski, Charlop, & Schreibman (1988)	n = 8 Ages 5–9.6	Multiple baseline across participants	Parent training in NLP (pivotal response intervention) at home and in clinic	1. Parent verbalizations 2. Child vocalizations 3. Frequency of echolalia	Posttreatment increases in parents' requests for vocalizations. Increases in the children's verbal responsiveness in both clinic and generalization setting (home).
Schreibman, Kaneko, & Koegel (1991)	n = 19 (parents of children with autism)	Comparison of two groups randomly assigned to two parent training conditions	Individual target behaviors (ITB) teaching vs. PRT	Parental affect (scored by naïve observers)	Parents who were trained in PRT displayed significantly more positive affect than parents trained in ITB.
Koegel, Koegel, & Surratt (1992)	n = 3 Ages 3.4–4.6	Repeated reversals design with order of conditions and number of sessions varied within and across children	Analogue vs. PRT on the teaching of target sounds and words	1. Disruptive behavior 2. Target language responses	Increased responding and less disruptive behaviors occurred during NLP condition compared to analogue condition.
Stahmer (1995)	n = 7 Ages 4.3–7.2	Multiple baseline across participants	Modified PRT that used symbolic play as a target behavior	1. Symbolic play 2. Complexity of play behavior 3. Creativity of play 4. Generalization across toys, settings, and play partners	Increase in symbolic play and play complexity after symbolic play training. Generalization also occurred.
Koegel, Bimbela, & Schreibman (1996)	n = 17 Average age = 6	Comparison of two groups randomly assigned to two parent training conditions	Individual target behaviors (ITB) teaching vs. PRT	Dinnertime interactions scored for happiness, interest, stress, and communication style	ITB produced no significant influence on interactions. PRT led to more positive parent–child interactions.

Study	n / Ages	Design	Comparison	Dependent measures	Results
Koegel, Camarata, Koegel, Bentall, & Smith (1998)	n = 5 Ages 4.8–6	ABA with counterbalancing to control for order effects; random assignment to one of two conditions	Analogue vs. PRT teaching of target sounds	1. Correct production of target sounds in language samples 2. Intelligibility ratings	Significant gains in correct production of the target sound occurred in the PRT condition. Significant gains in speech intelligibility followed improvements in speech sounds during PRT intervention.
Koegel, Camarata, Valdez-Menchaca, & Koegel (1998)	n = 3 Ages 3.8–5.4	Multiple baseline across participants	Self-initiated question asking (pivotal response) ("What's that?")	1. Number of times child spontaneously used targeted question 2. Number of stimulus items child labeled correctly	Children consistently and spontaneously initiated "What's that?" which included generalization across settings. Significant increase in vocabulary (e.g., labels) after intervention.
Koegel, Koegel, Shoshan, & McNerney (1999) Phase 1	n = 6 Ages 3.1–3.10	Retrospective analysis of archival data	High vs. low child-initiated social interactions (pivotal response)	1. Language age (pre) 2. Number of initiations during 15-minute social play interactions (pre) 3. Pragmatic ratings (pre–post) 4. Social and community functioning (post) 5. Adaptive behavior scale scores (post)	Children with poor and favorable outcomes had comparable language ages and levels on the adaptive behavior scales at preintervention. Children with favorable outcomes exhibited considerably more spontaneous initiations at preintervention.
Koegel, Koegel, Shoshan, & McNerney (1999) Phase 2	n = 4 Ages 2.7–3.11	Clinical replication	PRT teaching of child-initiated social interactions	1. Language ages (pre) 2. Number of initiations (pre–post) 3. Pragmatics ratings (pre–post) 4. Adaptive behavior scale scores 5. Social and community functioning	Prior to intervention, all children exhibited few initiations, scored 9–12 months below chronological age on adaptive behavior scale, had inappropriate pragmatic ratings, had been recommended for special day class placement, and had no sustained peer relationships. After intervention, all children made considerable increases in the number of initiations. Scores on the adaptive behavior scales and pragmatics ratings were very close to chronological age. None of the children retained their diagnoses of autism after intervention, and none still qualified for special education services. They had grades at or above average, had social circles of typically developing peers outside of school, and participated in extracurricular activities without support.

example, data indicate that teaching approaches that specifically incorporate pivotal response motivational techniques have demonstrated that 85–90% of children under the age of 5 who have been diagnosed with autism can learn to use verbal communication as their primary mode of communication (Koegel, 2000); however, there is still a subpopulation of children who do not seem to learn functional expressive language with the techniques available today. More research regarding these children and the teaching of an initial lexicon is warranted. In addition, studies assessing the interrelationship between communication and other variables such as child age, disruptive behavior, repetitive behaviors, and so on, might enhance our research knowledge. Further information relating to implementation regarding the best settings, times, types, and amount of intervention may also provide valuable advances.

However, at this point in time, it is clear that intervention programs employing a pivotal response paradigm have been shown to result in an effective treatment delivery model, increasing the total amount of treatment available to the child and improving generalization of treatment gains. In addition, such pivotal response programs have resulted in decreases in parental stress, in part because interventions are blended into family routines and individually designed to match family values. Research has shown that not only do intervention programs influence parental stress, but parent stress may moderate child progress made in treatment (Robbins, Dunlap, & Plienis, 1991).

Given that we have found the standard procedures of pivotal response training to be effective, we are now investigating more effective means of individualizing interventions to meet family and child needs. Part of the individualization process has been to focus on "parent empowerment" as both an important goal of intervention and a dependent measure of intervention effectiveness. Further research is needed to find the most culturally sensitive means to increase parent participation, parental competence in treatment procedures, and overall parental empowerment.

Finally, we have shown that once children are motivated to respond to and initiate social communication and learning opportunities, we see concomitant achievement of developmental milestones. That is, we observe that parents are able to engage in naturally occurring teaching interactions, characteristic of interactions with typically developing children, once they are proficient in PRT techniques. Further research in this area may help us to fully understand the developmental trajectories of children with autism and the interventions needed to put the children on a typical developmental track. We are highly optimistic about the effects that such a data-based approach will have on the condition of autism and the quality of life for the families.

ACKNOWLEDGMENTS

Preparation of this chapter was supported in part by U.S. Public Health Service Research Grants MH28210 and MH065219 from the National Institute of Mental Health and U.S. Department of Education Grant 5830-257-LO-B.

REFERENCES

American Psychiatric Association. (1994). *Diagnostic and statistical manual of mental disorders* (4th ed.). Washington, DC: Author.
American Psychiatric Association. (2000). *Diagnostic and statistical manual of mental disorders* (4th ed., text rev.). Washington, DC: Author.

Burke, J. C., & Cerniglia, L. (1990). Stimulus complexity and autistic children's responsivity: Assessing and training a pivotal behavior. *Journal of Autism and Developmental Disorders, 20,* 233–253.

Carter, C. M. (2001). Using choice with game play to increase language skills and interactive behaviors in children with autism. *Journal of Positive Behavior Interventions, 3,* 131–151.

Chakrabarti, S., & Fombonne, E. (2001). Pervasive developmental disorders in preschool children. *Journal of the American Medical Association, 285,* 3093–3099.

Dunlap, G. (1984). The influence of task variation and maintenance tasks on the learning and affect of autistic children. *Journal of Experimental Child Psychology, 37,* 41–64.

Dunlap, G., & Koegel, R. L. (1980). Motivating autistic children through stimulus variation. *Journal of Applied Behavior Analysis, 13,* 619–627.

Kanner, L. (1943). Autistic disturbances if affective contact. *Nervous Child, 2,* 217–426.

Kazdin, A. E. (1977). Influence of behavior preceding a reinforced response on behavior change in classroom. *Journal of Applied Behavior Analysis, 10,* 299–310.

Kazdin, A. E. (1982). Symptom substitution, generalization, and response covariation: Implications for psychotherapy outcome. *Psychological Bulletin, 91,* 349–365.

Kazdin, A. E., & Weisz, J. R. (1998). Identifying and developing empirically supported child and adolescent treatments. *Journal of Consulting and Clinical Psychology, 66,* 19–36.

Koegel, L. K. (2000). Interventions to facilitate communication in autism. *Journal of Autism and Developmental Disorders, 30,* 383–391.

Koegel, L. K., Camarata, S. M., Valdez-Menchaca, M., & Koegel, R. L. (1998). Setting generalization of question-asking by children with autism. *American Journal on Mental Retardation, 102,* 346–357.

Koegel, L. K., & Koegel, R. L. (1995). Motivating communication in children with autism. In E. Schopler & G. Mesibov (Eds.), *Learning and cognition in autism: Current issues in autism.* (pp. 73–87). New York: Plenum Press.

Koegel, L. K., Koegel, R. L., & Brookman, L. I. (in press). Child-initiated strategies for improving communication and reducing severe behavior problems in children with autism. In E. Hibbs & P. Jensen (Eds.), *Psychosocial treatments for child and adolescent disorders.* Washington, DC: American Psychological Association.

Koegel, L. K., Koegel, R. L., Harrower, J. K., & Carter, C. M. (1999). Pivotal response intervention I: Overview of approach. *Journal of the Association for Persons with Severe Handicaps, 34,* 174–185.

Koegel, L. K., Koegel, R. L., Kellegrew, D., & Mullen, K. (1996). Parent education for prevention and reduction of severe problem behaviors. In L. K. Lynn & R. L. Koegel (Eds.), *Positive behavioral support: Including people with difficult behavior in the community* (pp. 3–30). Baltimore: Brookes.

Koegel, L. K., Koegel, R. L., Shoshan, Y., & McNerney, E. (1999). Pivotal response intervention II: Preliminary long-term outcome data. *Journal of the Association for Persons with Severe Handicaps, 24,* 186–198.

Koegel, L. K., Stiebel, D., & Koegel, R. L. (1998). Reducing aggression in children with autism toward infant or toddler siblings. *Journal of the Association for Persons with Severe Handicaps, 23,* 111–118.

Koegel, R. L., Bimbela, A., & Schreibman, L. (1996). Collateral effects of parent training on family interactions. *Journal of Autism and Developmental Disorders, 23,* 347–359.

Koegel, R. L., Camarata, S., Koegel, L. K., Ben-Tall, A., & Smith, A. E. (1998). Increasing speech intelligibility in children with autism. *Journal of Autism and Developmental Disorders, 28,* 241–251.

Koegel, R. L., Carter, C. M., & Koegel, K. L. (1998). Setting events to improve parent–teacher coordination and motivation for children with autism. In J. K. Luiselli & M. J. Cameron (Eds.), *Antecedent control: Innovative approaches to behavioral support* (pp. 167–186). Baltimore: Brookes.

Koegel, R. L., Dyer, K., & Bell, L. K. (1987). The influence of child-preferred activities on autistic children's social behavior. *Journal of Applied Behavior Analysis, 20*(3), 243–252.

Koegel, R. L., Koegel, L. K., & McNerney, E. K. (2001). Pivotal areas of interventions for autism. *Journal of Clinical Child Psychology, 30,* 19–32.

Koegel, R. L., Koegel, L. K., & Surratt, A. (1992). Language intervention and disruptive behavior in preschool children with autism. *Journal of Autism and Developmental Disorders, 22*(2), 141–153.

Koegel, R. L., O'Dell, M., & Dunlap, G. (1988). Producing speech use in nonverbal autistic children by reinforcing attempts. *Journal of Autism and Developmental Disorders, 18*(4), 525–538.

Koegel, R. L., O'Dell, M. C., & Koegel, L. K. (1987). A natural language teaching paradigm for nonverbal autistic children. *Journal of Autism and Developmental Disorders, 17*(2), 187–200.

Koegel, R. L., Schreibman, L., Good, A., Cerniglia, L., Murphy, C., & Koegel, L. K. (1989). *How to teach pivotal behaviors to children with autism: A training manual.* Santa Barbara: University of California Press.

Koegel, R. L., Schreibman, L., Loos, L. M., & Dirlich-Wilhelm, H. (1992). Consistent stress profiles in mothers of children with autism. *Journal of Autism and Developmental Disorders, 22*(2), 205–216.

Koegel, R. L., Schreibman, L., O'Neill, R. E., & Burke, J. C. (1983). Personality and family interaction characteristics of parents of autistic children. *Journal of Consulting and Clinical Psychology, 16,* 683–692.

Koegel, R. L., & Williams, J. A. (1980). Direct versus indirect response–reinforcer relationships in teaching autistic children. *Journal of Abnormal Child Psychology, 8*(4), 537–547.

Laski, K. E., Charlop, M. H., & Schreibman, L. (1988). Training parents to use the natural language paradigm to increase their autistic children's speech. *Journal of Applied Behavior Analysis, 21,* 391–400.

Lovaas, O. I., Koegel, R. L., Simmons, J. Q., & Long, J. S. (1973). Some generalization and follow-up measures on autistics children in behavior therapy. *Journal of Applied Behavioral Analysis, 6,* 131–166.

Matson, J. L., Benavidez, D. A., Compton, L. S., Paclawskyj, T., & Baglio, C. S. (1996). Behavioral treatment of autistic persons: A review of research from 1980 to the present. *Research in Developmental Disabilities, 17,* 433–465.

McClannahan, L. E., Krantz, P. J., & McGee, G. G. (1982). Parents as therapists for autistic children: A model for effective parent training. *Analysis and Intervention in Developmental Disabilities, 2,* 223–252.

Moes, D. (1995). Parent education and parenting stress. In R. L. Koegel & L. K. Koegel (Eds.), *Teaching children with autism: Strategies for initiating positive interactions and improving learning opportunities* (pp. 79–93). Baltimore: Brookes.

Moes, D. (1998). Integrating choice-making opportunities within teacher-assigned academic tasks to facilitate the performance of children with autism. *Journal of the Association for Persons with Severe Handicaps, 23,* 319–328.

Prizant, B. M. (1983). Language acquisition and communicative behavior in autism: Toward an understanding of the "whole" of it. *Journal of Speech and Hearing Disorders, 48,* 296–307.

Ritvo, E. R., & Freeman, B. J. (1978). National Society for Autistic Children definition of the syndrome of autism. *Journal of Autism and Childhood Schizophrenia, 8,* 162–167.

Robbins, F. R., Dunlap, G., & Plienis, A. (1991). Family characteristics, family training, and the progress of young children with autism. *Journal of Early Intervention, 15,* 173–184.

Romaniuk, C., & Miltenberger, R. G. (2001). The influence of preference and choice of activity on problem behavior: Review and analysis. *Journal of Positive Behavior Interventions, 3,* 152–159.

Santarelli, G., Koegel, R. L., Casas, J. M., & Koegel, L. K. (2001). Culturally diverse families participating in behavior therapy parent education programs for children with developmental disabilities. *Journal of Positive Behavior Interventions, 3*(2), 120–123.

Saunders, R., & Sailor, W. (1979). A comparison of three strategies of reinforcement on two-choice language problems with severely retarded children. *AAESPH Review, 4,* 323–333.

Schreibman, L., Kaneko, W. M., & Koegel, R. L. (1991). Positive affect of parents of autistic children: A comparison across two teaching techniques. *Behavior Therapy, 22,* 479–490.

Singer, G. H., Singer, J., & Horner, R. H. (1987). Using pretask requests to increase the probability of compliance for students with severe disabilities. *Journal of the Association for Persons with Severe Handicaps, 12,* 287–291.

Stahmer, A. C. (1995). Teaching symbolic play skills to children with autism using pivotal response training. *Journal of Autism and Developmental Disabilities, 25,* 123–141.

Williams, J. A., Koegel, R. L., & Egel, A. L. (1981). Response–reinforcer relationships and improved learning in autistic children. *Journal of Applied Behavior Analysis, 14,* 53–60.

20

Behavioral Family Systems Therapy for Adolescents with Anorexia Nervosa

Arthur L. Robin

OVERVIEW

Anorexia nervosa (AN) is a life-threatening eating disorder characterized in the *Diagnostic and Statistical Manual of Mental Disorders*, fourth edition, text revision (DSM-IV-TR), by (1) a refusal to maintain body weight at or above a minimally normal weight for age and height; (2) intense fear of gaining weight or becoming fat, even though the individual is underweight; (3) body weight/shape disturbance or denial of the seriousness of low body weight; and (4) the absence of three consecutive menstrual cycles in postmenarchal females (American Psychiatric Association, 2000). The prevalence of AN in 15- to 19-year-old girls has been reported to be 0.48% (Fischer et al., 1995), but the prevalence of eating disorders is lower and not clearly known among younger children (Robin, Gilroy, & Dennis, 1998). Over 90% of the postpubertal adolescents with AN are female, although the ratio of girls to boys with AN is lower in prepubertal children (Robin et al., 1998). The following two vignettes illustrate two common presentations of AN.

> Nicole, 17 years old, weighed 84 pounds at intake, was 5 feet 4 inches in height, had amenorrhea for five months, and restricted her food intake to approximately 750 calories per day (fruits, vegetables, rice cakes, and water, but no protein or fats). She will not increase her eating because she is very fearful of getting fat, particularly her thighs and hips. Nicole started dieting 1 year ago because she was self-conscious about her "chubby" appearance. She dropped from 135 to 84 pounds. She does not see what the big deal is about her health.

> Adam, 12 years old, weighed 97 pounds at intake, was 5 feet 4 inches in height, and had not gained any weight over the past 18 months as he grew several inches in height. He denied trying to diet but indicated that he was trying to eat in a more healthy way in order to achieve his goal of becoming a professional gymnast. He changed his eating habits to be a vegetarian and greatly restricted his overall caloric intake following a summer at gymnastics camp. Adam also worked out with weights for 2 hours and jogged 5 miles every day. When his pediatrician and parents asked him to eat more and exercise less, he refused, indicating it would ruin his health and prevent him from being a world-class gymnast. He expressed surprise that he was too thin, indicat-

ing he was trying to eat healthily, not diet. He denied any concerns about getting too fat or the shape of particular body parts.

Nicole represents the classic DSM-IV-TR female picture of AN. She has lost a substantial amount of weight, has a dire fear of gaining weight, has body image distortions, has amenorrhea, and denies the seriousness of her condition. Adam illustrates a common male picture of AN; he also illustrates how a youngster may display significant eating disorder symptomatology but not meet the full DSM-IV-TR criteria for AN. He has failed to gain weight as expected and has restricted his food intake, but he does not have body image distortions or classic fears of getting fat. Although he claims not to be dieting, he avoids eating the food necessary to be at a healthy weight for his height, age, and high activity level. He would fall within the DSM-IV-TR criteria for an eating disorder not otherwise specified (American Psychiatric Association, 2000). This category is defined as a partial or subclinical AN, yet there is nothing "subclinical" or "partial" about the magnitude of Adam's problems.

Adam and Nicole both have a determined food avoidance and distorted cognitions, and as a result they have slipped into states of physiological starvation. Yet they differ from each other in many regards, illustrating the heterogeneity of eating disorders in children and adolescents. Both youngsters can be successfully treated with the intervention outlined in this chapter. To understand and successfully treat such youngsters, it is important at the outset to understand the ways in which eating disorders in children and adolescents differ from eating disorders in adults (Fisher et al., 1995; Robin et al., 1998):

1. Many children with eating disorders do not meet the full DSM-IV-TR criteria for AN or bulimia nervosa (BN), necessitating a diagnosis of eating disorder not otherwise specified if one has to use the official diagnostic system.
2. Research has indicated that these children and adolescents who fail to meet the DSM-IV-TR criteria for AN or BN are as impaired physiologically, behaviorally, and emotionally as those who do meet the full criteria.
3. Fears and anxieties may be different in some children and adolescents from the classic fear of fatness or the classic shape and size distortions about body parts seen in adults. Children may have concrete fears of choking, contaminated food, unhealthy food, or vomiting.
4. Children and adolescents tend to achieve a more severe degree of emaciation when compared to adults with the same degree of weight loss because of differences in the distribution of adipose tissue. As a result, they may reach the later stages of starvation with accompanying depressive symptoms more rapidly.
5. The wide variability in rate, timing, and magnitude of both height and weight gain during puberty makes evaluation of the weight and menstruation criteria for AN difficult.

The major implication of these differences is that the practitioner should not wait to intervene until a child or adolescent meets the full DSM-IV-TR criteria for AN or BN.

Conceptual Model

A variety of interventions have been used to treat eating disorders in children and adolescents: inpatient hospitalization, partial hospitalization, individual dynamic therapy, individual cognitive-behavioral therapy, and family therapy. In a chapter of their treatment manual reviewing controlled outcome studies, Lock, LeGrange, Agras, and Dare (2001) cited eight random-assignment controlled outcome studies evaluating the effectiveness of these various treatments. Six of these studies included some form of family therapy. Family therapy proved to be the most effective intervention for adolescents with eating disorders in these studies, helping approximately two-thirds of the patients return to health. A key element of all the successful family therapy approaches was putting the parents in charge of getting their adolescents to eat.

This chapter describes behavioral family systems therapy (BFST). BFST takes place within the context of a multidisciplinary team where the therapist works side by side with a pediatrician and a dietician, either in the same setting or in different settings with regular communication. There are five goals to this multidisciplinary intervention: (1) restore the teenager's health–weight, menses, and the effects of starvation; (2) change the teenager's eating habits and attitudes in a more normal direction; (3) correct distorted body images and unrealistic fears of getting fat; (4) change maladaptive family interaction patterns which may be preventing the teenager from achieving the developmental tasks of adolescence; and (5) help the adolescent achieve age-appropriate individuation and autonomy.

The BFST model is not a model for the etiology of AN, which is thought to be multifactorial but a working model for treating AN. BFST starts with the premise that families do not cause AN and blame should be removed. Pragmatically, it has proven useful to combine behavioral, cognitive, and family systems perspectives and interventions to help adolescents and their parents overcome AN. From a family systems perspective, the appropriate hierarchy of parent-in-charge-of-child is reversed with regard to food and eating. The adolescent is eating or not eating as she[1] wishes, and her parents have little influence over her eating behavior; in fact, many parents go to extraordinary lengths to appease their adolescent in the hopes of getting her to eat. Furthermore, the parents are often divided as a couple and fighting each other rather than working as a team to help their daughter recover. At the same time, the physical effects of starvation, together with the distorted cognitions, render the adolescent helpless to change her own eating behavior (e.g., she is stuck in a downward spiral). The BFST therapist rereverses the hierarchy, putting the parents in charge of getting the adolescent to restart eating.

The parents are helped to work as a united team to help their daughter recover from AN. Strategic/structural family therapy techniques are used to accomplish these change in the hierarchy. The therapist then teaches the parents to use behavioral weight gain procedures, demonstrated to be effective in inpatient programs (Robin et al., 1998), to help their adolescent restart appropriate eating and to change eating habits. As the adolescent begins to eat more appropriately, it is necessary to overcome the many cognitive distortions that are part of the eating disorder. The therapist creatively applies cognitive restructuring for this purpose. When the adolescent reaches the designated target weight, the goals shifts to maintenance of weight and return of control over eating to the adolescent. The adolescent is helped to accomplish the normal developmental task of individuation from the family. An integrative combination of strategic/structural, behavioral shaping, cognitive restructuring, and problem-solving communication training techniques are used to facilitate this individuation process.

CHARACTERISTICS OF THE TREATMENT PROGRAM

Who Is Seen and in What Format

The identified teenager with AN and her parents (or legal guardians if other than parents) are seen in all phases of treatment. The treatment program can roughly be divided into four phases: (1) assessment, (2) control rationale, (3) weight gain, and (4) weight maintenance. In the first three phases, the adolescent and her parents are seen together on a weekly basis for virtually all of the sessions. Each session lasts 55 minutes. These phases take from 6 to 12 months, depending upon how much weight the adolescent needs to gain. In the fourth phase, sessions are scheduled twice per month. This phase typically takes 3 to 4 months. Siblings are invited to attend family sessions when an issue arises between the identified patient and the parent that involves the sibling (e.g., arguments between the identified patient and a sibling or inappropriate involvement of a sibling in the eating routine for the identified patient). The overall length of treatment varies from 9 to 16 months, depending on the amount of weight to be gained and severity of the eating disorder. (An unpublished treatment manual describing the four phases of the intervention is available from the author.)

Phase 1: Assessment—Content of Treatment and Skills Emphasized

The first three sessions constitute the assessment phase. The goal and content of this phase are to (1) establish rapport with the adolescent and the parents; (2) collect information concerning weight, eating, body image, individual, and family problems; (3) build the therapeutic team by arranging for pediatric medical and dietary evaluations and exchanging information with these professionals; (4) separate the illness from the person and remove blame from the patient and the parents for causing AN; and (5) obtain the family's commitment to a therapeutic contract which specifies how the family, adolescent, parents, physician, and dietician will work together as a team to help the adolescent overcome the eating disorder.

Clinical experience has taught us that families are best engaged in treatment when the adolescent and the parents are seen separately in the first session, then brought together for subsequent sessions. Meeting first with the adolescent, the therapist establishes rapport through reflective listening, open-ended questioning, and careful explanations. After a brief period of ice-breaking social conversation about the adolescent's interests, the therapist encourages the adolescent to relate her story of dieting and weight loss, fears and body dissatisfaction, family relationships, school, peers, and anything else the adolescent considers important. The therapist listens empathetically to the adolescent's story, conveying acceptance and helping the adolescent label and understand the core symptoms of anorexia as inevitable sequelae of starvation. At this time, listening attentively to the adolescent is more important than collecting or imparting information about the treatment program or the adolescent's eating disorder.

Afterward, the therapist weighs the adolescent, either in street clothes without shoes on, or if the therapist is working near a medical clinic, the therapist has the adolescent change into a hospital gown; the therapist explains that the weight taken at the sessions will serve as the official weight for the record. When the physician will be closely monitoring the adolescent's health status, the therapist defers to the physician to weigh the adolescent weekly and arranges to obtain the weight by e-mail or written slips given to the parents.

The therapist is more information oriented in the parental interview than in the adolescent interview. The therapist takes a history of the onset and course of the dieting, weight loss, eating habits and attitudes, previous treatment attempts, general medical and developmental histories, school and peer functioning, and family relations. Then, the therapist describes the team approach to treating eating disorders and outlines the roles of each team member: the pediatrician will set target weights, rates of weight gain, make decisions about the need for hospitalization, and conduct regular medical follow-ups; the dietician will provide information about the types and amounts of food to be eaten; and the therapist will deal with all other issues, including eating, distorted cognitions, affect, self-esteem, and family relations. Only a few points are made about BFST at this session: that the adolescent will mostly be seen together with her parents, that the therapy is action oriented with an initial focus on the parents helping their daughter to relearn normal eating patterns and a later focus on feelings and beliefs, and that although the family is not the cause of their daughter's AN, it is central to helping her overcome her eating disorder.

At the end of the session, the therapist asks the parents to schedule a physical examination with the pediatrician as well as an initial consultation with the dietician. The parents are told that the first thing they can do to help their daughter is to collect detailed information for the therapist by recording everything that the adolescent eats over the next week, using specially designed food records provided by the therapist.

The family is given the following self-report measures to complete at home and return at the second session: Eating Attitudes Test (teen and parent versions), Eating Disorder Inventory–2 (EDI-2) (teen), the Symptom Checklist 90—Revised (SCL90-R) for the parents to rate themselves, the Beck Depression Inventory (teen), a specially designed demographic questionnaire which assesses eating-disordered symptom history, the Child Behavior Checklist (parents), and the Parent Adolescent Relationship Questionnaire (PARQ—parents and adolescent). The Eating Attitudes Test (EAT-26; Garner, Olmsted, Bohr, & Garfinkel, 1982) consists of 26 items rated on a 6-point Likert scale tapping dieting behavior, bingeing and purging, and unusual eating habits such as cutting food into very small pieces. The EDI-2 (Garner, 1991) consists of 91 items rated on a 6-point Likert scale combined to form the following scales: Drive for thinness, bulimia, body dissatisfaction, perfectionism, ineffectiveness (feelings of general inadequacy, insecurity, and lack of control), interpersonal distrust (sense of alienation and reluctance to form close relationships), interoceptive awareness (difficulty recognizing and accurately identifying feelings and hunger sensations), maturity fears (wish to retreat to the security of the preadolescent years), impulse control, social insecurity, and asceticism. The PARQ is a multidimensional self-report measure of family relations independently completed by the adolescent, mother, and father. It contains scales assessing overt conflict, beliefs, and family structure (Robin, Koepke, & Moye, 1990). Two summary scores are particularly useful with eating-disordered families: (1) General Conflict—a factorially based linear composite of 45 items tapping Communication ("My mom puts me down"), Problem Solving ("We think of many good ideas to solve our problems"), and Warmth Hostility ("Quite honestly, I hate my Dad"); and (2) Conflict over Eating—the sum of 14 items assessing conflict and hostility concerning eating, mealtimes, and food ("I dread mealtimes with my daughter," "We argue often about food and eating").

The parents and teen are seen together for the second assessment session. First, the therapist collects the self-report measures. These are scored later and feedback is given during the third session. Next, the therapist examines the parents' food records. Discussing the food record serves as a springboard to learn about family interactions during mealtime. The therapist picks a representative meal and asks for a "blow by blow" description of what happened. Their description provides the further opportunity to assess parental teamwork, parent–child coalitions, and triangulated behavior. The adolescent's reactions to the meal opens up a host of issues regarding distorted cognitions about food, weight, shape, and family life. Even though there is not sufficient time to assess all these areas in depth, the therapist tries to collect sufficient information to build a mental picture of family process.

When time permits, the therapist also assesses the parents' families of origin and the parents' and adolescent's interactions with the grandparents. The therapist ends the session by reassigning the task of recording all of the adolescent's food intake.

In the third session, the therapist obtains the family's commitment to a therapeutic contract. The target weight, hospitalization weight, required weekly rate of weight gain, and any restrictions on exercise outlined by the physician are reviewed, along with the food plan provided by the dietician. The results of the self-report questionnaires are reviewed, reinforcing the need to undertake a comprehensive family intervention. The therapist indicates that there will need to be big changes in eating habits, beliefs and attitudes, feelings, and family relations in order to achieve these medical and nutritional goals, and that the therapist will take responsibility for helping the patient and the parents make these changes through weekly family therapy sessions. The therapist indicates that these changes will not be easy but he or she feels confident that the adolescent can recover from the eating disorder. The family is asked to make a commitment to attend weekly, and specific scheduling and fee arrangements are discussed.

Typically, the teenager expresses a great deal of anger and refuses to commit to making any changes in eating or weight gain. She tries to convince her parents that therapy is not necessary because she can make the necessary changes on her own. Feeling guilty but helpless, the parents are triangulated between a therapist holding out hope of change but demanding a commitment and their very angry teenager, who is refusing to participate in therapy. They may vacillate and have a difficult time making the necessary commitment to family therapy.

The therapist must convey respect and empathy for the plight of the angry adolescent but must continue to ascribe her behavior and attitudes to the effects of starvation, which are clouding her mind and causing her to resist the necessary treatment. The therapist reassures the parents that their daughter's reaction is not her fault but is normal and expected for the advanced stage of her illness. The therapist holds out hope for overcoming the AN and empathizes with the difficult position in which the parents find themselves but nonetheless relentlessly demands a commitment to participate in weekly family therapy sessions.

Under these circumstances most parents commit to therapy despite their adolescent's objections. Occasionally, a couple is unable to make this commitment. The therapist does not try to persuade them but, rather, goes along with their resistance, indicating that they know their daughter best and perhaps she will overcome this life-threatening eating disorder on her own. The session is then quickly terminated. Often, this raises the parents' anxiety, and within a few days they call the therapist and commit to the treatment program.

Phase 2: Control Rationale—Content of Treatment and Skills Emphasized

During this phase of intervention the therapist teaches the parents the skills necessary to take charge of refeeding their daughter. The phase starts when therapist presents the control rationale to the family and ends when the teenager starts eating and gaining weight on a regular basis. During this phase, the therapist deals with the family's reaction to the control rationale and uses strategic interventions to overcome their resistance, building a strong parental coalition to take charge of the teen's eating. In doing so, the therapist coaches the parents to develop a behavioral weight gain program designed to achieve the weekly weight goal established by the pediatrician and the daily food intake goals established by the dietician.

Before being willing to take this onerous step, the parents need to appreciate the value and importance of taking charge of their daughter's eating. It is usually necessary to heighten the parents' fears and anxieties about the life-threatening nature of AN and the adolescent's inability to change on her own before parents are willing to take charge. The effects of starvation and the teen's poor eating record are reviewed and related to the teenager's currently impaired functioning, noting how she is completely out of control of her own eating. The dire medical consequences of continued starvation, including death, are clearly reviewed, along with the failure of any previous treatment programs. The teenager often pleads, "I will change this time; give me one more chance." The therapist asks the parents to present the "evidence" to support the teen's assertion that she will change on her own, and it is quickly established that despite good intentions, the teen has been unable to make the necessary changes. At this point, parents usually agree that a new approach is needed to help their daughter.

Then, the therapist presents the metaphor of "food as medicine" as a nonblaming rationale for parental control over eating:

> "AN is a life-threatening disease. When a child is sick, we consult the doctor, who usually prescribes medicine. You have consulted the doctors, and food as been prescribed as the only medicine that can cure AN. But your child's disease causes her to fear taking the medicine that she so desperately needs. When a child is unable to take her medicine on her own for any other disease, her parents who love her give her the medicine. Similarly, in this case you are going to need to give your daughter her medicine (e.g., the food which she needs to recover). Temporarily, you will take over complete control of everything related to eating. You will plan her menu based upon the dietician's recommendations. You will do the shopping. You will weigh and prepare her food. You will present the food to her and sit with her to make sure she eats it all. You will record everything that she eats on the sheets I give you. You will praise and reward her for eating all of her food, and you will arrange for her to preserve her energy by not engaging in any activities if its proves too difficult for her to eat all of her food. I understand that his is a very big responsibility. I will help you work as a team to divide this responsibility between the two of you. When she approaches her target weight and demonstrates readiness to take back responsibility for her food and eating, I will help you gradually return it to her. I know that I am asking you to do something that is very difficult, but I also know how much you love your daughter and I feel completely confident that you can help her take the food that is her only medicine."

After giving the control rationale, the therapist asks each family member for his or her reactions. Most adolescents angrily object that they do not need any parental control and they will refuse to put up with it; some act out by throwing things at the therapist, threatening suicide, or storming out of the office. Most parents express disbelief, skepticism, despair, helplessness, and even open defiance at being asked to carry out a seemingly impossible task. Within a few moments, the parents and teen are united in a coalition against the therapist, perhaps the first time in a long time that they have been on the same side of an issue related to food and eating.

The therapist should listen attentively to each family member's concerns about the control rationale. The teenager's objections are empathetically acknowledged, but the therapist reiterates that through no fault of her own, starvation has clouded her mind and prevented her from eating in a healthy manner. She is reminded that her parents will only take control of her eating temporarily, until she is healthy again and can take care of her own eating. The parents' resistance is empathetically reframed as the natural apprehension and fear of a loving couple who want to heal their daughter but do not know how to go about it. The life-threatening consequences of failing to take control are reiterated. The therapist must sound completely confident that the parents can succeed with the coaching by the therapist. Strategically, the therapist "goes with the resistance," creatively finding a graceful path to navigate around it.

If the therapist perseveres in nondefensively listening to everyone's objections and patiently reiterating the need for parental control to restart eating, the majority of parents eventually come to agree. Some more immediately embrace the behavioral weight gain program and experience initial successes with it, strongly reinforcing their commitment to it and their confidence in the therapist. Others cave into pressure from their daughter to give them "one more chance" to prove she can "do it on her own." Over the next few weeks, the adolescents are typically unable to eat the required calories and gain weight on their own, the parents become very anxious, and they come to realize that external control is necessary.

When the parents do make the commitment to take charge of their daughter's eating, the therapist coaches them to develop a behavioral weight gain program. First, they are asked to deal with one meal per day, to gradually shape their behavior. They are asked to plan the following aspects of their daughter's eating: writing a menu for that meal based on the amounts of different food groups specified by the dietician, doing the shopping, weighing and preparing the food, supervising their daughter at the table, responding to her resistance to eat, recording what she ate, providing a positive incentive contingent upon the teen's finishing the entire meal, handling failure to finish the meal, and so on. The family goes home and implements the plan for the single meal per day, reporting back at the next session. If the single meal plan worked reasonably well, the therapist coaches the parents on extending the behavioral eating plan to all of the meals and snacks for the day. If it did not work, the difficulties are discussed, the plan is modified, and the parents again handle one meal per day for the next week.

As the parents experience success refeeding their daughter over the course of an entire day, the therapist further prompts them to designate positive incentives for completing eating each meal, as well as longer-term incentives for achieving 25%, 50%, 75%, and so on, of the required weight gain. Often, access to activities that were curtailed due to the weight loss can be used as incentives for achieving the later stages of weight gain. The adolescent is asked to provide her own list of possible incentives.

Phase 3: Weight Gain—Content of Treatment and Skills Emphasized

During the weight gain phase of BFST, the therapist teaches the family the skills necessary to "fine tune" the behavioral weight gain program, closing off any loopholes and continuing the program as the adolescent gradually gains weight and moves toward her target weight. Later in this phase, the therapist explores other issues, including cognitive distortions and family structure problems.

The sessions follow the same general format. At the beginning of each session, the adolescent is either weighed or the weight slip sent by the pediatrician is collected. Then, the therapist gives the teen approximately 15 minutes to discuss anything that she wants.

This ventilation period is important during this phase of therapy when the adolescent does not have a great deal of choice about the eating program.

Next, the food logs provided by the parents are reviewed, discussing any problems which arose, and also relating the food logs to any change in weight which took place. If the adolescent has gained weight and eaten most of the required food, the therapist praises her, makes sure her parents provided any rewards she earned, and inquires about her reactions to the weight gain. If she evidences any distorted cognitions about the weight gain, the therapist helps her challenge them. For example, some adolescents believe that eating one cookie will put on 5 pounds, or that all fats are unhealthy. The therapist may provide corrective nutritional information and/or go through a Socratic discussion challenging the logic of such distortions, helping the adolescent develop more accurate cognitions about the impacts of specific foods. The therapist also praises the parents for working effectively as a team, urges them to continue, and prompts them to anticipate and plan to overcome any difficulties which may arise during the next week.

If the adolescent has lost weight or stayed the same, the therapist analyzes with the family which of the following factors may have been operative: (1) she consumed an insufficient number of calories, even if the written records suggest otherwise; (2) she dumped or hid some of her food; (3) she exercised secretly; (4) she skipped snacks or lunch at school; (5) she did not eat all that was served and the parents did not notice it; (6) she ate low-calorie foods; (7) she took laxatives or vomited; (8) the written records were inaccurate or altered by the teenager; (9) parental teamwork is breaking down; (10) there is interference from other family issues (e.g., marital conflict or sibling issues); and (11) the consequences for failing to eat were not enforced. The remainder of the session is devoted to coaching the parents to work on an approach to overcoming the "loopholes" that were identified.

Because the dietician initially prescribed a relatively small number of calories, it is expected that the calories will need to be increased regularly. The therapist should directly consult the dietician and then send the family to talk to the dietician. A caloric increase should be requested when the teen has failed to gain weight for 1 week and the therapist is certain that the family has complied with the behavioral weight gain program. The dietician typically makes 100–300 calorie increases, distributed across food groups, meals, and snacks. Many patients consume 3,000–4,000 calories daily in order to gain 1 pound per week.

Eventually, the teen eats most of the required foods and gains weight regularly. Then, the therapist shift the focus of the sessions to non–food-related issues. Cognitive restructuring is introduced to correct distorted thinking about certain foods, body parts, or body size. Cognitive restructuring involves (1) identifying a distorted cognition, (2) challenging it logically, (3) suggesting a more appropriate cognition, (4) proposing an experiment to determine which cognition makes more sense based upon the evidence collected by the teen, and (5) reviewing the results of the experiment (Robin & Foster, 1989). An example follows:

> As Nicole gained weight, she became increasingly distraught about the change in her appearance. She felt her stomach was sticking out and that she looked "gross." The therapist asked Nicole to bring in pictures of herself before she began to diet, at various points afterward, and during weight gain. Nicole was asked to identify four people she trusted. They reviewed the pictures and selected the one which represented the "healthiest" appearance. Three of the four raters chose the picture in which Nicole was close to her target weight as "healthiest" and "most attractive." Nicole was taken aback. This gave her cause to reevaluate her self-perceptions.

About 50% of the time such cognitive restructuring exercises fail to change the adolescent's fixed cognitions, which may be impervious to evidence. Such exercises are considered successful if the adolescent expresses an intellectual willingness to consider plausible alternatives to her fixed, distorted belief, even if she emotionally cannot accept such alternatives. For distorted beliefs concerning the shape and size of various body parts and their relationship to food (e.g., "If I eat this cookie, my thighs will get larger"), measuring the body part is a helpful task. For distorted beliefs concerning "forbidden foods," the teen can be asked to "experiment" by eating a small amount of the forbidden food, evaluate her feelings, and weigh herself to be reassured that the food did not "make her fat."

During this phase of treatment, it is often helpful to permit the adolescent to resume small to moderate amounts of exercise, after consulting with the dietician and physician. Walking for 15 minutes after a meal is a common first step. Many teens feel less bloated after a short walk. Later, the teen can be given the choice to resume limited participation in athletic or performing arts activities (dancing, ice skating, etc.) if she agrees to compensate for burning extra calories by further increasing her food intake.

Phase 4: Weight Maintenance—Content of Treatment and Skills Emphasized

As the teen approaches her target weight, the weight-maintenance phase of BFST begins. The therapist teaches the parents the skills necessary to gradually return the responsibility for eating to the teen. It is important that this does not occur too rapidly and that the teen demonstrates healthy weight-maintenance behaviors. The dietician is consulted to reduce caloric intake to facilitate maintaining rather than gaining weight. The family's reaction to the gradual transfer of control sets the stage for additional cognitive restructuring interventions because parents may express ruinous fears of a relapse and adolescents may yearn for additional freedoms from control without having to demonstrate increased responsibility for healthy eating.

It is during this phase that the therapist simultaneously encourages (1) the adolescent to seek age-appropriate individuation and autonomy from her parents and (2) the parents to refocus their energies on their strengthening their marital bonds. Encouraging autonomy seeking naturally leads to rebellious behavior as eating-disordered families are absolutistic thinkers. The therapist employs problem-solving communication-training techniques (Robin & Foster, 1989) to help the parents and adolescents negotiate mutually acceptable resolutions to independence-related conflicts.

At the beginning of the weight-maintenance phase, a "comfort zone" of 3–5 pounds around the target weight is defined. If the teen goes above or below the comfort zone, the family agrees that is a source of concern and the return of control over eating is temporarily halted or partially reversed. But weight fluctuations within the comfort zone are treated as "random noise" during experimentation with gradual return of control. This procedure helps these absolutistic families avoid excessively ruinous cognitions and overreactions to minor fluctuations in weight.

The therapist helps the family delineate the steps for giving the adolescent more decision-making control over her eating. These steps may be written in the form of a behavioral contract. At first, the teenager might plan one of her meals, measure and prepare some of her food, eat a meal without supervision, or write down her own foods for the meal. Later, she might eat a meal without supervision, plan her menus for an entire day, eat several meals without supervision, and so on. Eventually, she may eat all her meals for a day without any parental intervention or monitoring. Maintenance of weight within the comfort zone and reports of the adolescent's eating attitudes and behaviors constitute the yardsticks used to measure the success of the behavioral contract. The inevitable setbacks which occur are handled with restraint, teaching parents to make a measured response rather than a rigid resumption of all parental controls.

The therapist recognizes that whereas the overt agenda is return of control over eating, the covert agenda is negotiating individuation in highly enmeshed families. Individuation issues need to be handled in a sensitive, gentle manner when parents and children have been enmeshed with each other for a lifetime. Helping the adolescent "individuate" appropriately from parental control over eating becomes a metaphor for helping her individuate emotionally and behaviorally from her parents. As soon as she responsibly manages her own eating and weight maintenance, the therapist moves on to a broader agenda of individuating from other parental controls.

The therapist addresses the broader agenda of individuation by giving the parents a "crash course" in adolescent development, emphasizing the importance of autonomy seeking, identity formation, peer relationships, dating, and planning for a future career. Discrimination training is undertaken to help the family distinguish between autonomy-seeking behaviors and rebellious behaviors (Robin & Foster, 1989). Such "discrimination training" may take the form of asking the family to brainstorm a list of all of the "independent" adolescent behaviors they can, then differentiating the items into "rebellious" versus "autonomous" categories.

The adolescent is assigned tasks to engage in more autonomous behaviors such as spending more time with peers and less time with parents. Parents are urged to spend more time with each other. For example, the adolescent may be asked to spend the night with a friend while the parents go out together.

When the teenager has maintained her weight within the 3-pound comfort zone for at least 3 months, the therapist plans for termination. The interval between sessions is lengthened to 1 month. The therapist coordinates termination with the pediatrician, who has been conducting periodic medical follow-ups. The therapist discusses methods of coping with possible relapses with the family. In the last few sessions, the changes which have occurred are reviewed, and the family is left with the framework that coping with AN may be a lifelong process, and that they could return for more therapy at any time in the future.

EVIDENCE FOR THE EFFECTS OF TREATMENT

The effectiveness of BFST for treating adolescents with AN was assessed by comparing it to a different form of therapy, ego-oriented individual therapy (EOIT; Robin et al., 1999). BFST was expected to produce greater change than EOIT on weight, return of menstruation, eating attitudes, and family interactions. EOIT was expected to produce greater change than BFST on depression, internalizing behavior problems, ego functioning, maturity fears, and perfectionism. These predictions were based on the respective emphasis placed by the therapists on various areas of functioning. The BFST therapists directly targeted weight, eating attitudes, and family interactions, whereas the EOIT therapists emphasized strengthening ego functioning and insight into the dynamics blocking eating.

Thirty-seven Caucasian girls meeting the DSM-III-R (American Psychiatric Association, 1987) criteria for AN were randomly assigned to either BFST or EOIT and to a therapist nested within each condition. The BFST group consisted of 19 girls (mean age =

14.9) and the EOIT group consisted of 18 girls (mean age = 13.4). The two BFST and three EOIT female therapists were highly experienced in their respective approaches.

Each patient and her family participated in a preassessment, an average of 15.9 months of therapy, a postassessment, and a 12-month follow-up assessment. The length of therapy was permitted to range from 12 to 18 months, to give the therapist some flexibility. Sessions occurred weekly for the first half of therapy and bimonthly afterward.

The pediatrician selected an appropriate target weight for each patient based on age, height, and pubertal status. The dietician outlined a balanced food plan based upon the diabetic exchange model. Throughout the study, 11 BFST and 5 EOIT patients were hospitalized because of acute medical danger. These hospitalizations usually took place shortly after the preassessment, upon entry into the study. These patients spent 1–4 weeks undergoing a structured inpatient refeeding program on an adolescent medicine unit. EOIT or BFST were provided during hospitalization.

The therapist followed the protocol outlined earlier in this chapter for BFST, using a written manual to guide them. The EOIT therapist also followed a written manual, outlining a focus on ego strength, coping skills, individuation from the nuclear family, identity formation, and the relationships of these issues to weight, eating, and body image. The adolescent was seen weekly for individual sessions. The therapist took the position that AN represents a maladaptive response to family, environmental, interpersonal, and intrapersonal stresses. By identifying and achieving insight into the connection between these stressors and eating-disordered behavior, the patient was taught to strengthen her inner resources and learn more adaptive coping mechanisms. As her ego strength improved and she learned to cope effectively with adverse life circumstances, the patient could choose to eat in a healthy manner and gain weight. The therapist asked the parents to refrain from exercising any control over the adolescent's eating. The EOIT therapists met bimonthly with the patient's parents. These sessions were designed to educate the parents about normal adolescent development, provide support and understanding, help them cope with the changes occurring in their adolescents, and prepare them to live with a more assertive, self-sufficient daughter.

To demonstrate fidelity, therapy sessions were audiotaped, and a representative sample of them were coded by a doctoral-level psychologist using a checklist of 18 items covering activities unique to BFST and 9 items covering activities unique to EOIT. The BFST therapists exhibited significantly higher BFST and lower EOIT scores than did the EOIT therapists.

Dependent measures were selected to tap the return to health, eating attitudes, ego strength, depression, internalizing behavior problems, and family interactions. Analyses of mean body mass index (BMI) data revealed that from pre- to postassessment the BFST girls improved more (mean BMI change = 4.7) than the EOIT girls (mean BMI change = 2.3). At postassessment, 66.7% of the BFST girls and 68.8% of the EOIT girls attained their target weights; 94% of the BFST girls had resumed and/or started menstruating, compared to 64% of the EOIT girls. The differences in favor of BFST on menstruation were significant. At 1-year follow-up 80% of the BFST girls and 68.8% of the EOIT girls attained their target weights; 93% of the BFST and 80% of EOIT girls were menstruating, and the difference between the two therapy conditions was no longer significant. Although both therapies facilitated a return to health, BFST resulted in greater weight gain and a greater likelihood of starting/restarting menstruation at postassessment. By follow-up, the differences in favor of BFST were no longer significant.

It may seem puzzling that, at postassessment, a greater percentage of BFST than EOIT girls resumed menstruation, even though comparable percentages of girls in both conditions achieved target weight. It is possible that the greater absolute weight gain achieved by girls in the BFST condition predisposed more of them to menstruate sooner than the girls in the EOIT condition; further research is necessary to explore this hypothesis.

Table 20.1 presents the pattern of significant results on measures of eating attitudes, depression and internalizing behavior problems, and ego functioning. Eating attitudes were assessed with the EAT-26, on which the adolescents rated their own attitudes and their mothers and fathers also rated their daughters' eating attitudes. Depression was assessed through the adolescents' self reports on the Beck Depression Inventory and Youth Self-Report Internalizing Behavior Problem score, as well as the mothers' and fathers' Internalizing Behavior Problem scores on the Child Behavior Checklist. There were significant improvements on all of these measures from pre- to postassessment and from preassessment to 1-year follow-up. There were no differences between BFST and EOIT on these measures.

The Interoceptive Awareness, Ineffectiveness, Interpersonal Distrust, Maturity Fears, and Perfectionism scales of the EDI-2 served as measures of ego functioning. Higher scores are more negative than lower scores on these scales. There were no significant changes on any of these scales from pre- to postassessment and no significant differences between BFST and EOIT. However, there were significant reductions on Interoceptive Awareness and Maturity Fears from preassessment to follow-up for both therapy conditions.

Self-report and observational measures of family interaction were collected. Self-reported family interaction was assessed through the PARQ, independently completed by parents and adolescent (Robin et al., 1990). The General Conflict and Conflict over Eating scores were used.

Observations of family interaction were collected by videotaping each family conducting two 10-minute discussions: (1) a discussion of a non–food-related disagreement and (2) a discussion of the adolescent's weight and eating difficulties. Two graduate stu-

TABLE 20.1. Pattern of Significant Results

	Significant pre–post change	Significant pre–follow-up change	Significant differences between BFST and EOIT (pre–post)
EAT-26			
Teen	Yes	Yes	No
Mother	Yes	Yes	No
Father	Yes	Yes	No
Beck Depression Inventory	Yes	Yes	No
Youth Self-Report Scale	Yes	Yes	No
CBC			
Mother	Yes	Yes	No
Father	Yes	Yes	No
EDI-2			
Interoceptive Awareness	No	Yes	No
Ineffectiveness	No	No	No
Interpersonal Distrust	No	No	No
Maturity Fears	No	Yes	No
Perfectionism	No	No	No

Note. EAT-26, Eating Attitudes Test–26; CBC, Child Behavior Checklist; EDI-2, Eating Disorder Inventory–2.

dents coded the videotapes with the Interaction Behavior Code (IBC), a global inferential coding system that yields positive and negative communication scores for each family member (Robin & Foster, 1989). The IBC consists of 31 items tapping negative communication (denying responsibility, criticizing, making demands, acquiescing, name calling) and 7 items tapping positive communication (making suggestions, praising, compromising, stating what the other person said). Twenty-two of the negative and all of the positive communication items are rated dichotomously as absent or present (0,1), and nine of the negative communication items are rated on a 3-point scale as absent, a little, and a lot (0, .5, 1). The observer watches an entire videotaped discussion and then does a single rating of the adolescent, the mother, and the father on each item. The scores are summed across items to obtain negative and positive communication scores for the adolescent, the mother, and the father.

The means of the coders' summary scores were used as the dependent measures. Reliability correlations between the coders averaged .93 for adolescents' scores, .95 for mothers' scores, and .96 for fathers' scores.

BFST and EOIT adolescents and their parents reported little General Conflict at preassessment (mean T scores ranged from 46 to 57). As a result, little change occurred from pre- to postassessment or from pre- to 1-year follow-up assessment. By contrast, BFST and EOIT adolescents and their parents reported severe Conflict over Eating at preassessment (mean T scores ranged from 73 to 93). There were large and significant changes from pre- to postassessment and from pre- to follow-up assessment on Conflict over Eating for adolescents, mothers, and fathers (mean postassessment scores ranged from 51 to 58). Interestingly, there were no significant differences in improvement between BFST and EOIT on Conflict over Eating.

On the observational measures, there were significant decreases in negative and significant increases in positive communication from pre- to postassessment for adolescents, mothers, and fathers. These improvements were evident in both the non–food- and food-related discussions. As with the PARQ, there were no significant differences in improvement between the BFST and EOIT groups.

The results of this study are consistent with the hypothesis that BFST is an effective intervention for adolescents with AN. However, the study did not include a no-treatment group or a control condition in which the patients received nonspecific therapy. As a result, the positive changes cannot definitively be attributed to the active components of BFST rather than to general therapeutic variables and nonspecific factors. We carefully considered whether no-treatment or attention-placebo controls could be used but eventually rejected such control conditions as unethical and not feasible in the case of a life-threatening illness such as AN. Instead, we compared BFST to a maximally different psychotherapy, EOIT, in a comparative psychotherapy outcome design. We included a sufficient number of subjects to give a moderately strong degree of power to detect a medium effect size.

The girls enrolled in BFST made significant gains on BMI, eating attitudes, depressive affect and internalizing behavior problems, observed interaction with their parents, and self-reported conflict over eating. By 1-year follow-up four-fifths of the BFST patients had attained the target weight specified as healthy by their pediatrician and 93% were menstruating. There were no improvements at postassessment on measures of ego functioning and only two significant improvements at follow-up.

Only two of the predicted differential treatment effects were found. BFST produced faster weight gain and greater return to menstruation than EOIT by postassessment, but this difference disappeared by 1-year follow-up. Most surprising, families in EOIT that never attended a conjoint family therapy session showed comparable gains on self-report and observational measures of conflict over eating and observed communication to those of families in BFST that attended conjoint therapy sessions for an average of 16 months. Clearly, it is not always necessary to target family interaction directly to change such interaction in families with an eating-disordered adolescent. Perhaps the return to health produced by both therapies indirectly helped reduce conflict over eating and improve family functioning, regardless of whether the family was seen conjointly in the therapy sessions.

SUMMARY AND CONCLUSIONS

Starting with the premises that an effective treatment for eating disorders must take into account the developmental stage of the patient and must include the family, this chapter has outlined the application of a behavioral family systems model to the treatment of adolescents with AN. The intervention proceeds logically through four phases. First, the therapist conducts a comprehensive assessment and builds motivation for the family to participate in a family-oriented intervention. Second, the therapist places the parents in charge of the adolescent's eating and helps them work as a team to implement a behavioral weight gain program at home. Third, the therapist helps the parents successfully refeed the adolescent until she reaches a healthy weight, introducing cognitive restructuring to combat distorted beliefs. Fourth, the therapist helps the parents return control over eating to the adolescent and helps the family negotiate adolescent individuation.

A controlled investigation comparing the effectiveness of BFST to a maximally different form of individual therapy was summarized. This study provided promising evidence that both of these therapies can restore health, change eating attitudes, reduce depressive affect, and improve family relations. However, ethical constraints precluded including no-treatment or attention-placebo controls, which are necessary to demonstrate that the active components of BFST are responsible for the changes.

Future investigators need to find ways to determine whether the active ingredients of BFST are responsible for positive changes. Perhaps comparisons using attention-placebo and wait-list controls can be conducted using patients with milder forms of AN or relying on single-subject designs such as multiple baselines. Future investigators also need to explore the factors which caused 20% of the girls not to reach their target weight in the present study and strengthen the interventions to increase its success rate.

The results of this controlled trial of BFST need to be considered within the broader context of other research on family therapy for AN. Three controlled outcome studies have demonstrated the effectiveness of the Maudsley integrative family therapy, which is similar to BFST (Eisler et al., 2000; LeGrange, Eisler, Dare, & Russell, 1992; Russell, Szmukler, Dare, & Eisler, 1987). At the present time, no other form of therapy for AN has been subjected to as much empirical scrutiny as family therapy. Thus, although there are many unanswered questions, clinicians can proceed to treat adolescents with AN with either BFST or similar family interventions with reasonable confidence that they are implementing the best evidence-based psychotherapy available at the present time.

NOTE

1. The female pronoun will be used for convenience throughout the remainder of the chapter, recognizing that eating disorders occur in males and females.

REFERENCES

American Psychiatric Association. (1987). *Diagnostic and statistical manual of mental disorders* (3rd ed., rev.). Washington, DC: Author.

American Psychiatric Association. (2000). *Diagnostic and statistical manual of mental disorders* (4th ed., text rev.). Washington, DC: Author.

Eisler, I., Dare, C., Hodes, M., Russell, G., Dodge, E., & LeGrange, D. L. (2000). Family therapy for adolescent anorexia nervosa: The results of a controlled comparison of two family interventions. *Journal of Child Psychology and Psychiatry and Allied Disciplines, 41,* 727–736.

Fisher, M., Golden, N. H., Katzman, D. K., Kreipe, R. E., Rees, J., Schebendach, J., Sigman, G., Ammerman, S., & Hoberman, H. M. (1995) Eating disorders in adolescents: A background paper. *Journal of Adolescent Health, 16,* 420–437.

Garner, D. M. (1991). *Eating Disorder Inventory 2 Manual.* Odessa, FL: Psychological Assessment Resources.

Garner, D. M., Olmsted, M. D., Bohr, Y., & Garfinkel, D. E. (1982). The Eating Attitudes Test: Psychometric features and clinical correlates. *Psychological Medicine, 12,* 671–878.

Le Grange, D., Eisler, I., Dare, C., & Russell, G. F. M. (1992). Evaluation of family treatments in adolescent anorexia nervosa: A pilot study. *International Journal of Eating Disorders, 12,* 347–357.

Lock, J., LeGrange, D., Agras, W. S., & Dare, C. (2001). *Treatment manual for anorexia nervosa.* New York: Guilford Press.

Robin, A. L., & Foster, S. L. (1989). *Negotiating parent–adolescent conflict: A behavioral family systems approach.* New York: Guilford Press.

Robin, A. L., Gilroy, M., & Dennis, A. B. (1998). Treatment of eating disorders in children and adolescents. *Clinical Psychology Review, 18,* 421–446.

Robin, A. L, Koepke, T., Moye, A. (1990). Multidimensional assessment of parent–adolescent relations. *Psychological Assessment: A Journal of Consulting and Clinical Psychology, 2,* 451–459.

Robin, A. L., Siegel, P. T., Moye, A. W., Gilroy, M., Dennis, A. B., & Sikand, A. (1999). A controlled comparison of family versus individual therapy for adolescents with anorexia nervosa. *Journal of the American Academy of Child and Adolescent Psychiatry, 38,* 1428–1429.

Russell, G. F. M., Szmukler, G. I., Dare, C., & Eisler, I. (1987). A evaluation of family therapy in anorexia nervosa and bulimia nervosa. *Archives of General Psychiatry, 44,* 1047–1056.

21

Development of Evidence-Based Treatments for Pediatric Obesity

Leonard H. Epstein

OVERVIEW

Obesity is an increasingly prevalent disorder of childhood. Pediatric obesity is associated with a number of negative health outcomes including type 2 diabetes and pediatric obesity tracks, so that obese children will become obese adults. Pediatric obesity is associated with an increase in morbidity and mortality after 50-year follow-up, independent of adult weight, suggesting that pediatric obesity initiates changes in disease processes that persist even if children lose weight during development. This increase in prevalence of pediatric obesity has led to an increasing appreciation for the need for evidence-based treatments for pediatric obesity.

There have been a large number of reviews of pediatric obesity treatment, including reviews that have focused on the identification of evidence-based treatments (Jelalian & Saelens, 1999). These reviews have documented that the family-based behavioral treatment that we have developed is associated with both short- and long-term effectiveness, is associated with positive physical and mental health benefits, and has been replicated in a variety of settings. Also in association with the increasing interest in pediatric obesity, we have been asked to review our interventions and the state of pediatric obesity treatment numerous times (e.g., Epstein, Myers, Raynor, & Saelens, 1998).

The research program that has been implemented to develop the pediatric obesity treatment has included a number of randomized trials, with the results of the first trial published slightly over two decades ago in 1980 (Epstein, Wing, Steranchak, Dickson, & Michelson, 1980). These randomized trials have been supplemented by a number of laboratory investigations that have enabled us to refine our treatment methods and attempt to understand mechanisms for some treatment effects. This chapter provides an opportunity to present the logic of the progression of the studies and how decisions were made that influenced the shape of our research program on treatment of pediatric obesity.

DEVELOPMENT OF THE FAMILY-BASED APPROACH

Our first obesity studies were on the topography of eating behaviors in obese children and nonobese children at lunchtime over a 6-month period. We found the eating behaviors of obese and nonobese to differ, and we found that slowing down the bite rate reduced consumption (Epstein, Parker, McCoy, & McGee, 1976). This study was followed by an intensive evaluation of food intake in six low socioeconomic status (SES) obese black children in a Head Start center during breakfast and lunch meals. Our research group spent a lot of time thinking about the best way to teach complex nutritional ideas to young Head Start children and came upon the idea of classifying all foods according to the traffic light, a concept these children understood that signaled go, wait, and stop. Children were reinforced for eating healthily during a meal or for being active before the meal. A decrease in caloric intake was observed during either treatment, but as might be expected, changes in food selection were only observed during the eating regulation procedures (Epstein, Masek, & Marshall, 1978). This study provided an empirical basis for interventions for pediatric obesity.

The first clinical trial was conducted using the traffic-light diet in combination with an exercise program to test the importance of using behavioral treatment methods for pediatric behavior change. Table 21.1 presents the groups, *n*, percent females, duration of treatment and follow-up, and results for all randomized studies. The majority of families in all studies were white and of lower-middle to middle SES.

The study compared a nutrition education program versus nutrition education plus behavior modification for overweight children, ages 6–12, and their mothers. Both groups were provided similar information, but the behavioral group also was provided the use of behavioral therapy procedures to prompt and reinforce habit change. Results over 5 months favored the behavioral group, and there was a strong relationship observed for weight losses between children and parents in the behavioral group (Epstein et al., 1980).

Our research group now felt we were ready to conduct a larger clinical trial that capitalized on our behavioral treatment program and the potential for maximizing treatment effects by including parents as active participants in treatment. Previous research had shown the influence of parental weight on child weight (Garn & Clark, 1976), which has been confirmed in newer research (Whitaker, Wright, Pepe, Seidel, & Dietz, 1997). We randomized families to one of three groups, parent + child targeted and reinforced for weight loss, child alone targeted and reinforced for weight loss, and a no-target control group (Epstein, Wing, Koeske, Andrasik, & Ossip, 1981). This design provided the opportunity to examine the role of parental involvement in pediatric obesity treatment. The results at the end of the 21-month trial favored the parent + child group in terms of weight loss. Based on this result, we were able to secure funding on other treatment outcome grants to continue follow-up of this cohort through 5 and 10 years after randomization. We found the maintenance of long-term effects at both follow-up time points, with the parent + child group showing better maintenance than the control group and the child-alone group in between (Epstein, Valoski, Wing, & McCurley, 1990). We also demonstrated that the decrease in high-calorie, low-nutrient foods ("red" foods in the traffic-light diet) was related to treatment success.

Based on this study, we have kept the combined parent + child treatment as a constant in all further treatment programs and have extended our analysis of the influence of the family on childhood weight control in many ways. When we were designing this study we initially conceptualized the design in terms of a 2 × 2 factorial, crossing child as the targeted participant with parent as the targeted participant. Our final design used three of the

TABLE 21.1. Treatment and Follow-Up Results

Authors	Age	Groups	n	% girls	Duration (Rx/FU)	Results
Epstein, Wing, Steranchak, Dickson, & Michelson (1980)	6–12	1. Behavior modification 2. Nutrition education	14	38.5	5/0	Rx: 1 < 2
Epstein, Valoski, Wing, & McCurley (1990, 1994)	6–12	1. Mother and child targeted 2. Child targeted 3. Nonspecific target	76	69.6	8/120	Rx: 1 = 2 = 3 FU: 1 < 3
Epstein, Wing, Koeski, Ossip, & Beck (1982)	8–12	1. Aerobic activity + diet 2. Lifestyle activity + diet 3. Aerobic activity 4. Lifestyle activity	51	78.4	6/17	Rx: 1 = 2 = 3 = 4 FU: 2, 4 < 1, 3
Epstein, Valoski, Wing, & McCurley (1994); Epstein, Wing, Koeske, & Valoski (1984)	8–12	1. Exercise + diet 2. Diet 3. Control	53	NR	6/120	Rx: 1, 2 < 3 FU: 1 = 2
Epstein, Wing, Koeske, & Valoski (1985); Epstein, Valoski, Wing, & McCurley (1994)	8–12	1. Programmed aerobic activity 2. Lifestyle activity 3. Calisthenics	41	60.0	12/120	Rx: 1 = 2 = 3 FU: 1, 2 < 3
Epstein, Wing, Penner, & Kress (1985)	8–12	1. Exercise + diet 2. Diet	23	100.0	12/0	Rx: 1 < 2
Epstein, Wing, Woodall, et al. (1985)	5–8	1. Behavior modification 2. Education	19	100.0	12/0	Rx: 1 < 2
Epstein, Wing, Koeske, & Valoski (1986); Epstein, Wing, Valoski, & Gooding (1987); Epstein, Valoski, Wing, & McCurley (1994)	8–12	1. Parent overweight 2. Parent normal weight	41	NR	12/120	Rx: 2 < 1 FU: 1 = 2
Epstein, McKenzie, Valoski, Klein, & Wing (1994)	8–12	1. Mastery criteria 2. No mastery criteria (yoked)	44	74.4	12/24	Rx: 1 < 2 FU: 1 = 2
Epstein et al. (1995)	8–12	1. Increase activity 2. Reduce sedentary behavior 3. Increase activity + reduce sedentary	61	73.0	4/12	Rx: 2 < 1 FU: 2 < 1, 3
Epstein, Paluch, Gordy, Saelens, & Ernst (2000)	8–12	1. Std Rx + parent/child problem solving 2. Std Rx + child problem solving 3. Std Rx	52	51.9	6/24	Rx: 1 = 2 = 3 FU: 2, 3 < 1

TABLE 21.1. *Continued*

Authors	Age	Groups	*n*	% girls	Duration (Rx/FU)	Results
Epstein, Paluch, Gordon, & Dorn (2000)	8–12	1. Decrease sedentary behavior: Low 2. Decrease sedentary behavior: High 3. Increase physical activity: Low 4. Increase physical activity: High	76	68.4	6/24	Rx: 1 = 2 = 3 = 4
Goldfield, Epstein, Kilanowski, Paluch, & Kogut-Bossler (2001)	8–12	1. Group treatment 2. Group + individual treatment	24	70.8	6/12	Rx: 1 = 2 FU: 1 = 2
Epstein, Paluch, & Raynor (2001)	8–12	1. Increase activity 2. Increase activity + reduce sedentary behavior	56	48.2	6/12	Rx: 1 = 2 FU: M1 < F1, F2

Note. < indicates that the means for that group are significantly lower than means for other groups; Std Rx, standard treatment; NR, not reported; M, males; F, females. Adapted from Goldfield, Raynor, and Epstein (2002). Copyright 2002 by The Guilford Press. Adapted by permission.

four cells, with the missing cell being parent-alone target. At the time we did not feel that we could recruit children if we did not provide treatment for them. Evaluation of research comparing targeting of the parent versus targeting of the child was not accomplished until a 1998 study by Golan, Weizman, Apter, and Fainaru, which demonstrated that targeting the parent provided better effects than targeting the child alone, though they did not include a parent + child group, which theoretically may be the most powerful intervention.

One of the general characteristics of our family-based treatment was to provide treatment for the obese parent. This meant that we would only include families in which there was both an obese child and an obese parent. Parental obesity is one of the main risk factors for the development of pediatric obesity (Whitaker et al., 1997), and it is possible that parent weight may exert an effect on short- or long-term treatment outcome. To evaluate this possibility, we randomized families with obese children and nonobese parents to groups that varied in child self-management or parental control. This factorial design also provided information on whether children responded differently on the basis of their training in self-management and whether the differences interacted with parent weight status. While there were no differential effects of child self-management or parent management, parent weight was related to weight control. Obese children of one or more obese parents were significantly more overweight than obese children of nonobese parents 5 years after beginning a family-based behavioral weight control program, due in part to differential rates of maintenance after the 6-month treatment was completed (Epstein, Wing, Koeske, & Valoski, 1986; Epstein, Wing, Valoski, & Gooding, 1987).

FOCUSING ON PHYSICAL ACTIVITY

After the success in studying the role of parents in childhood weight control, we then began a series of studies on the best way to implement physical activity in pediatric weight control. This interest came in part based on research on the difficulties of getting sedentary people to adopt an exercise program, on ideas presented by Kelly Brownell on incorporating activity into one's lifestyle, and on my own interest in activity cultivated by my exercise program. The primary function of increasing activity for weight loss is to burn calories, and we burn the same number of calories per mile whether we walk or run. Of course, we can do more miles if we run rather than walk, but from the perspective of caloric expenditure, it does not matter. An individual gets about the same expenditure from walking or running a mile. Part of the reason for the difficulty in being active is making time for a continuous bout of activity, while another part is the difficulty in getting to an exercise site. We developed a lifestyle activity program in which children and their parents earned points for calorie expenditure, but they had maximal flexibility in choosing activities and in the activity intensity. This program was compared to a highly structured aerobic exercise program. In addition, we crossed the activity with diet or no diet. The exercise programs differed in the flexibility of scheduling, type of exercise, and intensity. Lifestyle was associated with better long-term weight control effects, and better maintenance of fitness (Epstein, Wing, Koeske, Ossip, & Beck, 1982). Surprisingly, there were no effects of diet or no diet. We attributed the failure to find differences to the fact that all groups had the same education on the traffic-light diet. Though it differed in what behaviors were targeted and reinforced, the education may have been sufficient to get motivated participants to make dietary changes.

We followed this study with a second comparison of lifestyle exercise versus aerobic exercise, but in this study we added a low-expenditure calisthenics control group. Many of the exercise studies done at that time compared a complete exercise program with a no-treatment control, and we felt the need to provide a control group that controlled for time and expectations for those in active treatment. The control subjects self-monitored their exercise behavior, were praised for improvement, and increased goals (e.g., more toe touches) as they got better at doing calisthenics. Results show similar and significant weight changes across the exercise conditions during the year of treatment. However, during the follow-up, subjects in the lifestyle group showed better maintenance than those in the calisthenics group, with the aerobic group in between. At 10 years, both exercise groups were superior to the control group (Epstein, Valoski, Wing, & McCurley, 1994; Epstein, Wing, Koeske, & Valoski, 1985).

However, we remained perplexed about the similarity of exercise alone and diet plus exercise in the first study on lifestyle exercise (Epstein et al., 1982). We conducted two new studies to try to better understand whether the combination is better than either alone. In the first study, we compared diet versus diet plus exercise in a sample of obese children and found no differences in short- or long-term weight control for the children group (Epstein, Valoski, et al., 1994; Epstein, Wing, Koeske, & Valoski, 1984). In this study we provided equal education to both groups, so that both groups were informed about the importance of exercise, even though only one group was targeted and reinforced for being more active. To provide the best information on whether exercise adds to weight control, we developed a summer camp that allowed us to exercise with the children, removing the possibility of differences in adherence influencing outcome. The children who were provided supervised exercise, up to 3 miles of walking per day, showed larger decreases in percent overweight over the year of study than children in the diet-alone group. A significant improvement in fitness was observed only for children in the diet-plus-exercise group (Epstein, Wing, Penner, & Kress, 1985).

GENERALIZING TO YOUNGER CHILDREN
AND REFINING TREATMENT

We also have extended the treatment initially designed for 8- to 12-year-old children to 5- to 8-year-old children (Epstein, Wing, Woodall, 1985) and 2- to 5-year-old children (Epstein, Valoski, Koeske, & Wing, 1986). We did not continue our efforts to develop more interventions for younger children for two reasons. First, it was hard to recruit children this young. Both parents and pediatricians have the idea that children will outgrow their obesity, and parents are encouraged to wait and see. Second, in these studies we found maintenance to be challenging, as the children are rapidly moving through developmental stages, and it was hard to match the program to their stages. With the great increase in pediatric obesity, the development of programs for younger children is worth another look.

At this point in our research program, we decided to evaluate a teaching technique designed to enhance learning. In our first treatment studies our treatment manuals were designed around the concept of mastery, or personalized instruction. Research on personalized instruction has shown better knowledge acquisition and maintenance than with standard lecture formats, but this technology had never been tested for behavior change. It makes sense that the same principles might apply for behavior change, because effective behavior change for eating or activity may depend on sequential skill acquisition. We tested the hypothesis that families required to master behavioral changes may produce better outcomes than the same intervention without mastery. As predicted, results indicated that children in the mastery group had significantly better treatment outcomes than did children in the nonmastery group at 12 months, but these differences were no longer significant at 24 months (Epstein, McKenzie, Valoski, Klein, & Wing, 1994).

USING WHAT I HAVE LEARNED FROM BASIC SCIENCE

While I was engaged in a systematic research program on obesity treatment, my laboratory also was working on basic research on eating behavior and behavioral pharmacology of smoking. The eating research focused primarily on understanding the role of habituation on changes in responses to repeated sensory stimulation that occurs during eating. The idea of applying habituation theory was based on research in which I was involved with rats on using habituation theory as a way to understand the development of tolerance to nicotine (Caggiula et al., 1998). We completed a series of studies on habituation in eating along with theoretical conceptualization of how habituation may be involved in understanding the effects of increased variety on intake (Raynor & Epstein, 2001).

Along with basic research on habituation in animals and humans, I became interested in new research on behavioral choice theory or behavioral economics that was beginning in behavioral pharmacology. Behavioral choice theory attempts to understand how people make decisions about allocating their time among alternatives, based in part on the relative reinforcing value of the alternatives and access to them. We started to assess the relative reinforcing value of smoking versus other commodities (Epstein, Bulik, Perkins, Caggiula, & Rodefer, 1991) and then to apply this methodology to food (Lappalainen & Epstein, 1990) and physical activity (Epstein, Smith, Vara, & Rodefer, 1991). At the same time that we were doing this research, I became interested in research on television and obesity (Dietz & Gortmaker, 1985). Dietz and Gortmaker showed that television watching was a powerful risk factor for developing obesity, which could be related to increased eating in front of the television or the suppression of activity when watching television. It made sense that one of the reasons for the difficulty in increasing physical activity in obese youth is the competition between sedentary behaviors and physical activity. If obese children find sedentary behaviors to be reinforcing, it may be difficult to get them to choose to be active rather than maintain their sedentary behaviors. This idea led to the hypothesis that decreasing sedentary behaviors may be useful in increasing physical activity in obese youth.

We initiated a series of laboratory studies to determine parameters that influence the role of decreasing sedentary behaviors on physical activity. These studies have demonstrated that obese children find sedentary behaviors more reinforcing than nonobese youth, that nonobese young adults will choose to be active if physical activities are more accessible than sedentary behaviors, that reducing access to sedentary behaviors results in an increase in physical activity, that reinforcing a reduction in sedentary behavior is more effective than removing access to the sedentary behavior, that liking or preference for an activity does not always predict what activities a person will choose when provided the choice between active and sedentary alternatives, and that a greater variety of activity choices is more reinforcing than having only one activity available (Epstein & Roemmich, 2001).

Another part of the hypothesis that obese children find sedentary behaviors to be reinforcing is that one might be able to use sedentary behaviors to reinforce children for being more physically active. Based on a methodology we developed to interface an exercise bicycle with reinforcing sedentary behaviors such as watching a VCR or playing computer games, we showed that sedentary behaviors could be used to increase physical activity in the laboratory (Saelens & Epstein, 1998) and in the homes of obese children (Faith et al., 2001). We also showed that how often children engaged in a sedentary behavior predicted the reinforcing value (Saelens & Epstein, 1999). Finally, we showed that a system based on earning points for pedometer counts could serve as the basis for earning access to sedentary behaviors to increase physical activity, an example of a flexible, open-loop feedback system (Goldfield, Kalakanis, Ernst, & Epstein, 2000).

Hypotheses about the relationship between sedentary and physical activities were tested in two clinical outcome studies. In the first study (Epstein et al., 1995) obese youth were reinforced for being more active, for being less sedentary, or for the combination of the two. The children reinforced for reducing sedentary behavior showed a significantly greater decrease in percent overweight compared with the children reinforced for increased activity, with the combined group in between. At 12-month follow-up, the group reinforced for less sedentary behavior maintained its weight loss, whereas the combined group had gained weight and become equivalent to the group reinforced for activity. Children reinforced for reducing sedentary activity increased their preference for vigorous physical activity more than children reinforced for increasing physical activity, though both groups showed similar improvements in fitness. Improvements in weight control were due to increases in physical activity and decreases in energy intake study (Epstein et al., 1995) when targeted sedentary behaviors were reduced.

The second study replicated the basic comparison of reinforcing children for being more active or less sedentary, with the addition of testing for a dose–response effect (Epstein, Paluch, Gordy, & Dorn, 2000). Results indicate that children reinforced for reductions in sedentary activity showed similar reductions in percent overweight compared to children reinforced for increased physical activity, and the effects of dose and dose by group interaction were not statistically significant. Children allocated approximately one-third of the time freed up from targeted sedentary behaviors for physical activity and two-thirds for other sedentary behaviors (Epstein, Paluch, Gordy, & Dorn, 2000). We have recently found sex differences in response to reducing sedentary behaviors, with boys showing an enhanced response to the combination of reinforcing an increase in physical activity with a decrease in sedentary behaviors, whereas girls showed a decreased response to the combination compared to reinforcing increases in physical activity alone (Epstein, Paluch, & Raynor, 2001).

We have completed two studies designed to improve implementation of our treatment program. The first of these studies was designed to determine whether adding training in problem solving would improve the treatment for childhood obesity. Problem solving could be useful for identifying and solving potential situations that threaten adherence to diet and exercise protocols. Other investigators (Graves, Meyers, & Clark, 1988) had found that families receiving problem solving, a component of many behavioral treatments, had significantly better outcomes at 8-month follow-up than families not provided training in problem solving. We (Epstein, Paluch, Gordy, Saelens, & Ernst, 2000) randomized families to groups that received (1) our standard family-based behavioral weight-control program plus parent and child problem solving, (2) child problem solving, or (3) standard treatment with no additional problem solving. The standard group showed better weight control than the parent + child group through 2 years. We speculated that our standard treatment includes some problem solving, and the addition of more problem solving may have reduced time spent on other behavioral skills that were more important to weight control (Epstein, Paluch, Gordy, Saelens, & Ernst, 2000).

Our usual intervention includes both individual attention for each family as well as group treatment. We completed a study to evaluate whether we could improve the efficacy and cost-effectiveness of our standard treatment program if the intervention was delivered in a group. Results over 1 year showed no differences in percent overweight change for either the parent or child in the group versus group plus individual treatment, but the group treatment was more cost-effective in terms of changes in percent overweight per dollar spent in treatment delivery (Goldfield, Epstein, Kilanowski, Paluch, & Kogut-Bossler, 2001).

PSYCHOLOGICAL CHANGES THAT ACCOMPANY CHILDHOOD WEIGHT CONTROL

We have performed a number of secondary analyses in the process of completing our treatment studies. One set of analyses was designed to better understand how childhood obesity influences child behavior problems. There has been much theorizing about the role of child obesity causing pediatric behavior problems, but based on our interest in families, we were aware that parental psychopathology also could be a cause of pediatric psychopathology. We measured child and parent psychopathology in two studies that showed that both childhood obesity and parental psychopathology improved after treatment, and that parental psychopathology was a better predictor of child psychopathology than child obesity (Epstein, Klein, & Wisniewski, 1994; Epstein, Myers, & Anderson, 1996). When we studied the relationship between changes in pediatric obesity and parent psychopathology, we found that improved parental psychopathology was related to a different set of improvements in child psychological functioning than child obesity, showing the multidimensional nature of psychosocial functioning in obese children and multiple avenues for intervention to improve their psychosocial functioning (Epstein et al., 1996).

There is also considerable interest in the role that obesity treatment may play in eating disorders, as dieting is a risk factor for the development of eating disorders. We found decreases in psychological problems and improvements in behavioral competence for children and a reduction in distress, disturbed eating, and weight-related cognitions in parents after treatment. No significant changes were observed in eating disorder symptoms (Epstein, Paluch, Saelens, Ernst, & Wilfley, 2001).

GENERALIZABILITY OF TREATMENT PROCEDURES

Though we have shown a consistent pattern of results across our intervention studies, it is necessary to ensure that other laboratories can replicate these results. There are three main intervention methodologies that we have developed in our laboratories that have been tested in other laboratories, the traffic-light diet, lifestyle activity programs, and reducing sedentary behavior.

The Traffic-Light Diet

Our research team and others have done a lot of research using the traffic-light diet for preschool (Epstein, Valoski, et al., 1986) and preadolescent children (Epstein et al., 1998). The traffic-light diet is a structured eating plan used to meet age recommendations of the basic four food groups, and now the Food Guide Pyramid, to increase the nutrient density of the diet. The traffic-light diet groups foods into categories based on nutrient density. The current version classifies groups based on dietary fat: green foods (go) are foods with 0–1 grams of fat per serving; yellow foods (caution) contain 2–5 grams of fat per serving; and red foods (stop) consist of more than 5 grams of fat per serving or high simple carbohydrate content (e.g., candy).

The traffic-light diet when used as part of a comprehensive pediatric treatment is associated with significant decreases in obesity along with improvement in nutrient density (Valoski & Epstein, 1990) and eating patterns (Epstein et al., 1981) in preadolescent children. Reductions in low-nutrient-dense "red foods" have also been observed after treatment (Epstein et al., 1981), with greater weight losses for those who had larger decreases in intake of red foods (Epstein et al., 1981). Finally, use of the traffic-light diet resulted in decreased liking for high-fat/low-sugar, high-sugar/low-fat, and high-fat/high-sugar foods and a greater increase in rated palatability for low-fat/low-sugar foods for obese children receiving treatment than a group of nontreated nonobese children (Epstein et al., 1989).

Lifestyle Activity

We initiated research in lifestyle activity in the early 1980s to facilitate children getting enough physical activity. The focus in most exercise research at the time was on highly structured aerobic exercise, but in the 1990s it became clearer to many investigators that most people were not going to meet the guidelines for aerobic exercise, and alternatives were needed. In addition, investigators realized that the major benefits for becoming active were for sedentary people, who could benefit from small changes in physical activity (Haskell, 1994), and investigators had begun to show fitness and health benefits from breaking down one long activity bout into several smaller bouts (DeBusk, Stenestrand,

Sheehan, & Haskell, 1990). The Centers for Disease Control and the American Society for Sports Medicine responded with new recommendations for physical activity, increasing the flexibility of types of activity and activity intensity and breaking down activity into smaller units (Pate et al., 1995). Several studies have tested versions of lifestyle activity in sedentary adults (Dunn et al., 1999) and obese adults (Andersen et al., 1999) with success compared to more structured methods. Though there are some differences in how lifestyle exercise interventions are defined across programs, this research has the potential to significantly change interventions for physical activity.

Reducing Sedentary Behavior

Based on research showing that TV watching was related to obesity, we developed intervention methods to reduce sedentary behaviors. Other investigators are beginning to test similar methods for prevention, rather than treatment, of pediatric obesity (Gortmaker et al., 1999; Robinson, 1999). The trial by Robinson (Robinson, 1999) is one of most successful trials in obesity prevention to date, and the primary behavior targeted in that study was reducing television watching. The method awaits generalization to adults.

DIRECTIONS FOR FUTURE RESEARCH

New Directions in our Research Program

Developing New and Innovative Treatments

One direction for our research program is to continue research in the development of more effective treatments. We are in the process of implementing new research on increasing the reinforcing value of alternatives to eating and are planning new studies to teach children to engage in alternatives to eating. We would like to extend our eating research to take advantage of the effects of reducing variety on intake, and we have completed laboratory research that suggests that stress may increase eating in children who are restrained eaters, and stress may shift children from choosing to be active to being sedentary. If stress is a major influence on eating and sedentary behaviors in youth, then intervention programs to reduce stress or better cope with stress may have a place as tools in obesity treatment. These studies continue the tradition of using laboratory studies to inform our clinical research.

Treating and Preventing Diabetes

A second direction for our research program is to begin to treat and prevent type 2 diabetes in youth. The epidemic of obesity in youth has led to drastic increases in hyperinsulimia and type 2 diabetes (Sinha et al., 2002). Reducing body weight will reduce insulin resistance and prevent diabetes in those at risk for diabetes and improve glycemic control in those with diabetes. The generalization of our treatment of obese children without diabetes to those at risk due to insulin resistance or to those with diabetes may provide some unique challenges. Many of these children will be minority children and will be adolescents. We will have to modify our current treatment to accommodate these changes in subject characteristics.

In addition, there may be challenges in recruiting enough hyperinsulinimic children or children with diabetes for groups, which may necessitate treating these children individually. That will reduce much of the cost–benefit of group treatment and may influence treatment efficacy. There is little research on group versus individual treatment in adults (Hayaki & Brownell, 1996), and none to our knowledge in youth. Treatment effects could be improved by providing more individualized treatment, but treatment effects may be reduced by not having the group to provide some accountability for behavioral change and group process in problem solving.

New Directions in Pediatric Obesity Treatment

As interest in pediatric obesity has been increasing, new approaches to obesity treatment are being developed. One of the least studied components of pediatric obesity treatment is the methods for improving eating control. Two new approaches to eating control are being evaluated. Ludwig et al. (1999) have demonstrated that low glycemic index diets can help reduce caloric intake, and he is in the process of evaluating low glycemic index diets, controlling for caloric intake, on pediatric obesity. In a different approach to eating regulation, Susan Johnson has shown that children differ in their ability to respond to regulate intake in relation to preloads (Johnson & Birch, 1994), and that children can be trained to self-regulate energy intake (Johnson, 2000). This research has the potential to teach children to adjust intake in relationship to previous eating, which could have a powerful influence on total caloric intake.

There is an increasing interest in alternatives to traditional, structured exercise programs based on the positive effects shown for lifestyle exercise (Andersen et al., 1999; Dunn et al., 1999; Epstein et al., 1982; Epstein, Wing, Koeske, & Valoski, 1985) and reducing sedentary behaviors (Epstein, Saelens, Myers, & Vito, 1997; Epstein et al., 1995; Gortmaker et al., 1999; Robinson, 1999). However, there are many benefits to structured exercise programs, and new approaches to achieving aerobic fitness (Gutin & Cucuzzo, 1995; Gutin, Cucuzzo, Islam, Smith, & Stachura, 1996) and resistance training (Treuth, Hunter, Pichon, Figueroa-Colon, & Goran, 1998) may lead to new ways to increase physical activity in obese youth.

The typical obesity treatment program focuses on the child, but new research has suggested that targeting only the parent is superior to targeting only the child (Golan et al., 1998). Research designed to understand the benefits of treating the parent and child is important, and the role of parent and child will change as a function of child age and development (Epstein, Wing, & Valoski, 1985).

New approaches to pharmacological intervention for child and adult obesity represent a major focus of research, and it is likely that new drugs will be available that affect eating, activity, or metabolic processes that can influence weight loss in youth. Behavioral researchers will need to understand the best way to combine behavioral and pharmacological interventions to maximize the effectiveness of both intervention approaches (Epstein, Roemmich, & Raynor, 2001).

SUMMARY AND CONCLUSIONS

Family-based behavioral treatment for pediatric obesity is a treatment approach designed to help obese children change their eating and physical activity behaviors by combining eating and activity and behavior change components in the context of a family-based treatment. The program has been extensively tested and replicated over 20 years, with research evaluating treatment effects over both short and long follow-up periods ranging up to 10 years after randomization. The family-based model has been used across multiple age groups and has served as the platform for investigations to improve treatment efficacy studying variables ranging from parent weight to the role of lifestyle activity and the role of group + individual versus group-alone interventions. Investigators have replicated the effects of the dietary and activity interventions in treatment and prevention programs.

The effects of the family-based behavioral intervention extend beyond changes in eating, exercise, and body weight to psychological factors. Research suggests that degree of psychological problems in the obese children is a function of both child weight and parental psychological problems, and treatment results in improvements in child psychological problems and behavioral competence and reduction in parent psychological problems and distress with treatment. The combination of improvements in weight, weight-related physiological outcomes such as glycemic control, and improvements in behavioral competence and reductions in psychological problems represents outcomes that can lead to improved physical and mental health in obese youth provided behavioral family-based treatments. Research continues to fine-tune the interventions and make them more user-friendly and applicable to larger numbers of families with obese children, and to extend the treatment to obese children with comorbid medical conditions.

ACKNOWLEDGMENTS

The research reported in this chapter is based on over 20 years of research and has benefited from the help of many postdoctoral, graduate, and undergraduate students. I have learned a lot about the research process in over two decades, but the learning curve is steepest in the beginning. That is when I benefited the most from my collaborations, and the collaborator who was most helpful as I learned to do clinical research was Rena Wing. Rena was a marvelous collaborator, and has remained a productive independent researcher. Tony Caggiula taught me to think (and, I hope, write) like a basic researcher, and Ken Perkins opened my eyes to new areas in behavioral pharmacology that served as the basis for much of our research on behavioral economics. The research reported in the chapter was supported by a series of grants awarded to me by the National Institutes of Child Health and Human Development and the National Institute for Diabetes and Digestive and Kidney Diseases. National Institutes of Health Grants HD 39792 and HD 39778 supported the preparation of this chapter.

REFERENCES

Andersen, R. E., Wadden, T. A., Bartlett, S. J., Zemel, B., Verde, T. J., & Franckowiak, S. C. (1999). Effects of lifestyle activity vs. structured aerobic exercise in obese women: A randomized trial. *Journal of the American Medical Association, 281,* 335–340.

Caggiula, A. R., Donny, E. C., Epstein, L. H., Sved, A. F., Knopf, S., Rose, C., McAllister, C. G., Antelman, S. M., & Perkins, K. A. (1998). The role of corticosteroids in nicotine's physiological and behavioral effects. *Psychoneuroendocrinology, 23,* 143–159.

DeBusk, R. F., Stenestrand, U., Sheehan, M., & Haskell, W. L. (1990). Training effects of long versus short bouts of exercise in healthy subjects. *American Journal of Cardiology, 65,* 1010–1013.

Dietz, W. H., & Gortmaker, S. L. (1985). Do we fatten our children at the television set? Obesity and television viewing in children and adolescents. *Pediatrics, 75,* 807–812.

Dunn, A. L., Marcus, B. H., Kampert, J. B., Garcia, M. E., Kohl, H. W., & Blair, S. N. (1999). Comparison of lifestyle and structured interventions to increase physical activity and cardiorespiratory fitness: A randomized trial. *Journal of the American Medical Association, 281,* 327–334.

Epstein, L. H., Bulik, C. M., Perkins, K. A., Caggiula, A. R., & Rodefer, J. (1991). Behavioral economic analysis of smoking: Money and food as alternatives. *Pharmacology, Biochemistry and Behavior, 38,* 715–721.

Epstein, L. H., Klein, K. R., & Wisniewski, L. (1994). Child and parent factors that influence psychological problems in obese children. *International Journal of Eating Disorders, 15,* 151–158.

Epstein, L. H., Masek, B. J., & Marshall, W. R. (1978). A nutritionally based school program for control of eating in obese children. *Behavior Therapy, 9,* 766–788.

Epstein, L. H., McKenzie, S. J., Valoski, A., Klein, K. R., & Wing, R. R. (1994). Effects of mastery criteria and contingent reinforcement for family-based child weight control. *Addictive Behaviors, 19,* 135–145.

Epstein, L. H., Myers, M. D., & Anderson, K. (1996). The association of maternal psychopathology and family socioeconomic status with psychological problems in obese children. *Obesity Research, 4,* 65–74.

Epstein, L. H., Myers, M. D., Raynor, H. A., & Saelens, B. E. (1998). Treatment of pediatric obesity. *Pediatrics, 101,* 554–570.

Epstein, L. H., Paluch, R. A., Gordy, C. C., & Dorn, J. (2000). Decreasing sedentary behaviors in treating pediatric obesity. *Archives of Pediatrics and Adolescent Medicine, 154,* 220–226.

Epstein, L. H., Paluch, R. A., Gordy, C. C., Saelens, B. E., & Ernst, M. M. (2000). Problem solving in the treatment of childhood obesity. *Journal of Consulting and Clinical Psychology, 68,* 717–721.

Epstein, L. H., Paluch, R. A., & Raynor, H. A. (2001). Sex differences in obese children and siblings for family-based obesity treatment. *Obesity Research, 9,* 746–753.

Epstein, L. H., Paluch, R. A., Saelens, B. E., Ernst, M. M., & Wilfley, D. E. (2001). Changes in eating disorder symptoms with pediatric obesity treatment. *Journal of* Pediatrics, 139, 58–65.

Epstein, L. H., Parker, L., McCoy, J. F., & McGee, G. (1976). Descriptive analysis of eating regulation in obese and non-obese children. *Journal of Applied Behavior Analysis, 9,* 407–415.

Epstein, L. H., & Roemmich, J. N. (2001). Reducing sedentary behavior: Role in modifying physical activity. *Exercise and Sport Science Reviews, 29,* 103–108.

Epstein, L. H., Roemmich, J. N., & Raynor, H. A. (2001). Behavioral therapy in the treatment of pediatric obesity. In D. Styne (Ed.), *Pediatric clinics of North America* (pp. 981–993). Philadelphia: Saunders.

Epstein, L. H., Saelens, B. E., Myers, M. D., & Vito, D. (1997). Effects of decreasing sedentary behaviors on activity choice in obese children. *Health Psychology, 16,* 107–113.

Epstein, L. H., Smith, J. A., Vara, L. S., & Rodefer, J. S. (1991). Behavioral economic analysis of activity choice in obese children. *Health Psychology, 10,* 311–316.

Epstein, L. H., Valoski, A., Koeske, R., & Wing, R. R. (1986). Family-based behavioral weight control in obese young children. *Journal of the American Dietetic Association, 86,* 481–484.

Epstein, L. H., Valoski, A. M., Vara, L. S., McCurley, J., Wisniewski, L., Kalarchian, M. A., Klein, K. R., & Shrager, L. R. (1995). Effects of decreasing sedentary behavior and increasing activity on weight change in obese children. *Health Psychology, 14,* 109–115.

Epstein, L. H., Valoski, A., Wing, R. R., & McCurley, J. (1990). Ten-year follow-up of behavioral family-based treatment for obese children. *Journal of the American Medical Association, 264,* 2519–2523.

Epstein, L. H., Valoski, A., Wing, R. R., Perkins, K. A., Fernstrom, M., Marks, B., & McCurley, J. (1989). Perception of eating and exercise in children as a function of child and parent weight. *Appetite, 12,* 105–118.

Epstein, L. H., Valoski, A. M., Wing, R. R., & McCurley, J. (1994). Ten year outcomes of behavioral family-based treatment for childhood obesity. *Health Psychology, 13,* 373–383.

Epstein, L. H., Wing, R. R., Koeske, R., Andrasik, F., & Ossip, D. J. (1981). Child and parent weight loss in family-based behavior modification programs. *Journal of Consulting and Clinical Psychology, 49,* 674–685.

Epstein, L. H., Wing, R. R., Koeske, R., Ossip, D. J., & Beck, S. (1982). A comparison of lifestyle change and programmed aerobic exercise on weight and fitness changes in obese children. *Behavior Therapy, 13,* 651–665.

Epstein, L. H., Wing, R. R., Koeske, R., & Valoski, A. (1984). Effects of diet plus exercise on weight change in parents and children. *Journal of Consulting and Clinical Psychology, 52,* 429–437.

Epstein, L. H., Wing, R. R., Koeske, R., & Valoski, A. (1985). A comparison of lifestyle exercise, aerobic exercise and calisthenics on weight loss in obese children. *Behavior Therapy, 16,* 345–356.

Epstein, L. H., Wing, R. R., Koeske, R., & Valoski, A. (1986). Effect of parent weight on weight loss in obese children. *Journal of Consulting and Clinical Psychology, 54,* 400–401.

Epstein, L. H., Wing, R. R., Penner, B. C., & Kress, M. J. (1985). Effect of diet and controlled exercise on weight loss in obese children. *Journal of Pediatrics, 107,* 358–361.

Epstein, L. H., Wing, R. R., Steranchak, L., Dickson, B., & Michelson, J. (1980). Comparison of family based behavior modification and nutrition education for childhood obesity. *Journal of Pediatric Psychology, 5,* 25–36.

Epstein, L. H., Wing, R. R., & Valoski, A. (1985). Childhood obesity. *Pediatric Clinics of North America, 32,* 363–379.

Epstein, L. H., Wing, R. R., Valoski, A., & Gooding, W. (1987). Long-term effects of parent weight on child weight loss. *Behavior Therapy, 18,* 219–226.

Epstein, L. H., Wing, R. R., Woodall, K., Penner, B. C., Kress, M. J., & Koeske, R. (1985). Effects of family-based behavioral treatment on obese 5–8-year-old children. *Behavior Therapy, 16,* 205–212.

Faith, M. S., Berman, N., Heo, M., Pietrobelli, A., Gallagher, D., Epstein, L. H., Eiden, M. T., & Allison, D. B. (2001). Effects of contingent television on physical activity and television viewing in obese children. *Pediatrics, 107,* 1043–1048.

Garn, S. M., & Clark, D. C. (1976). Trends in fatness and the origins of obesity. *Pediatrics, 57,* 443–456.

Golan, M., Weizman, A., Apter, A., & Fainaru, M. (1998). Parents as exclusive agents of change in the treatment of childhood obesity. *American Journal of Clinical Nutrition, 67,* 1130–1135.

Goldfield, G. S., Epstein, L. H., Kilanowski, C. K., Paluch, R. A., & Kogut-Bossler, B. (2001). Cost effectiveness of group and mixed family-based treatment for childhood obesity. *International Journal of Obesity, 25,* 1843–1849.

Goldfield, G. S., Kalakanis, L. E., Ernst, M. M., & Epstein, L. H. (2000). Open-loop feedback to increase physical activity in obese children. *International Journal of Obesity and Related Metabolic Disorders, 24,* 888–892.

Goldfield, G. S., Raynor, H. A., & Epstein, L. H. (2002). Treatment of pediatric obesity. In T. A. Wadden & A. J. Stunkard (Eds.), *Handbook of obesity treatment* (pp. 532–555). New York: Guilford Press.

Gortmaker, S. L., Peterson, K., Wiecha, J., Sobol, A. M., Dixit, S., Fox, M. K., & Laird, N. (1999). Reducing obesity via a school-based interdisciplinary intervention among youth: Planet Health. *Archives of Pediatrics and Adolescent Medicine, 153,* 409–418.

Graves, T., Meyers, A. W., & Clark, L. (1988). An evaluation of problem-solving training in the behavioral treatment of childhood obesity. *Journal of Consulting and Clinical Psychology, 56,* 246–250.

Gutin, B., & Cucuzzo, N. (1995). Physical training improves body composition of black obese 7-to 11-year-old girls. *Obesity Research, 3,* 305–312.

Gutin, B., Cucuzzo, N., Islam, S., Smith, C., & Stachura, M. E. (1996). Physical training, lifestyle education, and coronary risk factors in obese girls. *Medicine and Science in Sports and Exercise, 28,* 19–23.

Haskell, W. L. (1994). Health consequences of physical activity: Understanding and challenges regarding dose–response. *Medicine and Science in Sports and Exercise, 26,* 649–660.

Hayaki, J., & Brownell, K. D. (1996). Behaviour change in practice: Group approaches. *International Journal of Obesity and Related Metabolic Disorders, 20*(Suppl. 1), S27–S30.

Jelalian, E., & Saelens, B. E. (1999). Empirically supported treatments in pediatric psychology: Pediatric obesity. *Journal of Pediatric Psychology, 24,* 223–248.

Johnson, S. L. (2000). Improving preschoolers' self-regulation of energy intake. *Pediatrics, 106*(6), 1429–1435.

Johnson, S. L., & Birch, L. L. (1994). Parents' and children's adiposity and eating style. *Pediatrics, 94,* 653–661.

Lappalainen, R., & Epstein, L. H. (1990). A behavioral economics analysis of food choice in humans. *Appetite, 14,* 81–93.

Ludwig, D. S., Majzoub, J. A., Al-Zahrani, A., Dallal, G. E., Blanco, I., & Roberts, S. B. (1999). High glycemic index foods, overeating, and obesity. *Pediatrics, 103,* E26.

Pate, R. R., Pratt, M., Blair, S. N., Haskell, W. L., Macera, C. A., Bouchard, C., Buchner, D., Ettinger, W., Heath, G. W., King, A. C., Kriska, A., Leon, A. S., Marcus, B. H., Morris, J., Paffenbarger, R. S., Patrick, K., Pollock, M. L., Rippe, J. M., Sallis, J. F., & Wilmore, J. H. (1995). Physical activity and public health: A recommendation from the Centers for Disease Control and Prevention and the American College of Sports Medicine. *Journal of the American Medical Association, 273,* 402–407.

Raynor, H. A., & Epstein, L. H. (2001). Dietary variety, energy regulation and obesity. *Psychological Bulletin, 127,* 325–341.

Robinson, T. N. (1999). Reducing children's television viewing to prevent obesity: A randomized controlled trial. *Journal of the American Medical Association, 282,* 1561–1567.

Saelens, B. E., & Epstein, L. H. (1998). Behavioral engineering of activity choice in obese children. *International Journal of Obesity, 22,* 275–277.

Saelens, B. E., & Epstein, L. H. (1999). The rate of sedentary activities determines the reinforcing value of physical activity. *Health Psychology, 18,* 655–659.

Sinha, R., Fisch, G., Teague, B., Tamborlane, W. V., Banyas, B., Allen, K., Savoye, M., Rieger, V., Taksali, S., Barbetta, G., Sherwin, R. S., & Caprio, S. (2002). Prevalence of impaired glucose tolerance among children and adolescents with marked obesity. *New England Journal of Medicine, 346,* 802–810.

Treuth, M. S., Hunter, G. R., Pichon, C., Figueroa-Colon, R., & Goran, M. I. (1998). Fitness and energy expenditure after strength training in obese prepubertal girls. *Medicine and Science in Sports and Exercise, 30,* 1130–1136.

Valoski, A., & Epstein, L. H. (1990). Nutrient intake of obese children in a family-based behavioral weight control program. *International Journal of Obesity, 14,* 667–677.

Whitaker, R. C., Wright, J. A., Pepe, M. S., Seidel, K. D., & Dietz, W. H. (1997). Predicting obesity in young adulthood from childhood and parental obesity. *New England Journal of Medicine, 337,* 869–873.

22

Behavioral Treatment for Enuresis

Arthur C. Houts

OVERVIEW

Based on principles of learning and conditioning, urine alarm treatment for simple bedwetting is one of the oldest triumphs of modern behavior therapy. Urine alarm treatment is by far the most effective current treatment and costs considerably less than alternative medication treatments (Houts, 2000; Houts, Berman, & Abramson, 1994; Mikkelsen, 2001). This chapter reviews over 20 years of work to improve this basic behavior therapy and to make it more widely available. We also discuss factors that have impeded the dissemination of this treatment. Our approach is called full-spectrum home training (FSHT). Psychologists should collaborate with pediatricians and family doctors to offer this treatment.

Monosymptomatic Primary Enuresis

Bedwetting is a problem for 1 out of every 10 secondary school-age children. The prevalence at 6 years old is about 15% and declines to about 1% among 18-year-olds. Only 15 of every 100 can be expected to "outgrow" the problem in a year. Many will have to deal with the interference for years. Continued bedwetting leads to restricted social activities, embarrassment about a family secret, and possibly diminished confidence and interpersonal comfort. Given that a 4-month course of urine alarm treatment can permanently fix the problem in about 75% of these children, this treatment should be pursued once a child is 6 years old and poised for important emotional and social developmental milestones. In 20-plus years, my students and I have screened, treated, or supervised more than 1,500 cases. I have never met or heard of a child who preferred to keep wetting. The unfortunate fact is that most parents do not know what to do, and many get bad advice from the professionals they consult.

Of the 7 to 10 million bedwetting children in the United States, about 85% are monosymptomatic primary enuretics (MPEs). They have no medical problems, they wet only at night, and they have never been dry for at least 6 consecutive months. MPEs are ideal candidates for behavioral treatment. Children who have daytime wetting need more medical attention and may enter behavioral treatment when the daytime wetting is resolved. Children who have onset or secondary bedwetting also need more careful medical screening and evaluation for distress associated with the return of bedwetting. Definitions of secondary enuresis vary, but most consider bedwetting to be secondary if the child has been consistently dry for 6 months or longer and then has resumed regular bedwetting. Provided these secondary enuretic children have no current complications, they may also be successfully treated with FSHT.

All children referred for treatment should receive a basic physical examination and urinalysis from either their pediatrician or their family doctor. Consultation with a pediatric urologist can be useful to obtain a bladder and renal sonogram to rule out structural problems. Again, 90% will have no medical complications, but no one wants to have a child fail behavioral treatment because an easily curable infection was overlooked.

Active Avoidance Learning and the Urine Alarm

All children start out wetting the bed, and some fail to stop. Most stop without special help. On average, children attain daytime control of urination at 2½ years old, and nighttime control generally follows within 1 year. When a child continues regular bedwetting beyond 4½ years old, the child may have missed a developmental window for acquiring the responses needed to be dry at night. For practical reasons, behavioral treatment is generally not instituted until a child is 5 years old or older. Children acquire nighttime control either by waking up and going to the bathroom or by inhibiting urination at the first signals of a full bladder. Learning either response is facilitated by the natural discomfort of a wet bed. If for any number of reasons (e.g., sleeping for long periods and habituating to the discomfort of a wet bed) a child repeatedly fails to respond to the aversive conditions of a wet bed, the child will fail to learn the avoidance responses needed to maintain a dry bed. Continued bedwetting, then, is a failure to learn how to be dry from the naturally occurring conditions of development. From a biobehavioral perspective, MPE is caused by an interaction between delays in physical development that are genetically transmitted and behavioral histories that can either facilitate or further delay those active avoidance responses needed to maintain a dry bed (Houts, 1991; Lovibond, 1963).

Urine alarm treatment is one way to re-create the conditions that lead a child to perform the active avoidance response of inhibiting urination during sleep. The alarm is an aversive stimulus that produces a conditioned avoidance response of contracting the pelvic floor along with the external sphincter of the bladder neck. This active avoidance response is maintained by negative reinforcement. As long as the response is made, the child avoids having to wake and avoids the wet bed. This model is consistent with findings from nighttime recording of pelvic floor activity. Norgaard observed that when nighttime wetting was avoided, children aborted detrussor contractions by spontaneously contracting the muscles of the pelvic floor (Norgaard, 1989). In contrast, episodes of wetting without arousal were preceded by relaxation of the pelvic floor. In other words, when nighttime wetting was avoided, children were inhibiting bladder contractions by spontaneously contracting the muscles of the pelvic floor.

As applied to the urine alarm, the pelvic floor activity that occurs when a child either arouses to or sleeps through the sensation of a full bladder is a conditioned response, obtained by startling the child with the urine alarm. Specifically, the sound of the alarm may startle the child, thus causing contraction of the muscles of the pelvic floor. Over time, this physiological response becomes conditioned as the child's body responds to a full bladder and associated contractions with pelvic floor contraction in order to avoid being startled by the alarm and having to awaken. We obtained indirect evidence for this formulation in a study of children who completed daytime pelvic floor electromyography (EMG) assessments over the course of urine alarm treatment. Compared to those who failed to become completely dry, those who did become dry showed a steady increase in average peak voltage over the 16-week course of treatment even though their initial muscular response was weaker. In other words, the EMG assessments confirmed that muscle conditioning did in fact occur in those children who became dry with urine alarm treatment. Responders as compared to nonresponders appeared to acquire more pelvic floor reactivity and responsiveness (Scott, 1993). These findings support the view that the urine alarm works by training the child to make an inhibitory pelvic floor response during sleep. More direct confirmation can be obtained if future investigations assess pelvic floor reactivity during sleep as urine alarm treatment progresses.

Bladder Capacity and Maintenance of Dry Nights

Some bedwetting may be due to developmental delays in bladder capacity. In our original formulation of FSHT, we regarded this problem as a complicating factor rather than a primary cause of bedwetting. Subsequent evidence suggests that there may be a small proportion whose bedwetting is due primarily to the fact that their bladders cannot accommodate the volume of urine they produce at night. These are likely to be children who wet multiple times each night, and they are likely to be that small proportion who actually do fail to produce normal amounts of antidiuretic hormone at night. We have continued to use retention control training or bladder stretching exercises to address this problem. Others have used desmopressin acetate (DDAVP) medication to provide synthetic antidiuretic hormone, thereby reducing the volume of urine produced at night (Bradbury & Meadow, 1995). Whether one approaches this from the standpoint of increasing capacity or reducing the volume produced, the evidence is clear that such approaches alone are not sufficient to end bedwetting (Houts et al., 1994). The alarm is essential.

If nothing is done to prevent relapse, resumption of bedwetting after successful urine alarm treatment may be as high as 40% within a year. In FSHT we address the problem by building in overlearning as a relapse-reduction procedure. In our early studies, we followed the standard procedure of having the child consume 16 ounces of water immediately before going to bed. This happened after the child attained 14 dry nights in a row and continued until the child attained another 14 in a row. We replicated the previous findings of cutting the relapse rate in half, from 40% down to 20% (Young & Morgan, 1972). Recently, we modified the overlearning procedure to gradually increase the amount of water consumed before bedtime. This gradual overlearning has reduced the relapse rate in half once again, from 20% down to just less than 10%. Urine alarm treatment without some specific measure to prevent relapse is not the best treatment. Overlearning is a practical way to solve this limitation, and gradual overlearning is most effective.

Family Involvement

As with almost any child problem, behavioral treatment for bedwetting requires concerted and cooperative effort from the entire family. Most treatment failures are due to noncompliance with the procedures, which can occur for a variety of reasons. The most demanding part of FSHT is training a child to wake to the alarm within the first 4 weeks of treatment. Many children require parental assistance to wake up. Parents have to be committed to waking the child and requiring the child to get out of bed before turning off the alarm. A family environment of cooperation and firm resolve is essential. Children, too, have to be ready to do the hard work of getting up whenever the alarm sounds.

Fortunately, most MPEs come from families that have the resources and skills to implement behavioral treatment. Put another way, enuresis is not an epidemiological marker for family dysfunction. Obviously, in cases in which there is significant marital discord, extreme distress in the primary caretakers, chaotic family structure, parental neglect or abuse, and significant child conduct disorder, such problems must be resolved before implementing behavioral treatment for bedwetting. Routine use of screening instruments for marital distress and child conduct disorder can identify such problematic cases. We have used the Locke–Wallace Marital Adjustment Test (Locke & Wallace, 1959) and the Child Behavior Checklist (Achenbach, 1996). Such measures can provide normative-based assessments of marital satisfaction and child externalizing problems.

In FSHT we use a behavioral contracting procedure between parents and children to promote cooperation and to clarify family rules for assisting the child. Siblings are included in the family contract so that they will know how to help and what to avoid. In extended families and blended families, all are included in the contracting process provided they spend significant time with the child in the nighttime. Provided that there is consistency and follow-through in each household, children who share multiple households can be successful. As with any behavioral intervention implemented by parents and caretakers, it is essential that the adults cooperate to provide structure and support.

CHARACTERISTICS OF THE TREATMENT PROGRAM

FSHT includes four components: (1) basic urine alarm treatment, (2) cleanliness training, (3) retention control training, and (4) overlearning. The components are presented in an integrated manual for parents to follow, and a contract between parents and children forms the basis for implementing the treatment.[1]

The Family Support Agreement

Table 22.1 reproduces the Family Support Agreement. Parents and children complete this as a trainer illustrates what to do for each step. Children are instructed to follow the rule to get out of bed and stand up before turning off the alarm. Parents are told never to turn off the alarm for the child. The steps involved in cleanliness training are displayed on a wall chart (Daily Steps to a Dry Bed) placed in the child's room. The chart also displays a record of progress and is colored in as either wet or dry for each day. Parents are instructed to have the child go through with the full procedure of remaking the bed even if the sheets are not wet, something that typically happens in the latter part of training with newer body-worn alarms. Some children are difficult to arouse in the first 4 weeks. It is imperative that the child be awakened so that the child turns off the alarm. Even if this means that a parent must share the room with the child in the early phase of alarm treatment, training the child to awaken to the alarm is crucial. Children can do some rather remarkable things in their sleep, and it is important to give parents an easy way to determine if their child is truly awake. Short-term memory tasks such as choosing a pass-

TABLE 22.1. Family Support Agreement of FSHT

1. _____ AND _____ agree to do the training just like it is described in order to reach the goal of a dry bed.

2. Everyone agrees to follow the program for at least 84 days (12 weeks). Children who wet more than once a night will probably take longer to be completely dry.

3. The whole family agrees not to punish, scold, ridicule or even say anything negative about "bedwetting" during the training.

4. Both parents and child understand that training is most effective when the child is not overtired or stressed. Therefore _____ AND _____ agree that _____ p.m. is a reasonable bedtime, and _____ agrees to go to bed at that time every night.

5. NO RESTRICTIONS ON LIQUIDS. _____ will be allowed to drink as much liquid as desired at all times.

6. Parents and family agree to provide support, help and understanding to _____. They will praise him/ her when dry and provide encouragement that progress will be made. However, they understand that the training itself includes sufficient pressure and agree they will not urge him/her to try harder or do better.

7. Parents and family agree not to complain about the effects of the training on them or about the urine alarm, but to support and help instead. _____ also agrees not to complain about the training and to cooperate fully.

8. The family will provide a relatively stress-free environment at home during training. During the training, parents will not ask the child to do extra jobs around the house.

9. _____ AND _____ agree to participate in Self-Control Training once a day during the hours of _____ and _____ as explained in the Parent Guide.

   Parents will give _____ in money for each success according to the Reward Schedule for Self-Control Training.

10. _____ agrees to follow the procedure of Cleanliness Training as outlined on the wall chart and to put wet sheets and underwear in _____. Parents agree to keep clean sheets and clean underwear in the _____ in the child's room for him/her to use when remaking the bed.

11. Parents agree to wake _____ immediately if the buzzer rings and he/she does not wake up. IT IS ESSENTIAL THAT THE PERSON RESPONSIBLE FOR WAKING THE CHILD WILL BE ABLE TO HEAR AND BE AWAKENED BY THE ALARM. NOTHING ELSE SHOULD BE DONE TO WAKE THE CHILD DURING THE NIGHT. The alarm must do this.

12. Parents agree to check the batteries regularly and to have replacement batteries ready when needed. Parents will also check the absorbent pockets for wear and replace these when needed.

13. _____ AND _____ agree that ONLY _____ WILL TOUCH THE ALARM, except for alarm testing as described above.

14. Parents agree to assume all responsibilities associated with training for a dry bed as spelled out in the Parent Guide. _____ agrees to follow the Daily Steps to a Dry Bed outlined on the wall chart.

15. OVERLEARNING. When _____ has been dry for 14 consecutive nights, the Overlearning procedures will be followed until the child is dry for 14 more nights in a row. Overlearning will be explained when the child gets 14 dry nights in a row.

16. It is understood that every child has an occasional wet bed, especially when sick or under stress. DO NOT WORRY ABOUT THIS. TELL YOUR CHILD NOT TO WORRY.

_____	_____
(Child's Signature)	(Parent's Signature)
_____	_____
(Parent's Signature)	(Witness or Other Family Member)

Note. Parents and children complete this form during demonstrations of how each step is to be carried out. Explanations of the procedures are provided at each step. Completing all 16 items takes about 90 minutes.

word each night before bedtime or asking the child to spell a familiar word backwards are simple ways to determine whether the child is fully awake.

Retention control training is done once a day, and the child is given money for postponing urination for increasing amounts of time in a step-by-step fashion up to a 45-minute holding time. The total amount of money the child receives for reaching all 15 3-minute incremented goals is $6.25. Children are encouraged to save the money in a prominent place to remind them of their accomplishments. Parents may have difficulty monitoring this activity and often need assistance with scheduling the procedure. Retention control training ends when the child attains the 45-minute goal, typically within 3 weeks.

The first goal of treatment is to attain 14 consecutive dry nights in a row. This takes an average of 8–12 weeks. With children who wet more than once a night, the average time to this first goal is 16–20 weeks. Overlearning begins immediately and is an essential ingredient for preventing relapse.

Our gradual overlearning begins by determining a maximum amount of water. The maximum is 1 ounce for each year of age plus 2 ounces. For example, the maximum amount for an 8-year-old child is 10 ounces. Children then begin by drinking 4 ounces of water 15 minutes before bedtime. If they remain dry for 2 nights while drinking 4 ounces, the amount increases to 6 ounces. If they remain dry for 2 nights at 6 ounces, the water is increased to 8 ounces. The water increases continue in this fashion, 2 ounces more for every 2 consecutive dry nights, until the child's maximum reached. The child continues to drink this maximum until he or she attains 14 consecutive dry nights. In the event a child wets, and most do at least once, a simple rule is followed. The child goes back to whatever amount was consumed on the immediate last dry night and continues with that amount until he or she remains dry 5 nights in a row. If the child is not already at the maximum, the procedure continues as before, increasing by 2 ounces for every 2 dry nights. The goal remains 14 dry nights in a row during overlearning. Some children end up having all 14 of those dry nights at the maximum amount, but this is not required for the relapse prevention effect.

Optional Waking Schedule

Occasionally, it may be necessary to disrupt the child's sleep routine with a waking schedule to achieve the 14-consecutive-dry-nights goal. Parents are told to wake their child hourly using a minimal amount of prompting throughout the first night. Each time the child is awakened, he or she is praised for a dry bed and encouraged to void in the toilet. Any time the child wets the bed and consequently activates the alarm, the cleanliness training program is followed. The second night the child is awakened only once, 3 hours after falling asleep. From the second night forward, the waking schedule continues with the child being awakened only once each night. Following a dry night, the parents wake the child 30 minutes earlier than the previous night. If the child wets during the night, the time of waking remains the same as the previous night. The nightly waking schedule ends when the scheduled time for awakening the child is 30 minutes immediately following bedtime. The waking schedule resumes only if the child has 2 or more wet nights in 7 days. When resumption is necessary, the waking schedule begins at 3 hours after bedtime and decreases in the same manner (Azrin, Sneed, & Foxx, 1973; Bollard & Nettelbeck, 1982). The waking schedule is not a routine part of FSHT and is only indicated when there are extreme difficulties in training a child to awaken to the alarm.

Minimal Visit and Multiple Visit Protocols

We have implemented this treatment in single-visit and dual-visit protocols with comparable results. In the single-visit protocol, the entire program is covered in one 90-minute session during which parents and children complete the Family Support Agreement and observe a demonstration for how to implement each component. In the dual-visit protocol, we cover the first nine items of the Family Support Agreement, which takes about 30 minutes. We devote the other 30 minutes to building rapport and presenting information to the family about the problem of bedwetting. This information emphasizes the learning basis of the therapy and the fact that learning the new skills will take time and patience on the part of the whole family. In the second 60-minute visit we review the preceding week's records for retention control training and demonstrate the alarm. The family then continues retention control training and begins home implementation of the urine alarm.

Regardless of how the treatment is introduced, follow-up contact is important. We have achieved good results with minimal contact, such as having biweekly phone contact. Somewhat better results can be expected with more therapist contact. This can take the schedule of two initial visits followed by a 30-minute visit within the first 2 weeks of starting the urine alarm. Thereafter, half-hour visits can be scheduled about every 3 weeks to provide encouragement and to solve minor problems. We have also implemented the protocol in which the start of overlearning triggers a return visit. Much depends on the circumstances of the particular child and family. FSHT can be implemented with as few as one or two visits. Rarely have I ever conducted the treatment with more than six visits over the course of 16–20 weeks.

Group and Individual Session Formats

FSHT has been successfully delivered in both group and individual therapy formats. As summarized later, we have replicated the effectiveness of group-administered FSHT in a series of five studies. With the exception of differing relapse rates due to different forms of overlearning in these five trials, outcomes were comparable. In these studies, families attended group training sessions held in university classrooms large enough to accommodate up to 10 families at a single training demonstration. Due to developmental differences and the fact that some older children feel embarrassed in the presence of much younger children, we typically formed groups separately for children 12 years old and older. Presentations to adolescents differ in terms of how much the child is placed in charge of implementing the behavioral procedures. In most cases, these young people are highly motivated and want to "train themselves" with minimal assistance from adults.

Individual administration of FSHT has been conducted by numerous practitioners who have requested and used the treatment materials over the past 20 years.[2] In that same period, I have collected effectiveness data on individual administration using both single-visit and dual-visit initial training sessions. Those outcome data are presented here and suggest results comparable to those achieved via group administration of the FSHT protocol.

The decision to proceed with individual as opposed to group administration of FSHT is largely practical and economical. Many solo practitioners may not have access to a classroom-style facility to conduct groups attended by as many as 30 people. Also, insurance reimbursement for behavioral treatment is highly variable, and some plans may dictate individual as opposed to group therapy or offer financial incentives for one as opposed to the other. One of the true tragedies of the current U.S. healthcare system is that third-party providers almost always reimburse for medication treatments that are more expensive and less effective, and they may not provide any reimbursement for behavioral treatment.

Reinforcing Accomplishments and Reducing Frustrations

Although we have shown that effective behavioral treatment can be delivered in a cost-efficient manner using minimal contact and group delivery, it is important to note that our study protocols always included regular contact with the child and family during the course of treatment, even if that contact was confined to phone consultations. Again, the major weakness of any behavioral treatment is lack of compliance often due to the difficulty of implementing the treatment procedures with particular cases. General therapeutic skills and practical problem solving are needed to forestall noncompliance and premature dropout.

A focus on reinforcing accomplishments during treatment is helpful. Children who wet multiple times each night get easily discouraged. These families need to understand that it will take 12 to 16 weeks as opposed to the average of 8 to 12 weeks for the child to achieve the first 14 consecutive dry nights. Also, multiple wettings mean multiple awakenings with all the attendant work. Informing such children that their first goal is to get from multiple wettings to a single wetting episode each night adjusts their expectations and prevents some of the frustration.

Pointing out that progress can be measured by monitoring the size of wet spots helps parents and children to focus on the process and recognize that even though every night has been a "wet night," the child is responding more readily to the alarm. As the size of the wet spot gets smaller and smaller, the child is learning to make the active avoidance response sooner and sooner. Dry nights are sure to follow. In focusing on the goal of attaining 14 consecutive dry nights, parents and children often need to be reminded of the overall picture. Even though a child may not have reached the 14-night goal, he or she may have been 90% dry for the past 6 weeks. This can give the family a more positive perspective and encouragement to proceed. The goal of attaining 14 dry nights in a row can be frustrating, especially when a child gets 13 in a row and then wets on the 14th night. I tell children that of some 1,500 cases I have seen, no one has ever failed to be dry if he or she got 13 in a row and then wet. All those children went on to complete the treatment.

Many children enjoy the challenge of overcoming bedwetting, and it is easy to engage their competitive spirit to positive ends. Some bring their wall charts to each follow-up visit to show off their progress. Others set goals of beating the 42-day record for completing FSHT. As long as their goals are not outlandish and beyond reach, this energetic approach to getting rid of the problem is useful because the child's motivation can be directed to accomplishing the daily tasks of behavioral treatment.

Parents often want to add other incentives to the FSHT program, and this is not typically a good idea. What can be helpful is to redirect this urge to teach the parents to use contingent praise for completion of the various tasks involved in behavioral treatment. Praising children for their hard work of waking to the alarm, remaking the bed, and taking the soiled linens to the laundry is directly beneficial. Outcome-related rewards such as a new mattress or new bed upon completion of the program can be helpful but are not essential. We emphasize the inherent attraction of no longer wetting the bed, and children understand instantly that this is a big reinforcer.

Relapse Prevention and Follow-up

Carrying out the overlearning procedure can be especially challenging for children who have struggled and finally attained the first 14 dry nights in a row. Children and their parents often fear the prospect of overlearning because they fear that once a child wets again, the child will never recover and be dry at night. We typically tell such parents and children that overlearning is designed precisely to show them that their fear is unwarranted. In this regard it is important to emphasize that almost all children wet at least once during overlearning. The process of having a programmed relapse can produce the effect of building confidence in both parents and child.

Overlearning is introduced by citing the data to the parents and child. The chance of a relapse without overlearning is 4 out of 10. In contrast, the chance of relapse is less than 1 out of 10 if the child does the gradual form of overlearning. The benefit of doing overlearning far outweighs the time and effort to complete it. Occasionally, a child simply cannot complete overlearning (i.e., he or she cannot get 14 consecutive dry nights during the drinking procedure). Although our outcome trials have been conducted under rigorous procedures that required completion of overlearning to be counted a treatment success, in the effectiveness work based on clinical flexibility, I have suspended overlearning if a child has not completed it within 8 weeks. In such cases, the child stops the nighttime drinking and simply continues with the alarm until he or she attains 14 consecutive dry nights without the drinking. The child then proceeds to follow-up. This does not seem to lead to any worse outcome and causes me to suspect that the benefit of overlearning as a relapse prevention procedure may be as much psychological as it is physiological. The added water load before bedtime forces almost all children to wet at least one night. When they go on to overcome this "setback," they gain new confidence in their ability to maintain a dry bed. This may also contribute to their confidence to accept invitations to sleep over away from home, a practice that is strongly encouraged once the treatment is completed.

Follow-up in FSHT has been for 1 year or more. In both the efficacy data and the effectiveness data, we have followed children for 3 months, 6 months, and 1 year. In the outcome studies we did not offer retreatment in the event of relapse because we were interested in estimating the relapse rates. In data collection efforts, our focus has been on relapse prevention rather than retreatment of relapsers, a procedure strongly recommended for clinical practice.

In clinical applications, we have offered retreatment in the event a child wet four or more times in 14 days. Parents and children were instructed to contact the clinic in the event of a relapse and to reinstate the alarm until the child was dry for 14 consecutive nights. Such retreatment permanently stops the recurrence in over 95% of cases.

One other note about follow-up bears mentioning. Children and families follow-up with clinicians long after the follow up period has passed. Over the past 20 years, I have received numerous postcards, letters, and greetings from parents and former adolescent clients who have themselves become parents. Helping a family overcome a child's bedwetting problem is rewarding work, and the children and their families are typically grateful to have solved the problem.

EVIDENCE FOR THE EFFECTS OF TREATMENT

We have been fortunate to have collected both efficacy and effectiveness data on FSHT. When compared to urine alarm procedures without any ancillary procedures such as retention control training and overlearning, FSHT is an improvement over the urine alarm alone. In fact, it is not good practice to use the urine alarm without some form of relapse prevention. Our component's breakdown analysis of FSHT suggested that the addition of retention-control training to the package was helpful in getting the child to the first 14 dry nights in a row. Children who did the retention training as compared to those who did not attained the 14-night goal faster (Houts, Peterson, & Whelan, 1986). This is important in terms of motivating the family and speeding progress toward the ultimate goal of complete cessation of bedwetting.

Controlled Outcome Trials in Group Format

Figure 22.1 summarizes 1-year follow-up results from six observations of FSHT. Four of these are from published studies and are indicated by their respective dates of publication (Houts, Liebert, & Padawer, 1983; Houts et al., 1986; Houts, Whelan, & Peterson, 1987; Whelan & Houts, 1990). The 1991 sample shows FSHT outcomes from an unpublished randomized clinical trial comparing FSHT to imipramine and oxybutynin. The 137 cases labeled 2000 have accumulated in our private enuresis clinic over a period of 14 years and represent effectiveness data from a clinical practice.

Based on the five efficacy trials, about three of every four children treated with FSHT can be expected to stop bedwetting at the end of the average of 12 weeks needed to complete the treatment. It is important to remember that these data were obtained under research protocol conditions in which flexibility of procedures was highly constrained. Further, these samples did not include secondary enuretics and children with clinically significant behavioral problems such as conduct disorder and attention-deficit/

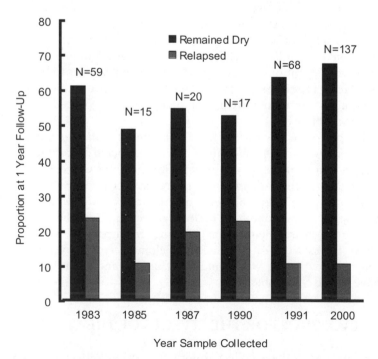

FIGURE 22.1. Mean percentage of children who remained dry or relapsed at 1-year follow-up with full-spectrum treatment for five samples. N = total sample size. "Relapse" was defined as 2 or more wet nights in 1 week.

hyperactivity disorder (ADHD). Single-parent households were represented in these data, as were low-income families. However, the samples did not include families with marked marital discord or clinically significant family dysfunction. Although these demographic limitations constrain the applicability of findings, it also should be remembered that these samples are quite representative of bedwetting children, most of whom do not have these additional problems.

At the 1-year follow-up, 6 of every 10 children are permanently dry. The lower relapse rates observed in the 1991 and 2000 samples were from children who did our gradual overlearning where they increased nighttime drinking in 2-ounce increments adjusted for their age. In the other samples, overlearning was done in the original fashion of having children consume 16 ounces of water regardless of age. We now consistently find that slightly less than 10% of children relapse using the gradual overlearning procedure.

Effectiveness Outcomes in Individual Format

In the case of FSHT, effectiveness data mirror the efficacy data. The 137 cases from our private enuresis clinic were referred by pediatricians and pediatric urologists. More than in the research trials, this sample contained children with additional problems, most often ADHD. Such children were typically receiving stimulant medication and varying degrees of supportive behavior therapy either through the schools or from another practitioner. The issues in dealing with such children are the same when dealing with children who have other behavioral problems. Successful behavioral treatment for bedwetting requires child compliance with the procedures and supportive and cooperative parents. Parents who use coercive parenting and engage in repeated struggles with a noncompliant child cannot expect to be successful with FSHT. In fact, I tell them that I will not provide the treatment until they first clear up the other problems so that the child has a good chance for success with the bedwetting treatment.

In this context, I have also treated a number of secondary enuretics, children who resumed wetting after a period of 6 months or more of continuous continence. Again, excepting oppositional behavior and family dysfunction and discord, these children also respond well to FSHT and achieve outcomes comparable to those achieved by monosymptomatic primary enuretics. The issue with secondary enuresis is not the history of continence followed by recurrence of bedwetting. Instead, the issue is the family environment and ancillary child behavior problems. Absent the correlated child behavior and family difficulties, secondary enuretic children are good candidates for FSHT.

Important Research Directions

In FSHT, we have not completely solved the problem of relapse, but we have come some distance in preventing relapse after successful treatment with the urine alarm. One thing that is needed is a quantitative study of the effects of retreatment of relapses. We may well be able to claim that behavioral treatment permanently cures over 90% of MPEs who follow through with the full treatment program. As it now stands, we can safely claim that most coveted outcome for about 70–75% of such cases.

There are true nonresponders to behavioral treatment. When one sets aside those cases in which the child defeats the alarm device and the parents fail to provide support and assistance, there are still some 10–15% of cases that do not respond despite the fact that they carry out the treatment to the fullest. What we need, and what we are not likely ever to get because there is no glory in it, is an intensive study of true treatment failures. This would be beneficial on the obvious front of improving treatment and screening for behavioral treatment. It would also be useful from an etiological point of view. Like most every other problem in the field of behavior, bedwetting is most likely the outcome of multiple causal pathways. Classifying the fallout from failure to respond to behavioral treatment could shed some light on the types of causal pathways not adequately addressed by urine alarm treatment. For example, some children never learn to awaken to the alarm. Such children may require a different type of alarm that is louder and might even provide tactile stimulation through vibration. A pioneer in the field, Dan Doleys once told me that he never had a child fail to awaken to the alarm because he used his own alarms built by a lab tech. These alarms used old school bells (D. Doleys, personal communication, April 30, 1990). Oddly enough, the first urine alarm was not an alarm at all but a spring-loaded metal bed that catapulted the child across the room when urine closed the pad contacts and activated a solenoid that released the bed frame (Mowrer, 1980). Waking the child at the correct time is both practically and theoretically important. Surely some of the nonresponders to behavioral treatment fail to arouse to the alarm, and methods for improving arousability are important to pursue. Technological innovations, behavioral additions such as the waking schedule, and pharmacological methods are all worth pursuing.

Another important type of failure is the child that continues multiple wetting and never moves to single-episode wetting. These children are most likely that subgroup which has a deficit in the natural production of antidiuretic hormone. They are also good candidates for combining behavioral treatment with synthetic antidiuretic hormone (Bradbury & Meadow, 1995; Sukhai, Mol, & Harris, 1989).

The role of airborne allergies and food allergies also merits further investigation. There are occasional references to the co-occurrence of these problems with bedwetting, but systematic investigations are lacking. With all of the aforementioned problems, the difficulty is the low base rate. It is difficult to accumulate a sufficient sample for study of the mechanisms relating such difficulties to bedwetting.

HISTORY AND THE FUTURE

Behavioral treatment of childhood enuresis with the urine alarm is one of the best examples of a highly effective intervention for a widespread problem where the intervention has been based on laboratory-derived principles of learning and conditioning. As one of the oldest forms of 20th century behavior therapy, the object lesson offered by the history of this treatment is important for the 21st century. To understand where we are and where we might go, it is important to appreciate the history of psychological and medical treatment for enuresis. This history reflects the larger issues for empirically supported psychological treatments more generally. Will children of the 21st century be medicated for their difficulties to the exclusion of alternative and adjunctive behavioral interventions? What is it about our culture in the United States that makes pharmacotherapy so attractive and so easily sold? What does it take to make a treatment available once it has been shown to be effective?

History of Urine Alarm Treatment

At the time that Mowrer faced the challenge of designing a solution to bedwetting, he was part of a group of Yale psychologists who were attempting to translate Hullian learning theory into clinically relevant terms. In the height of the Great Depression even a Yale professor could not earn enough to make ends meet, so Mowrer and his wife took up residence in a home for misfit boys, many of whom wet the bed. As house parents, the burden of 12 or so wet beds every night was surely enough adversity to give birth to some invention. From the impracticality, not to mention the danger, of the spring-loaded bed, Mowrer reasoned his way to the urine alarm. Some version of the urine alarm that uses moisture pads placed on the bed has been in use since the first publication by the two Mowrers in 1938 (Mowrer, 1980; Mowrer & Mowrer, 1938). The Mowrers did not get a patent on the device, nor did they copyright the procedures in written manuals or books. In fact, they did not pursue the subject of enuresis beyond their seminal 1938 publication.

Patents were, however, obtained by several commercial manufacturers in the United States, and from the early 1940s to the present, various versions of the urine alarm device have been available from the Sears catalogue and from such chain department stores as J. C. Penney and Montgomery Ward. In the early 1950s, several companies were formed in the United States to sell treatment for bedwetting, and these companies featured their own alarm devices, which were typically "leased" to the family for an exorbitant price. The business model for these companies, some still in existence today, is to place sales personnel in certain regions and then blanket the region with advertisements. A salesman then comes to the home in response to returned postcards and attempts to sell the family a treatment program. Today the contract costs about $2,000. The point is, these companies are still in business today, some 50 years later.

Where are the psychologists? Throughout the 1940s, theoretical interest in bedwetting took hold not in the United States but in the United Kingdom. Among the graduates of the first class of clinical psychologists trained at the Maudsley program organized by Eysenck were a number of investigators who went on to do empirical work in the field of conditioning treatment for enuresis. As an intellectual center for behavior therapy, this program attracted a number of students and postdoctoral fellows from around the world, thus spreading the word about conditioning treatment. The net effect of these developments is that within the National Health Service of the United Kingdom and throughout much of Australia, urine alarm treatment for enuresis is widely available. Intellectual interest in the principles of classical conditioning and avoidance learning spawned a keener awareness of conditioning treatment of enuresis and provided a solution to a problem that medical professionals had little success in treating.

By way of contrast, developments in the United States followed a different course. Interest in the problem of enuresis as a "laboratory" for testing various conditioning formulations did not take hold. Compared to the British and Australian empirical publications, relatively little work was conducted in the United States until the mid-1970s, when Azrin and his colleagues challenged the idea that the urine alarm worked by methods of classical conditioning (Azrin et al., 1973; Azrin & Thienes, 1978). When others failed to replicate the Azrin results and showed instead that the urine alarm was an essential component to successful behavioral treatment, the theoretical dispute about classical conditioning was largely settled (Bollard & Nettelbeck, 1982).

As graduate students in the late 1970s at Stony Brook University (then the State University of New York at Stony Brook), we enjoyed debates about classical versus operant conditioning explanations for urine alarm treatment. We followed the "experiments" (we did not call them clinical trials) with theoretical interest to see how the issues would be resolved by data. In retrospect, this intellectual interest in models of conditioning was probably atypical and was certainly short-lived in the broader scheme of training programs in the United States. Within a decade, everything and everyone went "cognitive," so much so that a fellow graduate student who was interested in the theoretical implications of enuresis treatment and who had since gone on to teach at the University of Illinois remarked to me that he had to give up his interest because graduate students responded to the subject matter like a "wet blanket." Today, it is extremely rare to find a clinical psychology graduate student who has any interest in basic research in classical or operant conditioning, and most have little or no knowledge of the relevant literature. In my own department, there is no graduate-level course in learning, and this is fairly typical throughout the United States. The point is that unlike the British and Australian histories, in the United States there has never really been sustained intellectual interest in the problem of enuresis. This has contributed to the relative lack of widespread availability of urine alarm treatment from properly trained professionals.

Another important part of the historical picture concerns the role of medical professionals and the pharmaceutical industry in treatment for bedwetting.

Recent History of Pharmaceutical Treatment

Prior to the introduction of DDAVP into the United States in 1989, the modal treatment recommended by medical doctors was to do nothing and wait for the child to outgrow the problem. If treatment was offered, most often it was an antidepressant, imipramine hydrochloride, which carried risks of poisoning and adverse cardiovascular events in overdose. Moreover, this treatment was not effective. Nevertheless, the medical community was generally not educated about behavioral treatment and among those few who were, providers were not readily available to deliver the treatment. Behavioral treatment was never integrated into primary care of enuretic children in the manner that had happened in the United Kingdom and Australia.

With the introduction of DDAVP into the culture of American medicine, this new and much safer medication offered primary care physicians the option to provide a treatment that was safe and that might be effective. As it turns out, the evidence clearly favors urine alarm treatment over DDAVP, but this has been practically negated by the powerful advertising campaigns of the drug company involved. The selling of DDAVP as a treatment for bedwetting is instructive, and to the extent that pharmaceutical companies can successfully sell medications for other problem behaviors, it does not bode well for the future of psychological treatments more generally. What is so fascinating about the case of treatment for enuresis is that an inferior and more expensive treatment has become the de facto standard of care even in a scientific climate that features "evidence-based medicine" and an economic climate that features "cost containment." How did this happen?

Pharmaceutical advertising has become very sophisticated. The obvious influences are easily recognized. Medical doctors in training receive gifts of all types. Physicians in practice are routinely visited by representatives who provide free samples, coffee mugs, pens, and even dinners and cruises called seminars. What is less obvious is the advertising that takes place in the form of studies and publications. When we examine the literature on enuresis over the past 15 years, there is an elephant in the library. The manufacturer of DDAVP has sponsored numerous publications and special issues of journals. The manufacturer has spent millions of dollars to conduct and publish research, much of which was designed to provide a rationale for the use of the product. The message is subtle but clear: Use the product instead of the urine alarm. What is left out of their messages is more telling than what is in them. Manufacturer materials refer to the inconvenience of urine alarm treatment and emphasize the safety of long-term use of DDAVP. They even question the durability of urine alarm treatment, as if we do not know fully well that urine alarm treatment is far more durable than DDAVP. Promoters of DDAVP routinely visit pediatricians. There is no comparable promotion for urine alarm treatment.

Promotion alone, however, does not account for the business success of DDAVP. Having the right cultural niche is also important, and this has been provided in the United States by popular culture and by the rise of managed health care.

Popular Culture Disinformation and Managed Care

Another influence on misconceptions about treatment for bedwetting comes through popular culture in television advertisements for special underpants, a euphemism for diapers. Diaper manufacturers remind parents to discuss the problem with the child's doctor and point out that the doctor will tell them there are no guarantees with any treatment. The idea that wearing diapers might further habituate a child to the sensations of a wet bed that might otherwise prompt waking and learning to be dry is never mentioned. In fact, waiting until the child is 11 to 15 years old is the main message of the diaper purveyors. After all, the sooner a child stops bedwetting, the sooner their product is no longer needed. No wonder parents are confused. Television advertisements convey the message that wearing diapers is normal for an adolescent who wets the bed.

In addition to such confusing messages within popular culture, there is the influence of managed care on which treatments are supported for bedwetting. Managed care companies routinely pay for prescription medicines, and they often question "nonmedical" services. Most insurance plans have different reimbursement rates for care provided under mental health as opposed to physical health. Hence, psychologists who provide treatment for bedwetting receive a lower rate of reimbursement. Thus, even when behavioral treatment for bedwetting is covered by third-party payers, the immediate contingencies for parents are such that it is cheaper for the parents to get the more expensive and less effective medication treatment with DDAVP. These market forces have led to expanded ignorance of behavioral treatment on the part of both parents and professionals.

Where Can We Go from Here?

Twenty years ago, I imagined that we might have an efficient delivery system for successful behavioral treatment of enuresis (Houts et al., 1983). We are far from that, but I remain hopeful. Several things are needed to bring about change in the routine treatment of bedwetting children.

First, behavioral treatment needs a sponsor that can compete with the pharmaceutical and diaper companies. The obvious organization is the American Psychological Association (APA). Psychologists developed urine alarm treatment, and they remain the most likely providers who have the requisite background to implement it successfully in both simple and complex cases. The APA or some division within the APA such as Pediatric Psychology should work together with the requisite medical associations to develop and publish a set of treatment guidelines for the care of enuretic children.

Second, through its accredited training programs, the APA should provide incentives for the teaching of behavioral treatment to new psychologists in training. Training programs may need to revamp their curricula so that students receive direct instruction in empirically supported child therapies, and the APA could facilitate this revamping with both carrot and stick. Providing programs with the training materials and publishing those materials on the Internet would make them widely available. Accreditation reviews can require evidence that students are instructed in empirically based therapies such as behavioral treatment for enuresis.

Third, advertising is clearly important. Organizations such as the APA can work with manufacturers of urine alarms to promote behavioral treatment. This can be done through print and media advertising.

Finally, adequate education of primary providers, mostly primary care physicians and pediatricians, remains to be accomplished. Hearing once vaguely about alarm treatment as a third-year medical student is no match for the constant bombardment of promotional materials from the pharmaceutical company once the student goes on to practice medicine. Psychologists and medical educators need to collaborate to find ways to convey to medical students the importance of research methodology in the assessment of claims for treatment efficacy. This includes the publication in medical journals of primary studies of behavioral treatment, something that has been sadly rare.

SUMMARY AND CONCLUSIONS

Bedwetting is a problem for some 5 to 7 million secondary school-age children in the United States. This problem can be solved in most cases with some form of urine alarm treatment. FSHT is a behavior treatment that has been tested in several clinical trials and shown to be efficacious. This treatment has also been used in clinical settings and has been demonstrated to be effective. A key feature of FSHT is that it contains a modified overlearning procedure to prevent relapse, and this gradual approach to overlearning is both effective and practical.

Although it is of considerable theoretical interest to document how the urine alarm works, this type of investigation involving all-night sleep studies is expensive and unlikely to be pursued. Hypotheses regarding the role of antidiuretic hormone in bedwetting have been investigated extensively because the pharmaceutical companies that manufacture synthetic antidiuretic hormone have a vested interest in such studies. Despite such extensive study, there is little reason to believe that the etiology of bedwetting is some defect in production of naturally occurring antidiuretic hormone. At best such an etiological hypothesis might be true for about 10% of bedwetting children who wet multiple times each night.

In the larger scheme of healthcare delivery, the problem with behavioral treatment for bedwetting is that the treatment is not being delivered to children and families. There are economic and social structural barriers to making this treatment widely available. Unlike medication treatments and stop-gap approaches such as diapers, behavioral treatment for enuresis has no corporate backing. There is no sales force for behavioral treatment, and there is no advertising campaign. Behavioral treatment for bedwetting needs some form of institutional backing and promotion. A logical place for this to happen is with the APA, because psychologists have developed behavioral treatment, and APA is the most likely group trained to implement it. Ironically, the APA is currently engaged in a massive campaign to obtain prescribing privileges for psychologists. Regardless of what one thinks about the general issue of prescribing privileges for psychologists, obtaining such privileges for treatment of bedwetting would be a step backward. The history of treatment for bedwetting has some interesting lessons to teach regarding the relative role of medications as contrasted with conditioning-based behavior therapies. At least in the case of bedwetting treatment, behavior therapy is the treatment of choice. Whether this will hold for other child problems remains to be seen. What is abundantly clear from the example of bedwetting is that establishing the superiority of one treatment over all others is no guarantee that the best treatment will be delivered in a market-driven healthcare economy.

ACKNOWLEDGMENTS

Partial support for this research was provided by a Centers of Excellence grant from the state of Tennessee to the Department of Psychology, University of Memphis, and also by National Institute of Health Grant R01 HD21736 to Arthur C. Houts.

NOTES

1. The 33-page manual for parents and wall chart for children is available on request from Arthur C. Houts, Department of Psychology, 202 Psychology Building, University of Memphis, Memphis, TN 38152. Telephone (901) 678–4685. E-mail *ahouts@bigfoot.com*. The cost is $5 for postage and handling.

    An affordable and durable body worn urine alarm, Wet Stop, is available from Palco Laboratories, 8030 Soquel Avenue, Santa Cruz, CA 95062; tel: (800) 346–4488.
2. I have maintained a list of professionals who requested the manual, and over the past 20 years this includes about 130 names. Unfortunately, I did not have the foresight to create a research network of practitioners who might report back their outcomes with FSHT. This is certainly possible with the advent of information technology and the Internet.

REFERENCES

Achenbach, T. M. (1996). *Manual for the Child Behavior Checklist 4–18 1991 profile*. Burlington, VT: Child Behavior Checklist.

Azrin, N. H., Sneed, T. J., & Foxx, R. M. (1973). Dry bed: A rapid method of eliminating bedwetting (enuresis) of the retarded. *Behaviour Research and Therapy, 11*, 427–434.

Azrin, N. H., & Thienes, P. M. (1978). Rapid elimination of enuresis by intensive learning without a conditioning apparatus. *Behavior Therapy, 9*, 342–354.

Bollard, J., & Nettelbeck, T. (1982). A component analysis of dry-bed training for treatment for bedwetting. *Behaviour Research and Therapy, 20*, 383–390.

Bradbury, M. G., & Meadow, S. R. (1995). Combined treatment with enuresis alarm and desmopressin for nocturnal enuresis. *Acta Pediatrica, 84*(9), 1014–1018.

Houts, A. C. (1991). Nocturnal enuresis as a biobehavioral problem. *Behavior Therapy, 22*, 133–151.

Houts, A. C. (2000). Commentary: Treatments for enuresis: Criteria, mechanisms, and health care policy. *Journal of Pediatric Psychology, 25*(4), 219–224.

Houts, A. C., Berman, J. S., & Abramson, H. A. (1994). The effectiveness of psychological and pharmacological treatments for nocturnal enuresis. *Journal of Consulting and Clinical Psychology, 62*, 737–745.

Houts, A. C., Liebert, R. M., & Padawer, W. (1983). A delivery system for the treatment of primary enuresis. *Journal of Abnormal Child Psychology, 11*, 513–519.

Houts, A. C., Peterson, J. K., & Whelan, J. P. (1986). Prevention of relapse in full-spectrum home training for primary enuresis: A components analysis. *Behavior Therapy, 17*, 462–469.

Houts, A. C., Whelan, J. P., & Peterson, J. K. (1987). Filmed vs. live delivery of full-spectrum home training for primary enuresis: Presenting the information is not enough. *Journal of Consulting and Clinical Psychology, 55,* 902–906.

Locke, H. J., & Wallace, K. M. (1959). Short marital adjustment and prediction tests: Their reliability and validity. *Marriage and Family Living, 21,* 251–255.

Lovibond, S. H. (1963). The mechanism of conditioning treatment of enuresis. *Behaviour Research and Therapy, 1,* 17–21.

Mikkelsen, E. J. (2001). Enuresis and encopresis: ten years of progress. *Journal of the American Academy of Child and Adolescent Psychiatry, 40*(10), 1146–1158.

Mowrer, O. H. (1980). Enuresis: The beginning work—What really happened. *Journal of the History of the Behavioral Sciences, 16,* 25–30.

Mowrer, O. H., & Mowrer, W. M. (1938). Enuresis: A method for its study and treatment. *American Journal of Orthopsychiatry, 8,* 436–459.

Norgaard, J. P. (1989). Urodynamics in enuretics I: Reservoir Function. *Neurourology and Urodynamics, 8,* 199–211.

Scott, M. A. (1993). *Facilitating pelvic floor conditioning in primary nocturnal enuresis.* Unpublished doctoral dissertation, University of Memphis, Memphis.

Sukhai, R. N., Mol, J., & Harris, A. S. (1989). Combined therapy of enuresis alarm and desmopressin in the treatment of nocturnal enuresis. *European Journal of Pediatrics, 148*(5), 465–467.

Whelan, J. P., & Houts, A. C. (1990). Effects of a waking schedule on the outcome of primary enuretic children treated with Full-Spectrum Home Training. *Health Psychology, 9,* 164–176.

Young, G. C., & Morgan, R. T. T. (1972). Overlearning in the conditioning treatment of enuresis: A long-term follow-up study. *Behaviour Research and Therapy, 10,* 419–420.

23

Brief Strategic Family Therapy for Hispanic Youth

Michael S. Robbins, José Szapocznik,
Daniel A. Santisteban, Olga E. Hervis,
Victoria B. Mitrani, and Seth J. Schwartz

OVERVIEW

Brief strategic family therapy (BSFT) was developed in response to the increased number of Hispanic adolescents in Miami involved with drugs in the early 1970s. This problem was particularly alarming because Hispanics were also not availing themselves of existing services. National trends suggest that Hispanic adolescents tend to exhibit levels of substance abuse (Substance Abuse and Mental Health Services Association, 2001), school failure (Fuligni, 1997), and unsafe sexual contact (Centers for Disease Control and Prevention, 2001) that surpass those of non-Hispanic whites and are comparable to those of African Americans. To address this problem, the Spanish Family Guidance Center (now the Center for Family Studies) was established at the University of Miami, Florida. The first goal of the program of clinical research was to identify and/or develop a culturally appropriate treatment intervention for behavior problem Cuban youths. After conducting a series of studies examining the values of the Cuban population, structural family therapy (cf. Minuchin, 1974; Minuchin & Fishman, 1981) was adopted as the Center's core approach, and structural theory and therapy have provided the foundation for every clinical development and innovation of the Center's work in culturally diverse contexts (Szapocznik, Scopetta, & King, 1978; Szapocznik & Williams, 2000). Through a series of clinical research studies, the structural approach has been refined to meet the needs of the diverse Hispanic community in Miami. Over time, the approach has also been modified to include treatment methods that are both strategic (i.e., problem focused and pragmatic) and time-limited. In doing so, the structural approach has evolved into a time-limited approach that combines both structural and strategic interventions. This approach, BSFT, has become the central model used by the Center to work with Hispanic families with behavior problem youth.

Conceptual Model and Assumptions of BSFT

BSFT is based on the fundamental assumption that the family is the "bedrock" of child development (Szapocznik & Coatsworth, 1999). That is, the family is viewed as the primary context in which children learn to think, feel, and behave. Family relations are believed to play a pivotal role in shaping child and adolescent development and behavior, and consequently they are a primary target for intervention. BSFT recognizes that the family itself is part of a larger social system and—in much the same way as a child is influenced by his or her family—the family is influenced by the larger social system in which it exists (Bronfenbrenner, 1977, 1979, 1986). This sensitivity to contextual factors begins with an understanding of the important influence of peers, school, and the neighborhood on the development of children's behavioral problems. However, in BSFT this *contextualism* also includes a focus on parents' relationships to children's peers, schools, and neighborhoods as well as a focus on the unique relationships that parents have with individuals and systems outside the family (e.g., work and Alcoholics Anonymous). At the broadest contextual level, BSFT recognizes the part that cultural factors play in the development and maintenance of behavior problems.

BSFT has been shaped through a systematic program of research and clinical practice conducted over the past 30 years. The structural orientation of BSFT draws on the work of Minuchin (Minuchin, 1974; Minuchin & Fishman, 1981; Minuchin, Rosman, & Baker, 1978), and the strategic aspects of BSFT are influenced by Haley (1976) and Madanes (1981). However, through a rigorous and continuous interplay among theory, research, and application, BSFT has been systematically modified to work specifically with behavior problem youth. BSFT is best articulated around three central constructs: system, structure/patterns of interactions, and strategy (Szapocznik & Kurtines, 1989).

System

A system is an organized whole comprised of parts that are interdependent or interrelated. A family is a system comprised of individuals whose behaviors affect other family members. Because such behaviors have occurred thousands of times over many years, family members become accustomed to the behavior of other family members. These behaviors synergistically work together to organize a family's system.

Structure

A central characteristic of a system is that it consists of parts that interact with each other. The set of repetitive patterns of interactions that are idiosyncratic to a family is called the family's structure. A maladaptive family structure is characterized by repetitive family interactions that persist despite the fact that these interactions fail to meet the needs of the family or its individual members. A maladaptive family structure is viewed as an important contributor to the occurrence and maintenance of behavior problems, such as conduct problems and drug abuse. BSFT specifically targets those family structures (e.g., patterns of interaction) that have been shown in the research literature to be predictors of drug abuse and related antisocial behaviors (cf. Szapocznik & Coatsworth, 1999).

Strategy

The third fundamental concept of BSFT, strategy, is defined by interventions that are practical, problem-focused, and deliberate. Practical interventions are selected for their likelihood to move the family toward desired objectives. For example, a therapist can choose to emphasize one aspect of a family's reality (e.g., that a drug-abusing youth is in pain) as a way to foster a parent–child connection, or another aspect (e.g., "this youth could get killed or overdose at any moment") as a way to heighten the parent(s)' sense of urgency. This pragmatically constructed reframing is done in lieu of portraying the entire reality of a situation. Such a practical selective focus is done, in part, in an effort to create movement outside or beyond the family's habitual and maladaptive patterns of interaction.

The problem-focused aspect of BSFT refers to targeting family interaction patterns that are the most directly relevant to the symptomatic behavior. Although families with behavior problem youth usually have multiple problems, targeting only those patterns of interactions linked to the development and maintenance of the symptomatic behavior contributes to the brevity of the intervention. For example, a couple's ability to parent is likely to be targeted because of its direct link to problem behaviors. However, the couple's sexual problems in their marital relationship might not be targeted in this brief therapy model. As such, intervention strategies are deliberate and are specifically intended to help the family shift from one set of interactions that maintain symptomatic behaviors in the youth (e.g., conflicted parent–child relationship) to another set of interactions that will reduce symptomatic behaviors (e.g., more effective parental monitoring and supervision).

CHARACTERISTICS OF THE TREATMENT PROGRAM

Treatment Population

BSFT has been implemented in research settings with a variety of populations. Client families are generally of low to moderate income, and the target youth is generally between 6 and 18 years of age. In studies of younger children, presenting problems have included behavioral disturbances at home or in school; in studies of adolescents, the list of presenting problems tends to include more serious delinquent behavior, along with alcohol, marijuana, and other drug use. Early research on BSFT was conducted at a time that the Hispanic population in Miami was almost exclusively of Cuban origin (e.g., Szapocznik, Rio, et al., 1989). In more recent studies, however (e.g., Santisteban et al., 1997; Santisteban, Muir-Malcolm, Mitrani, & Szapocznik, 2002), families have been from more varied ethnic backgrounds, including Nicaraguans, Colombians, Hondurans, and Puerto Ricans.

Goals and Main Themes of the Treatment Program

BSFT is predicated on several key assumptions: (1) changing the family is the most effective way of changing an individual, (2) changing an individual and then returning him or her to a detrimental or negative environment does not allow the individual changes to remain in place, and (3) changes in one central or powerful individual can result in changes in the rest of his or her family. For both individual and family change to be successful and maintained over time, BSFT proposes a treatment model that simultaneously addresses both domains. Therefore, BSFT focuses on changing individual behavior and experiences in a contextual frame (i.e., the family). Table 23.1 lists the specific change goals targeted in BSFT.

TABLE 23.1. Change Goals of BSFT

Structural level	Specific goals
Family	Increased parental figures' involvement with one another and improved balance of involvement of the parent figures with the child
	Improved effective parenting, including successful management of children's behavior
	Improved family cohesiveness, collaboration, and affect and reduced family negativity
	Improved "appropriate" bonding between children and parents
	Improved family communication, conflict resolution, and problem-solving skills
	Correct assignment and effective performance of the roles and responsibilities of the family
Individual child/adolescent	Reduced behavior problems
	Improved self-control
	Reduced associations with antisocial peers
	Reduced substance use
	Development of prosocial behaviors
	Bonding to family
	Good school attendance, conduct, and achievement

Who Is Seen and in What Format

BSFT sessions typically take place once a week for approximately 8–12 weeks. Sessions may occur more frequently around crises times because these are opportune moments for change. Sessions run 1 to 1½ hours. BSFT can be implemented in a variety of settings, including community social services agencies, mental health clinics, health agencies, and family clinics.

BSFT involves the whole family in treatment. BSFT engagement interventions (see later) are used for treatment-resistant families or family members. Services can be provided in the office or at the family's home.

Content of the Treatment; Sequence of Therapy Sessions

BSFT is a structured, problem-focused, directive, and practical approach. As such, BSFT follows a prescribed process format. However, the family process format is flexible in that it is adapted to the content of each family's central concerns.

The first step in BSFT—joining—is to establish a therapeutic alliance with each family member and with the family as a whole. This requires that the counselor accept and respect not only each individual family member in his or her behavior but also the way in which the family as a whole is organized. Interventions track individual family members' beliefs and emotions but are delivered with sensitivity to the processes that the family presents early in treatment.

Steps 2–5—diagnosis—involve diagnosing family strengths and weaknesses and developing a treatment plan. Step 2 involves identifying the symptom and the family relations surrounding it. This is done by encouraging and permitting the family to behave as it would usually behave if the counselor were not present. That is, encouraging family members to speak with each other about the concerns that bring them to therapy (in contrast to encouraging family members to tell the counselor their concerns). When family members speak with each other, they are likely to do so in their usual way of behaving/relating.

From the observations in step 2, the therapist is able to proceed with steps 3 and 4—diagnosis of both family strengths and problematic relations. Emphasis is placed on those family's problematic relations that are linked to the youth's problem behaviors, or that interfere with the parents' (or parent figures') ability to correct the youth's problem behaviors. For example, family members may not speak directly with each other, or when they speak their communications may be vague so that it would be difficult for other family members to know exactly what is being requested. Other examples of family problem relations that are assessed include alliances of one parent or parent figure with the problem youth against another parent or parent figure; appropriate involvement of parent figures with the problem youth; effective and ineffective conflict resolution styles (conflict denial, avoidance, diffusion, discussion, and resolution); extent to which family problems are perceived as shared versus lodged in a single individual (e.g., child may misbehave, but mother may be depressed, thereby interfering with her effective behavior management); and developmental appropriateness of family roles (Do children have too much or too little responsibility?; Do parents abdicate parental responsibility?).

Step 5 is to develop a treatment plan that systematically addresses the problems that are directly linked to the youth's problem behaviors. The treatment plan is strategic in that the most relevant problems that are identified in step 4 are the primary targets of intervention. In addition, the treatment plan strategically addresses problems that are relatively easier to change in early sessions to create positive therapeutic experiences for family members. All interventions are planned to capitalize on each family's and individual family member's unique strengths, identified in step 3.

Step 6—restructuring—involves the implementation of those change strategies needed to transform family relations from problematic to effective and mutually supportive. In this work the therapist is planful, problem-focused, direction-oriented (i.e., from problematic to competent interactions), and practical. Change strategies used include transforming the meaning of interactions through cognitive restructuring interventions called reframes. Reframes are intended to modify the negative affect of frustrating family interactions into more positive affect that improves communication and increases competence. Other change interventions include (1) directing, redirecting, or blocking communication; (2) shifting family alliances; (3) placing parents in charge; (4) helping families to develop conflict resolution skills; (5) developing effective behavior management skills; and (6) fostering parenting and parental leadership skills. For example, in the case of a family in which the mother is enmeshed (overinvolved) with the adolescent and disengaged from the father, the therapist might ask the mother and father to discuss disciplinary issues. When the adolescent tries to interfere in the discussion (which typically occurs in this type of family), the therapist might react with a statement such as, "Juan, wait. You will have your turn to speak. It is really important for Mom and Dad to have a chance now to talk about these important things." This sort of therapist intervention blocks the adolescent's interference in the parent dyad, and provides the mother and father with the opportunity to interact directly. During these interactions, maladaptive behaviors like blaming can be corrected by the therapist. When blaming is stopped or transformed by reframing in a positive light, parents are able to complete a discussion and/or make important decisions together.

EVIDENCE FOR THE EFFECTS OF TREATMENT

A systematic program of research has documented the positive impact of BSFT with behavior problem children and adolescents, including reductions in conduct problems, association with antisocial peers and drug use, and improvements in family functioning.
Studies have also provided evidence for the effectiveness of specialized engagement
strategies in increasing rates of engagement and retention of families seeking treatment
and in working with one family member to change family interactions and achieve successful treatment outcomes. This program of research has included youth from across the
age range: children (ages 6–11), early adolescents (12–14), and adolescents (13–18).

Children

With children, the predominant presenting complaint at our Center has been behavior
problems such as acting out, aggression in the company of peers, and attention difficulties. The goal of BSFT with this group of youth is to modify those family interactions
that are linked to the youth's current conduct problems. Modification of these patterns
of interaction is desired for two reasons: (1) to reduce current conduct and family problems and (2) to decrease the youth's risk for developing more serious problems (e.g., drug
abuse) during adolescence.

In a study examining the efficacy of BSFT with children (Szapocznik, Rio, et al.,
1989), 69 Hispanic behavior problem 6- to 11-year-old boys were randomly assigned to
one of three treatment conditions: (1) BSFT, (2) individual psychodynamic child-centered
psychotherapy, and (3) a recreational control condition. Individual psychodynamic child
therapy (Adams, 1974; Cooper & Wanerman, 1977) was chosen because it was the treatment of choice for therapists who worked with emotionally and behaviorally troubled
Hispanic children in the Miami area. The recreational control condition was comprised of
structured recreational activities and was used to control for attention placebo effects. Rigorous observational measures revealed that therapists adhered to their respective treatment conditions and that the treatments were significantly different from each other.

The results of this study revealed several important findings. First, the recreational
control condition was significantly less effective in retaining cases than the two treatment
conditions, with over two-thirds of all dropouts occurring in the control condition. Second, both BSFT and individual psychodynamic child therapy were more effective than
the recreational control group in reducing behavior problems (parent- and child reports)
as well as improving child psychodynamic functioning. However, no significant differences between the two intervention groups were observed on these variables. Third,
BSFT was significantly more effective than individual child psychodynamic therapy in
protecting family functioning at the 1-year follow-up (see Figure 23.1). In particular, in
the individual psychodynamic child therapy condition, a significant deterioration of family functioning was observed at the 1-year posttermination follow-up. In contrast, a significant improvement in family functioning at the 1-year follow-up was observed in
BSFT. These findings provided support for assumption that changing family processes
help to sustain treatment gains over time.

Early Adolescents

In our clinical work with early adolescent populations, we have found that the primary presenting problems are mild to moderate behavior problems at home or at school (e.g., disci-

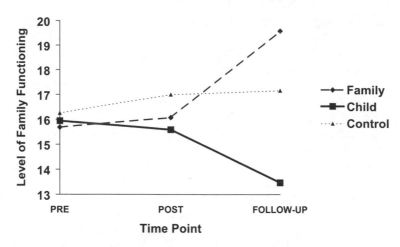

FIGURE 23.1. Comparison of family functioning at pretest, posttest, and 1-year follow-up for youth assigned to BSFT, individual child therapy, and recreational control group. From Szapocznik, Rio, et al. (1989). Copyright 1989 by the American Psychological Association. Reprinted by permission.

pline and fighting). Thus, the targets of BSFT with early-adolescent populations are similar to the targets with children. However, the intervention targets that are identified and the strategies implemented are adjusted to the developmental needs of early adolescence.

In a study conducted by Santisteban et al. (1997), data from 122 early adolescents (ages 12–14) who received BSFT and for whom all outcome data were available were examined to evaluate the impact of BSFT on reducing existing behavior problems and preventing future drug use. Although this study used only a one-group design rather than a more desirable comparison/control condition design, its results were consistent with the larger body of research findings on BSFT. For example, results suggested that BSFT was associated with reductions in both conduct problems and socialized aggression, and with improvements in family functioning. Further, reductions in conduct disorder and socialized aggression were associated with decreased likelihood of initiating substance use at a 9-month follow-up. An additional finding with respect to drug use was that, for those youth who had already initiated drug use at intake, overall substance use was significantly decreased between intake and termination.

Adolescents

Clinical work with adolescents (ages 12–18) typically involves addressing more serious delinquent behavior, drug use, and association with deviant peer networks, as well as behavior problems and family problems. In a clinical trial study, Santisteban, Coatsworth, et al. (2002) randomly assigned 126 Hispanic adolescents with externalizing problems (e.g., violent or disruptive behavior, drug use, and trouble with police) and their families to BSFT or a group-control condition. The group control condition was a participatory-learning group intervention in which adolescents were encouraged to discuss and solve problems among themselves with the guidance and help of a facilitator. The role of the group facilitator involved encouraging group cohesion, disseminating information regarding the detrimental effects of criminality and drug use, and maintaining a therapeutic atmosphere with regard to addressing problematic events in the group members' lives.

Adolescent participants in the study ranged in age from 12 to 18, with 87% between the ages of 13 and 17 ($M = 15.6$ years). 77% of the adolescent participants were male. Rigorous adherence procedures demonstrated that therapists adhered to their respective treatment conditions, and that there was minimal overlap between the conditions. Consistent with this study's focus on behavior problems, at intake the majority of the sample (94%) scored in the clinical range on one or both of the two behavior problem scales from the Revised Behavior Problem Checklist (RBPC; Quay & Peterson, 1987): Conduct Disorder (aggression and acting out) and Socialized Aggression (delinquency in the company of peers).

Of the original 126 participants, 79 adolescents and families completed treatment and were compared on pre–post change (BSFT = 52; group control = 27). Results indicated that adolescents in the BSFT condition showed significantly greater reductions in conduct disorder and socialized aggression than youth in the group-control condition. An analysis of clinically significant change was conducted on these two scales using the twofold criteria recommended by Jacobson and Traux (1991). The results of the analyses of clinical significance suggest that a substantially larger proportion of BSFT cases demonstrated clinically significant improvement (see Figure 23.2). While 39 of the 52 (75%) BSFT cases had clinical-level conduct disorder scores at intake, 18 (46%) of the 39 made reliable improvement and 2 (5%) showed reliable deterioration. In contrast, within the group control condition, only 2 (11%) of the 18 cases with clinical Conduct Disorder scores showed reliable change and both evidenced deterioration in functioning. With regard to Socialized Aggression, 42 (81%) BSFT cases and 18 (67%) group counseling cases were above clinical levels at intake. Of the clinical level cases at intake, 16 (38%) of BSFT cases showed reliable change, while only 2 (11%) did so in the group

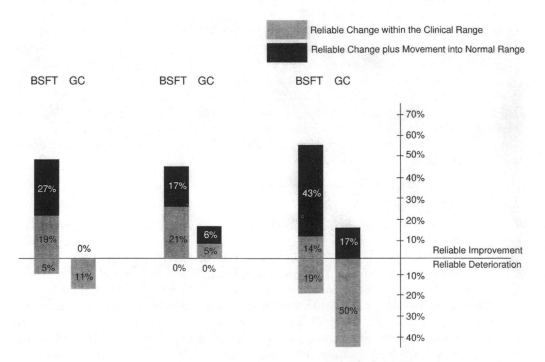

FIGURE 23.2. Reliable improvement or deterioration in conduct disorder, socialized aggression, and marijuana use for youth assigned to BSFT versus group counseling.

control condition. 7 (17%) BSFT cases recovered to nonclinical levels, while only 1 case (6%) from the group control condition recovered to nonclinical levels.

Analyses were also conducted to examine whether the interventions had a differential impact on alcohol and marijuana use, the two substances of choice at intake. Results indicated that BSFT was no more effective in reducing alcohol use than was the group control condition. However, BSFT was significantly more effective in reducing marijuana use than was the group control condition.

To investigate whether there were clinically meaningful changes in patterns of drug use, four use categories defined in the substance use literature were created (e.g., Brook et al., 1998; Tsuang et al., 1999). The categories are based on the number of days using marijuana in the 30 days prior to the intake and termination assessments: abstainer (0 days), weekly user (1–8 days), frequent user (9–16 days), and daily user (17 or more days). The analysis of clinically meaningful change in marijuana use showed that 16 participants in the BSFT condition, and 4 in the group control condition, changed categories. Of the 16 BSFT cases that showed change, 12 showed improvement and 4 showed deterioration. Of the 4 group control cases that showed change, 1 showed improvement and 3 showed deterioration. Adolescents who were not using at intake but started to use by termination were classified as deteriorators.

Exploration of the Role of Changes in Family Interactions in Reducing Behavior Problems

One of the most important products in the program of outcome research on BSFT has been the development of the Structural Family Systems Ratings (SFSR; Hervis, Szapocznik, Mitrani, Rio, & Kurtines, 1991; Szapocznik et al., 1991). This observational measure provides a means for identifying patterns of family interaction that are theoretically parallel to the clinical conceptualizations of BSFT therapists. The development and validation of this measure have made it possible to explore the presumed role of changes in family interactions in BSFT and to compare the effectiveness of BSFT to alternative interventions in bringing about improvements in family functioning.

One study in which the SFSR has been used involved examining the possibility that families entering the study with relatively "better" and "worse" family functioning could be responding differently to the family intervention. In this study, the Santisteban, Coatsworth, et al. (in press) sample was partitioned into two groups: "better baseline family functioning at intake" and "worse baseline family functioning at intake" based on a median split. Examination of the patterns of change (see Figure 23.3) show that for families classified as "worse baseline family functioning," BSFT cases demonstrated significantly greater pre- to-posttreatment improvement in family functioning compared to group therapy cases. In particular, BSFT cases showed significant improvements in family functioning, whereas group cases shown no improvement. A different picture emerged for the "better family functioning" group. For this group, there was also a significant condition × time interaction. However, analyses demonstrated that BSFT cases showed no significant change in family functioning, whereas group therapy cases showed a statistically significant deterioration in family functioning.

BSFT with Specialized Engagement Strategies

Previous research has demonstrated that a large proportion of families that seek treatment for drug-abusing adolescents are never engaged in therapy (cf. Szapocznik et al.,

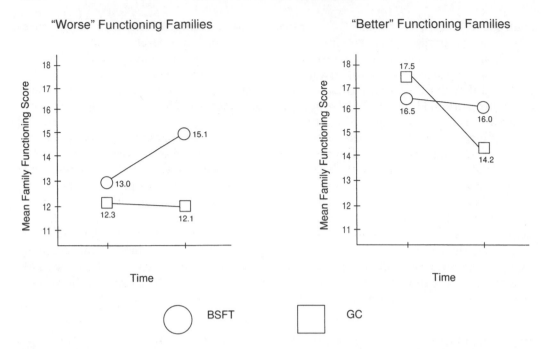

FIGURE 23.3. Changes in family functioning (SFSR) for family therapy and control conditions by intake levels of family functioning.

1988). In response to this problem, a set of specialized engagement procedures was developed (Szapocznik, Perez-Vidal, Hervis, Brickman & Kurtines, 1990; Szapocznik & Kurtines, 1989). Based on BSFT principles, this approach conceptualizes treatment "resistance" as interactional; therefore, failure to engage in therapy is best understood by identifying the same maladaptive family interaction patterns that also maintain the symptom in the family. As a result, BSFT includes specialized engagement strategies designed to modify these maladaptive interactions and bring the family into treatment. Examples of engagement strategies include allying with the adolescent (if the adolescent is the primary source of the "resistance") or asking the mother (or whoever else makes the initial call) for permission to talk to the most "resistant" family member.

The effectiveness of these procedures, BSFT–engagement, has been tested in three separate studies (Coatsworth, Santisteban, McBride, & Szapocznik, 2001; Santisteban et al., 1996; Szapocznik et al., 1988). In the first study (Szapocznik et al., 1988), 108 Hispanic families with behavior problem adolescents (who were suspected of, or were observed, using drugs) were randomly assigned to one of two conditions: Engagement as usual (i.e., the control condition) and BSFT–engagement (i.e., the experimental condition). Once engaged in treatment, all youth received BSFT. In the engagement-as-usual condition, client families were approached in a way that resembled as closely as possible the kind of engagement that usually takes place in outpatient centers (determined by a survey of community agency responses to a parent's call for help with a drug-abusing adolescent). In the experimental condition, client families were engaged using specialized engagement techniques developed to overcome the family patterns of interactions that interfered with engagement in family therapy treatment. Engagement was defined as the conjoint family (minimally the identified patient and his or her parents and siblings living in the same household) coming into the office—usually the first visit was for an intake assessment.

Treatment integrity guidelines and checklists were developed for both conditions, and six levels of engagement effort were identified (see Szapocznik et al., 1988, for details). Treatment integrity analyses revealed that interventions in both conditions adhered to guidelines and that the two conditions were clearly distinguishable by the level of engagement effort applied.

The effectiveness of BSFT–engagement module was measured using two criteria: (1) engaging client families to attend the intake session, and (2) retaining the client families to the completion of treatment. The results of the study revealed that 42% of the families in the engagement-as-usual condition were successfully engaged into treatment. In contrast, 93% of the families in the BSFT–engagement condition were engaged into treatment. Of the engaged cases, 59% (13) of the engagement-as-usual condition versus 83% (43) of the BSFT–engagement condition completed treatment. Thus, in the intent to treat analyses conducted for those randomized into the study, 25% (of the 52) in the engagement-as-usual condition and 77% (of the 56) in the BSFT–engagement condition were successfully terminated.

The second study (Santisteban et al., 1996) was a replication of the previous engagement study, and it explored factors that might moderate the effectiveness of the engagement intervention. In contrast to the previous engagement study, Santisteban et al. (1996) more stringently defined the success of engagement in terms of client families that attended the intake session *and* the first therapy session (i.e., minimally two office visits). Participants were 193 Cuban Hispanic and non-Cuban Hispanic families were randomly assigned to one experimental and two control conditions. The experimental condition was BSFT–engagement whereas the control conditions were BSFT with engagement as usual and group counseling with engagement as usual. Engagement as usual involved no specialized engagement strategies.

In the BSFT–engagement condition, 81% of the families (42 of 52) were successfully engaged, whereas in the two engagement control conditions combined, 60% (84 of 141) of the families were successfully engaged. The overall rates of this study appear lower than those of the previous study due to the more stringent criteria for engagement. However, when the less stringent criterion for engagement (i.e., attending intake) from the previous Szapocznik et al. (1988) study were used to compare the BSFT–engagement conditions from both studies there were no significant differences between the two experimental conditions on the rates of engagement.

A second major finding of the replication study was that the effectiveness of BSFT–engagement procedures was moderated by the type of Hispanic cultural/ethnic identity. Among the non-Cuban Hispanics (composed primarily of Nicaraguan families as well as Colombian, Puerto Rican, Peruvian, and Mexican families) assigned to the BSFT–engagement condition, the rate of engagement was high (93%) compared to the lower rate of the Cuban Hispanic sample assigned to the BSFT–engagement condition (64%). This differential finding is of particular interest because the majority of participants in the first study were Cuban. More recent findings (Mitrani et al., 2002) suggest that increasing levels of disengagement in more acculturated Cuban families may have been responsible for the lower rates of engagement with more acculturated Cubans in the second study. The results of the clinical analysis of engagement failures, strongly support the idea that therapeutic interventions must be responsive to the constantly evolving population–contextual conditions (Szapocznik & Kurtines, 1993).

A third study (Coatsworth et al., 2001) tested the ability of BSFT to engage and retain adolescents and their families, when compared to a community control condition. In this study, BSFT had been modified to fully incorporate the engagement module, as it is currently used. An important aspect of this study was that the control condition—community control—was not developed and implemented by the investigators. As such, the control intervention (e.g., usual engagement strategies) was less subject to the influence of the investigators. Findings in this study, as in previous studies, showed that BSFT was significantly more successful in engaging cases (43/53; 81%) than the community control (31/51; 61%). Likewise, among those engaged, a higher percentage of BSFT cases (31/43; 71%) retained compared to the community control (13/31; 42%). In the BSFT condition 58% of randomized cases completed treatment (31 of 53) compared to 25% (13 of 51) in the community control condition. A risk-ratio analysis revealed that families randomized into BSFT were 2.3 times more likely *both* to engage and to retain than families randomized to community control.

An interesting moderator emerged in the analyses. In the BSFT condition, families of children who showed more severe conduct problem scores were more likely to remain in treatment than were families of children whose conduct problem scores were less severe. The opposite pattern was evident in the community comparison condition, with families that retained in treatment showing *lower* intake levels of conduct problems scores than families that dropped out. These findings are particularly important because they suggest that youth who are most in need of services are more likely to stay in BSFT than in traditional community treatments.

Working with One Family Member

Recognizing that therapists are not always successful in engaging family members into treatment, our center has developed a procedure that is able to achieve the goals of BSFT (changes in maladaptive family interactions and symptomatic adolescent behavior) without requiring the whole family to be present in treatment. This approach, one-person BSFT (Szapocznik, Foote, Perez-Vidal, Hervis, & Kurtines, 1985; Szapocznik & Kurtines, 1989; Szapocznik, Kurtines, Perez-Vidal, Hervis, & Foote, 1990), capitalizes on the systemic concept of complementarity, which suggests that when one family member changes, the rest of the system responds by either restoring the family process to its old ways or adapting to the new changes (Minuchin & Fishman, 1981). One-person BSFT operates similarly to conjoint (traditional) BSFT in that family interactional patterns are the focus of treatment. The therapist focuses exclusively on family interactions and not on the individual adolescent. The goal of one-person BSFT is to change the drug-abusing adolescent's participation in maladaptive family interactions that include him or her. These changes often create a family crisis as the family attempts to return to its old ways. We use the opportunity created by crises to engage reluctant family members.

A major clinical trial was conducted to compare the efficacy of one-person BSFT to conjoint BSFT (Szapocznik, Kurtines, Foote, Perez-Vidal, & Hervis, 1983, 1986). An experimental design was achieved by randomly assigning 72 Hispanic families with a drug-abusing 12–17-year-old adolescent to the one-person or conjoint BSFT modalities. Both conditions were designed to use exactly the same BSFT theory, so that only one variable (one person vs. conjoint meetings) would differ between the conditions. The most significant difference was that the one-person condition was restricted to fewer than two conjoint sessions and the conjoint condition was restricted to fewer than two individual sessions. Analyses of treatment integrity revealed that interventions in both conditions adhered to guidelines, and that the two conditions were clearly distinguishable. The results showed that one-person was as efficacious as conjoint BSFT in significantly reducing youth drug use and behavior problems as well as improving family functioning (Szapocznik et al., 1983, Szapocznik, Kurtines, et al., 1986). When juxtaposed with the findings of our research cited earlier (Szapocznik, Rio, et al., 1989), these findings suggest that an individual modality, conceptualized in family terms (Szapocznik et al., 1983, Szapocznik, Kurtines, et al., 1986), can bring about improvements in family functioning, whereas an individual modality conceptualized in individual terms (Szapocznik, Rio, et al., 1989) can result in deterioration of family functioning.

DIRECTIONS FOR FUTURE RESEARCH

The aforementioned studies occurred as the clinical research team at the Spanish Family Guidance Center/Center for Family Studies responded to the most salient challenges encountered by the Hispanic community in Miami. The findings of each study contributed significantly to refinements of the clinical model, including the development and validation of an entire module (e.g., engagement strategies). At present, research on BSFT is focused on three areas: effectiveness research, process research, and expanding the intervention to target the adolescent's social ecology.

Effectiveness Research

As is the case throughout the mental health and drug abuse field, there is a substantial gap between the interventions validated in research studies and the interventions implemented in community settings. Thus, the next critical step in our program of research is test the effectiveness of BSFT in community treatment sites and to establish a mechanism to train BSFT on a large scale. To facilitate effectiveness trials and the dissemination of BSFT, the Center for Family Studies has established a Training Institute. One of the first products of the Training Institute was the completion of an updated version of the *BSFT Manual* (Szapocznik, Hervis, & Schwartz, 2002). The revised manual presents BSFT with the most recent clinical developments supported by efficacy findings and was written specifically for clinicians in community treatment settings as opposed to clinicians on clinical trials. The treatment manual will be available from the authors, or from the National Institute on Drug Abuse (*www.nida.nih.gov*) beginning in the summer of 2002. The Training Institute is currently involved in training therapists from community agencies across the country. The training process has been standardized and includes a didactic/interactive power point presentation, review of videotapes, and review/supervision of active cases. The Training Institute is also in the process of developing procedures for credentialing therapists. This process will have specific guidelines for monitoring fidelity and competence. The next wave of studies currently in the initial steps of review will examine the effectiveness of BSFT when carried out in community settings. This work would be carried out through National Institute on Drug Abuse's Clinical Trials Network, in which the Center for Family Studies leads a node.

Process Research

A second area of ongoing and future research studies involves examining the clinical interior of BSFT to identify processes that are related to successful and unsuccessful outcomes. Process studies are fundamental in model development and therapist training, and the results of these studies are immediately applicable to practicing clinicians. The rich theoretical base about the change process as well as the detailed definitions and examples contained in the treatment manual about joining, diagnosing, and restructuring family interactions provide a solid foundation for the design and implementation of process studies. Moreover, the Center for Family Studies has maintained a videotape library that contains thousands of tapes of therapy sessions collected as part of several clinical research studies. This database provides a unique opportunity for linking in-session processes to treatment outcomes. Currently, a process study is under way that is focused on identifying aspects of BSFT that may be related to retention in treatment. This "state-of-the-science" study examines videotapes of therapy sessions to identify therapeutic processes that predict retention in family therapy. Specifically, this study examines the therapist role as a change agent in family therapy by examining interventions that have an impact on family members' behaviors presumed to be directly related to retention in treatment. Two specific processes are examined: therapeutic alliance and within-family negativity. Future research studies are planned for linking changes over the course of treatment to changes in behavior problems.

Expanding BSFT to Target the Adolescent's Social Ecology

Research identifying multicausal pathways in the development of adolescent behavior problems (Dishion, French, & Patterson, 1995; Hawkins, Catalano, & Miller, 1992) and our own clinical work with adolescents with severe disruptive behavior disorders has led us to develop and test an ecological version of BSFT. In this BSFT–ecological version, increased recognition of the critical role of peers in the development and maintenance of antisocial behavior has required interventions that strategically target relationships that directly and indirectly influence the adolescent's peer relationships. This expansion into the family ecosystem is consistent with BSFT theory, which explicitly recognizes that the family itself is part of a larger social system and—as a child is influenced by his or her family—the family is influenced by the larger social system in which it exists. However, in this intervention, structural ecosystems therapy (the proper name of BSFT–ecological), the basic principles that have guided BSFT to modify within-family interactions have been systematically articulated to target interactions in other social ecological contexts.

The ecological framework for structural ecosystems therapy is based on the theoretical work of Urie Bronfenbrenner (1977, 1979, 1986). Consistent with Bronfenbrenner's organization of the social ecology of the adolescent, interventions focus on four levels of systems that affect youth's developmental trajectories: microsystems, mesosystems, exosystems, and macrosystems. *Microsystems* refer to systems that include the youth directly. The most prominent of these systems for youth with behavior problems, and which our intervention emphasizes, are the family, peer, school, and juvenile justice systems. *Mesosystems* are created from the relationship between the microsystems that contain the youth. In structural ecosystems therapy, the primary mesosystemic relationships involve parents' interactions with the youth's peer, school, and justice systems. *Exosystems* are those systems that include a member of a microsystem but not the target youth directly. Examples of exosystems are a gang to which a peer member may belong or the social support network of a parent. These exosystems, through their impact on the peer and the parent, respectively, may have an indirect impact on the target youth *Macrosystems* are defined by the large social forces and systems that have broad impact, such as the law; as well as by the cultural blueprints that pervade a family's social environment, such as the belief that parents are less valuable to society because they do not speak English.

In an ongoing clinical trial study, 190 African American and Hispanic adolescents and their families were randomized to one of three conditions. The experimental condition—structural ecosystems therapy—is compared to two controls: BSFT, restricted to within family, and community referral control. The experimental condition expands the use of BSFT's structural diagnostic approach to the adolescent's social ecology including family, family–school, family–peer, family–juvenile justice, and parent support systems. The experimental condition also extends the use of BSFT techniques of joining, diagnosis, and restructuring to their application in systems other than the family. Thus, in working with the family–school subsystem, for example, the therapist joins both the family and the school representatives, and restructures the interactions between them.

SUMMARY AND CONCLUSIONS

The primary goal of the Spanish Family Guidance Center/Center for Family Studies in the University of Miami Center for Family Studies has been to identify and develop a culturally appropriate intervention for Hispanic youth with behavior problems. BSFT continues to be adapted through a program of research that involves the rigorous and continuous interplay among theory, research, and application.

As a family intervention, the focus of BSFT is not the child or adolescent but the entire family system. A central tenet of BSFT is that problematic family interactions play a key role in the evolution and maintenance of behavior problems. The strategic, problem-focused aspect of BSFT refers to targeting those maladaptive family interaction patterns that are the most directly relevant to the symptomatic behavior.

BSFT was developed from within a Hispanic perspective and recognizes the influence of cultural factors in the development and maintenance of behavior problems. BSFT was first used to target specific problematic interactions that developed as a result of differential rates of acculturation between parents and youth, as well as generic maladaptive patterns of family interactions. Our training of clinicians pays specific attention to Hispanic-specific family processes. We have, for example, described how characteristics of Hispanic families affect their functioning along structural family dimensions (Santisteban, Muir-Malcolm, et al., 2002; Santisteban & Mitrani, 2003). In addition, we have developed BSFT-based interventions, not presented here, that use bicultural Hispanic/American contents (cf. Szapocznik, Santisteban, et al., 1986; Szapocznik, Santisteban, Rio, Perez-Vidal, & Kurtines, 1989).

Research on the efficacy of BSFT or of specific BSFT modules has documented the positive impact of BSFT with behavior problem children, early adolescents, and adolescents, including reductions in conduct problems, delinquency, and drug use and improvements in family functioning. In addition to the immediate impact on behavior problems, BSFT has been shown to reduce variables that increase the likelihood of initiation and maintenance of substance abuse.

Six of these studies reported findings from randomized trials. Two of these studies, one with children and one with adolescents, compared BSFT to a different modality. The child study compared BSFT to an individual child psychodynamic condition, whereas the adolescent study compared BSFT to a group counseling modality. In each case the comparison modality was selected because it was widely used in our community with that specific population at the time of the study. One study investigated a one-person version of BSFT. Three of these studies have provided evidence for the effectiveness of specialized engagement strategies in increasing rates of engagement and retention of families seeking treatment. The initial study of BSFT–engagement and its replication used a laboratory-run control condition. In contrast, the third study used a real community setting control for engagement.

One of the most important products in the program of BSFT research has been the development of the SFSR (Hervis et al., 1991). The development and validation (Szapocznik et al., 1991) of this measure made it possible to assess the efficacy of the BSFT interventions on repetitive maladaptive patterns of family interaction measured along structural domains.

Present and future research are focused on BSFT effectiveness, processes, and an expanded ecological version of BSFT. Because of the gap between interventions validated in university laboratories and the interventions implemented in community settings, the next logical step in BSFT research is to conduct effectiveness trials in community settings, an effort that is currently in its early stages. To make this possible and to disseminate BSFT to other sites, a Training Institute was established and a brief *BSFT Manual* (Szapocznik et al., 2002) was published by the National Institute on Drug Abuse. A system for credentialing BSFT therapists is under development that will include techniques for assessing therapist competence and treatment fidelity. A second area of ongoing and future research studies involves examining the inner clinical workings of BSFT to identify processes that are related to successful and unsuccessful outcomes. Other current expansions of the BSFT research program include the development and testing of an ecosystemic version of BSFT for African American and Hispanic drug-abusing adolescents.

REFERENCES

Adams, P. L. (1974). *A primer of child psychotherapy.* Boston: Little, Brown.

Bronfenbrenner, U. (1977). Toward an experimental ecology of human development. *American Psychologist, 32,* 513–531.

Bronfenbrenner, U. (1979). Contexts of child rearing: Problems and prospects. *American Psychologist, 34,* 844–850.

Bronfenbrenner, U. (1986). Ecology of the family as a context for human development: Research perspectives. *Developmental Psychology, 22,* 723–742.

Brook, J. S., Brook, D. W., de la Rosa, M., Duque, L. F., Rodriguez, E., Montoya, I. D., & Whiteman, M. (1998). Pathways to marijuana use among adolescents: Cultural/ecological, family, peer, and personality influences. *Journal of the American Academy of Child and Adolescent Psychiatry, 37,* 759–766.

Centers for Disease Control and Prevention. (2001). *HIV/AIDS among Hispanics in the United States.* Atlanta, GA: CDC-P Division of HIV/AIDS Prevention.

Coatsworth, J. D., Santisteban, D. A., McBride, C. K., & Szapocznik, J. (2001). Brief strategic family therapy versus community control: Engagement, retention, and an exploration of the moderating role of adolescent symptom severity. *Family Process, 40,* 313–332.

Cooper, S., & Wanerman, C. (1977). *Children in treatment.* New York: Brunner/Mazel.

Dishion, T. J., French, D. C., & Patterson, G. R. (1995). The development and ecology of antisocial behavior. In D. Cicchetti & D. J. Cohen (Eds.), *Developmental psychopathology, vol. 2: Risk, disorder, and adaptation. Wiley series on personality processes* (pp. 421–471). New York: Wiley.

Fuligni, A. J. (1997). The academic achievement of adolescents from immigrant families: The roles of family background, attitudes, and behavior. *Child Development, 68,* 351–363.

Haley, J. (1976). *Problem solving therapy.* San Francisco: Jossey-Bass.

Hawkins, J. D., Catalano, R. F., & Miller, J. Y. (1992). Risk and protective factors for alcohol and other drug problems in adolescence and early adulthood: Implications for substance abuse prevention. *Psychological Bulletin, 112,* 64–105.

Hervis, O. E., Szapocznik, J., Mitrani, V. B., Rio, A. T., & Kurtines, W. M. (1991). *Structural family systems rating: A revised manual* [Technical report]. Spanish Family Guidance Center, Department of Psychiatry, University of Miami School of Medicine, Miami, FL.

Jacobson, A., & Traux, P. (1991). Clinical significance: A statistical approach to defining meaningful change in psychotherapy research. *Journal of Consulting and Clinical Psychology, 59,* 12–19.

Madanes, C. (1981). *Strategic family therapy.* San Francisco: Jossey-Bass.

Minuchin, S. (1974). *Families and family therapy.* Cambridge, MA: Harvard University Press.

Minuchin, S., & Fishman, H. C. (1981). *Family therapy techniques.* Cambridge, MA: Harvard University Press.

Minuchin, S., Rosman, B. L., & Baker, L. (1978). *Psychosomatic families: Anorexia nervosa in context.* Cambridge, MA: Harvard University Press.

Mitrani, V. B., Schwartz, S. J., Santisteban, D. A., Robbins, M. S., Perez-Vidal, A., & Szapocznik, J. (2002). *The role of family functioning in family therapy outcomes among Hispanic behavior-problem adolescents.* Unpublished manuscript.

Quay, H. C., & Peterson, D. R. (1987). *Manual for the Revised Behavior Problem Checklist.* (Available from H.C. Quay, Department of Psychology, P. O. Box 248185, University of Miami, Coral Gables, Florida.)

Santisteban, D. A., Coatsworth, D., Perez-Vidal, A., Kurtines, W. M., Schwartz, S. J., & Szapocznik, J. (in press). The efficacy of brief strategic family therapy in modifying adolescent behavior problems and substance use. *Journal of Family Psychology.*

Santisteban, D. A., Coatsworth, D., Perez-Vidal, A., Mitrani, V., Jean-Gilles, M., & Szapocznik, J. (1997). Brief structural/strategic family therapy with African American and Hispanic youth. *Journal of Community Psychology, 25,* 453–471.

Santisteban, D., & Mitrani, V. B. (2002). The influence of acculturation processes on the family. In K. M. Chun, P. B. Organista, & G. Marín (Eds.), *Acculturation: Advances in the theory, measurement, and applied research.* Washington, DC: American Psychological Association.

Santisteban, D. A., Muir-Malcolm, J. A., Mitrani, V. B., & Szapocznik, J. (2002). Integrating the study of ethnic culture and family psychology intervention science. In H. A. Liddle & D. A. Santisteban (Eds.), *Family psychology: Science based interventions* (pp. 331–351). Washington, DC: American Psychological Association.

Santisteban, D. A., Szapocznik, J., Perez-Vidal, A., Kurtines, W. M., Murray, E. J., & LaPerriere, A. (1996). Efficacy of intervention for engaging youth and families into treatment and some variables that may contribute to differential effectiveness. *Journal of Family Psychology, 10,* 35–44.

Substance Abuse and Mental Health Services Association. (2001). *1999 Monitoring the Future survey and results.* Washington, DC: Department of Health and Human Services.

Szapocznik, J., & Coatsworth, J. D. (1999). An ecodevelopmental framework for organizing the influences on drug abuse: A developmental model of risk and protection. In M. D. Glantz & C. R. Hartel (Eds.), *Drug abuse: Origins and interventions* (pp. 331–366). Washington, DC: American Psychological Association.

Szapocznik, J., Foote, F. H., Perez-Vidal, A., Hervis, O. E., & Kurtines, W. (1985). *One-person family therapy.* Coral Gables, FL: Miami World Health Organization.

Szapocznik, J., Hervis, O. E., & Schwartz, S. (2002). *Brief strategic family therapy for adolescent drug abuse.* Rockville, MD: National Institute on Drug Abuse.

Szapocznik, J., & Kurtines, W. M. (1989). *Breakthroughs in family therapy with drug abusing and problem youth.* New York: Springer.

Szapocznik, J., & Kurtines, W. (1993). Family psychology and cultural diversity: Opportunities for theory, research and application. *American Psychologist, 48,* 400–407.

Szapocznik, J., Kurtines, W., Foote, F., Perez-Vidal, A., & Hervis, O. (1983). Conjoint versus one person family therapy: Some evidence for the effectiveness of conducting family therapy through one person. *Journal of Consulting and Clinical Psychology, 51,* 889–899.

Szapocznik, J., Kurtines, W. M., Foote, F., Perez-Vidal, A., & Hervis, O. (1986). Conjoint versus one-person family therapy: Further evidence for the effectiveness of conducting family therapy through one person. *Journal of Consulting and Clinical Psychology, 54,* 395–397.

Szapocznik, J., Kurtines, W., Perez-Vidal, A., Hervis, O., & Foote, F. (1990). One-person family therapy. In R. Wells & V. Giannetti (Eds.), *Handbook of brief psychotherapies: Applied clinical psychology* (pp. 493–510). New York: Plenum Press.

Szapocznik, J., Perez-Vidal, A., Brickman, A., Foote, F. H., Santisteban, D. A., Hervis, O. E., & Kurtines, W. M. (1988). Engaging adolescent drug abusers and their families in treatment: A strategic structural systems approach. *Journal of Consulting and Clinical Psychology, 56,* 552–557.

Szapocznik, J., Perez-Vidal, A., Hervis, O. E., Brickman, A., & Kurtines, W. (1990). Innovations in family therapy: Strategies for overcoming resistance to treatment. In R. A.Wells & V. J. Giannetti (Eds.), *Handbook of brief psychotherapies. Applied clinical psychology* (pp. 93–114). New York: Plenum Press.

Szapocznik, J., Rio, A. T., Hervis, O. E., Mitrani, V. B., Kurtines, W. M., & Faraci, A. M. (1991). Assessing change in family functioning as a result of treatment: The structural Family Rating Systems Scale (SFSR). *Journal of Marital and Family Therapy, 17,* 295–310.

Szapocznik, J., Rio, A. T., Murray, E., Cohen, R., Scopetta, M. A., Rivas-Vasquez, A., Hervis, O. E., & Posada, V. (1989). Structural family versus psychodynamic child therapy for problematic Hispanic boys. *Journal of Consulting and Clinical Psychology, 57,* 571–578.

Szapocznik, J., Santisteban, D., Rio, A., Perez-Vidal, A., & Kurtines, W. M. (1989). Family effectiveness training: An intervention to prevent drug abuse and problem behavior in Hispanic adolescents. *Hispanic Journal of Behavioral Sciences, 11,* 3–27.

Szapocznik, J., Santisteban, D., Rio, A., Perez-Vidal, A., Kurtines, W. M., & Hervis, O. E. (1986). Bicultural effectiveness training (BET): An intervention modality for families experiencing intergenerational/intercultural conflict. *Hispanic Journal of Behavioral Sciences, 6,* 303–330.

Szapocznik, J., Scopetta, M., & King, O. E. (1978). Theory and practice in matching treatment to the special characteristics and problems of Cuban immigrants. *Journal of Community Psychology, 6,* 112–122.

Szapocznik, J., & Williams, R. A. (2000). Brief strategic family therapy: Twenty-five years of interplay among theory, research and practice in adolescent behavior problems and drug abuse. *Clinical Child and Family Psychology Review, 3,* 117–135.

Tsuang, M. T., Lyons, M. J., Harley, R. M., Xian, H., Eisen, S., Goldberg, J., True, W. R., & Faraone, S .V. (1999). Genetic and environmental influences on transitions in drug use. *Behavior Genetics, 29,* 473–479.

24

Narrative Therapy for Hispanic Children and Adolescents

ROBERT G. MALGADY AND GIUSEPPE COSTANTINO

OVERVIEW

The need for mental health services that address the problems of high-risk behavior and increased substance abuse among ethnic minority children and adolescents is widely acknowledged in the early prevention and mental health treatment literature (e.g., Botvin & Malgady, 1998; Hatterer & Malgady, 2000; Rogler, Malgady, & Rodriguez, 1989). According to the National Comorbidity study (Kessler, McGonagle, & Zhao, 1994), Hispanic youth present the highest prevalence rates of depression and comorbid substance abuse relative to all other ethnic groups based on the Diagnostic Interview Schedule (Robins, Helzer, Croughan, & Ratcliff, 1981; Malgady, Rogler, & Tryon, 1992). Similarly, Vega, Zimmerman, Warheit, Apospori, and Gil (1993) found high prevalence rates of drug use among Hispanic adolescents. One study, with therapeutic implications, indicated that adherence to more traditional Hispanic cultural values was associated with lower risk of drug use among Hispanic youth (Pumariega, Swanson, Holzer, Linskey, & Qintero-Salinas, 1992).

Substance abuse and high-risk behavioral interventions have been empirically tested in treatment outcome research with large samples of minority youth, especially Hispanics, in school-based inner-city settings (Botvin, Baker, Dusenbury, Botvin, & Diaz, 1995; Botvin, Baker, Dusenbury, Tortu, & Botvin, 1990). Much of this research has involved the presentation of adaptive role models with whom Hispanic children and adolescents can readily identify, thus bridging the cultural distance they often reportedly experience when receiving mainstream health care services. Culturally competent mental health and treatment services have been made available by matching consumers with health care providers of the same ethnicity; by tailoring the theoretical orientation of services to Hispanic cultural values, beliefs, and mores (e.g., familism, spiritualism, and *respecto*); and by introducing ethnic and cultural narratives and imitative role play directly into the therapeutic process (Brizer, Costantino, & Malgady, 2001; Costantino, Malgady, & Rogler, 1986; Rogler, Malgady, Costantino, & Blumenthal, 1987).

This chapter describes evidence-based treatment outcome research on culturally competent narrative interventions for Hispanic children and adolescents. These studies consist of treatment services provided in clinical settings and among school-based populations.

CHARACTERISTICS OF THE TREATMENT PROGRAM

The treatments were developed as narrative therapies using cultural role modeling and presented through a videotaped modality. The narrative modalities were varied according to children's and adolescents' ages. For young children in kindergarten to third grade, *cuentos* (Puerto Rican folktales) were illustrated in pictures and stories about adaptive and maladaptive behavior, which were read aloud by therapists and the children's mothers. This process was videotaped and played back to the children and their mothers for role playing, which was reinforced verbally and with tokens. For young adolescents in grades eight and nine, treatments were designed to have an impact on high-risk indicators such as anxiety and depression symptomatology, acting-out behavior, ethnic identity, and self-esteem (e.g., Costantino, Malgady, & Rogler, 1986, 1994; Malgady, Rogler, & Costantino, 1990). Biographies of "heroic" role models were presented and discussed by therapists in conjunction with the adolescents' self-identification experiences; these interactions were videotaped and therapeutically discussed in small-group sessions. A similar intervention was developed for prevention of substance use and abuse among white, African American, and Hispanic youth, 15–25 years old. This intervention focused on the involvment of family members and significant others in the treatment process to enhance disclosure of behavior problems, drinking and substance abuse frequency, and likelihood of seeking treatment services (Brizer et al., 2001; Hatterer & Malgady, 2000; for related work, see also Szapocznik, Kurtines, & Santisteban, 1994).

HISPANICS AND MENTAL HEALTH

The growth rate of the Hispanic population in the United States is more than seven times that of any other ethnic population (U.S. Bureau of the Census, 1994), the largest concentrations being Mexican and Central Americans in the Southwest, Puerto Ricans and Dominicans in the Northeast, and Cubans in the Southeast. This has been attributed by demographers to high birth rates, youthful age distribution, (twice as many Hispanics under age 18 compared to non- Hispanic whites), and high levels of immigration (Mann & Salvo, 1985). For example, more Hispanics reside in New York City than in any other city in the United States, composing over one- quarter of the city's population (New York City Board of Education, 1993; New York City Department of City Planning, 1992). Recent reports in New York City, for example, portray the Hispanic population as a high-risk group, with school achievement rates far lower and dropout rates much higher than those of their white and Asian American counterparts ("The racial gap . . . ," 2002).

Yet there are vast patterns of socioeconomic, family structural, and cultural similarities and differences among these Hispanic groups (Malgady, 1994), and treatment strategies have yet to take subcultural issues into consideration. A challenge to culturally sensitive therapists is to construct treatment modalities that have differential validity for

Hispanic subgroups, including Mexican Americans, Central and South Americans, Cubans, and Puerto Ricans.

Cross, Bazron, Dennis, and Isaacs (1989) and Bernal and Castro (1994) estimated that 40% of the clients in the mental health delivery system are members of ethnic minority groups, compared to only 3–16% of service care providers, depending on their specialty. Thus, Vargas and Willis (1994) lamented the paucity of research and theoretically driven descriptions of culturally sensitive interventions in sharp contrast to the growing mental health needs of ethnic minority populations.

NARRATIVE THERAPY

Despite considerable attention to problems regarding the delivery of mental health services to Hispanics, such as underutilization of services (Rodriguez, 1987), premature dropout rates from psychotherapy (Sue, Fujino, Hu, Takeuchi, & Zane, 1991), and allegations of ineffective treatment modalities (Padilla, Ruiz, & Alvarez, 1975; Rogler et al., 1987), there has been little research evaluating the effectiveness of psychotherapy for Hispanics and even less attention to outcomes of services for children or adolescents.

The more general literature on Hispanics, largely focused on Mexican American adults, somewhat less on Puerto Ricans, implicates cultural distance between the typically low socioeconomic status (SES), Spanish-dominant Hispanic client and the middle-class, English-speaking non-Hispanic therapist as the root of psychotherapeutic calamity. Those populations increasing in number, the Central and South American Hispanic, are especially underrepresented in the mental health research literature. The recognition of cultural conflict not only between the client and therapist but also between Hispanic clients' cultural values and the orientations embodied in mainstream health care services has prompted considerations of cultural "sensitivity" (Rogler et al., 1987) or cultural "responsiveness" (Sue, 1988), or cultural "competence" (American Psychological Association, 1990) in the provision of mental health services.

In an early study, Costantino et al. (1986) introduced Puerto Rican folktales (adapted to reflect Anglo cultural values and settings) into a therapeutic modality to treat young, high-risk children; Malgady et al. (1990) based a modeling therapy modality on heroic Puerto Rican characters with older adolescents; Costantino et al. (1994) used a narrative therapy model with young adolescents.

These therapeutic interventions were all conducted in a group therapy format, by bilingual/bicultural clinical psychologists in a mental health clinic within a major urban Hispanic community. Treatments were conducted over standardized 50-minute sessions; closure was reached by mutual accord of the child, family member, and therapist. Thus, the efforts of bicultural approaches to treatment were to shape adaptive behavior by bridging cultural conflict and any language barriers, with a sense of *respecto* for family, personal, and cultural values. Standardization of treatments were ensured by creating manuals for uniform adherence to the structure of treatment formats:

- Greeting and establishing rapport and rules of order.
- Introduction of group members and reasons for attending the session.
- Presentation of *cuentos,* biographies, or stories.
- Self-disclosure and discussion and mutual reinforcement.
- Role playing and videotaping, discussion of videotapes, and verbal reinforcement.
- Closure and token reinforcement.

The majority of programmatic, culturally sensitive treatment outcome research efforts for Hispanic youth have been conceptualized, in the broadest sense, in the narrative process and rooted in social learning theory principles such as immitative role modeling. The specific treatment modalities within narrative modeling interventions have varied depending on developmental considerations.

Narrative psychotherapy has gained acceptance as a culturally sensitive treatment modality (Howard, 1991). Some cognitive psychologists (e.g., Bruner, 1986; Mair, 1988) maintain that identity development occurs as a result of life-story construction. Howard (1991) conceptualized psychopathology as an incoherent story with an incorrect ending; thus, the goal of successful psychotherapy is to restructure a child or adolescent's cognitions, underlying behavior leading to risk taking and substance abuse, in a coherent story with a correct ending. Further, he describes the technique of storytelling as the most adept process in understanding culturally diverse individuals and in conducting cross-cultural psychotherapy.

CUENTO THERAPY

Intervention

In a study of a culturally sensitive treatment intervention with 5- to 8-year-old children, Costantino et al. (1986) developed a storytelling modality based on Puerto Rican *cuentos,* or folktales, as a modeling therapy. The characters in folktales were posed as peer models conveying the theme or moral of the stories. The stories were selected from a vast array of Puerto Rican children's literature with the consideration of captivating children's attention to the models, which is critical to the first stage of the modeling process. Second, the models were adapted to present attitudes, values, and behaviors that reflect adaptive responses to the designated targets of therapeutic intervention, such as acting out, anxiety symptoms, and low self-esteem. The folktales were adapted to bridge both Puerto Rican and Anglo cultural values and settings. Reinforcement of children's imitation of the models through active role playing facilitated social learning of adaptive responses which were targeted in the stories' themes. Thus, the treatment was rooted in the children's own cultural heritage, presented in a format with which they could readily identify and imitate, and therapeutically aimed to affect psychosocial adjustment.

Sessions took place in a group therapy room at the clinical site, with participants seated in a circle with child–mother dyads sitting together. Two *cuentos* were read by the therapist at each session, alternatively along with the child and mother. To balance gender, one *cuento* had a female and one a male as the main character of the story. Personal experiences of the participants were shared and verbally reinforced. Subsequently, the participants enact the *cuentos* through role playing and videotaping, and reinforcement then followed. Following is an excerpt from one of the Puerto Rican *cuentos.*

"The Little Boy Who Wanted to Become a Big Man"

Not too long ago, there was a boy called Juanito who did not want to go to school. One day, he told his parents: "I'm sick and tired of being treated like a boy, I'm old enough to do want I want to." His parents were sad. His mother said: "You're too little, you can't leave us. . . . I would get sick from worrying about you." His father added: "Son, wait until you finish school, you're too young. Don't you know what happened to your grandfather? He left school and couldn't get a good job . . . They all called him Donkey Juan [Juanito el Burrito]." The little boy Juanito left anyway, but he had a hard time to find places to sleep and had no money to buy food. He realized he was better off at home, but was afraid to return. Then he met Mister Fox and Mister Dog, who promised him a home and food. They promised him a bag of gold. But they wanted him to steal it from someone's house. A neighbor saw the three of them and called "Police, Police!" The police came and caught Juanito, but not the other two. Crying, the boy wanted to go home. He felt bad but was happy because it was a Hispanic police officer taking him home. As he climbed the stairs to his apartment, he heard his parents crying because they missed him. He realized that his parents still loved him. From that day on he went to school, learned his lessons, and listened to his parents . . . on the way to becoming a man.

In this treatment intervention, children were screened for presenting emotional and behavior problems in school and at home, and the most symptomatic were selected for inclusion in the study. The presenting problems were symptoms of anxiety, depression, and conduct disorders, at the threshold of diagnostic criteria according to the third edition, revised, of the *Diagnostic and Statistical Manual of Mental Disorders* (DSM-III-R; American Psychiatric Association, 1987). Their low SES and high rate of single-parent household composition (60% female-headed households) also characterized these children as representing a high-risk population.

Evidence for the Effects of Treatment

The effectiveness of the *cuento* intervention was determined by comparing treatment outcomes with respect to a second folktale condition in which the same stories were not adapted to bridge cultural conflict, a mainstream (art/play) intervention, and an attention-only waiting-list control group. The evaluation of treatment outcomes indicated that the bicultural folktale intervention led to significantly more improvement in social judgment and reduction in anxiety symptomatology relative to both comparison groups at the immediate posttest after 20 sessions and at a 1-year follow-up posttest.

Further analysis revealed that the folktale intervention was most effective with younger children, 5–6 years old. Debriefing interviews conducted with 7–8-year-old children revealed that they viewed some of the *cuentos* as "childish." This developmental consideration prompted the development of another narrative modeling modality that was appropriate for older children and adolescents.

HERO/HEROINE THERAPY

Intervention

Another modeling intervention for older children and adolescents was based on "heroic" adult role models (Malgady et al., 1990). A major rationale underlying this treatment was the frequency of single-parent households, typically headed by young mothers. This suggests that Puerto Rican children and adolescents often lack intact adult role models with whom they can identify, and therefore adaptive values and behaviors of appropriate gender to imitate during the later child and early adolescent years.

This narrative modeling intervention was based on stories of heroic male and female Puerto Ricans in an effort to bridge the bicultural, intergenerational, and identity conflicts faced by Puerto Rican adolescents. The modality, which was implemented with 12–14-year-old adolescents, enhanced the relevance of therapy for adolescents by exposing them to successful male and female adult models in their own culture, fostering ethnic pride and identity as a Puerto Rican, and modeled achievement-oriented behavior and adaptive coping with the stress common to life in the urban Hispanic community, such as poverty, minority status, and racial prejudice. In this intervention, adolescents were screened for conduct behavioral problems in school and at home, low self-esteem, and phobic and anxiety symptoms. The participants selected for inclusion were threshold cases but did not meet DSM-III-R diagnostic criteria for caseness.

Historical inquiry showed that there was a large pool of male candidates as heroes in Puerto Rican history, representing diverse occupations and achievements. Female characters were less well documented in Puerto Rican history and tended to be more contemporary and less variable in endeavors. Nonetheless, 10 male heroes and 10 female heroines were thus selected by a panel of psychologists and sociologists, an historian, and a Puerto Rican literary expert.

Following is an abbreviated biography of a female heroic character from Puerto Rican history.

"Angelita Lind"

Angelita Lind was born in 1959 in the town of Patillas in Puerto Rico. She had six brothers and sisters. Angelita was one of the fastest runners in the history of Puerto Rico's sports. She had a strong need for friends as a child and found out that the best students had the most friends. Because she was only average, she became the class clown to make friends. Her mother would dress her and fix her hair every morning, but she would mess herself up to act like a clown. Soon she found out that this did not make her any friends.

When she was in the seventh grade, she would run from school to her grandmother's house to eat lunch—3 miles away. Then she would run back another 3 miles to school—day after day. She then started studying her homework and became a good student too, like her new friends.

Later, Angelita went to college in Puerto Rico where she became a famous sports star and also an excellent student. One day, when she was running a race—and winning—another runner bumped into her and she fell down. She was very sad that she didn't win the race and that she let down her country. She said, "There is an invisible wall in front of us all the time, and we have to be strong enough to knock it down to get what we want." Thinking like this and overcoming her hardships, she achieved her goals and the respect of the people of Puerto Rico.

Evidence for the Effects of Treatment

Therapeutic outcomes were assessed relative to an attention-control group participating in an after-school dropout program. Statistical analyses of treatment effectiveness indicated that the culturally sensitive modeling intervention decreased anxiety symptomatology and increased Puerto Rican identity. However, treatment interacted with household composition and participants' gender. The role models promoted greater ethnic identity in the absence of a male adult in the adolescents' households—but only among male adolescents. Female adolescents evidence greater Puerto Rican identification than males regardless of treatment, possibly due to stable maternal identification. Similarly, the role models promoted greater self-esteem among male and female adolescents from female-headed households. However, the self-image of females from intact families diminished in the process. The heroic role models presented in treatment may have aroused conflicting feelings about their real parents' daily functioning. Comparison of idealized and real-life adult models through the process of identification thus may have led to lower self-esteem. This process may have been promoted among females participants because the female role models presented in treatment often represented untraditional female sex roles.

Interviews with research participants provided information consistent with this interpretation of developmental interaction effects. Male adolescents in father-absent households expressed feelings of identification with male models, regardless of their family context. Males also preferred sports figures and had little appreciation of female role models' accomplishments. Female adolescents seemed to have a different perspective and were dismayed by certain role models' altruistic and patriotic acts that disrupted family harmony. Although a research panel selecting the role models judged these stories to be among the most heroic, adolescent females were disturbed by themes of family separation (e.g., a painter leaving his family to study in Spain and a political party leader sending his family away while struggling for independence). The considerations that affect treatment outcomes emphasize the importance of social context in calculating the mental health value of culturally sensitive interventions. These findings also prompt a need for research on how the integrity and quality of intrafamilial relationships may mediate, as well as moderate, treatment outcomes. For instance, intact parental household structure, extended family networks, father visitation, and complete father absence pose a multitude of scenarios for further study. Thus, the infrastructure of the household, in combination with quality-of-life issues, presents an array of independent variables which may have a significant impact on the need for, utilization of, and effectiveness of psychotherapeutic interventions for Hispanic children and adolescents.

TEMAS STORYTELLING THERAPY

Intervention

Another intervention developed was also a narrative modality with older children and young adolescents, 9–11 years old, composed of an ethnically and culturally diverse group consisting of Puerto Ricans, Dominicans, and Central and South Americans (Costantino et al., 1994). The participants were screened for DSM-III-R symptomatology with structured clinical interviews. The most prevalent symptoms were associated with conduct, anxiety, and phobic disorders. The upper quartile of symptomatic cases were included in the study (though none satisfied DSM caseness criteria).

The intervention consisted of a storytelling modality based on pictures depicting Hispanic cultural elements (e.g., traditional foods, games, gender roles), family scenes, and neighborhoods (e.g., bodegas) in urban settings. The pictures were selected from the stimulus cards of the "Tell-Me-A-Story" (TEMAS) Thematic Apperception Test (Costantino, Malgady, & Rogler, 1988). Pictures portrayed multiracial Hispanic characters engaged in interpersonal situations in a variety of home, city, and school settings.

Small-group therapy sessions (averaging five to seven children each) were conducted by bilingual/bicultural clinical psychologists in three phases over a 50-minute duration.

In the first phase, group members collaborated to develop a composite story about a particular picture, identifying the characters, setting, what is happening, and the resolution of the story. In the second phase, group members shared their personal experiences as related to the composite story and the therapist verbally reinforced adaptive behaviors and themes expressed in their personal narratives. Maladaptive narratives were discussed by members seeking alternative, more adaptive resolutions of interpersonal conflict. This engaged the youth in self-disclosure of personal conflict in their lives, how they coped, and reinforced the internalization of adaptive models of coping strategies. In the third phase, participants dramatized the composite story by performing the roles of the characters in the pictures. Verbal reinforcement of imitative target behaviors was administered by the therapist and peers. The psychodrama was videotaped and played back for critical review and discussion of appropriate behavior. The narrative intervention was compared to an attention-control group that engaged in psychoeducational discussion sessions. These sessions were of equivalent duration, also conducted by bilingual/bicultural therapists in the clinical setting.

Evidence for the Effects of Treatment

Results indicated that there was no significant reduction of depression symptomatology, but there were significant decreases in conduct disorder and phobic symptoms. More interesting, there were significant interaction effects as a function of the age factor such that treatment effects were enhanced among the younger adolescents. Thus, it would appear that younger adolescents more readily identify psychologically with cultural role models. Perhaps by the time adolescents mature, bordering on young adulthood, they are relatively more inured to the therapeutic message of this type of intervention.

FAMILIES IN CRISIS

Intervention

Another culturally sensitive treatment intervention was developed for Hispanic and African American families surrounding a crisis due to an adolescent family member's alcohol and substance abuse and high-risk sexual behavior (Hatterer & Malgady, 2000). This modality presented a 20-minute movie of a Hispanic family and another of an African American family interacting at "the dinner table" regarding an adolescent's problems with drugs and alcohol, high-risk sexual behavior, and personality functioning. The youth targeted in the intervention was a user of illicit substances and had recently been incarcerated for criminal possession.

The movies depicted high-risk settings, including a parental figure with a history of substance abuse and criminal activity, urban settings, and poverty-level existence. The youth was helped by discussions with family members, such as the parents and, in particular, an older sibling. The goal of the intervention was to induce the adolescent at risk to seek a preventive intervention program available in the community. The narrative ended on a positive note with the individual agreeing to seek treatment and a list of services available in the actual community.

A comparison group of African American, Hispanic, and white youth viewed a comparable length videotape on a related topic of smoking cessation. The control group's videotape did not portray ethnic minority characters.

Evidence for the Effects of Treatment

Participants were pre- and posttested with a variety of instruments measuring substance use and abuse and high-risk behavior. Although the study's main target was to establish help-seeking behavior and to open a "dialogue" between the adolescent and significant others, there were significant effects on the reduction of alcohol intake and use of illicit substances (cocaine, marijuana, heroin, inhalants, etc.). Substance use and intention to seek help were assessed by a self-report questionnaire, administered in the adolescents' preferred language by a bilingual/bicultural clinician.

Consistent with the hypothesis of the study, posing ethnically matched models in a family narrative in an impoverished urban setting had the intended effect of promoting help seeking. Perhaps the most interesting finding was that Hispanic adolescents were most likely to opt for speaking with a family member regarding substance abuse, consistent with the Hispanic cultural value of familism. Conversely, African American participants were more like to choose to speak with someone outside their family. Moreover, these treatment outcomes were persistent at 3- and 12-week follow-up assessments.

Given the positive treatment outcomes of this research, pilot studies were later undertaken (L. Hatterer, personal communication, August 2001) to implement the intervention through a closed-circuit television station reaching over 10,000 viewers.

SUMMARY AND CONCLUSIONS

The introduction of Hispanic cultural elements into the treatment process is a promising approach to treat emotional and behavioral problems and substance abuse among Hispanic children and adolescents. Special developmental considerations can be introduced into therapy protocols as a function of participants' ethnicity, age, and gender. Clearly, however, further research is warranted inquiring how culturally sensitive services can be implemented more effectively given that dynamic processes may intervene to enhance or impede their effectiveness. A major objective of future research should be to focus on the dynamics of familial context of male and female Hispanic youngsters to make gender- and family-specific refinements in treatment protocols as they are developmentally arrayed.

Most research on Hispanic substance abuse has been conducted on Mexican Americans; thus, future research must broaden its generalizability to other Hispanic subgroups, particularly to the influx of relatively unacculturated immigrants. Similarly, little research has been devoted to children or adolescents, who are critical to reach in the early developmental years. Comparison groups with various diagnoses according to the fourth edition of the DSM (DSM-IV; American Psychiatric Association, 1994) that are comorbid with substance abuse also need to be studied, in terms of both different main effects of treatment interventions and moderator and mediator effects.

REFERENCES

American Psychiatric Association. (1987). *Diagnostic and statistical manual of mental disorders* (3rd ed., rev.). Washington, DC: Author.

American Psychiatric Association. (1994). *Diagnostic and statistical manual of mental disorders* (4th ed.). Washington, DC: Author.

American Psychological Association. (1990). *Guidelines for providers of psychological services to ethnic, linguistic, and culturally diverse populations.* Washington, DC: Author.

Bernal, M. E., & Castro, F. (1994). Are clinical psychologists prepared for service and research with ethnic minorities? Report of a decade of progress. *American Psychologist, 49,* 797–805.

Botvin, G. J., & Malgady, R. G. (1998). Alcohol and marijuana use among rural youth: Interaction of personality and social factors. *Addictive Behaviors, 23,* 379–387.

Botvin, G. J., Baker, E., Dusenbury, L., Botvin, E., & Diaz, T. (1995). Long-term follow-up results of a randomized drug abuse prevention trial in a white middle-class population. *Journal of the American Medical Association, 273,* 1106–1112.

Botvin, G. J., Baker, E., Dusenbury, L., Tortu, S., & Botvin, E. (1990). Preventing adolescent drug abuse through a multimodal cognitive-behavioral approach: Results of a 3-year study. *Journal of Consulting and Clinical Psychology, 58,* 437–446.

Brizer, D., Costantino, G., & Malgady, R. G. (2001). *Preventive intervention of substance abuse among Hispanic adolescents.* Washington, DC. Substance Abuse and Mental Health Administration.

Bruner, J. (1986). *Actual minds, possible worlds.* Cambridge, MA: Harvard University Press.

Costantino, G., Malgady, R. G., & Rogler, L. H. (1986). Cuento therapy: A culturally sensitive modality for Puerto Rican children. *Journal of Consulting and Clinical Psychology, 54,* 739–746.

Costantino, G., Malgady, R. G., & Rogler, L. H. (1988). *The TEMAS thematic apperception test: Technical manual.* Los Angeles: Western Psychological Services.

Costantino, G., Malgady, R. G., & Rogler, L. H. (1994). Storytelling-through-pictures: Culturally sensitive psychotherapy for Hispanic children and adolescents. *Journal of Clinical Child Psychology, 23,* 13–20.

Cross, T. L., Bazron, B., Dennis, K. W., & Isaacs, M. R. (1989). *Towards a culturally competent system of care.* Washington, DC: CAASP Technical Assistance Center, Georgetown University.

Hatterer, L. J., & Malgady, R. G. (2000). *Urban drug abuse risk assessment and prevention.* Washington, DC: National Institute of Drug Abuse.

Howard, G. S. (1991). Culture tales: A narrative approach to thinking, cross-cultural psychology, and psychotherapy. *American Psychologist, 46,* 187–197.

Kessler, R. C., McGonagle, K. A., & Zhao, S. (1994). Lifetime and 12-month prevalence of DSM-III psychiatric disorders in the United States. *Archives of General Psychiatry, 51,* 8–19.

Mair, M. (1989). *Between psychology and psychotherapy.* London: Routledge.

Malgady, R. G. (1994). Hispanic diversity and the need for culturally sensitive mental health services. In R. G. Malgady & O. Rodriguez (Eds.), *Theoretical and conceptual issues in Hispanic mental health* (pp. 227–247). Melbourne, FL: Krieger.

Malgady, R. G., Rogler, L. H., & Costantino, G. (1990). Hero/heroine modeling for Puerto Rican adolescents: A preventive mental health intervention. *Journal of Consulting and Clinical Psychology, 58,* 469–474.

Malgady, R. G., Rogler, L. H., & Tryon, W. W. (1992). Issues of validity in the Diagnostic Interview Schedule. *Journal of Psychiatric Research, 26,* 59–67.

Mann, E. S., & Salvo, J. J. (1985). Characteristics of new Hispanic immigrants to New York City: A comparison of Puerto Rican and non-Puerto Rican Hispanics. *Research Bulletin* (Hispanic Research Center, Fordham University), *8*(1–2).

New York City Board of Education. (1993). *Immigrant enrollment in the public schools.* New York: Division of Public Affairs.

New York City Department of City Planning. (1992). *Demographic profiles: A profile of New York City's community districts from the 1980 & 1990 censuses of population and housing* (No. 92–32). New York: Author.

New York State Office of Mental Health. (1994). *Primary diagnoses of all children in CDF database.* Albany, NY: Author.

Padilla, A. M., Ruiz, R. A., & Alvarez, R. (1975). Community mental health services for Spanish-speaking/ surnamed population. *American Psychologist, 30,* 892–905.

Pumariega, A. J., Swanson, J. W., Holzer, C. E., Linskey, A. O., & Qintero-Salinas, R. (1992). Cultural context and substance abuse in Hispanic adolescents. *Journal of Child and Family Studies, 1,* 75–92.

The racial gap in test scores. (2002, March 28). *New York Times,* pp. C21–22.

Robins, L., Helzer, J., Croughan, J., & Ratcliff, G. (1981). The NIMH Diagnostic Interview Schedule: Its history, characteristics, and validity. *Archives of General Psychiatry, 38,* 381–389.

Rodriguez, O. (1987). *Hispanics and human services: Help-seeking in the inner city* (Monograph No. 14). Bronx, NY: Hispanic Research Center, Fordham University.

Rogler, L. H., Malgady, R. G., Costantino, G., & Blumenthal, R. (1987). What does culturally sensitive mental health services mean? The case of Hispanics. *American Psychologist, 42,* 565–570.

Rogler, L. H., Malgady, R. G., & Rodriguez, O. (1989). *Hispanics and mental health: A framework for research.* Melbourne, FL: Krieger.

Sue, S. (1988). Psychotherapeutic services for ethnic minorities. *American Psychologist, 43,* 301–308.

Sue, S., Fujino, D. C., Hu, L. T., Tackeuchi, D. T., & Zane, N. W. S. (1991). Community mental health services for ethnic minority groups: A test of the cultural responsiveness hypothesis. *Journal of Consulting and Clinical Psychology, 59,* 533–540.

Szapocznik, J., Kurtines, W., & Santisteban, D. A. (1994). The interplay of advances among theory, research and application in family interventions for Hispanic behavior-problem youth. In R. G. Malgady & O. Rodriguez (Eds.), *Theoretical and conceptual issues in Hispanic mental health* (pp. 155–180). Melbourne, FL: Krieger.

U.S. Bureau of the Census. (1994, March). *Current population reports, population characteristics.* Washington, DC: Author.

Vargas, L. A., & Willis, D. J. (1994). Introduction to thespecial section: New directions in the treatment and assessment of ethnic minority children and adolescents. *Journal of Clinical Child Psychology, 23,* 2–4.

Vega, W. A., Zimmerman, R. S., Warheit, G. J., Apospori, E., & Gil, A. G. (1993). Risk factors for early adolescent drug use in four ethnic and racial groups. *American Journal of Public Health, 83,* 185–189.

III

CONCLUSIONS AND FUTURE DIRECTIONS

25

Concluding Thoughts

Present and Future of Evidence-Based Psychotherapies for Children and Adolescents

JOHN R. WEISZ AND ALAN E. KAZDIN

The chapters in this volume reveal a remarkable blend of intelligence, creativity, and perseverance—sheer hard work by clinical scientists dedicated to the pursuit of treatments that work for children and adolescents. In this volume, these scientists have summarized important work on a variety of intervention programs, highlighted critical ethical and legal issues, spelled out the need for a solid developmental foundation, and offered historically informed and insightful perspectives on the developing "frontier" of evidence-based practice.

Collectively, these authors convey a great deal about the state of the art in youth treatment research. In this respect, the chapters nicely complement what we know about general trends from meta-analyses of published trials (e.g., Kazdin, Bass, Ayers, & Rodgers, 1990; Weisz, Weiss, Alicke, & Klotz, 1987; Weisz, Weiss, Han, Granger, & Morton, 1995). The meta-analyses have shown fairly consistently that the average treated youngster shows better outcomes after treatment than at least 75% of comparable youngsters placed in control groups; the effects are relatively specific to the problems and disorders targeted in treatment, not just general improvements in overall adjustment (Weisz et al., 1995), and they hold up well, at least across the 5- to 6-month periods characteristic of most follow-up assessments (Weisz et al., 1987, 1995). The chapters in this book take us beyond these general characterizations, describing specific treatments that produce such respectable effects, summarizing the evidence on those treatments, and characterizing the familial, developmental, theoretical, historical, ethical, and legal context of treatment development and testing, and youth mental health care.

COVERAGE OF CONDITIONS AND TYPES OF DYSFUNCTION

The descriptions tell us a good deal about the breadth of coverage of youth problems and dysfunction in current treatment research. Tested treatments have now been developed to address multiple internalizing conditions within the anxiety–depression spectrum, multiple externalizing conditions ranging from chronic disobedience and aggression to the disruptive behavior disorders, autism and related developmental disorders, habit problems such as enuresis and obesity, anorexia nervosa, and some forms of substance misuse. Indeed, the problems and disorders for which evidence-based treatments now exist encompass the concerns that bring the great majority of children and adolescents into clinical care.

That said, there are certainly troubling problems that remain relative orphans in the treatment development domain. More than 200 disorders listed in the fourth edition of the *Diagnostic and Statistical Manual of Mental Disorders* (DSM-IV; American Psychiatric Association, 1994) can be applied to children or adolescents (Kazdin, 2000b), and for most of these we lack well-tested treatments. For example, treatment of bulimia nervosa in youth has received relatively little research attention (but see Foreyt, Poston, Winebarger, & McGavin, 1998, for descriptions of primarily adult approaches that might be adapted for adolescents). With only a few exceptions (see, e.g., Azrin, Donohue, Besalel, Kogan, & Acierno, 1994; Malgady & Costantino, Chapter 24, this volume), empirically supported treatments for substance-abusing youth are rare, particularly for users of harder drugs such as cocaine. Also with few exceptions (e.g., Borduin, Henggeler, Blaske, & Stein, 1990), the literature lacks successes in the treatment of youthful sex offenders. And despite attempts by several research teams, we still lack interventions for suicidal youth that clearly reduce the risk of further attempts (see Miller & Glinski, 2000; Weisz & Hawley, 2002).

Finally, some of our field's success stories have boundary conditions that restrict their benefits in significant ways; for example, psychosocial treatment success with attention-deficit/hyperactivity disorder (AD/HD) has been largely limited to preadolescents, and some of the most beneficial parent training programs for conduct problems and disorder also may not travel so well up the developmental ramp into adolescence. In fact, one author of a widely used behavioral parent training program argues that adolescents should *not* be considered candidates for the program, that they often do not respond well, and that their reaction may exacerbate family conflict (Barkley, 1997, p. 5). Thus, while evidence-based treatments exist for most of the conditions that propel the largest numbers of youth into treatment, the majority of relevant DSM-IV disorders are not yet covered, and some of the treatments for highly prevalent conditions may not work equally well across the age spectrum. In summary, there is a good deal to like about current coverage across domains of dysfunction, but a good deal of work remains to be done, as noted in Table 25.1.

COVERAGE OF THEORETICAL PERSPECTIVES
ON YOUTH TREATMENT

The evidence-based psychotherapies encompass several of the theoretical perspectives that have guided youth treatment historically, but certainly not all the relevant theories. Behavioral (operant, classical, and modeling) approaches are common among the tested treatments, as are cognitive-behavioral applications; and psychodynamic and family systems perspectives are evident in some treatments (see e.g., Mufson & Dorta, Chapter 9, this volume; Robin, Chapter 20, this volume). But numerous other schools of therapy are missing from the roster. A similar pattern is evident in meta-analyses of published treatment outcome research (e.g., Kazdin, Bass, et al., 1990; Weisz et al., 1987, 1995), with

TABLE 25.1. Challenges for Future Research on Evidence-Based Psychotherapy

1. Expand coverage to forms of dysfunction that lack empirically tested treatments.
2. Address boundary conditions that constrain tested treatments (e.g., broadening the age range within which treatments produce benefit).
3. Broaden the array of theoretical models tested, encompassing more of the treatments widely used in practice.
4. Test an enriched array of treatment packaging and delivery models, to address well-known complexities (e. g., comorbidity, episodic conditions, and heterogeneity within conditions).
5. Extend scope and duration of outcome assessment to include youth functioning, consumer perspectives, system impact, and effects on family members.
6. Intensify research on how therapist behavior and the therapeutic relationship relate to treatment benefit.
7. Delineate the effective range of treatments in regard to youth and family clinical and demographic characteristics.
8. Use dismantling and related approaches to identify necessary and sufficient conditions of treatment benefit.
9. Use multiple strategies (mediation analysis and beyond) to identify mechanisms of change that explain why treatments work.
10. Develop and test treatments under clinical practice conditions, to foster robust treatment design and evidence on effectiveness in clinical care.

more than 70% of published studies testing behavioral and cognitive-behavioral treatments.

A problem posed by this state of affairs is that the nonbehavioral treatments models, those least favored in the research literature, are actually the models used most widely in clinical practice (see, e.g., Kazdin, Siegel, & Bass, 1990; Weersing, Weisz, & Donenberg, 2002). The treatment models that service providers use and trust certainly warrant more attention in clinical trials than they have received to date. The disparity between the scope of evidence and the scope of practice is illustrated by a recent count identifying more than 500 named therapies used with children and adolescents (see Kazdin, 2000b). Only a tiny percentage of those therapies have been subjected to any empirical test. It is clear that researchers who seek to broaden the array of empirically tested treatment models will find no shortage of candidates.

INTERVENTION DELIVERY STRATEGIES AND MODELS

Across the various intervention programs, one sees a growing array of models for getting treatment content to the child and family. To be sure, the most common model follows the tradition of talking to the therapist during weekly office visits, but investigators have pushed the boundaries with tests of treatments in which core concepts and skills training are embedded in videotaped vignettes for parents (see Webster-Stratton & Reid, Chapter 13, this volume) or stories or videos for youth (see Malgady & Constantino, Chapter 24, this volume; Webster-Stratton & Reid, Chapter 13, this volume), treatment in which therapists coach parents as they interact with their children (see Brinkmeyer & Eyberg, Chapter 12, this volume), home-based behavioral training using a urine alarm for enuresis (Houts, Chapter 22, this volume), approaches using summer camp as a treatment medium (e.g., Epstein, Chapter 21, this volume; Pelham & Hoza, 1996), intervention providing behavioral training and support for foster parents (see Chamberlain & Smith, Chapter 16, this volume), treatment supplements in the form of post-therapy booster sessions (see Clarke, DeBar, & Lewinsohn, Chapter 7, this volume), a peripatetic therapist-in-the-youth's-environment model (see Henggeler & Lee, Chapter 17, this volume), and an intensive approach in which children spend 40 hours per week in discrete trials training (see Lovaas & Smith, Chapter 18, this volume). This array makes it evident that treatment researchers are concerned not only with what contents (concepts, experiences, skills) to include in their interventions but how best to package and present those contents.

While the array of treatment packaging and delivery strategies is impressive in work completed to date, it seems likely that continued creativity will be needed in the future to address the variety of ways youth dysfunction presents in relation to treatment (see Kazdin, 2000b; Kazdin & Weisz, 1998; Weisz, Huey, & Weersing, 1998). The episodic, recurring nature of many youth conditions may need to be addressed via models that encompass regular periodic monitoring of the child's status (analogous to the 6-month dental checkup or the yearly physical) with treatment resumed as needed (cf. Clarke et al., Chapter 7, this volume). The likelihood that not all youth diagnosed with the same disorder will manifest all symptoms of that disorder, or need all the same treatment elements, suggests the potential value of modular treatment strategies (see Chorpita, 2002). As an example, some youths treated for depression do not manifest marked cognitive distortion, and others seem to have strong social skills; for such youth, a treatment program in which cognitive modules and social skills training were optional might make for enhanced efficiency.

An important counterargument is that even those without major deficits in a particular domain may profit from treatment focused on that domain. An intriguing challenge for treatment planning and design is that there is no essential match between the causal pathway into and current characteristics of an individual's problem or disorder, on the one hand, and the treatment that is most likely to be effective, on the other. As an example, children may develop aggressive or delinquent behavior in ways that are not primarily caused by parental behavior, yet intervention focused on parent behavior may be quite effective in changing the children's behavior. Thus, while modular approaches to treatment design may have potential benefits, the benefits may remain elusive for some time, because we know so little about how best to match treatments and treatment elements to individual youngsters.

As a third illustration of how our treatment delivery models may need to be stretched, we note that most of the evidence-based treatments are focused on single conditions or homogeneous clusters of them. By contrast, most treated children do not manifest only one problem or diagnosis, or even one at a time (Angold, Costello, & Erkanli, 1999), and even conditions that may seem quite different superficially, such as depression and conduct disorder, show rather high rates of co-occurrence. The fact that different problems and diagnoses co-occur so regularly suggests a need for models to guide blending and combining elements of distinct treatments for different conditions. This promises to be a challenging task, one that could engage some of the best minds in the field for many years.

SCOPE AND DURATION OF OUTCOME ASSESSMENT
IN TREATMENT RESEARCH

The body of evidence surveyed in this book illustrates how outcome assessment has expanded in scope, intensity, and rigor over the years. In the best research, child dysfunction is now assessed from multiple perspectives, often including youth, parent, and teacher report, and ideally including direct observation of treated youth's behavior. Formal diagnostic assessment is often included now, in part to assess the clinical significance of treatment-related change. Increasingly, such measures of problems, symptoms, and diagnoses, are complemented by assessments of real-world functioning—grades and school behavior reports, for example, and arrests, when relevant. Beyond the treated youth, assessments focus increasingly on dispersion of treatment benefit—for example, increases in parents' child management skills, parenting confidence, parental stress and mental health, and even changes in marital satisfaction associated with changes in child behavior. And consumer satisfaction with treatment is making its way into the outcome literature as well.

While the increasing breadth and intensity of outcome assessment is a positive feature, some leaders in the field have encouraged further broadening. For example, Hoagwood, Jensen, Petti, and Burns (1996) have argued for tapping such system-related outcomes as the extent to which treatment reduces the use of other mental health services. We would add that there is also room for expansion in the *duration* of outcome assessment. In meta-analyses (Weisz et al., 1987, 1995), only about a third of the published studies have included any assessment other than immediate posttreatment. And for that third, the mean follow-up lag time was 5–6 months after the end of treatment. As a consequence, we know relatively little about the long-term holding power of the effects generated by most treatments, and thus little about whether or when there may be a need for treatment supplements, booster sessions, and the like to maintain gains.

UNDERSTANDING OF HOW THERAPIST BEHAVIOR AND THE THERAPEUTIC RELATIONSHIP RELATE TO BENEFIT

The treatment outcome research literature is particularly strong in describing principles and procedures to apply in treatment but weak in helping therapists build a warm, empathic relationship and a strong working alliance with children and their families (see Shirk & Russell, 1996). This gap is striking in light of the widespread belief that quality of the therapeutic relationship or alliance is important to success in most treatment encounters. Indeed, many child therapists rate the therapeutic relationship as more important than the specific techniques used in treatment (Kazdin, Siegel, & Bass, 1990; Motta & Lynch, 1990; Shirk & Saiz, 1992), and some treated children may agree, even those treated with evidence-based treatments. Kendall and Southam-Gerow (1996), for example, found that children treated for anxiety disorders using the Coping Cat program rated their relationship with the therapist as the most important aspect of treatment.

What we lack thus far is a strong body of evidence that (1) clearly defines what a positive therapeutic relationship is, (2) establishes how best to measure it, (3) identifies therapist characteristics and behaviors that foster it, and (4) tests the extent to which such a relationship actually predicts outcome when evidence-based treatments are used. It seems inherently useful, at any time, to learn all we can about therapist behavior and therapist–youth interactions that predict good treatment outcomes; but it seems especially timely to do so in relation to structured, manualized treatments, which may call for a special set of skills. As an example, effective use of such treatments may require multitasking therapists who can maintain attention to a structured treatment plan, remain responsive to what youth and parents bring to the session, find ways to connect the treatment agenda to the youngster's real-life concerns, nurture a warm relationship, and make sessions lively and fun. Tests of these and other speculations on therapist–process–outcome connections would be an exciting addition to the research agenda in the years ahead.

IDENTIFYING THE EFFECTIVE RANGE OF TREATMENTS

The youth treatment outcome literature is much stronger in demonstrating benefit than in identifying the boundary conditions that constrain benefit. For each treatment, we need to know as much as possible about the range of youth and family clinical and demographic characteristics within which the treatments are helpful and outside of which effects diminish. Even the best-supported treatments are beneficial for some conditions and some youth but not others, with benefit potentially limited by comorbid conditions, age, socioeconomic status, ethnicity, family configuration, or other clinical and demographic factors; but, with a relatively small number of exceptions, research to date has left us relatively uninformed about such constraints. Racial, ethnic, and cultural factors, for example, are embedded but unexamined in most of our treatment outcome research (Kazdin, Bass, et al., 1990; Weisz et al., 1998), and this makes it difficult to know how robust most treatment effects are across various population groups.

Given the relative youth of our field, it is not surprising that most tested treatments lack provisions for dealing with broad variations in language, values, customs, childrearing traditions, beliefs and expectancies about child and parent behavior, and distinctive stressors and resources associated with different cultural traditions. But it does seem possible that the interplay between such factors and treatment characteristics may influence the relationship between child/family and therapist, the likelihood of treatment completion versus dropout, and the outcome of the treatment process (Weisz et al., 1998). We need more research assessing the extent to which treatment persistence, process, and outcome are moderated by race, ethnicity, culture, and a variety of other child and family characteristics.

UNDERSTANDING THE NECESSARY AND
SUFFICIENT CONDITIONS FOR TREATMENT BENEFIT

Among the diverse tested treatments, a substantial subset are omnibus or multicomponent in form, packing a variety of concepts and skills into one program, with termination considered appropriate only when all the components have been covered. For some of these treatments, all the elements may well be needed, but often the evidence base is too poorly developed to make clear just which elements are truly necessary or whether a subset of them might actually be sufficient to produce most of the benefit possible from the treatment. Indeed, it is the absence of such a clear picture that often stimulates development of multicomponent interventions; new concepts and skills are added when in doubt, because it seems that they may help and probably cannot hurt.

One result of this process may be treatments that have a good deal of fat, elements that do not actually contribute substantially to the outcomes achieved. As a matter of principle, given the time and expense associated with treatment, we need treatments that are as fat-free and efficient as possible. Indeed, treatments that fall short of this goal are apt to clash with the current emphasis (in real-world clinical care) on managing costs and professional time. Increasing treatment efficiency will likely enhance the attractiveness of the interventions to practitioners, improve the teachability of the procedures, and increase the likelihood that they will reach the children and families that need them. Of course, many of the elements of treatment may not enhance outcome directly but may still be important to retain. For example, some elements of treatment may contribute to or enhance the acceptability of treatment, minimize dropout rates, or increase patient and therapist compliance with the treatment regimen. Such elements of treatment may serve as the spoonful of sugar that makes the medicine go down and be important to retain.

In our field, a traditional pathway to understanding which treatment elements are actually contributing to outcomes is *dismantling* research, in which different treatment components are broken apart and tested separately. In principle, such research should provide the key to understanding necessity and sufficiency in the evidence-based treatments. But the task is complex when many elements are involved in the same treatment, because the number of combinations multiplies quickly. And, of course, different subgroups of youth may differ from one another in their responsiveness to different subsets of treatment components. All of this means that the dismantling process may be particularly challenging for some of the more complex treatments. But the potential benefits make the job worth doing.

IDENTIFYING MECHANISMS OF CHANGE THAT EXPLAIN WHY TREATMENTS WORK

The job of making treatments more efficient could be greatly simplified by an understanding of the specific change processes that make the treatments work. But a close review of youth treatment research reveals much more about what outcomes are produced than about what actually *causes* the outcomes (Kazdin, 2000a, 2000b; Shirk & Russell, 1996; Weersing & Weisz, 2002). This is understandable for at least two reasons. First, simple logic dictates that we find out *whether* a treatment works before turning to *why*. Second, figuring out *why* (i.e., what the causal mechanisms are) is not a simple task. But, temporal order and difficulty notwithstanding, we need to take on the task. If we fail to identify core causal processes, we risk a proliferation of treatments administered rather superstitiously "because they work," but without an understanding of the change processes that must be set in motion to produce results. And we risk the inclusion of therapy components that add to treatment burden without actually contributing to change.

To understand *how* the treatments actually work, we need a new generation of research on mechanisms underlying change. One element of this process (but *only* one) is testing hypothesized mediators of outcome. Data-analytic procedures for mediation testing have been well described (Baron & Kenney, 1986; Holmbeck, 1997), and the raw material needed for such procedures exists in many treatment investigators' data sets, albeit in a rather dormant state. A recent review (Weersing & Weisz, 2002) noted that 63% of clinical trials in the areas of anxiety, depression, and disruptive behavior included measures of potential mediators in their designs. The figures ranged from 22% for studies of learning-based treatments for anxiety to 91% of parent training studies. But only 6 of the 67 studies surveyed had included any formal mediation test. Evidently, there is a great deal of untapped potential in data that have already been collected.

The modest number of mediational analyses that have been carried out thus far illustrates the potential this work has for refining our understanding. Huey, Henggeler, Brondino, and Pickrel (2000), for example, found that decreased affiliation with delinquent peers mediated reductions in delinquent behavior among youth treated with multi-systemic therapy. And Eddy and Chamberlain (2000) found that improved family management skills and reductions in deviant peer associations mediated the effects of their behaviorally oriented treatment foster care program on adolescent antisocial behavior. More disappointing, but quite important, were Kolko, Brent, Baugher, Bridge, and Birmaher's (2000) failure to find that changes in cognitive distortions mediated the effect of cognitive-behavioral therapy on self-rated depression (see Weersing & Brent, Chapter 8, this volume). A case could be made that findings failing to support a popular mediational hypothesis are in some respects more important than supportive findings because they may steer us away from unfounded assumptions and open our minds to new possibilities that warrant attention. We need more analyses focused on hypothesized change processes in other evidence-based treatments. Failure to rigorously test for mediation limits the field in a significant way, creating an environment within which faulty notions about the nature and causes of change may sprout and thrive.

While mediation tests have real value, a case can be made that such tests alone cannot yield a complete understanding of causal mechanisms and change processes. Critical logical and design issues may well need to be addressed to fill out the picture, and this will likely require going beyond prevailing methods of mediator detection. For present purposes, let us note that with increased understanding of the mechanisms underlying therapeutic change, the prospects will increase for us to (1) understand and address impediments, stalls, and failures in treatment; (2) train therapists by teaching them what change processes they need to effect rather than simply what techniques to use; and (3) identify cross-cutting principles that can be used in designing, refining, and possibly combining interventions.

UNDERSTANDING OF EVIDENCE-BASED TREATMENTS IN RELATION TO CLINICAL PRACTICE

The research challenges identified thus far strike us as exciting opportunities to improve on work that is already inspiring. And we see the treatments described in this book as promising methods for improving the mental health and adaptation of children and adolescents. But not all who share our interest in quality mental health care share our enthusiasm for evidence-based treatments (see, e.g., Garfield, 1996; Havik & VandenBos, 1996). Many mental health care professionals have genuine concerns that this new generation of manual-guided treatments is neither relevant to the work they do nor appropriate for the clients they treat. The specific concerns are diverse, but among those frequently mentioned are that (1) the use of prescriptive, manualized treatments limits creativity and innovation and turns therapists into mere technicians who memorize and follow cookie-cutter procedures; (2) manual adherence will interfere with development of a productive therapeutic relationship and constrain the therapist's ability to individualize treatment; (3) the treatments have only been tested with simple cases with low levels of psychopathology and may not work with more severe cases; (4) the treatments tend to focus on single problems or disorders and thus may not work with comorbid cases; and (5) the complexity and volatility of clinically referred individuals and their families make each session unpredictable and a predetermined series of session plans unworkable (for details on some of these arguments, focused especially on evidence-based treatments for adults, see Addis & Krasnow, 2000; Addis, Wade, & Hatgis, 1999; Garfield, 1996; Havik & VandenBos, 1996).

Some of these concerns may be exaggerated, and certainly not all of them fit all evidence-based treatments equally well. But it would be a mistake to simply dismiss the points. At a minimum, we need to understand the concerns that make many practitioners reluctant to use these treatments so that we can grasp and address impediments to dissemination in practice settings. But we also need to attend to the concerns because there may be elements of truth in some of them; indeed, most of the concerns can be construed as empirical questions that need research attention. In this respect, differences between researcher and practitioner perspectives can be valuable heuristically.

Differences between the perspectives of treatment researchers and treatment providers may be understood partly in relation to the distinction—in psychosocial and medical research—between efficacy and effectiveness. In *efficacy designs,* experimental control is used to test treatment impact under carefully arranged idealized conditions designed to maximize treatment effects—for example, with clients carefully screened and selected, with potentially troubling comorbidities excluded, with treatment carried out by a select group of therapists who are paid by the researcher and trained to deliver the target treatment as perfectly as possible, and with arrangements designed to keep therapists functioning at their best and treated clients engaged. In *effectiveness designs,* the aim is to assess intervention effects under ordinary clinical conditions, with treatment delivered to "average" or representative patients or clients, by "average" or representative practitioners, working under conditions that reflect typical practice realities (e.g., full caseloads and clinic productivity pressures). Of course, the efficacy–effectiveness distinction is best construed as a multidimensional continuum, spanning the degree to which treated youth, therapists, settings, and so on, are representative of those in clinical practice. Given the nature of the research conducted to date, most of what we know about the evidence-based treatments is clustered at the *efficacy* end of the continuum.

This state of affairs presents a real problem from the perspective of many practitioners. The apparent gap between the conditions prevailing in most treatment research and the conditions of actual youth mental health practice raises questions about whether the resultant treatments would work well in a practice context (Weisz & Weiss, 1993). The gap is likely to include characteristics of the treated individuals (e.g., youth in the clinic may be more severely disturbed, more likely to meet criteria for a diagnosis, more likely to have numerous comorbidities, and less motivated for treatment), their families (e.g., more parental psychopathology, family life event stressors, and perhaps even maltreatment), reasons for seeking treatment (e.g., not recruited from schools or through ads, but referred by caregivers because of unusually serious problems or family crisis, or even court ordered), the settings in which treatment is done (e.g., more financial forms to complete, more bureaucracy, and sometimes a less welcoming approach in the clinic), the therapists who provide the treatment (e.g., not graduate students or research assistants hired by and loyal to the adviser and committed to his or her treatment research program, but rather staff therapists who barely know the treatment developer or the tested treatment, and who may prefer different treatment methods), the incentive system (e.g., not paid by the treatment developer to deliver his or her evidence-based treatment with close adherence to the manual, but paid by the clinic to see many cases and with no method prescribed), and the conditions under which therapists deliver the treatment (not graduate students' flexible time, but strict productivity requirements, paperwork to complete, and little time to learn a manual or adhere closely to it).

Such differences between psychotherapy in most clinical trials and psychotherapy in actual clinical practice constitute several reasons why practitioners might question the relevance of the evidence to their own clinical practice. The differences could also be viewed as a nascent agenda for treatment researchers. Indeed, the real-world factors that experimentalists might view as a nuisance (e.g., child comorbidity, parent pathology, life stresses that produce no-shows and dropouts, and therapists with heavy caseloads) and thus attempt to avoid (e.g., by recruiting and screening cases, applying exclusion criteria, and hiring their own therapists) or control may in fact be precisely what we need to include, to understand, and to address, if we are to develop psychosocial treatment protocols that work well in practice (Weisz, in press-a, in press-b). Treatments that cannot cope with these real-world factors may not fare so well in practice, no matter how efficacious they are in well-controlled laboratory trials.

Thus, another critical direction for research on evidence-based psychotherapies to move is toward clinical practice. Testing treatments under conditions more and more like those of actual practice in mental health service settings may be a way to build especially robust treatments and a way to build an evidence base that supports their use in everyday clinical care.

OVERVIEW AND CONCLUSIONS

We have come a long way, as a field, from the early days. Many years passed between Aristotle's speculations on catharsis in the arts (*Poetics*, 350BCE; *Politics* VIII, 350BCE) and Sigmund Freud's work on the case of little Hans and Freud's psychoanalysis of his daughter Anna, in the early 1900s (see Kazdin & Weisz, Chapter 1, this volume). But child psychotherapy accelerated quickly through the 20th century, propelled in part by a new behavioral perspective. Emblematic of this new approach, Mary Cover Jones (1924a, 1924b) used modeling and "direct conditioning" to help a 2-year-old, Peter, overcome his fear of a white rabbit. By midcentury, evidence from actual studies of youth treatment had begun to accumulate, but reviews (e.g., Levitt, 1957, 1963) offered highly pessimistic conclusions about what those studies showed.

Undeterred by the bad news, intrepid investigators increased both the quality and pace of research over the ensuing decades, with an output of more than 1,500 youth treatment outcome studies by the year 2000 (see Kazdin, 2000a). As one index of the quality of that output, the *Journal of Clinical Child Psychology* devoted an entire issue, in 1998, to articles reporting on 27 youth treatments meeting multiple criteria for the status of "empirically supported psychosocial interventions" (see Brestan & Eyberg, 1998; Kaslow & Thompson, 1998; Lonigan, Elbert, & Johnson, 1998; Ollendick & King, 1998; Pelham, Wheeler, & Chronis, 1998). And now, in this book, we bring together descriptions of evidence-based treatments for young people, and the evidence on those treatments, written by the authors who know those treatments best.

In this final chapter, we note several characteristics of the treatments and the evidence that are particularly admirable, including breadth of coverage of important youth problems and disorders, a creative array of treatment delivery models, an increasingly rich mix of informants and measures in outcome assessment, and recently expanded attention to moderators of treatment outcome. But we also find areas in which change is needed and topics that need attention in future research. Among these, we note orphan conditions—most youth-relevant categories in DSM-IV, in fact—for which treatment development and testing are sorely needed. We also note a need to extend treatment outcome research to the treatment models, or schools of therapy, that are widely used in clinical practice but quite poorly represented in the research literature thus far. We note how little is currently known about the ways therapist behavior and the therapeutic relationship relate to treatment persistence and outcome, particularly in the new world of manual-guided treatments. We stress the critical importance of mediation tests, to identify the mechanisms of action that explain why treatments work. And we emphasize the need to understand evidence-based treatments in relation to clinical practice, with more of the research on treatments carried out under conditions such as those practitioners confront; this change could both strengthen our treatments and increase the likelihood that they will be used in everyday clinical care in service settings.

Viewed in historical perspective, the trajectory of research on child and adolescent treatment is quite remarkable, particularly in recent decades. The clinical scientists who have contributed to this book are a significant part of that trajectory, and their accounts in this book are both enlightening and inspiring. There are laurel wreaths all around for the leaders who have brought us to this significant point in treatment research. But there is little time for resting on laurels. A great deal of work remains to be done.

REFERENCES

Addis, M. E., & Krasnow, A. D. (2000). A national survey of practicing psychologists' attitudes toward psychotherapy treatment manuals. *Journal of Consulting and Clinical Psychology, 68,* 331–339.

Addis, M. E., Wade, W. A., & Hatgis, C. (1999). Barriers to dissemination of evidence-based practices: Addressing practitioners' concerns about manual-based psychotherapies. *Clinical Psychology: Science and Practice, 6,* 430–441.

American Psychiatric Association. (1994). *Diagnostic and statistical manual of mental disorders* (4th ed.). Washington, DC: Author.

Angold, A., Costello, E. J., & Erkanli, A. (1999). Comorbidity. *Journal of Child Psychology and Psychiatry, 40,* 57–87.

Azrin, N. H., Donohue, B., Besalel, V. A., Kogan, E. S., & Acierno, R. (1994). Youth drug abuse treatment: A controlled outcome study. *Journal of Child and Adolescent Substance Abuse, 3,* 1–16.

Barkley, R. A. (1997). *Defiant children: A clinician's manual for assessment and parent training.* New York: Guilford Press.

Baron, R. M., & Kenny, D. A. (1986). The moderator–mediator variable distinction in social psychological research: Conceptual, strategic, and statistical considerations. *Journal of Personality and Social Psychology, 51,* 1173–1182.

Borduin, C. M., Henggeler, S. W., Blaske, D. M., & Stein, R. J. (1990). Multisystemic treatment of adolescent sexual offenders. *International Journal of Offender Therapy and Comparative Criminology, 35,* 569–578.

Brestan, E. V., & Eyberg, S. M. (1998). Effective psychosocial treatments of conduct-disordered children and adolescents: 29 years, 82 studies, and 5,272 kids. *Journal of Clinical Child Psychology, 27,* 180–189.

Chorpita, B. F. (2002). Treatment manuals for the real world: Where do we build them? *Clinical Psychology: Science and Practice, 9,* 431–433.

Eddy, J. M., & Chamberlain, P. (2000). Family management and deviant peer association as mediators of the impact of treatment condition on youth antisocial behavior. *Journal of Consulting and Clinical Psychology, 68,* 857–863.

Foreyt, J. P., Poston, W. S. C., Winebarger, A. A., & McGavin, J. K. (1998). Anorexia nervosa and bulimia nervosa. In E. J. Mash & R. A. Barkley (Eds.), *Treatment of childhood disorders* (2nd ed., pp. 647–691). New York: Guilford Press.

Garfield, S. L. (1996). Some problems associated with "validated" forms of psychotherapy. *Clinical Psychology: Science and Practice, 3,* 218–229.

Havik, O. E., & VandenBos, G. R. (1996). Limitations of manualized psychotherapy for everyday clinical practice. *Clinical Psychology: Science and Practice, 3*, 264–267.

Hoagwood, K., Jensen, P. S., Petti, T., & Burns, B. J. (1996). Outcomes of mental health care for children and adolescents: I. A comprehensive conceptual model. *Journal of the American Academy of Child and Adolescent Psychiatry, 35*, 1055–1063.

Holmbeck, G. N. (1997). Toward terminological, conceptual, and statistical clarity in the study of mediators and moderators: Examples from the child-clinical and pediatric psychology literatures. *Journal of Consulting and Clinical Psychology, 65*, 599–610.

Huey, S. J., Jr., Henggeler, S. W., Brondino, M. J., & Pickrel, S. G. (2000). Mechanisms of change in multisystemic therapy: Reducing delinquent behavior through therapist adherence and improved family and peer functioning. *Journal of Consulting and Clinical Psychology, 68*, 451–467.

Jones, M. C. (1924a). A laboratory study of fear: The case of Peter. *Pedagogical Seminary, 31*, 308–315.

Jones, M. C. (1924b). The elimination of children's fears. *Journal of Experimental Psychology, 7*, 382–390.

Kaslow, N. J., & Thompson, M. P. (1998). Applying the criteria for empirically supported treatments to studies of psychosocial interventions for child and adolescent depression. *Journal of Clinical Child Psychology, 27*, 146–155.

Kazdin, A. E. (2000a). Developing a research agenda for child and adolescent psychotherapy. *Archives of General Psychiatry, 57*, 829–835.

Kazdin, A. E. (2000b). *Psychotherapy for children and adolescents: Directions for research and practice.* New York: Oxford University Press.

Kazdin, A. E., Bass, D., Ayers, W. A., & Rodgers, A. (1990). Empirical and clinical focus of child and adolescent psychotherapy research. *Journal of Consulting and Clinical Psychology, 58*, 729–740.

Kazdin, A. E., Siegel, T. C., & Bass, D. (1990). Drawing on clinical practice to inform research on child and adolescent psychotherapy: Survey of practitioners. *Professional Psychology: Research and Practice, 21*, 189–198.

Kazdin, A. E., & Weisz, J. R. (1998). Identifying and developing empirically supported child and adolescent treatments. *Journal of Consulting and Clinical Psychology, 66*, 19–36.

Kendall, P. C., & Southam-Gerow, M. A. (1996). Long-term follow-up of a cognitive-behavioral therapy for anxiety-disordered youth. *Journal of Consulting and Clinical Psychology, 64*, 724–730.

Kolko, D., Brent, D., Baugher, M., Bridge, J., & Birmaher, B. (2000). Cognitive and family therapies for adolescent depression: treatment specificity, mediation and moderation. *Journal of Consulting and Clinical Psychology, 68*, 603–614.

Levitt, E. E. (1957). The results of psychotherapy with children: An evaluation. *Journal of Consulting Psychology, 21*, 189–196.

Levitt, E. E. (1963). Psychotherapy with children: A further evaluation. *Behaviour Research and Therapy, 60*, 326–329.

Lonigan, C. J., Elbert, J. C., & Johnson, S. B. (1998). Empirically supported psychosocial interventions for children: An overview. *Journal of Clinical Child Psychology, 27*, 138–145.

Miller, A. L., & Glinski, J. (2000). Youth suicidal behavior: Assessment and intervention. *Journal of Clinical Psychology, 56*, 1131–1152.

Morrow-Bradley, C., & Elliott, R. (1986). Utilization of psychotherapy research by practicing psychotherapists. *American Psychologist, 41*, 188–197.

Motta, R. W., & Lynch, C. (1990). Therapeutic techniques vs. therapeutic relationships in child behavior therapy. *Psychological Reports, 67*, 315–322.

Ollendick, T. H., & King, N. J. (1998). Empirically supported treatments for children with phobic and anxiety disorders. *Journal of Clinical Child Psychology, 27*, 156–167.

Pelham, W. E., Wheeler, T., & Chronis, A. (1998). Empirically supported psychosocial treatments for attention deficit hyperactivity disorder. *Journal of Clinical Child Psychology, 27*, 190–205.

Shirk, S. R., & Russell, R. L. (1996). *Change processes in child psychotherapy: Revitalizing treatment and research.* New York: Guilford Press.

Shirk, S. R., & Saiz, C. C. (1992). Clinical, empirical, and developmental perspectives on the therapeutic relationship in child psychotherapy. Special Issue: Developmental approaches to prevention and intervention. *Development and Psychopathology, 4,* 713–728.

Weersing, V. R., & Weisz, J. R. (2002). Mechanisms of action in youth psychotherapy. *Journal of Child Psychology and Psychiatry, 43,* 3–29.

Weersing, V. R., Weisz, J. R., & Donenberg, G. R. (2002). Development of the Therapy Procedures Checklist: A therapist-report measure of technique use in child and adolescent treatment. *Journal of Clinical Child and Adolescent Psychology, 31,* 168–180.

Weisz, J. R. (in press-a). Milestones and methods in the development and dissemination of child and adolescent psychotherapies: Review, commentary, and a new deployment-focused model. In E. D. Hibbs & P. S. Jensen (Eds.), *Psychosocial treatments for child and adolescent disorders: Empirically based approaches* (2nd ed.). Washington, DC: American Psychological Association.

Weisz, J. R. (in press-b). *Psychotherapy for children and adolescents: Evidence-based treatments and case examples.* Cambridge, UK: Cambridge University Press.

Weisz, J. R., & Hawley, K. M. (2002). Developmental factors in the treatment of adolescents. *Journal of Consulting and Clinical Psychology, 70,* 21–43.

Weisz, J. R., Huey, S. J., & Weersing, V. R. (1998). Psychotherapy outcome research with children and adolescents: The state of the art. In T. H. Ollendick & R. J. Prinz (Eds.), *Advances in clinical child psychology* (Vol. 20, pp. 49–91). New York: Plenum Press.

Weisz, J. R., & Weiss, B. (1993). *Effects of psychotherapy with children and adolescents.* Newbury Park, CA: Sage.

Weisz, J. R., Weiss, B., Alicke, M. D., & Klotz, M. L. (1987). Effectiveness of psychotherapy with children and adolescents: A meta-analysis for clinicians. *Journal of Consulting and Clinical Psychology, 55,* 542–549.

Weisz, J. R., Weiss, B., Han, S. S., Granger, D. A., & Morton, T. (1995). Effects of psychotherapy with children and adolescents revisited: A meta-analysis of treatment outcome studies. *Psychological Bulletin, 117,* 450–468.

Author Index

Subject Index